UNIVERSITY OF
BRADFORD

Library

REFERENCE ONLY

This book must not be
removed from the library

Dictionary of
Toxicology

Second Edition

Editors
Ernest Hodgson, Richard B. Mailman
and Janice E. Chambers

Assistant Editor - Robert E. Dow

Dictionary of
Toxicology

Second Edition

Editors
Ernest Hodgson, Richard B. Mailman
and Janice E. Chambers

Assistant Editor - Robert E. Dow

Published in the United Kingdom by
MACMILLAN REFERENCE LTD, 1998
25 Eccleston Place, London, SW1W 9NF
and Basingstoke

Companies and representatives throughout the world.

http://www.macmillan-reference.co.uk

Distributed in the UK and Europe by
Macmillan Direct,
Brunel Road, Houndmills,
Basingstoke,
Hampshire, RG21 2XS, England

ISBN 0-333-547004

A catalogue record for this book is available from the British Library.

Published in the United States and Canada by
GROVE'S DICTIONARIES INC, 1998
345 Park Avenue South, 10th Floor
New York, NY 10010-1707, USA

ISBN 1-56159-216-1

Typeset by Hodgson Williams Associates,
Tunbridge Wells, Kent

Printed and bound in the UK by
BPC Information Ltd, Exeter, Devon

Contents

Preface

In the preface to the first edition, we noted that *"a [new] reference work, especially in a field where no comparable work exists, represents an enormous investment of time, energy and enthusiasm. Despite a desire to continually refine and improve the end product, practical considerations (including the need to conserve the Editors' resources) demand a stopping point."* Somewhat naively, we thought that the second edition would be markedly easier, not realizing that the decisions on which entries needed to be rewritten, added, or culled would make this job equally daunting (and equally difficult to finalize). Despite our limitations, the first edition was very well received in the toxicology community, and we hope that this volume also will be useful to our colleagues.

This work was assisted markedly by many people. Specific accolades are due the editorial assistance of Mr. Robert E. Dow of the University of North Carolina. Rob provided magnificent organizational skills, true diligence, and excellent editorial input at critical times in the conduct of this project. His efforts deserve the special recognition of inclusion on the title page. As with the first edition, the members of Toxicology programs at our three Universities were generous with their time, and both this and the first edition benefited from the input of the dozens of knowledgeable contributors who are acknowledged on pages following. Specific thanks also are accorded to Ms. Theresa Brooks of the University of North Carolina at Chapel Hill for excellent assistance with both editions and to Dr. Mechelle Lewis of the University of North Carolina at Chapel Hill for assistance with chemical structures. Finally, we acknowledge the patience and guidance of Macmillan Reference Ltd in helping to make us persevere at times when our other professional responsibilities made concluding this project a daunting task.

Thanks are expressed to Macmillan Reference Ltd for permission to abstract and adapt entries from other dictionaries to which they hold the copyright. They include: Allaby, M. Macmillan Dictionary of the Environment, 3rd edn. (Macmillan Reference Books, London, 1989); Hibbert D.B. and A.M. James, Macmillan Dictionary of Chemistry, (Macmillan Reference Books, London, 1987); Maclean, N., Macmillan Dictionary of Genetics and Cell biology (Macmillan Press, London, 1987). The authors and editors of these dictionaries served the scientific community well; hopefully, we may see new editions of their works.

Ernest Hodgson, Raleigh, North Carolina, USA
ernest_hodgson@ncsu.edu

Janice E. Chambers, Mississippi State, Mississippi, USA
chambers@novell.cvm.msstate.edu

Richard B. Mailman, Chapel Hill, North Carolina, USA
rmailman@css.unc.edu

June, 1998

Contributors

Alley, Earl G.
Mississippi State Chemical Laboratory
Mississippi State University
Mississippi State, MS 39762

Benson, William H.
Research Institute of Pharmaceutical Sciences
School of Pharmacy
University of Mississippi, MS 38677

Berndt, William O.
Office of Vice-Chancellor and Graduate Studies
University of Nebraska Medical Center
Omaha, NB 68105

Bouldin, Thomas W.
Departments of Pathology and Ophthalmology
University of North Carolina School of Medicine
Chapel Hill, NC 27514

Brimfield, Alan
United States Army Medical Research Institute of
Chemical Defense
Aberdeen Proving Ground, MD

Brown, Leslee D.
Murfreesboro, TN

Brown, Lewis R.
Department of Biological Sciences
Mississippi State University
Mississippi State, MS 39762

Browne, Jerry
University of North Carolina School of Medicine
Chapel Hill, NC 27514

Carl, Philip
Department of Pharmacology
University of North Carolina School of Medicine
Chapel Hill, NC 27514

Champlin, Franklin R.
Department of Biological University
Mississippi State University
Mississippi State, M 39762

Chambers, Howard
Department of Entomology and Plant Pathology
Mississippi State University
Mississippi State, MS 39762

Chambers, Janice E.
Center for Environmental Health Studies
College of Veterinary Medicine
Mississippi State University
Mississippi State, MS 39762-9825

Cockerham, Lorris G.
SITEK Research Laboratories
Rockville, MD 20850

Collins, Robert K.
Student Health Center
Mississippi State University
Mississippi State, MS 39762

Conly-Danehower, Sue
Glaxo-Wellcome, Inc.
Research Triangle Park, NC 27709

Cook, Jon C.
Dupont-Haskell Laboratory
Elkton Road
Newark, DE 19711

Cox, Nancy M.
Department of Animal and Dairy Science
Mississippi State University
Mississippi State, MS 39762

Crofton, Kevin M.
Neurotoxicology Division,
U.S. Environmental Protection Agency
Research Triangle Park, NC 27711

Dauterman, Walter C. (deceased)
Department of Toxicology
North Carolina State University
Raleigh, NC 27695

Diehl, Walter J.
Department of Biological Sciences
Mississippi State University
Mississippi State, MS 39762

Downer, Donald N.
Department of Biological Sciences
Mississippi State University
Mississippi State, MS 39762

Fishbein, Laurence
Environ Corporation
1000 Potomac St., NW
Washington, DC 20007

Goldstein, Joyce E.
National Institute of Environmental Health
Sciences
Research Triangle Park, NC 27709

Guthrie, Frank E. (deceased)
Department of Toxicology
North Carolina State University
Raleigh, NC 27695

Graham, Doyle
Department of Pathology
Vanderbilt University Medical Center
Nashville, TN 37232-2562

Grissom, Raymond E.
Agency for Toxic Substances and Disease Registry
Atlanta, GA 30333

Harkness, John E.
College of Veterinary Medicine
Mississippi State University
Mississippi State, MS 39762

Hodgson, Ernest
Department of Toxicology
North Carolina State University
Raleigh, NC 27695

Hodgson, Mary E.
Department of Epidemiology
School of Public Health
University of North Carolina, Chapel Hill
Chapel Hill, NC 27599

Kilts, Clinton D.
Department of Psychiatry
Emory University Medical Center
Atlanta, GA

Kimbrough, Renate D.
Institute for Evaluating Health Risks
Washington, DC

Kinsler, Steven
Agency for Toxic Substances and Disease Registry
Atlanta, GA 30333

Kizer, John S.
Department of Medicine
University of North Carolina School of Medicine
Chapel Hill, NC 27514

Lawler, Cindy P.
Neuroscience Center and Toxicology Curriculum
University of North Carolina School of Medicine
Chapel Hill, NC 27599-7250

Leidy, Ross B.
Pesticide Residue Research Laboratory
North Carolina State University
Raleigh, NC 27695

Lemley, Ann T.
Department of Textiles and Apparel
Cornell University
New York College of Human Ecology
Ithaca, NY 14853

Levi, Patricia E. (retired)
Department of Toxicology
North Carolina State University
Raleigh, NC 27695

Lewandowski, Margaret
BASF
Research Triangle Park, NC 27709

Lewis, Mark H.
Department of Psychiatry
University of Florida Health Science Center
Gainesville, FL 32610-0256

Light, Kim E.
Center for Addiction Studies
University of Arkansas for Medical Sciences
College of Pharmacy
Little Rock, AR 72205

Lipton, Morris A. (deceased)
Departments of Psychiatry and Biochemistry and
Nutrition
University of North Carolina School of Medicine
Chapel Hill, NC 27514

Mailman, Richard B.
UNC Neuroscience Center
Departments of Psychiatry and Pharmacology
University of North Carolina School of Medicine
Chapel Hill, NC 27599-7250

Mileson, Beth
International Life Sciences Institute
Washington, DC 20036-4804

Morell, Pierre
Department of Biochemistry and Nutrition
University of North Carolina School of Medicine
Chapel Hill, NC 27514

Narahashi, Toshio
Department of Molecular Pharmacology
Northwestern University Medical School
Chicago, IL 60611

Nichols, David E.
Department of Medicinal Chemistry and Molecu-
lar Pharmacology
School of Pharmacy and Pharmaceutical Sciences
Purdue University
West Lafayette, IN 47907

Novicki, Deborah L.
Chiron Corporation
Walpole, MA

Perry, Jerome J.
Department of Microbiology
North Carolina State University
Raleigh, NC 27695

Perez-Reyes, Mario
Departments of Psychiatry
University of North Carolina School of Medicine
Chapel Hill, 27514

Peterson, Gary
Departments of Psychiatry and Psychology
University of North Carolina
Chapel Hill, NC 27514.

Pruett, Stephen B.
Department of Cellular Biology and Anatomy
Louisiana State University Medical Center
Shreveport, LA 71130

Schultz, T. Wayne
Department of Animal Science
College of Veterinary Medicine
University of Tennessee
Knoxville, TN 37901

Shih, Tony M.
US Army
Medical Research Institute of Chemical Defense
Aberdeen Proving Ground, MD 21010

Silver, Ivin S.
Glaxo-Wellcome, Inc
Research Triangle Park, NC 27709

Smith, Gary
Department of Pathology
University of North Carolina School of Medicine
Chapel Hill, NC 27514

Tynes, Ronald E.
Sandoz Biotechnology
Basel
Switzerland

Vore, Mary
Department of Pharmacology
University of Kentucky College of Medicine
Lexington, KY 40536

Waggoner, Charles A.
Department of Chemistry
Mississippi State University
Mississippi State, MS 39762

Walker, Quentin David
Department of Pharmacology
Duke University Medical Center
Chapel Hill, NC 27514

Wargin, William
Glaxo-Wellcome Research Center
Research Triangle Park, NC

Wax, Charles L.
Department of Geology and Geography
Mississippi State University
Mississippi State, MS 39762

Weisburger, John H.
Naylor Dana Institute for Disease Prevention
American Health Foundation
Valhalla, NY 10595

Wilkinson, Christopher F.
Jellinek, Schwartz and Connolly, Inc.
Arlington, VA 22209

Williams, Gary M.
Division of Pathology and Toxicology
Naylor Dana Institute for Disease Prevention
American Health Foundation
Valhalla, NY 10595

Wise, Dwayne A.
Department of Biological Sciences
Mississippi State University
Mississippi State, MS 39762

Young, John F.
National Center for Toxicological Research
Division of Reproductive and Developmental
Toxicology
Jefferson, AR 72079

Introduction

Entries in a technical directory are neither intended for, nor often used by, specialists needing information related to the research areas in which they are expert. In fact, such scientists are usually quite capable of writing these items, or, at the very least, will have no need to read them. From time to time, however, most of us require information that while within the scope of the science of toxicology, is somewhat removed from our own specialties. An encyclopedia or dictionary (such as this volume) should offer a starting point for such needs. Of greater importance may be the goal of bringing to graduate and undergraduate students, and to scientists in other disciplines, the terms and concepts of toxicology. The entries in this volume, and their cross references, should form for such individuals a useful starting point, with the list of general references providing further information and serving as a bridge to the scientific literature. While many of the entries in this volume are related directly to the broad vista encompassed by toxicology, others (particularly certain anatomical, biochemical, pathological, and physiological terms) are provided to give background information that a toxicologist (neophyte or otherwise) might require. Such entries stress the relationship to toxicology, rather than their importance to the discipline from which they are drawn.

From the first edition, The Macmillan Dictionary of Toxicology made use of microcomputer technology, facilitating both the creation of the document, as well as additions and corrections. Ultimately, this information can best serve the scientific community if it were readily available "on-line", e.g., on the World Wide Web. We hope that the publisher can facilitate such a goal, and as such, we recognize the need to keep the content of this work dynamic. This type of work is likely to contain both errors and omissions, we continue to welcome corrections, additions, and criticism from our readers. Suggestions for new entries, revisions or modifications of existing entries, missing cross-references, etc., can be communicated to any of the editors, or via the book's website – www.macmillan.co.uk/science/dictionaryof toxic.htm.

A word about the choice of spelling may be appropriate. We feel that arguments about this subject generate more heat than light, and we were influenced to use American spelling primarily because of the national origin of the editors. In those cases in which the difference would affect the alphabetized position of the entry (e.g., oestrus versus estrus; haem versus heme), we have included the British spelling as a cross reference.

Finally, the list of general references is not intended to be exhaustive. The selection is quite arbitrary, and the list is intended only as a source of further information on subjects mentioned in the dictionary entries. Other excellent works could be added, and the list also will be revised in subsequent editions. Entries in certain listed reference works, however, are listed by their accession numbers as cross-references for entries in this dictionary. For example, entries in Lewis, R.J. Hazardous Chemicals Desk Reference (2nd ed., Van Nostrand Reinhold, New York, 1991) are cross-listed as HCDR followed by the number used in that work. Toxicological Profiles are a series of comprehensive toxicological profiles from the Agency for Toxic Substances and Disease Registry (ATSDR; US Public Health Service). Each item is about a single compound or a small group of related compounds, and is cross-referenced as ATSDR, followed by the month and year of publication. A list of these profiles is provided in the reference section.

A

AAALAC. *See* AMERICAN ASSOCIATION FOR ACCREDITATION OF LABORATORY ANIMAL CARE.

AAAS. *See* AMERICAN ASSOCIATION FOR THE ADVANCEMENT OF SCIENCE.

AACT. *See* AMERICAN ACADEMY OF CLINICAL TOXICOLOGY.

2-AAF. *See* N-2-ACETYLAMINOFLUORENE

AAFS. *See* AMERICAN ACADEMY OF FORENSIC SCIENCES.

AAG. *See* α_1-ACID GLYCOPROTEIN.

AAPCC. *See* AMERICAN ASSOCIATION OF POISON CONTROL CENTERS.

AAS. *See* SPECTROMETRY, ATOMIC ABSORPTION.

Abakabi disease. *See* TRICOTHECENES.

ABCW extrapolation. A method for extrapolating germ cell mutation tests from species to species. The name is derived from the authors of the initial paper (Abrahamson, Bender, Conger & Wolf, Nature 245, 461 (1973)). Based on the results of published studies on the effects of ionizing radiation, the extrapolation is performed by normalizing the mutation rate to the amount of DNA in the haploid genome of the species in question. Attempts to extend the ABCW hypothesis to chemical mutagens have been less successful, and the original hypothesis has been challenged even with regard to ionizing radiation. It appears that this extrapolation is of considerable historical importance and is useful for qualitative

assessments, but it is not appropriate for quantitative extrapolations. *See also* EXTRAPOLATION; EXTRAPOLATION, TO HUMANS; SPECIES EXTRAPOLATION.

ABFT. *See* AMERICAN BOARD OF FORENSIC TOXICOLOGY.

abiotic. Nonliving; in toxicology used primarily for the nonliving parts of ecosystems, or of the environment in general.

ABMT. *See* AMERICAN BOARD OF MEDICAL TOXICOLOGY.

abnormal base analogs. Exogenous (xenobiotic) analogs of the bases normally found in DNA. They are potent mutagens and many were originally developed as drugs for cancer therapy. As anticancer drugs, their effectiveness results from their ability to produce lethal mutations in rapidly dividing cancer cells. 5-Bromouracil, 5-fluorouridine, 2-aminopurine and 6-mercaptopurine are examples of mutagenic base analogs. Incorporation into DNA results in mispairing during the

5-Bromouracil

5-Fluorodeoxyuridine (Floxuridine)

next replication cycle, giving rise to altered (mutant) DNA. Since these chemicals are mutagens and carcinogens, the toxic hazard attendant upon their use is high; however, the life-threatening nature of the disease justifies the use of drugs with a small therapeutic index. *See also* CARCINOGENESIS; DNA; 6-MERCAPTOPURINE; MUTATION; THERAPEUTIC INDEX.

abnormal development, consequences. Death, malformation, growth retardation or functional disorders can occur as consequences of abnormal development. The embryo is not usually damaged by most agents prior to differentiation; however, a sufficiently high dose may result in death of the embryo. The time of organogenesis is the most sensitive time for induction of specific malformations, whereas structural defects at the tissue level, growth retardation or functional deficits are most likely to occur from damage during the fetal period. Structural defects are the main criteria used in estimating teratological risks since they are more obvious. However, functional disorders may be as incapacitating and result in as great a mortality rate among offspring as morphological abnormalities. *See also* TERATOGENESIS, CRITICAL PERIODS.

ABP. *See* ANDROGEN-BINDING PROTEIN.

ABPI. *See* ASSOCIATION OF THE BRITISH PHARMACEUTICAL INDUSTRY.

abrin (toxalbumin). A lectin composed of two polypeptide chains connected by a disulfide bridge. It is nearly identical to the toxin produced by the castor bean *(Ricinus communis)*. Abrin is found in the seed of the rosary pea *(Abrus precatorius)*, a common vine of the tropics. The LD50 in mice is 0.02 mg/kg, i.p. Ingestion of one chewed or broken seed can be fatal. It is a gastrointestinal toxin; one of the polypeptide chains binds to the intestinal cell membrane, allowing the other chain to enter the cytoplasm. Ribosomal protein synthesis is inhibited, resulting in cell death. Diarrhea associated with bloody mucus may begin as late as three days following ingestion of seeds with broken seed coats. Death may occur from loss of intestinal function and consequent alterations in plasma composition leading to secondary cerebral edema

and cardiac arrhythmia. Therapy for acute poisoning is to correct hypovolemia and electrolyte balance. *See also* CASTOR BEANS; LECTINS; RICIN.

absinthe. Alcoholic drink manufactured from wormwood *(Artemisia absinthum)*, similar to pastis, popular in late nineteenth and early twentieth centuries especially in France. It contained several neurotoxic extracts from the wormwood.

absorbance (*A*; optical density). A measure of the amount of radiation, at a particular wavelength, absorbed by a sample.

$$A = \log\left(\frac{I_0}{I}\right)$$

where I_0 is the radiation intensity incident upon the sample and I is the radiation intensity passing through the sample. *See also* ANALYTICAL TOXICOLOGY; BEER'S LAW; ELECTROMAGNETIC SPECTRUM; SPECTROMETRY.

absorbed dose. The amount of a chemical that enters the body of an exposed organism.

absorption. The uptake of water or dissolved chemicals by cells or organisms.

absorption factor. That fraction of a chemical coming into contact with an organism that is absorbed and enters the body of the organism.

absorption of toxicants. The processes involved in the movement of the toxicant from the exterior or the lumen of the portal of entry (i.e., skin, respiratory system or gastrointestinal tract) to the circulatory system (generally the blood, but can include the lymphatic system). Absorption of toxicants is generally a passive process, dependent upon the lipophilicity of the toxicant, but, in some cases, it involves active or facilitated transport. *See also* ACTIVE TRANSPORT; ENTRY MECHANISMS, ENDOCYTOSIS; ENTRY MECHANISMS, FILTRATION; ENTRY MECHANISMS, PASSIVE TRANSPORT; ENTRY MECHANISMS, SPECIAL TRANSPORT; FACILITATED TRANSPORT; PENETRATION; PENETRATION ROUTES, DERMAL;

PENETRATION ROUTES, GASTROINTESTINAL; PENETRATION ROUTES, PULMONARY; PERCUTANEOUS ABSORPTION.

absorption spectrum. *See* ELECTROMAGNETIC SPECTRUM.

ABT. *See* AMERICAN BOARD OF TOXICOLOGY.

ABVT. *See* AMERICAN BOARD OF VETERINARY TOXICOLOGY.

acaricides. Pesticides with specificity for mites, typically phytophagous mites in contrast to parasitic mites. A number of insecticides also display acaricidal activity. The acaricides include a diverse array of chemical structures. Common examples are dicofol and chlorobenzilate. *See also* DICOFOL.

Acarin. *See* DICOFOL.

acceptable daily intake (ADI). The estimated amount of a chemical (usually restricted to pesticides and food additives) that can be ingested daily, by humans, for an entire lifetime without causing appreciable adverse effects; it is expressed in mg/kg body weight/day. The ADI is obtained by dividing the no observed effect level (NOEL) by a safety factor (e.g., 10, 100 or 1000) that is intended to make allowance for possible differences in sensitivity between the animal test species and humans, as well as for interindividual variations within the human population. The term ADI was first used by the Joint FAO/WHO Expert Committee on Food Additives in 1961 and subsequently was adopted by the Joint FAO/WHO Expert Committee on Pesticide Residues (1962). The ADI constitutes a useful regulatory benchmark that is employed by international (e.g., FAO/WHO) and national (e.g., EPA, UK Advisory Committee on Pesticides and Other Toxic Chemicals) agencies for establishing tolerances for pesticide residues in raw agricultural and other commodities and for developing health advisory guidelines for such residues in potable water. For regulatory purposes, however, it is being replaced by the USEPA with the reference dose (RfD). *See also* NO OBSERVED EFFECT LEVEL; REFERENCE DOSE (RFD); SAFETY FACTOR.

accessory cells of immune system. *See* IMMUNE SYSTEM; MACROPHAGES/MONOCYTES.

accessory cells of testis. *See* SERTOLI CELLS.

accreditation. Certification of the expertise of individuals in toxicology or in various toxicological specialties. Accreditation is done by several organizations who establish standards and accredit on the basis of education, experience, accomplishments and/or successful completion of a written examination. *See also* AMERICAN BOARD OF FORENSIC TOXICOLOGY; AMERICAN BOARD OF MEDICAL TOXICOLOGY; AMERICAN BOARD OF TOXICOLOGY; AMERICAN BOARD OF VETERINARY TOXICOLOGY; AMERICAN COLLEGE OF TOXICOLOGY.

acesulphane K (Sumet). *See* SWEETENING AGENTS.

acetaldehyde (ethanal; ethylaldehyde; acetic aldehyde, CH_3CHO). CAS number 75-07-0. An organic compound used in the manufacture of paraldehyde, acetic acid, butanol, aniline dyes, synthetic rubber, and in the silvering of mirrors. It is also used in trace quantities in artificial flavors. It is produced physiologically in significant quantities in individuals taking disulfiram who have also ingested ethanol. The oral LD50 in rats is 1930 mg/kg and the inhalation LD50 in rats is 4000 ppm/4 hr. The primary toxic action is irritancy. Acetaldehyde interferes with mitochondrial oxygen consumption and energy production in rat liver. After inhalation, it causes irritation, nausea and vomiting. Skin and eye contact results in a burning sensation and severe irritation. The therapy after inhalation is to remove the victim to fresh air and give artificial respiration if breathing has stopped. Following eye contact, the eyes should be flushed with water; following skin contact, the skin should be washed with soap and water. *See also* DISULFIRAM.

acetaminophen (N-(4-hydroxyphenyl)acetamide; paracetamol; Tylenol®). CAS number 103-90-2. An analgesic and antipyretic drug. It is also used in the manufacture of azo dyes and photographic chemicals. The oral LD50 in mice is 338 mg/kg and the i.p. LD50 is 500 mg/kg. Acetaminophen is a hepatotoxicant at high doses following its metabolism to a toxic intermediate by cytochrome P450. The proposed toxic metabolite is acetimidoquinone. Following an overdose, detoxication by glutathione conjugation is saturated, leading to an increase in the concentration of the toxic metabolite that, in turn, binds to various hepatocellular constituents. Within hours sweating, anorexia, nausea and vomiting develop. In three to five days, jaundice, coagulation defects, hypoglycemia, renal failure and myocardiopathy may occur. If given within 12 hours of ingestion of an acetaminophen overdose, N-acetylcysteine appears to be effective in blocking the covalent binding of the toxic metabolite and the prevention of hepatotoxicity. Hinson, J.A. Rev. Biochem. Toxicol. 2, 103–129 (1980).

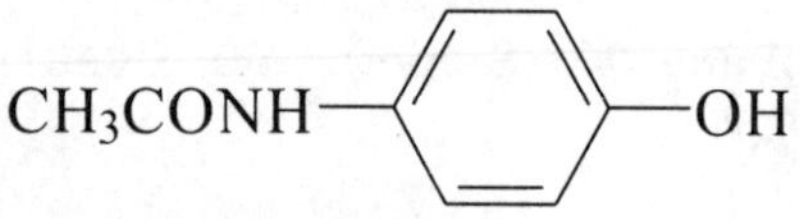

$$CH_3CONH \text{—} \bigcirc \text{—} OH$$

Acetaminophen

acetazolamide (N-(5-)aminosulfonyl)-1,3,4-thiadiazo-1,2-yl) acetamide; 5-acetamido-1,3,4-thiadiazole-2-sulfonamide; Diamox). CAS number 59-66-5. Acetazolamide is a carbonic anhydrase inhibitor used as a diuretic, including use in the treatment of lithium overdose and toxicity, and in the treatment of glaucoma. It is known to be teratogenic in mice and the effect is believed to be mediated via elevated maternal plasma CO_2 tension.

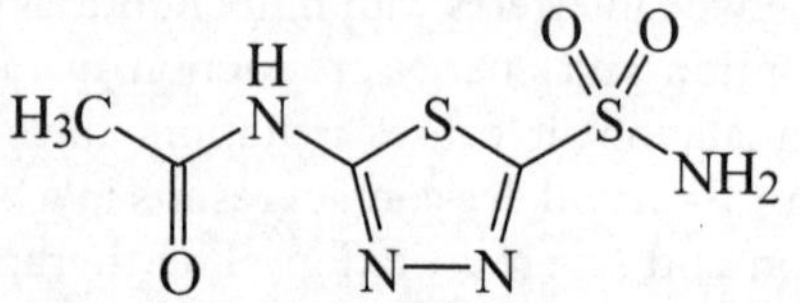

Acetazolamide

acetone. CAS number 67-64-1. A metabolic intermediate formed during the degradation of fats as well as a widely manufactured solvent and chemical intermediate. Acetone can be exhaled or further metabolized to acetate and, subsequently, to glucose. While acetone has a variety of irritant or chronic effects at high doses it does not appear to represent a serious chronic hazard. It has not been reported to be carcinogenic. Acetone is an inducer of cytochrome P450 2E1 (CYP 2E1) in

the liver of rodents regardless of the route of exposure. The mechanism is not well understood but appears to involve both increased protein synthesis and inhibition of protein kinase c.

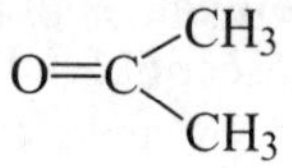

$$O = C \big\langle {}^{CH_3}_{CH_3}$$

Acetone

acetonylacetone. *See* 2,5-HEXANEDIONE.

***N*-2-acetylaminofluorene (2-AAF). CAS number 53-96-3.** Originally developed as an insecticide. Because of its effect as a potent bladder carcinogen, it is of importance as a model compound that has been studied intensively with regard to metabolic activation as a carcinogen and hepatotoxicant and the role of its metabolites in the subsequent processes of carcinogenesis. The primary metabolism of N-2-acetylaminofluorene is monooxygenation catalyzed by cytochrome P450. The reactions involved are either aromatic hydroxylation (a detoxication reaction) or N-hydroxylation (an activation). Interspecies variations in the cytochrome P450 isozymes catalyzing these reactions are held to explain interspecies differences in carcinogenic susceptibility. Subsequent phase II reactions, sulfate ester formation, acetylation and glucuronidation yield reactive metabolites that can react with nucleophilic substitutents on nucleic acids and proteins. Adducts of N-2-acetylaminofluorene with DNA bases (particularly the C-8 of guanine) have been identified. *See also* PHASE I REACTIONS; PHASE II REACTIONS.

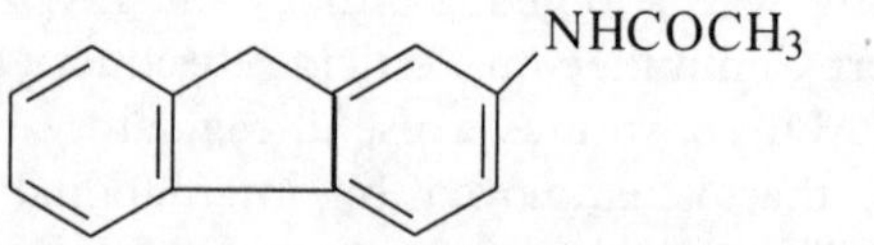

N-2-Acetylaminofluorene

acetylation. Acetylated derivatives of foreign exogenous amines are formed by N-acetyltransferase, an enzyme that utilizes acetyl CoA as the acetyl donor. This cytosolic enzyme has been purified from rat liver, but is known to occur in several organs, probably in multiple isozymic forms. Although a variety of groups on endogenous substrates may be acetylated, in xenobiotics only amino groups appear to function as acetyl group acceptors. Newborn mammals generally have low levels of the transferase activity, whereas genetically determined fast and slow acetylators occur in both rabbit and human populations. Slow acetylators are more susceptible to the effects of compounds detoxified by acetylation. The *N*-acetyltransferase(s) responsible for the acetylation of *S*-substituted cysteines, the last step in mercapturic acid formation, is found in the microsomes of kidney and liver. It is specific for acetyl CoA as the acetyl donor and is distinguished from other *N*-acetyltransferases by substrate specificity and subcellular location. *See also* ACYLATION; FAST AND SLOW ACETYLATORS; POLYMORPHISMS.

acetylator phenotype. Variation in the expression of *N*-acetyltransferase (NAT) isoforms in humans giving rise to two groups within any given population, fast and slow acetylators. Slow acetylators are more susceptible to the toxic effects of drugs that are detoxified by acetylation. *See also* ACETYLATION, FAST AND SLOW ACETYLATORS; POLYMORPHISMS.

acetylcholine (ACh). CAS number of chloride 60-31-1, of bromide 66-23-9. The choline ester of acetic acid. ACh is released in vertebrates as the neurotransmitter for cholinergic neurons in the CNS, as well as at several peripheral locations: somatic neurons innervating skeletal muscle (neuromuscular junctions); preganglionic neurons in both divisions of the autonomic nervous system; parasympathetic postganglionic neurons; and a few sympathetic postganglionic neurons. ACh is synthesized from choline and acetyl CoA by the mitochondrial enzyme choline acetyltransferase. Choline, but not ACh, is absorbed into nerve terminals by a specific, high-affinity, sodium- and energy-dependent process. This high-affinity uptake process is specific to cholinergic nerve terminals, is tightly coupled to ACh synthesis, is the rate-limiting step for ACh levels and is the target for some toxicants, such as hemicholinium-3. Cholinergic receptors (cholinoceptors), that mediate the effects of ACh, are generally classified as nicotinic or muscarinic, based on their binding preferences for nicotine and muscarine, respectively. Receptors can be blocked by such agents as *d*-tubocurarine, decamethonium, atropine and scopolamine. ACh is hydrolyzed to choline and acetate by acetylcholinesterase, that is an important target for a variety of toxic and therapeutic anticholinesterases, such as the nerve agents, carbamate, thiocarbamate and organophosphorus insecticides, and eserine. *See also* ACETYLCHOLINE RECEPTORS, MUSCARINIC AND NICOTINIC; ACETYLCHOLINESTERASE; ANTICHOLINESTERASES; CHOLINE ACETYLTRANSFERASE; ORGANOPHOSPHORUS INSECTICIDES.

$$CH_3-\overset{\overset{\displaystyle CH_3}{+|}}{\underset{\underset{\displaystyle CH_3}{|}}{N}}-CH_2CH_2-O-\overset{\overset{\displaystyle O}{||}}{C}-CH_3$$

Acetylcholine

acetylcholine receptors, muscarinic and nicotinic (cholinergic receptors; cholinoceptors). The receptors for the neurotransmitter acetylcholine (ACh) are classified into two major groups—muscarinic and nicotinic. The muscarinic receptors occur at autonomic effector cells and are stimulated by the alkaloid muscarine derived from certain mushrooms; these receptors mediate the effects of postganglionic parasympathetic neurons. Some muscarinic receptors also occur in autonomic ganglia and in cortical and subcortical neurons in the brain. Cholinergic agonists for muscarinic receptors include bethanechol and methacholine; the belladonna alkaloid atropine is an effective antagonist. Muscarinic receptors are subdivided into subtypes, such as M1 and M2 receptors, based on selective agonist/antagonist activities or binding affinities. The nicotinic receptors occur at autonomic ganglia and at the endplates of skeletal muscle and are stimulated by the alkaloid nicotine. Cholinergic agonists for nicotinic receptors include nicotine, and antagonists include *d*-tubocurarine, hexamethonium and some snake toxins. *See also* MUSCARINE; NICOTINE.

acetylcholine release. Acetylcholine (ACh) is released from the nerve terminals of cholinergic neurons in response to an action potential in the neuron (excitation-secretion coupling). Agents that enhance ACh release cause hyperexcitability of cholinergic pathways. Two natural toxins possessing this activity are black widow spider venom and β-bungarotoxin. *See also* BLACK WIDOW SPIDER VENOM; β-BUNGAROTOXIN.

acetylcholinesterase (AChE; acetylcholine acetylhydrolase; cholinesterase; EC 3.1.1.7). An enzyme that hydrolyzes the neurotransmitter acetylcholine (ACh) to choline and acetate, and thus terminates the action of ACh. It is found extensively throughout the nervous system, as well as in many non-nervous tissues. The enzyme contains two binding sites for ACh: an anionic site and an esteratic site, containing a serine residue that is the target for numerous organophosphorus and carbamate inhibitors. The inhibition of AChE by these anticholinesterases leads to an accumulation of endogenous ACh, and thus results in hyperactivation of cholinergic receptors. Symptoms of acute poisoning can include irritability, tremors, convulsions and predominately parasympathetic effects, with death usually the result of respiratory failure. The recovery of enzyme activity varies within the groups of anticholinesterases: the carbamates are sometimes considered "reversible" inhibitors because they are relatively transient, whereas the organophosphorus compounds are quite persistent, with some of these capable of aging and therefore causing permanent destruction of the enzyme. Since AChE is contained in erythrocytes, the assay of erythrocyte AChE activity can be used as a diagnostic tool to assess exposure to organophosphorus anticholinesterases. *See also* ACETYLCHOLINESTERASE, AGING; ANTICHOLINESTERASES; ACETYLCHOLINE RECEPTORS, MUSCARINIC AND NICOTINIC; CARBAMATE INSECTICIDES; CARBAMATE POISONING, SYMPTOMS AND THERAPY; NERVE GASES; ORGANOPHOSPHATE POISONING, SYMPTOMS AND THERAPY; ORGANOPHOSPHORUS INSECTICIDES.

acetylcholinesterase, aging. An event that occurs subsequent to the inhibition of acetylcholinesterase (AChE) by certain organic phosphates and phosphonates. Although the precise mechanism involved has not been established, it is apparently a simple hydrolysis of an alkoxy group on the phosphorus atom. Cleavage of the P-O-alkyl, rather than the P-O-AChE, bond yields an inhibited enzyme with a spontaneous recovery rate near zero and that is refractory to reactivation by oximes. Fortunately, the methoxy and ethoxy groups prevalent in commercial insecticides age rather slowly. The isopropoxy group (e.g., DFP

and sarin) ages within one to two hours, and the 1,2,2-trimethylpropoxy group (e.g., soman) ages within minutes. *See also* ACETYLCHOLINESTERASE.

acetylcholinesterase, in chronic toxicity testing. *See* CHRONIC TOXICITY TESTING.

acetylcholinesterase, inhibitors. *See* ANTICHOLINESTERASES.

acetylcholinesterase, reactivation. Acetylcholinesterase (AChE) that has been inhibited by a carbamate or organophosphorus (OP) anticholinesterase can be restored to normal functional capacity if hydrolysis removes the moiety carbamylating or phosphorylating the enzyme. This reactivation occurs spontaneously for both groups of anticholinesterases, with the reactivation of carbamates occurring much more rapidly than that of the OP compounds. The reactivation of OP-inhibited AChE can be enhanced by the use of oxime reactivators, such as *N*-methylpyridinium-2-aldoxime (2-PAM), provided that aging of the phosphorylated AChE has not occurred. *See also* ACETYLCHOLINESTERASE, AGING; ANTICHOLINESTERASES; *N*-METHYLPYRIDINIUM-2-ALDOXIME.

***N*-acetylcysteine conjugates.** *See* MERCAPTURIC ACIDS.

acetylene dichloride. *See* 1,2-DICHLOROETHENE.

acetylesterases. *See* HYDROLYSIS.

acetylethyltetramethyltetralin (AETT; polycyclic musk; musk tetralin; Versalide; Musk 36A; 1,1,4,4-tetramethyl-6-ethyl-7-acetyl-1,2,3,4-tetrahydronaphthalene). CAS number 83-29-9. A neurotoxic compound originally used in fragrance preparations, but now withdrawn from commercial use and thus primarily of historical interest. Blue tissue discoloration follows i.p. injection into rats and rabbits, but not monkeys, ostensibly from metabolism to a triketoindane. After acute intoxication, animals experience hyperexcitability, depression and then progressive tremors. In subchronic exposure, animals exhibit hyperexcitability and hyperirritability, intermittent arching of the back, ataxia, limb weakness, foot drop and eversion of the hindfeet. Morphological changes include early and widespread neuronal pigmentation, and, later, scattered neuronal degeneration, intramyelinic edema and segmental demyelination. The LD50s in female rats are 316 mg/kg (oral), 126 mg/kg (i.p.) and 584 mg/kg (unoccluded percutaneous). The mechanism of action is unknown. One sign of intoxication is a green-colored urine. There is no effective therapy.

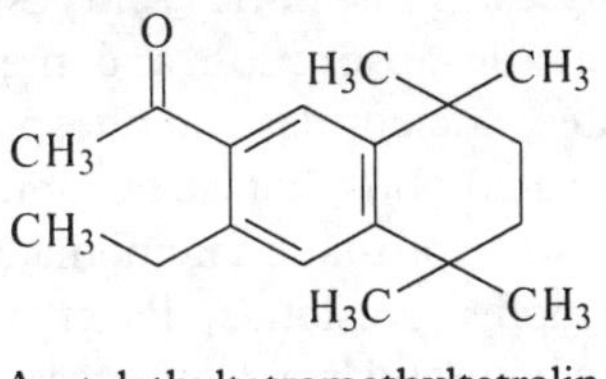

Acetylethyltetramethyltetralin

3-acetylpyridine (methyl pyridyl ketone). CAS number 350-03-8. An analog of nicotinamide that competes for incorporation into NAD. It has been used to chemically lesion the inferior olive nucleus, thereby eliminating climbing fibers within the cerebellar cortex. The loss of contacts to the Purkinje cells of the cerebellum from climbing fibers can seriously impair locomotor activity. In addition to the inferior olive, 3-acetylpyridine also induces neuropathological changes in areas CA3 and CA4 of the hippocampus, the lateral geniculate nucleus, pars compacta of the substantia nigra, supraoptic nucleus of the hypothalamus and the nucleus dorsalis of the raphe. Toxic effects of 3-acetylpyridine are thought to result from abnormal nucleotide synthesis following replacement of pyridine by 3-acetylpyridine. The compound has had particular utility in neurotoxicological studies (e.g., in which the climbing fibers were thought to be altered by toxicants).

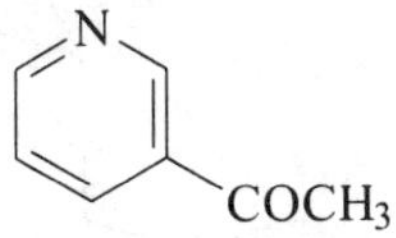

3-Acetylpyridine

acetylsalicylic acid. *See* ASPIRIN.

N-acetyltransferase. *See* ACETYLATION.

ACGIH. *See* AMERICAN CONFERENCE OF GOVERNMENTAL AND INDUSTRIAL HYGIENISTS.

ACh. *See* ACETYLCHOLINE.

AChE. *See* ACETYLCHOLINESTERASE.

acid activating enzyme. *See* AMINO ACID CONJUGATION.

acid/base balance. The ratio of acidic to basic ions in a solution. *In vivo* the acid/base balance is controlled physiologically, and disturbances, often resulting from the effect of toxicants, can have profound toxicological effects. Carbon dioxide is transported in the blood primarily as bicarbonate ions (HCO_3^-), the bicarbonate ion being formed in the red blood cell by carbonic anhydrase. The Henderson–Hasselbach equation illustrates the role of bicarbonate in maintaining blood pH at 7.4.

$$pH = pK_A + \log \frac{[HCO_3^-]}{[H_2CO_3]}$$

Thus disturbances in acid/base balance affect blood pH, giving rise to acidosis or alkalosis. *See also* ACIDOSIS, METABOLIC; ACIDOSIS, RESPIRATORY; ALKALOSIS, METABOLIC; ALKALOSIS, RESPIRATORY.

acid deposition. The wet and dry air pollutants that lower the pH of deposition and subsequently of the environment. Acid rain refers to the wet components. Acid rain has a pH of 4 or lower, compared with normal rain that has a pH of about 5.6. Sulfuric and nitric acids, from sulfur and nitrogen oxides, respectively, are the major contributors arising primarily from burning fossil fuels. High sulfur-content coal is responsible for much of the sulfuric acid. In regions where the buffering capacity of substrates is limited, the lakes have become acidic enough to kill fish and are unable to support fish populations. Contributing to this toxicity in fish is the fact that the acidic conditions concurrently release toxic metals (e.g., aluminum) into the water. In terrestrial ecosystems the acids also leach nutrients (e.g., sodium, potassium, calcium, magnesium) from the soil, resulting in a detrimental effect on tree growth.

α₁-acid glycoprotein (AAG; acute-phase reactant protein; orosomucoid). A low-molecular-weight (Mr = 40,000), anionic (pI =

2.7–3.5), polymorphic protein produced primarily by the liver. Approximately 45% of AAG is carbohydrate, consisting of hexose, hexosamine and sialic acid in equal proportions. Normal plasma concentration of AAG is 50–150 ng/ml, with a plasma half-life of five days. The clinical function of AAG is unknown. AAG is an acute-phase reactant, and plasma levels may be elevated as a consequence of acute physiological stress or from chronic inflammation. Decreases in AAG may occur secondary to severe malnutrition, severe hepatic damage and severe protein-losing gastroenteropathies. AAG binds many basic drugs through electrostatic interactions. *See also* PROTEIN BINDING; PLASMA PROTEINS.

acid mine drainage. Drainage from pyritic coal mines that is frequently acidic as a result of the chemical and bacterial oxidation of reduced iron and sulfur to ferric hydroxide precipitates and sulfuric acid, respectively. The acid drainage has killed fish and lowered the quality of drinking water. It also has the potential for leaching heavy metals into the water supply.

acidosis. A condition in which the pH of the blood is acidic beyond the normal range. Although acidosis can occur for reasons unrelated to toxic compounds, it may also result from the generation of an acidic metabolite (e.g., formic acid from methanol), by loss of base or by carbon dioxide retention. Therapeutically acidosis is treated by maintaining an adequate airway, artificial respiration to prevent carbon dioxide retention or by administering sodium bicarbonate, either i.v. or orally. *See also* ACIDOSIS, METABOLIC; ACIDOSIS, RESPIRATORY; ALKALOSIS; MAINTENANCE THERAPY, RESPIRATION; MAINTENANCE THERAPY, WATER AND ELECTROLYTE BALANCE.

acidosis, metabolic. A form of acidosis resulting from the generation of excess acid and the resultant disturbance of the acid/base balance. It occurs not only in diabetes and renal disease, but also following acid salt poisoning, methanol poisoning, etc. Characteristic signs are a decrease in blood bicarbonate and increased respiratory rate. *See also* ACIDOSIS.

acidosis, respiratory. A form of acidosis resulting from failure to expire carbon dioxide. It can occur in pneumonia, emphysema and congestive heart failure, but also with poisons causing lung edema and with narcotic depressants. It involves an increase in blood bicarbonate concentration. *See also* ACIDOSIS.

acid phosphatase. A lysosomal acid hydrolase that hydrolyzes phosphoric acid esters and is important in the absorption and metabolism of carbohydrates, nucleotides and phospholipids. Serum levels of acid phosphatase become elevated in cases of metastatic prostatic carcinoma, benign prostatic hypertrophy, prostatitis, Paget's disease and metastases to bone and liver from breast carcinoma.

acid rain. *See* ACID DEPOSITION.

acid soot (acid smut). Particles of carbon held together by water made acidic due to combination with sulfur trioxide. The carbon particles are emitted during combustion, with the soot particles being roughly 1–3 mm in diameter. Where oil-burning installations have metal chimneys, acid soot can acquire iron sulfate, which produces brown stains on materials and damages paintwork.

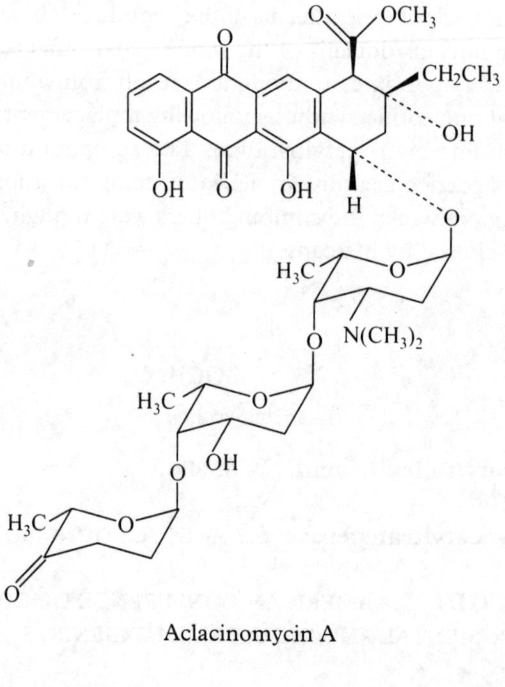

Aclacinomycin A

acinus. A number of secretory cells in an exocrine gland that secrete into a cavity; the smallest unit in a gland.

aclacinomycins. A family of antineoplastic antibiotics isolated from *Streptomyces galilaeus*. The major components (aclamycin A and aclamycin B) have LD50s in mice of 22.6 and 13.7 mg/kg, i.p., respectively.

ACM. *See* ADVISORY COMMITTEE ON MUTAGENESIS.

ACNFP. *See* ADVISORY COMMITTEE ON NOVEL FOOD AND PROCESSES.

aconitase. The enzyme that reversibly interconverts citric acid, *cis*-aconitic acid and isocitric acid in the citric acid (Krebs) cycle by dehydration and hydration reactions. Aconitase is the target for fluoroacetate, a potent rodenticide, that condenses with oxaloacetate to yield an aconitase inhibitor (fluorocitric acid), with resultant accumulation of citric acid and thus blockage of the citric acid cycle, leading to an inhibition of aerobic energy production. *See also* LETHAL SYNTHESIS.

aconitine (16-ethyl-1,16,19-trimethoxy-4-(methoxymethyl)aconitane-3,8,10,11,18-pentol 8-acetate 10-benzoate; Monkshood). CAS number 302-27-2. A toxic alkaloid that causes reflex bradycardia, induces arrhythmias and causes nausea, vomiting and weakness. A tingling, burning feeling on the lips, mouth, gums and throat is the first sign following ingestion. Aconitine acts on nerve axons by opening sodium channels, as well as by inhibiting complete repolarization of the membrane of myocardial tissue, causing repetitive firing. It is sometimes used to

Aconitine

produce cardiac arrhythmias in experimental animals. It also has an antipyretic action. The oral LD50 in mice is about 1 mg/kg. Procaine may be useful in reversing the toxic effects of aconitine.

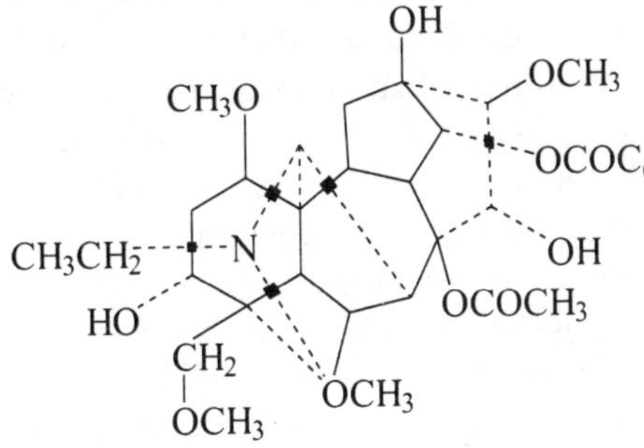

aconitum species. A genus of the family Ranunculaceae, *A. napellus* is the cultivated aconite, *A. columbianum* is a native of moist woodlands in western North America, *A. reclinatum* and *A. uncinatum* are native to the eastern USA, while *A. japonicum* and *A. carmichaelii* are oriental species that are used in oriental medicine. Aconitum species contain several C19 diterpenoid ester alkaloids that are potent poisons, including aconitine, mesaconitine and jesaconitine. Historically, aconite root has been used for homicides, as an arrow poison, and in medicine.

ACOP. Approved Code of Practice under UK's COSHH Regulation. The two original codes are "General ACOP" and "Carcinogens ACOP". *See also* COSHH.

acoustic startle response. *See* AUDITORY STARTLE; NEUROBEHAVIORAL TOXICOLOGY

ACP. *See* ADVISORY COMMITTEE ON PESTICIDES.

acquired immune deficiency syndrome (AIDS). A condition in humans in which the immune system suffers a progressive failure, leaving the victim susceptible to opportunistic infections. It is caused by the human immunodeficiency virus (HIV), a slow-acting retrovirus that invades and kills T_4 helper cells that are integral to the immune system. AIDS is believed to have occurred first in the late 1950s and was identified as a distinct medical condition in the early 1980s. It is believed to have originated in Africa, probably by several mutations of a virus transmitted from green monkeys to humans in an area where green monkeys are eaten; within a few years further mutations produced a number of distinct viral strains. Estimates of the number of infected persons who will develop the full range of symptoms varies widely, but in the absence of an effective antiviral drug the great majority of those who develop symptoms will die.

acridine (10-azaanthracene; dibenzo[*b,e*]-pyridine). CAS number 260-94-6. A compound occurring in coal tar that has been used in the manufacture of dyes and intermediates. Derivatives are used as antiseptics (e.g., acriflavin) and antimalarial drugs. Acridine is a strong irritant to mucous membranes and skin, and it causes sneezing on inhalation. Antimalarials may cause skin hyperpigmentation. A mutagen causes additions and deletions of base pairs, especially in plasmids and other extra-chromosomal DNA. The oral LD50 in rats is 2.0 g/kg and in mice is 0.5 g/kg.

Acridine

acridine orange (3,6-bis(dimethylamino) acridine). CAS number 494-348-2. A dye used to stain nucleic acids. It fluoresces at 530 nm when intercalated into double-stranded DNA, or at 640 nm when ionically bound to single-stranded DNA. It produces mutations, some involving reading frame shifts, other deletions or insertions, although its carcinogenicity is questionable. It is also known to be a dermal phototoxicant. *See also* ACRINIDINE; AMINOACRIDINES.

acrolein (acraldehyde; acrylaldehyde; acrylic aldehyde; aqualin; 2-propenal; allyl aldehyde; NSC 8819). CAS number 79-06-1. A chemical intermediate in the manufacture of methionine, glycerine, acrylic acid esters, glutaraldehyde and cycloaliphatic epoxy resins. It is used as an aquatic herbicide, biocide and slimicide. Acrolein is formed during partial combustion of organic material (e.g., in forest fires, urban fires, exhaust emissions and tobacco smoke). The oral LD50 in rats is 46 mg/kg and in mice is 28 mg/kg. The irritation threshold is 0.1 ppm, the TLV-TWA 0.1 ppm, TLV-STEL 0.3 ppm and IDLH 5 ppm. Acrolein reacts with critical sulfhydryl groups in lungs, heart, eyes, skin and the respiratory tract, and causes disruption of intermediary metabolism, impairment of DNA replication, inhibition of protein synthesis and mitochondrial respiration, hepatic periportal necrosis, and destruction of NADPH-cytochrome *c* reductase. In humans, it causes intense irritation of eye and mucous membranes of the respiratory tract. Direct contact leads to skin or eye necrosis, pulmonary edema, bronchitis, tracheobronchitis, severe gastrointestinal distress and/or lachrymation. Inhalation can lead to pneumonia and nephritis, degeneration of the bronchial epithelium leading to emphysema and focal calcification of the renal tubular epithelium. After acute poisoning, the subject should be removed from the contaminated area and should be administered oxygen with subsequent corticosteroid treatment for pulmonary inflammation. If acrolein is ingested, gastric lavage, saline cathartics, and demulcents should be used. Beauchamp, R.O. et al. CRC Crit. Rev. Toxicol. 14(4), 309–380 (1985).

$$CH_2=CHCHO$$

Acrolein

acrylaldehyde. *See* ACROLEIN.

acrylamide (acrylamide monomer; acrylic acid amide; propenamide; vinylformic acid). CAS number 79-06-1. Acrylamide is polymerized in the manufacture of paper and cardboard, and is used as a grouting agent and in modern biochemistry laboratories. Humans exposed to acrylamide monomer, but not its polymers, are vulnerable to neurotoxic injury. Although acute high doses can result in an encephalopathy that is apparently reversible, repeated smaller doses are cumulative and result in a distal sensorimotor axonopathy. The earliest signs are difficulty in walking and clumsiness of the hands. Distal deep tendon reflexes are lost, and sensory disturbances, such as numbness in feet and fingers are accompanied by objective loss of vibration sensation without objective changes in superficial sensation. Excessive sweating and contact dermatitis are common. Neurofilament-filled axonal swellings are less common than in γ-diketone or carbon disulfide intoxication. Degeneration of distal axons follows, especially in the long, large-diameter axons in the peripheral nervous system. Neurofilament-filled axonal swellings and axonal degeneration are seen to a lesser degree in the CNS. The oral LD50 is 150–180 mg/kg in rats, guinea pigs and rabbits. The mechanism of action is unknown, but suspected to be related to the reaction of the vinyl group with nucleophiles, such as thiols and amino groups. There is no therapy except removal from exposure.

$$CH_2{=}CHCONH_2$$
Acrylamide

acrylonitrile (vinyl cyanide; cyanoethylene; propene nitrile). CAS number 107-13-1. A designated probable carcinogen (IARC), hazardous substance (EPA), hazardous waste (EPA) and priority toxic pollutant (EPA). It is a slightly acrid, colorless liquid that is both explosive and flammable. Acrylonitrile is used as an intermediate in the manufacture of synthetic fibers, plastics, nitrile rubber and adhesives. The common routes of entry are inhalation and percutaneous absorption. Local effects of acrylonitrile include irritation of the eyes, and prolonged exposure may cause skin irritation. The effects of systemic exposure include nausea, vomiting, headache, etc., whereas exposure to high concentrations may cause weakness, asphyxia and death.

$$CH_2{=}CHCN$$
Acrylonitrile

ACT. *See* AMERICAN COLLEGE OF TOXICOLOGY.

ACTH (adrenocorticotropic hormone; adrenocorticotropin). A hormone secreted by the adenohypophysis in response to hypothalamic corticotropin-releasing hormone (CRH). ACTH stimulates the secretion of glucocorticoids and androgens from the zona fasciculata and the zona reticularis of the adrenal cortex, respectively, but does not stimulate the secretion of mineralocorticoids from the zona glomerulosa. ACTH secretion is increased in stress situations.

actinomycin D (Dactinomycin; Meractinomycin; Cosmegen). An antibiotic and antineoplastic produced by *Streptomyces parvullus*. The LD50 in mice is 2.0–2.4 mg/kg, i.p. Actinomycin D is a carcinogen that inhibits DNA-dependent RNA synthesis and DNA synthesis. It produces chromosomal breaks and translocations, by intercalation in double-stranded DNA between deoxyguanine residues with the peptide side chains in the minor groove. In humans, it produces bone marrow suppression, gastrointestinal toxicity and the possibility of anaphalaxis.

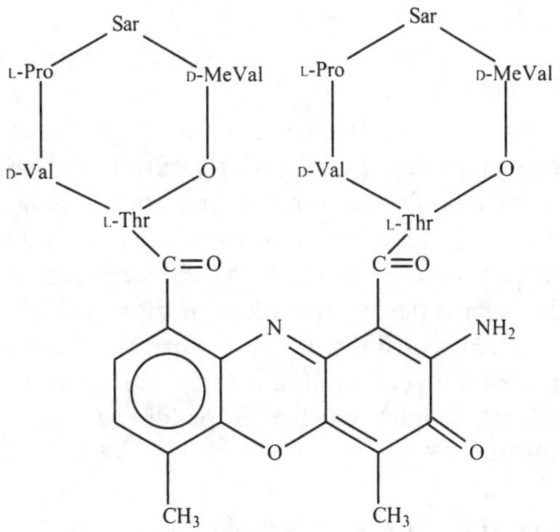

Actinomycin D

activated charcoal. Charcoal that, after pyrolysis during manufacture, has been subjected to steam or air at high temperature, thus making it an efficacious absorber of substances. It is used as an oral absorbent in treating oral intoxication from many substances.

activation (bioactivation). In toxicology, any metabolic reaction of a xenobiotic in which the product is more toxic than the substrate. Such reactions are most commonly monooxygenations, the products of which are electrophiles that, if not detoxified by phase II (conjugation) reactions, may react with nucleophilic groups on cellular macromolecules such as protein and DNA. *See also* PHASE I REACTIONS; PHASE II REACTIONS; REACTIVE INTERMEDIATES.

activation energy. The energy required, in addition to the change in free energy, to convert chemical reactants to products. Enzymes catalyze reactions by lowering the activation energy and thereby allow reactants (substrates) to be converted to products more quickly.

active avoidance. *See* CONDITIONED AVOIDANCE.

active oxygen (singlet oxygen). The highly reactive oxygen intermediates formed from the reduction of triplet state divalent oxygen or the spin inversion to the singlet state. The univalent reduction of diatomic oxygen (O_2) results in superoxide (O_2^-) formation. The divalent reduction of (O_2^-) results in (H_2O_2) formation. Trivalent reduction of oxygen yields the highly reactive hydroxyl radical $(OH^{\bullet})$. This extremely strong oxidant can also be formed in a metal-catalyzed Fenton-type reaction between (O_2^-) and (H_2O_2). Reactions of these compounds with organics could yield organic peroxy and alkoxy radicals, which are also often considered active forms of oxygen. Upon spin inversion of one of the electrons in the π-orbital, singlet oxygen is produced. *See also* SUPEROXIDE.

active site. Part of an enzyme that (1) specifically binds the substrate(s) and (2) catalyzes product formation. The active site consists of two or more often overlapping regions that recognize and bind the substrate(s) and then catalyze the ensuing reactions. The amino acids of each of these regions are not necessarily adjacent in the linear polypeptide(s), but may be brought together by the protein folding. The active site, whether occurring on the surface of the enzyme or buried in a cleft, usually occupies only a small percentage of the total surface of the enzyme molecule. The initial binding of the substrate involves the formation of non-covalent bonds (e.g., hydrogen bonds, ionic bonds, hydrophobic interactions) with chemical groups at the active site. During catalysis, covalent bonds may be formed, and then broken, as part of the reaction mechanism. Catalysis generally involves one or more of the following: optimal spatial alignment of the substrate(s) on the protein surface; distortion of bond angles and stretching of bond lengths or transfer of protons or electrons (acid/base catalysis). The chemical groups involved in catalysis include the chemically reactive sidechains of the amino acids histidine, lysine, arginine, serine, threonine, tyrosine, cysteine, glutamic acid and aspartic acid, and for some enzymes a coenzyme or cofactor. The active sites of many enzymes are targets for a number of toxicants. *See also* COVALENT BINDING; ENZYME; HYDROGEN BONDING; HYDROPHOBIC BONDING; VAN DER WAALS FORCES.

active transport. The various energy-requiring processes that permit the movement of chemicals across biological membranes. Active transport is important in toxicology primarily with regard to the excretion of toxicants (or, more importantly, their metabolic conjugation products) from the liver or the kidney. It is sometimes important with regard to entry (uptake) of toxicants, although this usually results from passive diffusion of lipophilic molecules. In a few cases, however, toxicants are absorbed by active transport because of their close similarity to either nutrients or endogenous metabolites (e.g., 5-fluorouracil is transported by the pyrimidine transport system, MPPT is transported by the dopamine transport system). Active transport systems have several properties in common: they require metabolic energy; they can be inhibited by chemicals that affect energy metabolism; they are selective in terms of the molecules transported; they are saturable; and they can transport chemicals against a concentration gradient. *See also* ABSORPTION OF TOXICANTS; ENTRY MECHANISMS, SPECIAL TRANSPORT; EXCRETION, ALIMENTARY; EXCRETION, HEPATIC; EXCRETION, RENAL; FACILITATED TRANSPORT.

acute exposure. *See* EXPOSURE, ACUTE.

acute-phase reactant protein. *See* α_1-ACID GLYCOPROTEIN.

acute toxicity. Toxicity manifested within a relatively short time interval after toxicant exposure (i.e., as short as a few minutes to as long as several days). Such toxicity is usually caused by a single exposure to the toxicant. *See also* ACUTE TOXICITY TESTING.

acute toxicity, clinical signs. The signs of intoxication displayed by the person or animal that has been exposed to a toxicant. These signs will include levels of activity such as restlessness, irritability, hyperreflexia, confusion, delirium, mania, self-injury, convulsions, coma or circulatory collapse; they will also include autonomic signs such as diarrhea, altered pupil size, gooseflesh, hyperactive bowel sounds, hypertension or hypotension, tachycardia or bradycardia, and lacrimation. Other signs can include insomnia, muscle cramps and yawning.

acute toxicity testing. In the past, such tests were usually concerned with lethality estimated by the LD50 or LC50 tests. At present acute tests include those for eye and skin irritation and sensitization and changes in autonomic and cardiovascular function. More comprehensive acute toxicity tests also include gathering data on cause of death (where applicable), symptomatology, specific organ effects, metabolism and mode of toxic action, as well as forming the basis for subsequent subchronic studies. *See also* ACUTE TOXICITY TESTING, FACTORS AFFECTING; DERMAL IRRITATION TESTS; DERMAL SENSITIZATION TESTS; EYE IRRITATION TESTS; LC50; LD50; PHOTOTOXICITY TESTS; TESTING VARIABLES, BIOLOGICAL; TESTING VARIABLES, NON-BIOLOGICAL; TOXICITY TESTING.

acute toxicity testing, alternate approaches. *See* LD50.

acute toxicity testing, factors affecting. Biological variables including: species; strain; sex; stage of reproductive cycle; age; diet; disease and stress that can affect the results of acute toxicity tests. Non-biological variables include: environmental conditions (temperature, humidity, light cycle); housing (cage design, bedding, population density and composition); hygiene; statistical design and randomization. The two classes of variables are related since many of the non-biological variables directly affect such biological variables as stress and disease. These variables also affect subchronic and chronic tests and must be carefully controlled to ensure reproducibility. *See also* ACUTE TOXICITY TESTING; LD50; TESTING VARIABLES, BIOLOGICAL; TESTING VARIABLES, NONBIOLOGICAL.

acycloguanosine. *See* ACYCLOVIR.

acyclovir (2-amino-1,9-dihydro-9-[(2-hydroxyethoxy)methyl]-6H-purin-6-one; acycloguanosine; Zovirax). CAS number 277-89-3. A synthetic acyclic nucleoside with inhibitory activity towards herpes viruses. In mice its oral LD50 is

Acyclovir

greater than 10,000 mg/kg and its i.p. LD50 is about 1000 mg/kg. Topical application may cause irritation, and i.v. administration may cause transient renal dysfunction. Acyclovir is phosphorylated by herpes-specific thymidine kinases, resulting in the formation of acyclo-GTP, that inhibits viral DNA polymerase 10–30 times more efficiently than it does cellular DNA polymerase. Acyclo-GTP is incorporated into viral DNA causing termination of strand synthesis.

acylation. Important phase II reactions of two general types: (1) acetylation by an activated conjugation agent, CoA; (2) a process consisting first of the activation of the foreign compound and the subsequent acylation of an amino acid to yield the amino acid conjugate. This type of conjugation is characteristic of exogenous carboxylic acids and amides. *See also* ACETYLATION; *N,O*-ACYLTRANSFERASE; AMINO ACID CONJUGATION; PHASE II REACTIONS.

acyl CoA:amino acid *N*-acyltransferase. *See* AMINO ACID CONJUGATION.

acyl CoA synthetase. *See* AMINO ACID CONJUGATION.

***N,O*-acyltransferase.** A recently described enzyme, believed to be important in the activation of carcinogenic arylamines. Arylamines are first *N*-oxidized and then, in some species, *N*-acetylated to arylhydroxamic acids. The *N*-acyl group of the hydroxamic acid is first removed by the *N,O*-acyltransacetylase and then transferred either to an amine to yield a stable amide or to the oxygen of the hydroxylamine to yield a reactive *N*-acyloxyarylamine. These highly reactive compounds form adducts with proteins and nucleic acids. *N,O*-Acyltransferase that has been purified from the cytosolic fraction of rat liver, increases the mutagenicity of compounds such as *N*-hydroxy-2-acetylaminofluorene when added to the medium in the Ames test.

ADAM. *See* MDMA.

adaptation to toxicants. The ability of an organism to show either insensitivity or decreased sensitivity to a chemical that normally causes deleterious effects. The terms resistance and tolerance are closely related and have sometimes been used interchangeably. The present consensus is that resistance refers to the situation in which a change in the genetic constitution of a population in response to selection by the stressor chemical enables a greater number of individuals to resist the toxic action than were able to resist it in the unselected population. Thus, an essential feature of resistance is its inheritance by subsequent generations. In microorganisms this frequently involves mutations and induction of enzymes by the toxicant; in higher organisms it usually involves selection for genes already present in the population at low frequency. Tolerance is reserved for those situations in which individual organisms acquire the ability to resist the effect of a toxicant, usually as a result of prior exposure. Tolerance may also be used for populations that have the genes for resistance at a high frequency before exposure. More often, however, this is known as natural resistance, in contrast to acquired resistance, derived by selection as described above. *See also* CROSS-RESISTANCE.

ADCC. *See* ANTIBODY-DEPENDENT CELLULAR CYTOTOXICITY.

addiction. The overwhelming desire or need to continue the ingestion of a xenobiotic even when such use has deleterious physical, psychological, or social/legal manifestations. *See also* ALCOHOL; AMPHETAMINES; COCAINE; DEPENDENCE; MORPHINE; NICOTINE; TOLERANCE.

additive effect. That situation in which the combined effect of two or more chemicals is equal to the sum of the individual effects. *See also* SYNERGISM AND POTENTIATION.

additives, food. *See* FOOD ADDITIVES.

adduct. A chemical moiety that has become covalently bound to a large molecule such as DNA or protein; the term may cover both the chemical and the portion of the macromolecule with which it is combined.

adducts, DNA. *See* DNA ADDUCTS.

adducts, protein. Covalent compounds resulting from the reaction of a toxicant with a protein. The term is usually used in connection with carcinogens bound to proteins, such as hemoglobin, that then can serve as biomarkers of exposure. *See also* PROTEIN BINDING.

adenocarcinoma. A malignant tumor arising from epithelium and comprising malignant cells characteristic of the tissue from which it arises. Unlike an adenoma, these specific tissue characteristics are often unrecognizable in the cancer cells due to profound degeneration of morphology accompanying malignant transformation. Thus, the tissue of origin of a disseminated adenocarcinoma often cannot be determined. *Compare* ADENOMA.

adenohypophysis (anterior hypophysis; anterior pituitary). The anterior portion of the hypophysis (pituitary), which secretes a variety of tropic hormones in response to the releasing factors (releasing hormones) secreted by the hypothalamus. The releasing factors reach the adenohypophysis via the blood in the hypothalamic–hypophyseal portal system. The hormones released are part of the hypothalamic–hypophyseal axis in which control of endocrine secretions of the adrenal cortex, the thyroid and the gonads, as well as general metabolic function, is exerted by the hypothalamus. Hormones of the adenohypophysis are follicle-stimulating hormone (FSH), luteinizing hormone (LH), thyroid-stimulating hormone (TSH), adrenocorticotropic hormone (ACTH), somatotropin (growth hormone) and prolactin.

adenoma. A benign (i.e., non-malignant) tumor arising from epithelium and containing cells characteristic of the tissue from which it arises. The term is most often applied to tumors of glands or of mucosal epithelium (e.g., the lining of the mouth, bronchial tree, intestines, etc.). *Compare* ADENOCARCINOMA.

adenosine-3′,5′-monophosphate. *See* CYCLIC AMP.

adenosine monophosphate (AMP). A nucleotide that is part of the ATP energy cycle that supplies energy to drive reactions that require input of free energy, such as muscle contraction. Free energy is liberated when ATP is hydrolyzed to AMP and pyrophosphate. The AMP can be recycled to ADP via adenylate kinase and oxidative phosphorylation.

$$AMP + ATP \rightarrow 2ADP.$$

See also CYCLIC AMP; ATP; ENERGY SUPPLY.

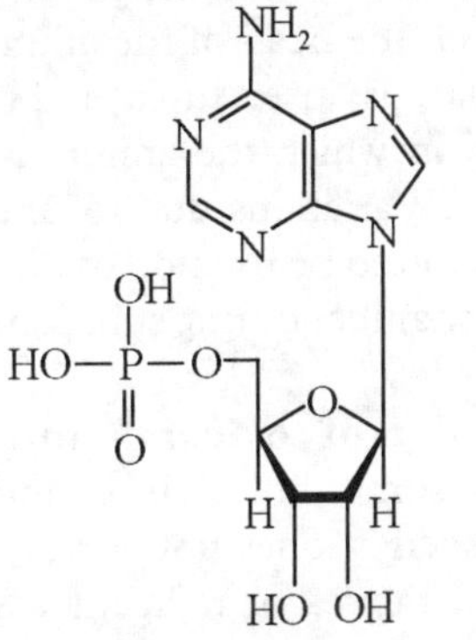

Adenosine monophosphate

adenosine 5′-phosphosulfate kinase. *See* SULFATE CONJUGATION.

adenosine 5′-triphosphatase. *See* ATPASE.

adenosine 5′-triphosphate. *See* ATP.

S-adenosylmethionine. CAS number **29908-03-0**. A reactive methionine derivative that donates the methyl group in the methylation of xenobiotics. *See also* METHYLATION; PHASE II REACTIONS.

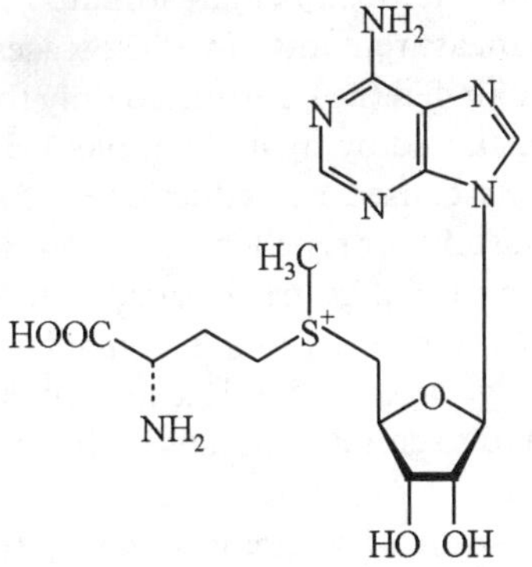

S-Adenosylmethionine

adenylate cyclase (adenylyl cyclase). The enzyme that synthesizes cAMP from ATP. Because of the role of cAMP as a second messenger, this enzyme plays a very important regulatory role and has sometimes been shown to be a site for toxicant action. In most well-characterized systems, the catalytic portion of the enzyme is activated or inhibited by guanine nucleotide-binding proteins (G proteins). Effects of the G proteins are initiated by the many members of seven-transmembrane spanning receptors that constitute the G protein-coupled receptor superfamily (GPCR), the latter providing the transduction mechanism by which the receptor change is transduced to the enzyme. *See also* CHOLERA TOXIN; CYCLIC AMP; G PROTEINS; PERTUSSIS TOXIN; RECEPTORS.

adenylyl cyclase. *See* ADENYLATE CYCLASE.

ADH (antidiuretic hormone). *See* VASOPRESSIN.

ADI. *See* ACCEPTABLE DAILY INTAKE.

adipose tissue. Fat tissue that stores fat reserves. Since so many xenobiotics are lipophilic, adipose tissue is a very likely storage location for xenobiotics. Adipose tissue can accumulate very large concentrations of xenobiotics in the process of bioaccumulation. It is unclear how readily xenobiotics stored in adipose tissue would be mobilized in starvation or weight loss, or during reproduction and lactation.

adjuvant. Literally, that which assists; can be used in pharmacy to describe a component of a prescription added to increase or speed up drug action. More commonly, the term is used, as in immunology and immunotoxicology, for foreign substances administered with an antigen to provoke a stronger immune response than would be obtained with the antigen alone. *See also* FREUND'S ADJUVANT.

administration of toxicants. *In vivo* testing requires the administration to animals of a known dose of the test chemical applied in a reproducible manner, and by a route of exposure similar to that expected of humans to the chemical in question or similar to the environmental exposure of natural populations. Both the nature and the degree of toxic effect may be affected by the route of administration because of effects at the portals of entry or to effects on pharmacokinetic processes. In order to identify the effects of handling and other stress, as well as the effects of the solvents or other carriers, treated animals are usually compared with both solvent-treated and untreated controls. *See also* ADMINISTRATION OF TOXICANTS, DERMAL; ADMINISTRATION OF TOXICANTS, IMPLANTATION; ADMINISTRATION OF TOXICANTS, INHALATION; ADMINISTRATION OF TOXICANTS, INJECTION; ADMINISTRATION OF TOXICANTS, ORAL; ADMINISTRATION OF TOXICANTS, PARENTERAL; ADMINISTRATION OF TOXICANTS, RECTAL.

administration of toxicants, dermal. Dermal administration is necessary for determination of the toxicity of chemicals taken up via the skin, as well as for determination of skin irritation and photosensitization. Test compounds are applied, either directly or in a suitable solvent, to the shaved skin of experimental animals. This technique is also referred to as skin painting. Since the animals must often be under restraint to prevent licking of the material, and thereby oral exposure, solvent and restraint controls are necessary. Skin irritancy tests may also be conducted on humans, using volunteer test panels.

administration of toxicants, implantation. The technique of surgical implantation, either subcutaneous or intramuscular, was developed for the testing of materials to be used in prostheses or other medical devices. It is now being developed, through the use of slowly soluble or biodegradable matrices, for controlled slow administration of clinical drugs or chemicals being tested for toxicity.

administration of toxicants, inhalation. Since the respiratory system is an important portal of entry, animals must be exposed to atmospheres containing potential toxicants for evaluation of toxicity. The generation and control of the physical characteristics of such contaminated atmospheres are technically complex and expensive in practice. The alternative (direct instillation into the lung via the trachea) presents problems of reproducibility and stress, and is often unsatisfactory. A complete inhalation test system contains an apparatus for the generation of aerosol particles, dusts or gas mixtures of defined composition and particle size, a chamber for the exposure of experimental animals and a sampling apparatus for the determination of the actual concentration within the chamber. Animals are usually exposed for a fixed number of hours per day and a fixed number of days per week. Exposure may be head-only, in which the head of the animal, wearing an airtight collar, is inserted into the chamber, or whole-body, in which the animal is placed inside the chamber. Variations due to unequal distribution are minimized by rotation of the position of the cages in the chamber during subsequent exposures.

administration of toxicants, injection. Except in the case of some clinical drugs and certain drugs of abuse, injection does not correspond to any of the expected modes of toxicant exposure. However, it may be useful in studies of mechanism or in quantitative structure–activity relationships (QSAR) studies in order to bypass absorption and permit rapid action. Injection methods include intravenous (iv), intramuscular (im), intraperitoneal (ip) and subcutaneous (sc). Infusion of toxicants over an extended period is also possible. *See also* QUANTITATIVE STRUCTURE–ACTIVITY RELATIONSHIPS.

administration of toxicants, oral. Compounds being tested for toxicity can be administered, either mixed in the diet or dissolved in drinking water, by gastric lavage, controlled-release capsules or gelatin capsules. In the first two cases a measured amount can be given or access can be *ad libitum*, with the dose being estimated from consumption measurements. In these cases controls should be pair-fed (i.e., permitted only the amount of food consumed by treated animals) since nutritional effects caused by reduction of food intake due to distasteful or repellent test materials is possible. In the case of gastric lavage the test material is administered directly to the stomach via a stomach tube or gavage needle. If a solvent is used it is administered to control animals in the same way.

administration of toxicants, parenteral. Parenteral administration denotes any route of delivery or uptake other than the gastrointestinal route, although common usage generally does not include uptake through the intact skin (percutaneous absorption) or the intact lung (inhalation).

administration of toxicants, rectal. Rectal administration is used only for the testing of pharmaceuticals normally administered as suppositories, not in other toxicity tests.

administration of toxicants, water column. An experimental technique for exposing aquatic organisms to toxicants by dissolving or suspending the toxicant in the water column of the experimental container (for example, an aquarium or vat). Non-water soluble toxicants may require a water-miscible vehicle. Physical methods, such as sonication, may be sufficient to suspend non-water soluble xenobiotics in the water column.

ADR. *See* ADVERSE DRUG REACTION; SUSPECTED ADVERSE DRUG REACTION.

adrenal gland (suprarenal gland). An endocrine gland that occurs cephalic to the kidney. It has two distinct layers, a cortex and a medulla, that have different embryological origins, different mechanisms of control and produce different chemical classes of hormones. The cortex produces two important classes of steroid hormones: the mineralocorticoids, primarily aldosterone, from the zona glomerulosa, that cause the excretion of sodium and the retention of potassium, and thereby influence water balance; and the glucocorticoids, that include cortisol (hydrocortisone) and corticosterone, from the zona fasciculata, that enhance gluconeogenesis (and thereby can deplete body protein), assist in combating long-term stress and exert an anti-inflammatory action. Also small amounts of sex steroids, mostly androgens, are secreted, but these low levels have no effects in males and exert some isolated effects in females (e.g., acne and development of axillary and pubic hair). The medulla secretes the catecholamines epinephrine and norepinephrine in response to stimulation by the sympathetic nervous system; these hormones help to combat short-term stress by contributing to the fight-or-flight mechanisms (e.g., increased heart rate, vasoconstriction and glycogen mobilization).

adrenal gland toxicity. Hypersecretion of the glucocorticoids resulting in Cushing's syndrome, characterized by changes in protein and carbohydrate metabolism, hyperglycemia, muscular weakness and hypertension. The immune response is suppressed and the body takes on a puffy appearance. These signs are also seen when patients receive glucocorticoids therapeutically for a prolonged time. Hypersecretion of the adrenal androgens results in the adrenogenital syndrome. In children this causes premature puberty, enlarged genitals, increased body hair and shortened stature upon reaching adulthood. In adult females, hirsutism results. Hypersecretion of the adrenal medulla can deplete the body's energy reserves. Prolonged stress can lead to disease because of the extended secretions of the medullary catecholamines and the glucocorticoids.

adrenaline. *See* EPINEPHRINE.

β-adrenergic antagonists (β-adrenergic blocking agents; β-blockers). A group of drugs that competitively inhibit the binding of catecholamines to β-adrenergic receptors. There are two general types of receptors: β_1 located in the heart; β_2 located in all other areas. β-Blockers are classified as cardioselective or non-selective with regard to their β_1/β_2 activity, but these are not absolute terms. They are also classified according to their lipid solubility. Hydrophilic β-blockers are poorly absorbed from the gut, are not extensively metabolized, have longer half-lives and do not readily cross the blood–brain barrier. They are used to treat hypertension, angina, vascular headaches, and arrhythmias, as well as in post-infarction cardioprotection. Their adverse reactions are largely based on their β_2-blocking properties and include bronchospasm, hypoglycemia and fatigue.

adrenocorticotropic hormone. *See* ACTH.

adrenogenital syndrome. *See* ADRENAL GLAND TOXICITY.

adriamycin. *See* DOXORUBICIN.

adsorption. Process by which chemicals are bound to a surface. Usually used for binding to soil or other nonliving particles but also, less often, for binding to cell surfaces.

adsorption assay. *See* ELISA.

advanced waste treatment. Any process for the treatment of waste that follows other physical, chemical or biological treatments and aims to improve the quality of effluent prior to reuse or discharge. The term often refers to the removal of nitrate and phosphate plant nutrients.

advection. Transport by motion of the air, water or other fluid. Advection has the same general meaning as convection, but is used particularly to refer to the horizontal transport by wind of something carried by the air (e.g., pollutants, heated air, fog, etc.).

adverse drug reaction (ADR, adverse drug event). Harmful events associated with the use of therapeutic drugs have been variously defined. WHO defines ADR as "a response to a drug which is noxious and unintended and occurs at doses used in man for the prophylaxis, diagnosis or therapy of disease, or for modification of physiological function." The USFDA and EEC definitions are more inclusive but deal with essentially the same problem. ADRs include many different effects of varying severity, however, it has been estimated that they may be responsible for 3–6% of all medical admissions and may cause as many as 160,000 deaths in US hospitals alone. *See also* SUSPECTED ADVERSE DRUG REACTION.

adverse effect. A pathological lesion, or a biochemical, metabolic or genetic change that affects the normal function of the organism, impairs the ability to adapt to environmental change, or causes a change in the genetic information transmitted to offspring.

Advisory Committee on Dangerous Pathogens. A UK committee set up in 1981 to advise UK government departments and the Health and Safety Commission on work with infectious microorganisms. The committee's recommen-

dations were published in Categorisation of Pathogens According to Hazards and Categories of Containment (Second edition, 1990).

Advisory Committee on Mutagenesis (ACM). Canadian expert committee to advise the Canadian government on the evaluation and regulation of chemical mutagens.

Advisory Committee on Novel Food and Processes (ACNFP). A UK expert committee that advises government ministers (Health and Food) on matters relating to the safety of novel foods, including food irradiation. Novelty may result from new processing or preparation techniques, the novelty of the food's role in diet, or because there is no history of its use in the UK.

Advisory Committee on Pesticides (ACP). A UK expert committee (set up under the Food and Environment Protection Act, 1985, s. 16(7)) that advises government ministers on matters relating to pesticides, including safety aspects of their authorization for use.

aerobic. With oxygen. Aerobic cells or organisms require oxygen and depend upon the pathways of aerobic respiration (i.e., glycolysis to pyruvate, tricarboxylic acid cycle and electron transport system) for their energy generation.

aerobic respiration. Process in living organisms that utilizes molecular oxygen for the release of energy during the degradation of nutrients, or metabolites derived from nutrients. The energy released is usually conserved as adenosine triphosphate (ATP), subsequently utilized in energy-requiring processes, although other high-energy intermediates are known. *See also* ANAEROBIC.

aerodynamic diameter. A standard for characterizing airborne particles that are not spherical in shape. It includes both density and aerodynamic drag, and is expressed as the diameter of a unit density sphere with the same terminal settling velocity as the particle in question, whatever its shape, size or density. This value is of particular interest in respiratory toxicology since it reflects the ease of deposition of all particles except the very small, the deposition of which is determined by particle size alone.

aerosol. A solid or liquid particle suspended in a gaseous medium and so small that its fall speed is small compared with the vertical components of air motion. Haze and cloud are the commonest atmospheric aerosols, with fall speeds much less than 10 mm/sec. Aerosols in the troposphere generally fall to the surface in a matter of hours or days; those in the stratosphere may remain there for months or years. Volcanoes are the major source of atmospheric aerosols, but human activities (e.g., cultivating dry soils, quarrying, industrial manufacturing, etc.) contribute about 30% of tropospheric aerosols. Tropospheric aerosols may act as condensation nuclei; some stratospheric aerosols, especially sulfate particles, have a climatic effect by increasing the Earth's albedo (whiteness or degree of reflection of incident light).

aerosol spray. A container in which a propellant (e.g., ammonia, butane or chlorofluorocarbons) is mixed with a substance (e.g., paint, perfume, hairspray, polish or wound dressing) and held under pressure. When the pressure is released the substance is propelled through a nozzle as a mist of aerosols. A more primitive version of the aerosol spray is the liquid atomizer, in which the propulsion pressure is produced by a small hand-operated pump.

A-esterase. Hydrolases that are calcium dependent and are capable of hydrolyzing organophosphorus triesters. Likely substrates are organophosphorus insecticides that are phosphates, the phosphate (oxon) metabolites of phosphorothionate insecticides, nerve agents and diisopropylfluorophosphate (DFP). The enzymes have been sometimes named for the substrate studied, such as paraoxonase or DFPase. *See also* HYDROLYSIS.

AETT. *See* ACETYLETHYLTETRAMETHYLTETRALIN.

affinity. The ability of a substance to bind to another substance. The term is usually used to refer to the likelihood of a substrate binding to an enzyme or a ligand binding to a receptor. *See also* ASSOCIATION CONSTANT; RECEPTOR.

affinity chromatography. *See* CHROMATOGRAPHY, AFFINITY.

affinity constant. *See* ASSOCIATION CONSTANT.

affinity labeling. A procedure for identifying or quantifying receptors by covalently binding a high affinity ligand to the receptor. This can be accomplished by either using a ligand possessing a chemical grouping capable of covalently binding to the receptor, or by allowing a cross-linking reagent to covalently bind to both the ligand and the receptor. Photoaffinity labeling uses a chemical moiety that can be activated by ultraviolet radiation.

aflatoxins. CAS number 1402-68-2. A family of mycotoxins produced by the mold *Aspergillus flavus* and related fungi; included among them are carcinogens and hepatotoxicants. Aflatoxins affect male reproductive capacity and growth rate in birds. They are the causative agents in the Turkey X disease. Aflatoxin B_1 is hepatotoxic and is one of the most potent carcinogens known, being active at dietary doses in the part per billion range. Aflatoxins are found as contaminants in both human foodstuffs and animal feed, particularly in corn and peanuts. The extent of aflatoxin contamination is a function of environmental conditions at the time of harvest and storage conditions. Although generally a liver carcinogen, there are species differences, mice being relatively insensitive and showing lung tumors on treatment. Aflatoxin B_1 (CAS number 1162-65-8) is oxidized by the cytochrome P450-dependent monooxygenase system to form a highly reactive epoxide. Carcinogenesis is believed to be initiated when this potent electrophile reacts with DNA, and hepatotoxicity when it reacts with proteins to cause either fatty liver or liver necrosis. Epidemiological studies in Africa and Asia indicate that it is a human liver carcinogen, although similar studies in North America where aflatoxin contamination is common are generally negative. More recent studies on the occurrence of hepatitis B virus indicate that the

Aflatoxin B_1

presence of this virus, endemic in many African and Asian populations, may potentiate aflatoxin carcinogenicity. *See also* ACTIVATION; MYCOTOXINS; REACTIVE INTERMEDIATES.

Agency for Toxic Substance and Disease Registry (ATSDR). A division of the US Public Health Service charged, under the Superfund Amendments and Reauthorization Act (SARA), an act that amended the Comprehensive Environmental Response, Compensation and Liability Act (CERCLA) of 1980, with the preparation and publication of toxicological profiles for hazardous substances most commonly found at facilities on the CERCLA National Priorities List and that pose the most significant potential threat to human health as determined by ATSDR and the US Environmental Protection Agency. Such profiles summarize the available adverse health effects and review the key peer reviewed literature. Each profile is first published as a draft for public comment, then as a revised document with updated versions as appropriate.

Agent Blue. A herbicide used to control vegetation in the Vietnam conflict; a solution of cacodylic acid employed in the short-term control of rice and other food crops. The concentration of cacodylic acid in Agent Blue is 0.37 kg/l. Bovey, R.W. & Young, A.L. The Science of 2,4,5-T and Associated Phenoxy Herbicides (Wiley, New York, 1980). *See also* CACODYLIC ACID.

Agent Orange. The most commonly used "defoliant" in the Vietnam conflict; a mixture of two commercial herbicides widely employed for a number of years in the brush control programs throughout the USA and for weed control in agriculture. Active ingredients of Agent Orange are the two *n*-butyl esters of 2,4-dichlorophenoxyacetic acid (2,4-D) and 2,4,5-trichlorophenoxyacetic acid (2,4,5-T) with concentrations of 0.50 and 0.53 kg/l, respectively. Of particular interest in Agent Orange is the contaminant of 2,4,5-T, 2,3,7,8-tetrachlorodibenzo-*p*-dioxin (TCDD, dioxin), sometimes said to be the most toxic chlorine-containing compound known. Bovey, R.W. & Young, A.L. The Science of 2,4,5-T and Associated Phenoxy Herbicides (Wiley, New York, 1980). Tucker, R.E. et al. (eds) Human and

Environmental Risks of Chlorinated Dioxins and Related Compounds (Plenum Press, New York, 1983). *See also* 2,4,5-T; TCDD.

Agent Purple. A herbicide used to control vegetation in the Vietnam conflict; a mixture of two herbicides employed in the control of forests, brush and broadleaf crops prior to its replacement by Agent Orange in 1964. Active ingredients of Agent Purple were the *n*-butyl esters of 2,4-dichlorophenoxyacetic acid (2,4-D) and 2,4,5-trichlorophenoxyacetic acid (2,4,5-T) plus the isobutyl ester of 2,4,5-T, with concentrations of 0.50, 0.31 and 0.22 kg/l, respectively. Bovey, R.W. & Young, A.L. The Science of 2,4,5-T and Associated Phenoxy Herbicides (Wiley, New York, 1980). *See also* 2,4,5-T; TCDD.

Agent White. A herbicide used to control vegetation in the Vietnam conflict; a mixture of two commercial herbicides employed for a number of years in the long-term control of forest and brush vegetation. Active ingredients of Agent White were the triisopropanolamine salt of 2,4-dichlorophenoxyacetic acid (2,4-D) and picloram, with concentrations of 0.24 and 0.07 kg/l, respectively. Bovey, R.W. & Young, A.L. The Science of 2,4,5-T and Associated Phenoxy Herbicides (Wiley, New York, 1980). *See also* PICLORAM.

aggregate risk. The sum of individual risks of adverse effects on an exposed population. It should be noted that the simple summation of risks, determined separately, into an aggregate may give an erroneous estimate. Risks may be additive, less than additive, or more than additive (synergistic).

aging, organophosphate inhibited cholinerasterase. See ACETYLCHOLINESTERASE, AGING.

aglycone. The xenobiotic fragment that combines with a carbohydrate, such as glucuronic acid, to form a conjugate (Phase II metabolite).

agonist. Compounds that exert their toxico- or pharmacodynamic effects by interacting with a receptor in the same fashion as the endogenous ligand for the receptor, thereby mimicking the action of the endogenous molecule. Agonists can be divided into two classes: direct-acting and indirect-acting. A direct-acting agonist is a toxicant or drug that directly interacts with the receptor site. An indirect-acting agonist exerts its action by increasing the concentration of the endogenous compound (e.g., by affecting vesicular storage or release of a neurotransmitter) that then activates the receptor. The potency of an agonist *in vitro* is typically expressed as its K_D or K_I, that is estimated from Scatchard or other kinetic equations. The K_M or K_D is inversely proportional to the affinity of the compound in question for its receptor site. *In vivo* the potency of an agonist can be expressed as the ED50. *See also* AFFINITY CONSTANT; DISSOCIATION CONSTANT; ENZYME KINETICS; RECEPTOR.

agranulocytosis. An absence of cells of the granulocytic series (neutrophils, eosinophils and basophils) in peripheral blood; in actual usage the term usually refers to a severe granulocytopenia. It is often a manifestation of leukemia or bone marrow toxicity due to radiation or chemicals, or an idiosyncratic manifestation to an administered therapeutic drug. Severity of granulocytopenia is based on the absolute neutrophil count. Because of the essential role of the neutrophils in the body's control of microbial invasion, neutrophil counts between 500–1000 per cubic millimeter represent a moderate risk of serious invasive infection, counts between 200–500 represent a serious risk and counts below 100–200 represent an almost certain risk. Neutropenia is often used as a synonym, but it is not a true synonym since it refers specifically to a decrease in neutrophils. *See also* APLASTIC ANEMIA.

Agricultural and Food Research Council. A UK government organization that supports research institutes throughout the UK. It also provides funds for academic research projects concerned with agricultural, horticultural and veterinary science, and food technology.

agricultural chemicals. Those chemicals used in agriculture that are designed to increase yield of food and fiber either by direct action on crop plants or domestic animals (e.g., fertilizers, plant growth regulators, etc.) or by controlling their diseases, pests, predators or competitors (e.g., fungicides, insecticides, rodenticides, etc.). In the latter case selectivity (i.e., toxicity to the pest with lower toxicity to non-target species) is a desired quality, and the development of such specific toxicants is an important function of comparative toxicology. Other chemicals, although not directly involved in increased production, are used to improve cost effectiveness in agriculture by improving handling and storage qualities of the harvested crop. Agricultural chemicals have the potential of contaminating soil and also water (from surface run-off and leaching into the ground water). In addition, exposure to agrochemicals in both workers and the public can occur because of residues on crops, air contamination resulting from spraying and drift, exposure during manufacture and formulations, and contamination from waste disposal sites. The persistence and bioaccumulation of the older organochlorine insecticides has been well recognized. Newer insecticides, such as the organophosphates, carbamates and synthetic pyrethroids, are more labile and less likely to cause ecological damage. Fertilizers can contribute to eutrophication and therefore alter ecological balance. Because of their actual or potential toxicity to non-target species, including humans, agricultural chemicals are regulated by law in many countries. *See also* ACARICIDES; FUNGICIDES; HERBICIDES; INSECTICIDES; MOLLUSCICIDES; NEMATOCIDES; PESTICIDES; POLLUTION, AGRICULTURAL CHEMICALS; RODENTICIDES.

Agricultural Chemicals Approval Scheme. *See* PEST INFESTATION CONTROL LABORATORY.

Agricultural (Poisonous Substances) Regulations. UK regulations published in 1966, with amendments in 1967 and 1969, that prohibit the carrying out of certain procedures involving the use of listed pesticides without the wearing of protective clothing. The poisonous substances covered under these regulations include 27 organophosphorus compounds, two organochlorine insecticides and three nitrophenol compounds.

Agrimet. *See* PHORATE.

agrochemicals. *See* AGRICULTURAL CHEMICALS.

agroecosystem. A specialized ecosystem resulting from agricultural practices, with the specific introduction and culturing of crop plant or animal species and the elimination of pest plant or animal species. Agroecosystems are important in toxicology because of the widespread use of pesticides and other agricultural chemicals and their possible dissemination into air, ground water, surface water and the food chain. *See also* ECOSYSTEMS.

AHH. *See* ARYL HYDROCARBON HYDROXYLASE.

Ah locus. A gene, or genes, controlling the trait of aromatic hydrocarbon (Ah) responsiveness. Aromatic hydrocarbons include: the polycyclics; the chlorinated dibenzo-*p*-dioxins (e.g., TCDD); dibenzofurans and biphenyls (PCBs); and the brominated biphenyls (PBBs). This trait, originally defined as induction of hepatic aryl hydrocarbon hydroxylase (AHH) activity following 3-methylcholanthrene treatment, is inherited by simple autosomal dominance in crosses and backcrosses between C57BL/6 (Ah-responsive) and DBA/2 (Ah-non-responsive) mice. It has been proposed that the Ah locus is composed of regulatory, structural and, perhaps, temporal genes. *See also* AH RECEPTOR.

Ah receptor (TCDD-binding protein). A protein coded by a putative regulatory gene of the Ah locus. The initial location of the Ah receptor is believed to be in the cytosol, although recent evidence suggests it may reside within the nucleus. Binding of aromatic hydrocarbons (Ah) to the Ah receptor of mice is a prerequisite for the induction of many xenobiotic-metabolizing enzymes, as well as two responses to 2,3,7,8-tetrachlorodibenzo-*p*-dioxin: epidermal hyperplasia and thymic atrophy. Ah-responsive mice (e.g., C57BL/6) have a high-affinity receptor, whereas the Ah-non-responsive mice (e.g., DBA/2) presumably have a low-affinity receptor. The Ah receptor is present in many species including humans, other primates and lower vertebrates. *See also* AH LOCUS.

AIDS. *See* ACQUIRED IMMUNE DEFICIENCY SYNDROME.

AIHA. *See* AMERICAN INDUSTRIAL HYGIENE ASSOCIATION.

air pollution. A serious problem in populated areas of industrialized nations and in other locations where, for example, excessive amounts of fossil fuels are burnt. Both the nature and source of air pollutants vary with the location: open country, remote from industry or heavy traffic, differs from the center of a large city or from an area downwind from a coal-fired power plant or other industry. In general, the principal air pollutants are carbon monoxide, oxides of nitrogen, oxides of sulfur, hydrocarbons and particulates. The principal sources are transportation, industrial processes, electric power generation, and the heating of homes and buildings. Of the organic constituents, hydrocarbons such as benzo[*a*]pyrene are produced by incomplete combustion and are associated primarily with the automobile. Hydrocarbons are usually not present at levels high enough to cause a direct toxic effect, but are important in the formation of photochemical air pollution. This is formed as a result of interactions between hydrocarbon and oxides of nitrogen in the presence of ultraviolet light, giving rise to lung irritants such as peroxyacetyl nitrate, acrolein and formaldehyde. Particulates are a heterogeneous group of particles, often seen as smoke, that are important as carriers of adsorbed hydrocarbons and as irritants to the respiratory system. The distribution of such particles in the atmosphere, as well as in the respiratory tract, is largely a function of their size. Respiratory system effects are the primary human health effects observed, with individuals possessing weak or immature respiratory and circulatory systems being at greatest risk. The known health effects of specific pollutants include: sulfur dioxide and sulfuric acid—bronchoconstriction and irritation of mucous membranes; nitrogen dioxide—pulmonary edema and hemorrhage; ozone—pulmonary edema and hemorrhage; carbon monoxid —headaches, dizziness and suffocation; lead—renal toxicity, impaired erythropoiesis, and nervous system damage (primarily in the fetus and young child); and dust and fibers—scarring or fibrosis in lungs. Environmental effects of air pollution include: injury to plants, including changes in color and growth, increased susceptibility to disease, death and ultimately replacement of species in ecosystems; chronic poisoning of domestic animals from ingestion of food contaminated with pollutants from air, primarily metals and fluoride (leading to fluorosis); damage to buildings, metal structures, rubber and other materials from acids and ozone; reduced visibility from particulates in smog; the "greenhouse effect" from elevated carbon dioxide concentrations; the formation of acid deposition, primarily from the presence of sulfuric and nitric acids, that causes toxicity to fish and forests. Stern, A.C. et al. Fundamentals of Air Pollution, 2nd edn (Academic Press, Orlando, 1984). *See also* ACROLEIN; AIR QUALITY INDEX; AIR QUALITY STANDARDS; CARBON MONOXIDE; FORMALDEHYDE; NITROGEN OXIDES; OZONE; PARTICULATES; PEROXYACETYL NITRATE; POLLUTION, EFFECT ON DOMESTIC ANIMALS; POLLUTION, EFFECT ON PLANTS; POLLUTION, EFFECT ON STRUCTURES; POLLUTION, ENERGY SOURCES; POLLUTION, EXHAUST EMISSIONS; POLLUTION, FOSSIL FUELS; POLLUTION, INDUSTRIAL PROCESSES; POLLUTION, PARTICULATES; POLYCYCLIC AROMATIC HYDROCARBONS; SULFURIC ACID; SULFUR OXIDES.

Air Quality Act, 1967. U.S. Federal law that empowered the Department of Health, Education, and Welfare to designate areas within which air quality was to be controlled, to set ambient air standards, to specify technologies to be used in pollution control and to prosecute offenders if local agencies fail to do so. Subsequently replaced by the Clean Air Act, administered by the Environmental Protection Agency. *See also* CLEAN AIR ACTS.

air quality index. A standardized system proposed by the Environmental Protection Agency (EPA) to give the public an indication of the degree of air pollution. The numbers of the index result from measurements of ozone, suspended particulates, sulfur dioxide and carbon dioxide. The descriptors associated with various index levels are: 0, no pollution; 100, standard; 200, alert; 300, warning; 400, emergency; 500, significant harm.

air quality standards. Legal standards of exposure to air pollutants that should not be exceeded in a given geographical area. The standard specifies both the concentration and the duration of exposure, and usually is below the threshold value.

air sampling. *See* SAMPLING, AIR.

airway. Any segment, such as the bronchial tubes, conducting air between the mouth and the alveoli. Also used to describe the entire route for air flow between mouth and alveoli.

airway resistance. The resistance to air flow caused by the airways between mouth and alveoli.

akathesia. *See* EXTRAPYRAMIDAL SIDE EFFECTS.

alachlor. *See* PHENOXYACETIC ACIDS.

ALAD (aminolevulinic acid dehydratase). *See* FREE ERYTHROCYTE PROTOPORPHYRIN.

Alar (daminozide; butanedioic acid mono-(2,2-dimethylhydrazide); *N*-(dimethylamino) succinamic acid; succinic acid 2,2-dimethylhydrazide). Plant growth regulator. Metabolized in mammals to 1,1-dimethylhydrazine. Banned for use in the USA on the basis of equivocal chronic feeding tests in rodents. While there was no evidence from properly conducted carcinogenicity tests that Alar was carcinogenic, the metabolite 1,1-dimethylhydrazine produced tumors at very high doses.

$$\text{HO}-\overset{\overset{\textstyle O}{\|}}{\text{C}}-\text{CH}_2\text{CH}_2-\overset{\overset{\textstyle O}{\|}}{\text{C}}-\text{NH}-\text{N}\overset{\textstyle \diagup \text{CH}_3}{\diagdown \text{CH}_3}$$

Alar

albumins. A group of proteins characterized by their heat coagulation characteristics and solubility in dilute salt solutions. Although found in most tissues and species, they are best known from mammalian blood. Serum albumins together form the most abundant class of blood proteins and are important in toxicology because of their role in the transport of toxicants. Although it is frequently stated that they are of primary importance in the transport of xenobiotics, this is based on experimental studies with drugs that often are less lipophilic than toxicants. Lipoproteins may be the principal transport proteins for lipophilic toxicants. Binding to albumin involves specific sites on the molecule and hydrophilic bonds, although hydrogen bonding and hydrophobic interactions may also play a role. Because of the large amount of albumin in blood, bound toxicants may represent a significant depot of transiently inactive toxicants in the body. *See also* BINDING; BINDING AFFINITY; BINDING SITES AND TRANSPORT; COMPETITIVE BINDING AND TRANSPORT; LIGANDS; LIPOPHILICITY; LIPOPROTEINS; PROTEIN BINDING.

albuminuria. *See* PROTEINURIA.

alcohol. A class of organic compounds containing one or more hydroxyl groups; the term alcohol is often used to refer specifically to ethanol (ethyl alcohol). *See also* ALCOHOLS; ETHANOL.

alcohol dehydrogenase (EC 1.1.1.1). An enzyme that catalyzes the conversion of alcohols to aldehydes or ketones.

$$RCH_2OH + NAD^+ \rightarrow RCHO + NADH + H^+$$

The reaction is reversible, and *in vitro* carbonyl compounds are reduced to alcohols. *In vivo*, however, the reaction proceeds in the direction of alcohol consumption, since aldehydes are further oxidized to acids. The enzyme is found in the soluble fraction of liver, kidney and lung, and is the most important enzyme involved in the metabolism of foreign alcohols. It is a dimer, the subunits of which can occur in several forms, thus giving rise to a large number of variants of the enzyme. It can use either NAD^+ or $NADP^+$ as a coenzyme, but the reaction proceeds more slowly with $NADP^+$. Since aldehydes are toxic and, because of their lipophilicity, not readily excreted, alcohol oxidation may be considered an activation reaction, the further oxidation of the aldehyde being detoxication. Primary alcohols are oxidized to aldehydes, *n*-butanol having the highest oxidation rate. Secondary alcohols are oxidized to ketones, but the rate is less than that for primary alcohols, and tertiary alcohols are not readily oxidized. This reaction should not be confused with the monooxygenation of alcohols, a cytochrome P450-dependent reaction that occurs in the microsomes. *Compare* MONOOXYGENASES. *See also* ACETALDEHYDE; DISULFIRAM; ETHANOL.

alcohol-related birth defects. *See* FETAL ALCOHOL EFFECT; FETAL ALCOHOL SYNDROME.

alcohols. Organic compounds with one or more hydroxyl (-OH) substituents on an aliphatic carbon atom(s); not to be confused with phenols in which the hydroxyl substituent is on an aromatic carbon atom. Alcohols are widely used and are frequently toxic. *See also* ALCOHOLS, ALIPHATIC; ALCOHOLS, AROMATIC; ALCOHOLS, POLYHYDROXY.

alcohols, aliphatic. Alcohols have a hydroxyl group (-OH) attached to a carbon atom, in lieu of a hydrogen atom, in an aliphatic hydrocarbon. They can be either branched or straight-chain, depending upon the position of the substituted carbon atom in the chain and are classified as primary, secondary and tertiary (e.g., primary, secondary and tertiary butanol). This group of compounds has extensive use as industrial solvents; only one of them, ethanol, is used as a beverage with potentially toxic effects. Others in the series are more toxic than ethanol and are not used for this purpose. *See also* ETHANOL; METHANOL.

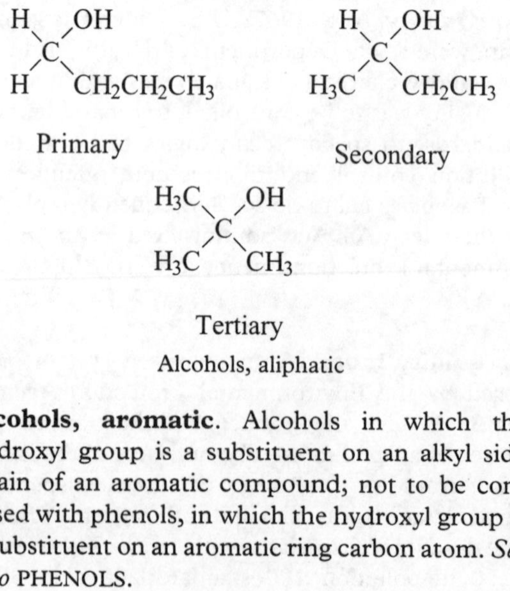

Primary

Secondary

Tertiary

Alcohols, aliphatic

alcohols, aromatic. Alcohols in which the hydroxyl group is a substituent on an alkyl side chain of an aromatic compound; not to be confused with phenols, in which the hydroxyl group is a substituent on an aromatic ring carbon atom. *See also* PHENOLS.

alcohols, polyhydroxy (glycols, polyhydric alcohols). Alcohols that contain two or more hydroxyl (-OH) groups attached to different aliphatic carbon atoms. They are widely utilized as heat exchangers, hydraulic fluids and in antifreeze preparations. Toxicity has been noted in both humans and experimental animals. *See also* ETHYLENE GLYCOL.

aldehyde and ketone reduction. Aldehydes and ketones are reduced not only by the reverse reaction of alcohol dehydrogenase, but also by aldehyde reductases. These enzymes are NADPH-dependent cytoplasmic enzymes of low molecular weight and have been found in liver, brain, kidney and other tissues. *See also* ALCOHOL DEHYDROGENASE; REDUCTION.

aldehyde dehydrogenase. An enzyme that catalyzes the formation of acids from aliphatic and aromatic aldehydes; the acids are then available as substrates for phase II conjugating enzymes.

$$RCHO + NAD^+ + O_2 = RCOOH + NADH + H^+$$

The enzyme from mammalian liver has been isolated, and a large number of aldehydes can serve as substrates. Aldehyde oxidase and xanthine oxidase are both flavoproteins that contain molybdenum. Their primary role, however, seems to be the oxidation of endogenous aldehydes formed as a result of deamination reactions. *See also* ALDEHYDE OXIDASE; PHASE II REACTIONS; XANTHINE OXIDASE.

aldehyde oxidase. A flavoprotein, also containing molybdenum, that is found in the soluble fraction of liver cells. Unlike aldehyde dehydrogenase, its primary role appears to be the oxidation of endogenous aldehydes. It is very similar to xanthine oxidase. *Compare* ALDEHYDE DEHYDROGENASE. *See also* XANTHINE OXIDASE.

aldehydes ($C_nH_{2n}O$). Organic compounds containing the group >C=O, designated by the suffix group [al] added to the name of the hydrocarbon from which it is derived (e.g., propanal). Aldehydes are reactive and intensely irritant to the respiratory system. Aldehydes in polluted air are formed as reaction products in the photooxidation of hydrocarbons and contribute to the irritant qualities of photochemical smog with formaldehyde and acrolein being the most important. They may be formed metabolically from the corresponding alcohol and are involved in the mechanism of alcohol toxicity, for example, acetaldehyde formed *in vivo* from ethanol and formaldehyde from methanol. *See also* ACETALDEHYDE; ACROLEIN; FORMALDEHYDE.

aldicarb (2-methyl-2-(methylthio)propanal O-[(methylamino)carbonyl]oxime; Temik). CAS number 116-06-3. A systemic carbamate insecticide, acaricide and nematocide for soil use with an extremely high level of acute toxicity. It has also become a contaminant of ground water in some regions because of its relatively high water solubility. The acute oral LD50 in male rats is 0.93 mg/kg and acute dermal LD50 in male rabbits is 5.0 mg/kg. The 96-hour LC50 in rainbow trout is 8.8 mg/ l. It is a neurotoxicant by virtue of its ability to inhibit acetylcholinesterase. Hallenbeck, W.H. & Cinningham-Burns, K.M. (eds) Pesticides and Human Health (Springer-Verlag, New York, 1985). *See also* CARBAMATE INSECTICIDES; CARBAMATE POISONING, SYMPTOMS AND THERAPY.

$$CH_3S-\underset{\underset{CH_3}{|}}{\overset{\overset{CH_3}{|}}{C}}-CH=NOCONHCH_3$$

Aldicarb

aldrin. *See* CYCLODIENE INSECTICIDES.

aliesterases. *See* CARBOXYLESTERASES.

alimentary excretion. *See* EXCRETION, ALIMENTARY.

aliphatic. Aliphatic compounds are carbon compounds with the carbon atoms in chains as opposed to ring structures. Aliphatic compounds may be straight or branched chain, saturated or unsaturated. In some cases carbon chains attached to ring structures are referred to as aliphatic substituents.

aliphatic amine, *N*-hydroxylation. *See* N-OXIDATION.

aliphatic amines. Aliphatic compounds with one or more carbon having amino ($-NH_2$) substituents.

aliphatic epoxidation. Many aliphatic and alicyclic compounds containing unsaturated carbon atoms are thought to be metabolized via transient epoxide intermediates. In some cases, such as the cyclodiene insecticide aldrin, the product is an extremely stable epoxide. Thus dieldrin, the epoxide derivative of aldrin, is the principal residue found in animals that have been exposed to aldrin. In the case of aflatoxin, the epoxide is believed to be the ultimate carcinogen, and in this case, therefore, aliphatic epoxidation is an activation reaction. Cytochrome P450 is the principal, and perhaps the only, enzyme involved in this reaction as it applies to xenobiotics. *See also* CYTOCHROME P450-DEPENDENT MONOOXYGENASE SYSTEM; EPOXIDES.

aliphatic hydrocarbons. A class of chemicals that contains non-cyclic derivatives of carbon and hydrogen. They may be saturated or unsaturated and have either straight or branched carbon chains. Members of the straight-chain saturated series are also known as alkanes or paraffins. The lower members (e.g., methane and ethane) are simple asphyxiants. Pentane, hexane, heptane and octane all cause CNS depression, dizziness and decreased coordination when inhaled. Hexane is known to cause a severe polyneuropathy in humans and experimental animals. Many industrial solvents contain a high proportion of aliphatic hydrocarbons, as do gasoline, kerosene and Stoddard's solvent. Many of the halogenated aliphatic hydrocarbons are much more toxic than the parent compounds. *See also* HALOGENATED HYDROCARBONS; HEXANE.

aliphatic hydroxylation. Simple aliphatic molecules such as *n*-butane, *n*-pentane, *n*-hexane, etc., as well as alicyclic compounds such as cyclohexane, are oxidized *in vivo* to alcohols. However, alkyl side chains of aromatic compounds are more readily oxidized, often at more than one position. For example, the *n*-propyl side chain of *n*-propylbenzene can be oxidized at any of the three carbons to yield 3-phenylpropan-1-ol ($C_6H_5CH_2CH_2CH_2OH$), benzylmethylcarbinol ($C_6H_5CH_2CHOHCH_3$) or ethylphenylcarbinol ($C_6H_5CHOHCH_2CH_3$). As far as is known, the enzyme involved in all aliphatic oxidations of xenobiotics is cytochrome P450. *See also* CYTOCHROME P450-DEPENDENT MONOOXYGENASE SYSTEM.

alkali. Corrosive or caustic alkaline substances. When ingested they cause chemical burns to the mouth, esophagus and stomach. Alkalis such as sodium and potassium hydroxide, ammonia, etc. are frequently found in the home as cleaning fluids, drain cleaners, etc.

alkaline. Having a pH higher than 7.0, i.e., between 7 and 14.

alkaline phosphatase (EC 3.1.3.1). An enzyme that hydrolyzes phosphate monoesters. It has an alkaline pH optimum. An elevation of its activity in the serum usually indicates obstructive jaundice, Paget's disease (osteitis deformans) or bone carcinoma.

alkaloids. Organic nitrogenous bases produced (with the exception of ergot alkaloids) by dicotyledonous plants. They occur as salts with organic hydroxy acids such as hydroxybutanedioic, 2-hydroxy-1,2,3-propanetricarboxylic, tannic and quinic (1,3,4,5-tetrahydroxycyclohexanecarboxylic) acids. They have potent pharmacological activity and form the basis of many drugs. The majority are very toxic both by inhalation and ingestion. They vary considerably in their chemical properties and constitution depending on the parent base: aryl-substituted amines, indole, pyridine, quinoline and isoquinoline. Most alkaloids are crystalline solids with a very bitter taste; they are sparingly soluble in water, but usually soluble in organic solvents such as ethanol, ether and trichloromethane. They are optically active, most being dextrorotatory; they have been used for the resolution of racemic acids into their enantiomorphs. They are basic, forming crystalline salts with acids; these are water soluble. Drug preparations are usually based on the salts (e.g., hydrochloride, bromide, sulfate). Alkaloids give precipitates with such reagents as phosphomolybdic acid, potassium mercury(II) iodide and potassium triiodide. Commercially the alkaloids are extracted from powdered plant material with alcohol, water or dilute acid, and then precipitated out on the addition of base. The crude extract, often containing a range of alkaloids, is purified by physical methods of separation including fractional crystallization, countercurrent distribution, adsorption and partition chromatography. There are a very large number of plant alkaloids, of which many are listed below. *See also* EPHEDRINE; MESCALINE; RICININE; NICOTINE; PIPERINE; CONIINE;

COCAINE; TROPINE; ATROPINE; HYOSCYAMINE; HYOSCINE; ERGOT ALKALOIDS; LYSERGIC ACID; NUX VOMICA ALKALOIDS; STRYCHNINE; BRUCINE; RESERPINE; YOHIMBINE; CINCHONA ALKALOIDS; CINCHONINE; QUININE; QUINIDINE; OPIUM ALKALOIDS; MORPHINE; CODEINE.

alkalosis. A condition in which the pH of the blood is alkaline beyond the normal range, usually above 7.8, due to a disturbance in the acid/base balance. *Compare* ACIDOSIS. *See also* ACID/BASE BALANCE; ALKALOSIS, METABOLIC; ALKALOSIS, RESPIRATORY.

alkalosis, metabolic. A form of alkalosis caused by severe vomiting and the resultant loss of hydrogen chloride or changes in potassium ion concentration, either of which may be due to a variety of poisons. It involves an increase in blood bicarbonate concentration. *See also* ALKALOSIS.

alkalosis, respiratory. A form of alkalosis caused by excessive expiration of carbon dioxide. It involves little or no change in blood bicarbonate concentration, but rather an increase in carbonic acid. It may be due to hyperventilation or poisoning with toxicants such as salicylate. *See also* ALKALOSIS.

alkenes. Hydrocarbons that possess a carbon–carbon double bond, formerly called olefins. The double bond provides the opportunity for epoxide formation, which could be a bioactivation reaction.

Alkeran. *See* MELPHALAN.

alkylating agents. Chemicals that can add alkyl groups to DNA, a reaction that can result either in mispairing of bases or in chromosome breaks. The mechanism of the reaction involves the formation of a reactive carbonium ion $\left(\text{e.g.,} CH_3^+\right)$ that combines with electron-rich bases in DNA. Thus alkylating agents such as N-dimethylnitrosamine are frequently carcinogens and/or mutagens. *See also* CARCINOGENESIS; MUTATIONS.

alkylating drugs. *See* ALKYLATING AGENTS.

alkylation. The substitution of a hydrogen atom in an organic molecule by an alkyl group. Alkylation, particularly of macromolecules, may lead to toxicity. *See also* ALKYL GROUP; ALKYLATING AGENT.

alkyl group. An organic substituent with the general formula C_nH_{2n+1}.

alkyl halides. Organic compounds of the general structure RX where R is an alkyl group and X is Cl, Br or I; examples include methyl bromide and methyl chloride. Fluorine is usually not considered with the other alkyl halides because of the very different properties of the fluorocarbons. Alkyl halides are frequently toxic, particularly those with short chain alkyl groups. *See also* METHYL BROMIDE; METHYL CHLORIDE.

alkylmercury. *See* METYHLMERCURY.

alkyl sulfonates. Surfactants used in synthetic detergents. Those with a linear molecular structure are degraded fairly readily by microorganisms; those with a branched structure (e.g., alkyl benzene sulfonate) are stable and resist biodegradation, causing foaming in water into which they are discharged. In the UK and most industrial countries commercial detergents sold for domestic use, but not necessarily those for industrial use, are biodegradable. Detergents are of concern in contamination of aquatic ecosystems.

allele. One of a pair of genes situated at the same location on homologous chromosomes that controls a specific inherited trait.

allergen. Any substance capable of eliciting an allergic response. *See also* ALLERGIC RESPONSE.

allergenicity. The potential of a compound to provoke an allergic response. *See also* ALLERGENICITY TESTING; ALLERGIC RESPONSE.

allergenicity testing. The most common methods for testing the allergenicity of a compound are the dermal sensitization tests. The radioallergosorbent test (RAST) can also be used to screen individuals for elevated levels of IgE specific for the tested allergen. A high level of IgE specific for that allergen would predict a type I, or anaphylactic, response to that compound. *See also* ACUTE TOXICITY TESTING; ALLERGIC RESPONSE; DERMAL SENSITIZATION TESTS; IMMUNOASSAY; PHOTOTOXICITY TESTS.

allergic response. The term has been used in several different ways. The broadest definition, and the one upon which the Gell and Coombs classification of allergic response is based, is that it is any immune response detrimental to the host (*see* Table 1). In this scheme, allergic responses are classified by the mechanism involved, rather than by the causative agent or symptoms produced. Consequently, many things not commonly thought of as allergic responses, such as systemic lupus erythematosis (SLE), serum sickness, tuberculosis and hemolytic anemia, are included. A narrower definition includes only those immediate hypersensitivity reactions, the local and systemic anaphylactic reactions that are produced by IgE antibodies. Although this definition includes common allergic responses, such as the rhinitis and asthma produced by pollens and danders, it does not include the delayed-type hypersensitivity reactions such as contact dermatitis caused by poison ivy, drugs, cosmetics and certain metals, or the immediate hypersensitivity reactions not mediated by IgE (*see* IMMEDIATE HYPERSENSITIVITY). Most environmental agents will produce either a type I or a type IV hypersensitivity reaction (*see* HYPERSENSITIVITY), the types most commonly referred to as allergic responses. For example, *Bacillus subtilis*, pesticides, food additives and drugs can produce both local and systemic anaphylactic reactions. Formaldehyde, antimicrobials used in cosmetics and poison ivy can all produce delayed-type hypersensitivity (*see* DELAYED HYPERSENSITIVITY). There are also a few notable environmental agents that produce type II and type III responses. The gold salts used in medicinal treatments and the mercury used in photography can cause type II and type III reactions, as can certain drugs (e.g., penicillin, quinidine, tetracycline). Many allergenic compounds can induce different types of responses depending on the conditions of exposure (e.g., concentration, route of exposure, genetic predisposition of the host, etc.). Toluene diisocyanate (TDI), a compound used in the manufacture of plastics and resins, can cause both pulmonary effects (asthma, a type I reaction) and dermal effects (contact dermatitis, a type IV reaction). In studies of workers and studies using a guinea pig model system, pulmonary effects were produced by TDI exposure at high concentrations, regardless of whether the initial exposure was through inhalation or contact. There is a strong component of autoimmunity in the reaction to TDI, as there is with many other environmental toxicants (*see* AUTOIMMUNITY). Many chemicals, drugs, metals and/or their metabolites are highly reactive and bind to or substantially alter native proteins. Often, these are low-molecular-weight compounds that are not allergenic in their native form, but as "altered-self" proteins can induce a substantial allergic response. These autoimmune reactions can be of any class. α-Methyldopa, used in treatment of essential hypertension, can modify red cell surface antigens and cause autoimmune-like hemolytic anemia. Hydralazine can produce an SLE-like syndrome. The actual allergen in penicillin allergy, that can cause anaphylactic shock, is thought to be the penicilloyl group, a biotransformation product of penicillin, conjugated to self or non-self proteins (e.g., gastrointestinal contents or manufactured contaminants). There is also an element of genetic predisposition in many allergic responses. For instance, family studies have shown that ragweed hay fever is more likely to occur in those individuals carrying various genetic markers. *See also* ANTIBODY-DEPENDENT CELLULAR CYTOTOXICITY; COMPLEMENT; MAST CELLS/ BASOPHILS.

allergic shellfish poisoning. Allergic reaction that can result in certain individuals after the ingestion of shellfish that contain powerful sensitizing agents. Such poisoning is rarely fatal.

allergy. Classically, an altered state of immune responsiveness to an antigen (protein, lipopolysaccharide, etc., of any substance capable of eliciting an immune response). Now common usage equates allergy and hypersensitivity, and refers to an enhanced immune reactivity. Thus, an allergic response is an unusually vigorous host reaction to an antigen. There are two fundamental types of allergic response. (1) Immediate—unusual sensitivity to an antigen manifested by a tissue reaction

Table 1   Gell and Coombs classification scheme of allergy

Classification	Mechanism	Targets	Examples
Type I—anaphylaxis	IgE bound to mast cell/ basophil triggers the release of soluble mediators (e.g., leukotrienes and vasoactive amines such as histamine), after contact with antigen, to produce local or systemic effects. The effects occur within minutes of the secondary challenge	Gastrointestinal tract (food allergies), skin (urticaria and atopic dermatitis), respiratory system (rhinitis and asthma)	Local effects—asthma, urticaria (hives), rhinitis, atopic dermatitis. Systemic effects—vascular shock, asphyxia
Type II—cytolytic	IgG and/or IgM directed against cells bind to the cells and result in the destruction of the cells via complement fixation, opsonization or antibody-dependent cellular cytotoxicity	Tissues of circulatory system (e.g., red blood cells, white blood cells), their progenitors, and the spleen	Haemolytic anaemia, leukopenia, lungs and kidneys (Goodpasture's disease)
Type III—immune complex cytolytic	Antigen/antibody complexes of a certain size deposit in various tissues and may then fix complement, resulting in inflammation and destruction of nearby tissue	Skin (systemic lupus erythematosis), joints (rheumatoid arthritis), kidneys (glomerular nephritis), lungs (hypersensitivity pneumonitis), circulatory system (serum sickness)	Systemic lupus erythematosis (SLE), glomerular nephritis, rheumatoid arthritis, serum sickness
Type IV—delayed-type hypersensitivity	Sensitized T cells induce a delayed-type hypersensitivity response. This response does not involve antibody. Effects generally appear 24–48 hr after exposure and peak 48–72 hr after exposure	Any organ, but especially skin (contact dermatitis)	Contact dermatitis, tuberculosis

occurring within minutes after an antigen combines with antibody. Anaphylaxis is an example. (2) Delayed—cell-mediated sensitivity manifested 24–48 hours after an antigen combines with antibody. Hypersensitivity to poison ivy is an example. *See also* ALLERGIC RESPONSE.

allometric scaling. Used in extrapolation between species, it relates various biological parameters to body weight, e.g., organ size, physiological functions. The general formula for this relationship is $P = aw^b$, where P is the parameter under consideration, a and b are constants and w is the body weight. It is generally true within a group of organisms of widely divergent body weight provided they have similar anatomy, physiology and metabolism, e.g., within the mammalia.

allometric scaling, and species extrapolation. Allometric scaling, as described above, has been used as a method of extrapolating toxicity, or toxic dose, from one species of mammal to another. Although generally appropriate, it has been suggested that inclusion of surface area as well as body weight permits a more accurate extrapolation.

allowable human daily intake. *See* ACCEPTABLE DAILY INTAKE.

alloxan. *See* PANCREATIC TOXICITY.

allyl alcohol (2-propen-1-ol; vinyl carbinol). Used in the manufacture of plastics, war gases and other allyl compounds. Causes severe irritation of eyes and mucus membranes, and is oxidized to the toxicant acrolein by alcohol dehydrogenase. Has been demonstrated to cause pancreatic and liver injury in the rat. These effects are probably due to the toxic metabolite acrolein.

$$CH_2=CHCH_2OH$$

allylisopropylacetamide. An irreversible inhibitor of cytochrome P450. It is first oxidized by the cytochrome to a reactive intermediate that binds covalently to the heme moiety of the cytochrome. The subsequent breakdown of the heme gives rise to characteristic pigments. This is an excellent example of a "suicide inhibitor". *See also* XENOBIOTIC METABOLISM, IRREVERSIBLE INHIBITION.

Allylisopropylacetamide

alpha-2μ-globulin. A low molecular weight protein synthesized exclusively by the rat and, as far as is known, no other species. The amount and nature of the isoforms of α-2μ-globulin are gender specific. The synthesis and high rate of excretion of α-2μ-globulin is correlated with the development of nephrotoxicity and renal tumors in the male chronically administered such compounds as *d*-limonene and unleaded gasoline. Because of the species and gender specificity of the expression of this protein, the detection of such rodent tumors in chronic testing protocols has little relevance to human cancer risk assessment.

alpha helix. *See* PROTEIN.

alpha particles. Heavy particles (i.e., helium nuclei) of ionizing radiation produced by some modes of radioactive decay (e.g., decay of plutonium) with little penetrative power, but damaging when in contact with living tissue such as occurs following inhalation or ingestion. *See also* IONIZING RADIATION.

alpha naphthylisothiocyanate. *See* α-NAPHTHYLISOTHIOCYANATE.

ALS. *See* AMYOTROPHIC LATERAL SCLEROSIS.

Aluminum (Al). CAS number 7429-90-5. An element that is abundant (about 8%) in the crust of the Earth. Because it is primarily eliminated by excretion, people with compromised kidney function may accumulate the metal. In kidney dialysis patients, this is a particular problem because the dialyzing solution may contain high concentrations of aluminum. This condition (dialysis encephalopathy or dialysis dementia) has symptoms that include impaired memory, EEG changes, dementia, aphasia, ataxia and convulsions. One possible mechanism of toxicity may be inhibition of hexokinases in the brain. The chelating agent deferoxamine has been used successfully in treating this condition. Strict limits on the amount of aluminum in the dialyzing solution produce dramatic decreases in the condition, thus preventing its occurrence. Fine particles of the metal may also cause lung fibrosis (aluminosis). Aluminum is one of the primary toxicants leached into surface water (and, therefore, water supplies) by acid deposition. In addition, accumulation of aluminum in the brain has been suggested to be an etiological factor in Alzheimer's disease and amyotrophic lateral sclerosis. In uncompromised animals, however, aluminum does not readily penetrate the gastrointestinal tract, suggesting that a genetic predisposition, and/or other plausible routes of penetration (e.g., nasal or respiratory) must be demonstrated before these hypotheses can be widely accepted. *See also* ALZHEIMER'S DISEASE; AMYOTROPHIC LATERAL SCLEROSIS.

alveolar clearance. Particles that reach the alveoli are cleared by two principal routes: (1) phagocytosis and removal either via the mucociliary process or via the lymphatic system; (2) dissolution of the particles, with the dissolved material passing either to the blood stream or the lymphatic system. *See also* ALVEOLUS.

alveolar macrophage. A cell-type in the lung that kills and engulfs (phagocytosis) microorganisms as well as secreting antimicrobial substances. The alveolar macrophage may also secrete enzymes involved in the lysis of lung tissue. *See also* ALVEOLUS; PHAGOCYTOSIS.

alveolar ventilation. The volume of fresh air available for exchange at the alveolar surface. It is equal to the volume entering the lung and the volume not exhaled during respiration. *See also* ALVEOLUS.

alveolus. In general, a small hollow or cavity (e.g., a tooth socket or depression in the gastric mucosa). The most important use of the term is for the terminal air sacs of the lung. The pulmonary alveoli are thin-walled hollow structures opening from an alveolar duct or sac. Each alveolus is approximately 250–350 μm in diameter, and estimates of the total number in the adult human vary from 100×10^6 to 500×10^6. The pulmonary capillaries pass between the alveoli with the blood air distance (capillary wall and alveolar wall) varying up to 2.5 μm. The large total alveolar surface area, up to 100 m^2 at maximum inspiration, not only provides the surface for exchange of oxygen and carbon dioxide, but also makes the alveolar surface an important portal of entry for volatile toxicants and/or for the elimination of volatile toxicants or volatile products of toxicant metabolism.

Alzheimer's disease. A neurological disorder of unknown etiology that has a characteristic progressive dementia, often accompanied by emotional disturbances. The condition is usually associated with defined pathology, most characteristic being plaques and tangles in the neurophil. Several neurotoxicological hypotheses have been suggested, including the involvement of metals such as aluminum or natural toxins such as quinolinic acid. *See also* ALUMINUM; CYCAD.

Amanita phalloides. *See* AMANITIN.

amanitin. **CAS number 11030-71-0**. A drug derived from the highly poisonous fungus *Amanita phalloides* (death cap). Alpha-amanitin, a cyclic octapeptide, is toxic because of its affinity for RNA polymerase II in eukaryotic cells. Since this enzyme is responsible for mRNA synthesis in the cell, the compound is a potent and selective inhibitor of mRNA synthesis. It is effective at concentrations below 1 μg/ml, and its specific action has made it useful in experimental biology. It is often used with actinomycin D to block RNA synthesis. *See also* RNA.

amaranth (E123; FD&C Red No. 2; trisodium salt of 1-(4-sulfo-1-naphthylazo)-2-naphthol-3,6-disulfonic acid). **CAS number 915-67-3**. A food color approved for use in several countries, including the EEC, but no longer in the USA. It is metabolized primarily by intestinal microflora to naphthionic acid, 1-amino-2-naphthol-3,6-disulfonic acid and 1,2-naphthoquinone-3, 6-disulfonic acid. Drug eruption has been reported with this compound, but the primary toxicological concern that resulted in delisting in the USA was the presence of tumors in female rats fed diets containing amaranth at 3% concentrations. *See also* FOOD COLORS.

Amaranth

ambient. Environmental or surrounding conditions. In environmental toxicology, used to describe the concentration of a toxicant in the environment of a living organism.

ambient air standard. A quality standard for air in a particular place defined in terms of pollutants. Industries discharging pollutants are required to limit emissions to levels that will not reduce the quality of air below the standard. The principle is used widely in the USA, but not generally in the UK.

American Academy of Clinical Toxicology (AACT). An organization of professionals active in clinical toxicology or teaching and/or research related to clinical toxicology. Its goals include advancing the study of problems relative to clinical toxicology, information exchange and accreditation of clinical toxicologists. AACT established the American Board of Medical Toxicology. *See also* ACCREDITATION; AMERICAN BOARD OF MEDICAL TOXICOLOGY.

American Academy of Forensic Sciences (AAFS). A society to encourage the study of all aspects of forensic science, including toxicology. It organizes national meetings.

American Association for Accreditation of Laboratory Animal Care (AAALAC). A non-profit-making corporation directed by a Board of Trustees, comprising representatives of 27 scientific and professional organizations. The Board appoints the 16 members of the Council on Accreditation, that, on invitation, conducts site visits for the purpose of accrediting laboratory animal care facilities and programs. AAALAC, founded in 1965, encourages optimal care for laboratory animals by a mechanism of peer review, periodic site visits and specific recommendations. Recently renamed Association for the Assessment and Accreditation of Laboratory Animal Care (AAALAC). *Compare* ANIMALS (SCIENTIFIC PROCEDURES) ACT.

American Association for the Advancement of Science. A US professional society whose members are from all branches of science, medicine and engineering. Organizes annual meetings of international scope consisting of specific sessions with subject matter corresponding to that of the specialty sections as well as general sessions stressing integrative approaches and the philosophy of science. Perhaps best known as the publisher of the journal *Science*, one of the premier journals of peer reviewed research reports and reviews.

American Association of Poison Control Centers (AAPCC). Establishes standards for poison control and information centers and procures information on the composition of commercial products that may cause accidental poisonings and on the acute toxicity of toxicants.

American Board of Forensic Toxicology. Certifies (accredits) forensic toxicologists on the basis of education, experience and formal examination.

American Board of Medical Toxicology (ABMT). Established in 1975 by the American Academy of Clinical Toxicology and incorporated as a separate organization in 1980. Certifies

(accredits) physicians in medical toxicology. Certification is designed to assure competence in the evaluation and treatment of patients poisoned by drugs and other xenobiotics. *See also* ACCREDITATION; AMERICAN ACADEMY OF CLINICAL TOXICOLOGY.

American Board of Toxicology (ABT). A board in the United States that certifies diplomates in general toxicology following successful passage of a written examination. Recertification occurs at 5-year intervals. The Executive Office is in Raleigh, North Carolina, USA

American Board of Veterinary Toxicology (ABVT). Associated with the American Veterinary Medical Association and establishes standards for accreditation as a veterinary toxicologist.

American College of Toxicology (ACT). A US professional society whose members are toxicologists from all specialities, although preponderantly those in or associated with regulatory toxicology. It organizes meetings, publishes a newsletter and journal and accredits toxicologists.

American Conference of Governmental and Industrial Hygienists (ACGIH). A non-governmental organization in the USA, important primarily for the development and publication of threshold limit values to airborne toxicants in the workplace. *See also* THRESHOLD LIMIT VALUES, CEILING; THRESHOLD LIMIT VALUES, SHORT-TERM EXPOSURE LIMIT; THRESHOLD LIMIT VALUE, TIME-WEIGHTED AVERAGE.

American Industrial Hygiene Association (AIHA). Professional society of industrial hygienists devoted to the study of factors affecting the safety and health of industrial workers.

American Society for Testing and Materials (ASTM). Society devoted to the development and publication of methods for the testing of materials, including tests for toxicity. Since 1977 they have published a series of volumes based on papers presented at their annual symposia on aquatic toxicology. They include symposia sponsored by the

ASTM Committee on Pesticides and by the ASTM Committee on Biological Effects and Environmental Fate.

Ames test. An *in vitro* test for mutagenicity and, by implication, carcinogenicity, using mutant strains of the bacterium *Salmonella typhimurium*, that can be used as a preliminary screen of chemicals for assessing potential carcinogenicity. A variety of bacterial strains are available that cannot grow in the absence of histidine because of metabolic defects in histidine biosynthesis. Mutagens and presumed carcinogens can elicit mutations in which the strains regain their ability to grow in a histidine-deficient medium. The test can also be performed in the presence of the S9 fraction from rat liver to allow metabolic activation of promutagens (procarcinogens). There is a high, although not absolute, correlation between bacterial mutagenicity and carcinogenicity of chemicals. *See also* BACTERIAL MUTAGENESIS; MUTATION; PROKARYOTE MUTAGENICITY TESTS; S-9 FRACTION.

amethoprim. *See* METHOTREXATE.

amidases. *See* HYDROLYSIS.

amine oxidases. The most important function of amine oxidases other than the flavin-containing monooxygenase appears to be the oxidation of biogenic amines formed during normal processes. Two of these amine oxidases—monoamine oxidase and diamine oxidase—are concerned with the oxidative deamination of both endogenous and exogenous amines. The flavin-containing monooxygenase, formerly described as an amine oxidase, has a wide xenobiotic substrate specificity since it also oxidizes both organic sulfur and organic phosphorus compounds. *See also* DIAMINE OXIDASE; FLAVIN-CONTAINING MONOOXYGENASE; MONOAMINE OXIDASES.

amines. Organic derivatives of ammonia in which one (primary), two (secondary) or three (tertiary) hydrogen atoms are replaced by alkyl or aryl groups. A fourth group may be added to give a quaternary ammonium salt. The lone pair on the nitrogen atom makes amines bases. Alkylamines are all stronger bases than ammonia ($pK_b > 4$), with $R_2NH > RNH_2 > R_3N$. Aromatic amines are very weak bases ($pK_b > 9$). The amino group is found widely in biologically important molecules (e.g., amino acids, alkaloids and some vitamins). The smell of rotting fish is due to amines produced by bacteria.

amino acid. Organic compounds containing both carboxyl (-COOH) and amino ($-NH_2$) groups. Over 100 amino acids have been isolated and identified from natural sources, but only about 20 α-amino acids (with $-NH_2$ and -COOH attached to the same carbon atom) form the building blocks of proteins. These contain (i.e., except glycine) at least one asymmetric carbon atom with the L-configuration. Condensation of the $-NH_2$ of one amino acid with the -COOH of another gives an amide bond (-CONH-), leading to peptides and proteins. They are used as a food additives (e.g., monosodium glutamate (MSG)) or as dietary supplements. Essential amino acids are necessary nutritional factors for survival; they are not synthesized in the body and must be supplied from external sources. Amino acids are amphoteric, forming hydrochlorides and sodium salts; in solution the zwitterion is predominant. *See also* PROTEINS; PEPTIDE.

amino acid antagonists. Chemical analogs of amino acids or other chemicals that interfere with the uptake, metabolism or function of amino acids. Amino acid analogs may also be incorporated into proteins, affecting the subsequent functioning of the protein. Amino acid antagonists include ethionine, azaserine, *p*-fluorophenylalanine and asparagine, and their effects may be seen in such toxic events as teratogenesis, hepatotoxicity, etc. *See also* ETHIONINE.

amino acid conjugation. A type of acylation reaction in which exogenous carboxylic acids are activated to form S-CoA derivatives in a reaction involving ATP and CoA. The CoA derivatives formed acylate the amino group of an amino acid:

RCOO⁻ + ATP + CoASH →
  RCOSCoA + PPi + AMP

RCOSCoA + R'NH₂ → CoASH + RCONHR'

Glycine and glutamate are the most common acceptor amino acids in mammals, but other amino acids may be utilized including ornithine in reptiles and birds, and taurine in fish. The mitochondrial activating enzyme is one of a class of enzymes known as the ATP-dependent acid CoA ligases (AMP). It has also been known as acyl CoA synthetase and acid activating enzyme, although it appears to be identical to the intermediate-chain-length fatty acyl CoA synthetase. Two acyl CoA:amino acid N-acyltransferases have been purified from liver mitochondria. One utilizes benzoyl CoA, isovaleryl CoA and tiglyl CoA, but not phenylacetyl CoA, malonyl CoA or indoleacetyl CoA. The other utilizes phenylacetyl CoA and indoleacetyl CoA, but is inactive toward benzoyl CoA. The enzymes are not specific for glycine, but both utilize glycine at a faster rate than other amino acids. Bile acids are also conjugated, primarily with taurine, by a similar sequence of reactions. *See also* ACYLATION; PHASE II REACTIONS.

aminoacridines. When an amino group is substituted in the 3-, 6- or 9- positions of an acridine molecule, a strong base is obtained as a result of delocalization of the positive charge on the cation. Only acridines that are highly ionized at physiological pH (e.g., proflavine, 9-aminoacridine) and that have a critical minimum area of flatness are active as antiseptics. The flat acridine ring is believed to be held by aromatic forces to corresponding flat purine and pyrimidine rings in microbial DNA. Interaction of the positively charged amino groups with the phosphate anions results in stiffening of the helical structure of DNA.

4-aminoazobenzene (4-(phenylazo)benzenamine). **CAS number 60-09-3**. Suspected human (group 2B) carcinogen. Carcinogenic in rodents, mutagenic. It is used as a dye for varnish, wax products, oil stains and styrene resins. *See also* AMINOAZO DYES.

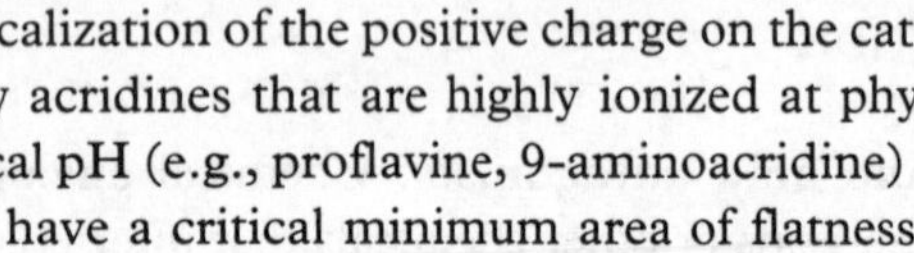

Aminoazobenzene

aminoazo dyes. Azo compounds are comprised of aromatic rings coupled by linkages consisting of two nitrogen atoms, the azo bond (-N=N-). These compounds are often colored and can be used as dyestuffs; many of them are also amino compounds. Aminoazo compounds, as a group, have long been known to act as carcinogens, and 4-dimethylaminoazobenzene (butter yellow) is a classic carcinogen for experimental studies. Direct blue 6 is an example of a complex aminoazo dye. *See also* AZO COMPOUNDS.

o-aminoazotoluene. **CAS number 97-56-3**. A known carcinogen similar in structure to many food colors used throughout the world. *See also* AMINOAZO DYES; AZO COMPOUNDS; FOOD COLORS.

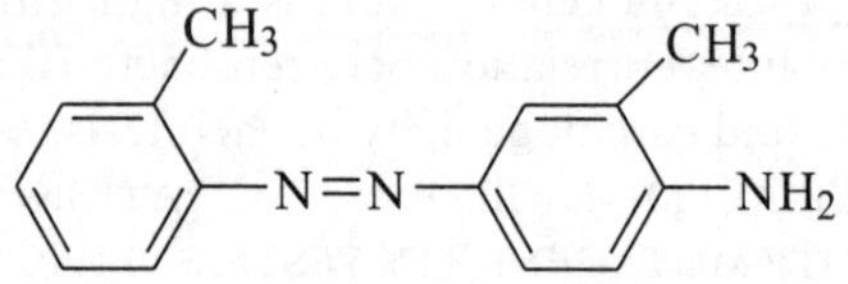

o-Aminoazotoluene

aminobenzene. *See* ANILINE.

p-aminobenzoic acid. *See* ANTIMETABOLITES; *p*-AMINOHIPPURATE, IN RENAL FUNCTION.

2-aminobiphenyl. *See* 4-AMINOBIPHENYL.

4-aminobiphenyl. **CAS number 92-67-1**. A designated human carcinogen (IARC) and hazardous waste (EPA). Formerly used as a rubber antioxidant and dyestuff intermediate, it is now used only as a research carcinogen. It was established that exposure of humans for as little as 133 days could give rise to bladder cancer, the latent period being 15–35 years. The isomer 2-aminobiphenyl is neither mutagenic nor generally carcinogenic. Activation of 4-aminobiphenyl appears to be via N-oxidation and N-glucuronide formation. The N-glucuronide is unstable in the acidic conditions of the urinary bladder, giving rise to reactive species.

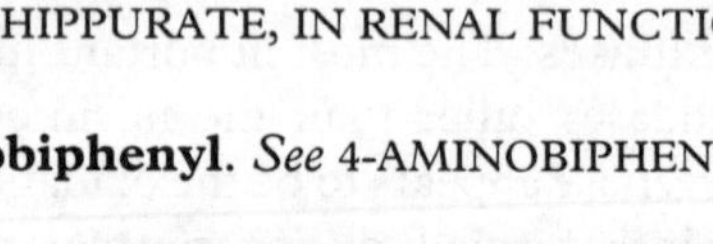

4-Aminobiphenyl

4-aminobutyric acid. *See* GABA.

γ-aminobutyric acid transaminase (GABA-T; γ-aminobutyrate-α-ketoglutarate aminotransferase; EC 2.6.1.19). An enzyme located in mitochondria that is responsible for the degradation of GABA by transfering its amino group to α-ketoglutaric acid (an intermediate in the Krebs cycle), yielding succinic semialdehyde and glutamic acid. Due to the high mitochondrial concentration of succinic semialdehyde dehydrogenase, succinic semialdehyde is rapidly converted to succinate that re-enters the Krebs cycle. Glutamic acid is decarboxylated by glutamic acid decarboxylase (GAD) to form GABA. The production of succinic acid from GABA is a part of the so-called GABA shunt pathway. GABA-T (Mr = 109,000) like GAD requires pyridoxal phosphate as a cofactor. *See also* GABA; GLUTAMIC ACID DECARBOXYLASE.

amino compounds. Organic compounds in which an amino group ($-NH_2$) is a substituent on a carbon atom. The amino group may itself be substituted (e.g., in peptide bonds), and amino groups are so widespread, both in endogenous body constituents and in toxicants, that generalizations about their specific importance to toxicology can come only from consideration of specific groups of compounds. The amino acids are clearly essential to life, and amino acid analogs such as ethionine are toxic. Many groups of amino compounds, such as aniline and its derivatives, are toxic, while others are relatively harmless. *See also* ANILINE; ETHIONINE.

4-aminofolic acid. *See* AMINOPTERIN.

aminoglycosides. *See* ANTIBIOTICS.

***p*-aminohippurate, in renal function.** *p*-Aminohippuric acid is the glycine conjugate of *p*-aminobenzoic acid. It is excreted by the organic anion transport system of the renal tubule, and its renal clearance is used as a measure of kidney function, specifically secretory activity of the nephron. Measurement of renal extraction of *p*-aminohippurate is used in the estimation of renal blood flow. *See also* NEPHRON; NEPHROTOXICITY.

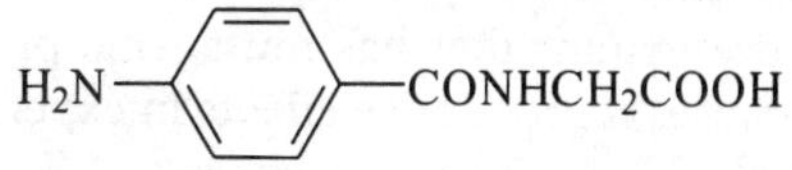

$$H_2N-\!\!\!\left\langle\;\right\rangle\!\!\!-CONHCH_2COOH$$

p-Aminohippuric acid

aminolevulinic acid dehydratase. *See* FREE ERYTHROCYTE PROTOPORPHYRIN.

DL aminomalonyl-D-alanine isopropyl ester. *See* SWEETENING AGENTS.

aminonaphthalenes. *See* β-NAPHTHYLAMINES.

aminonitriles. *See* LATHYRISM.

4-amino-PGA. *See* AMINOPTERIN.

2-aminophenol. *See* AMINOPHENOLS

3-aminophenol. *See* AMINOPHENOLS.

4-aminophenol. *See* AMINOPHENOLS.

aminophenols. Aminophenols are widely used as photographic developers and as intermediates in the manufacture of azo and sulfur dyes. They are compounds that contain a phenolic hydroxyl and an amino substituent on a benzene ring. They readily undergo redox reactions and are readily oxidized in air. Important aminophenols include the following:

2-aminophenol (*o*-aminophenol, 2-amino-1-hydroxybenzene, 2-hydroxyaniline). CAS number 95-55-6. Hair and fur dye, intermediate in sulfur and azo dye manufacture. It causes the formation of methemoglobin both *in vivo* and *in vitro*, and has mutagenic properties and causes reproductive effects in experimental animals.

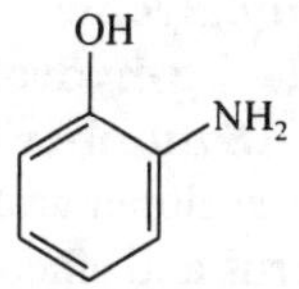

2-Aminophenol

3-aminophenol (*m*-aminophenol, 3-amino-1-hydroxybenzene, 3-hydroxyaniline). CAS number 591-27-5. Intermediate in dye and *p*-aminosalicylic acid manufacture. It is a skin and eye irritant that has mutagenic properties and causes reproductive effects in experimental animals.

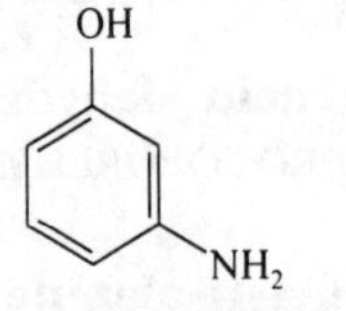

3-Aminophenol

4-aminophenol (*p*-aminophenol, 4-amino-1-hydroxybenzene, *p*-hydroxyaniline). CAS number 123-30-8. Photographic developer, intermediate in azo and sulfur dye manufacture and used as a dye for hair and feathers. Dermal contact may cause skin sensitization and dermatitus, inhalation may cause asthma. It causes the formation of methemoglobin both *in vivo* and in vitro, and causes kidney damage via a purative benzoquinoneimine intermediate.

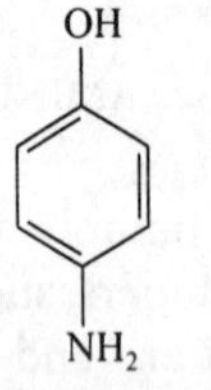

4-Aminophenol

2,4-diaminophenol. CAS number 95-86-3. Used in dye manufacture, in hair and fur dyeing and in tests for formaldehyde and ammonia.

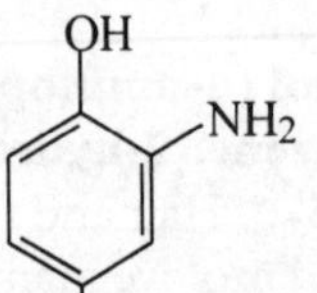

2,4-Diaminophenol

4-hydroxyphenylglycine (*N*-4-hydroxyphenylglycine; *p*-hydroxyphenylaminoacetic acid). CAS number 122-87-2. Used as a photographic developer and in the determination of phosphorus and silicon.

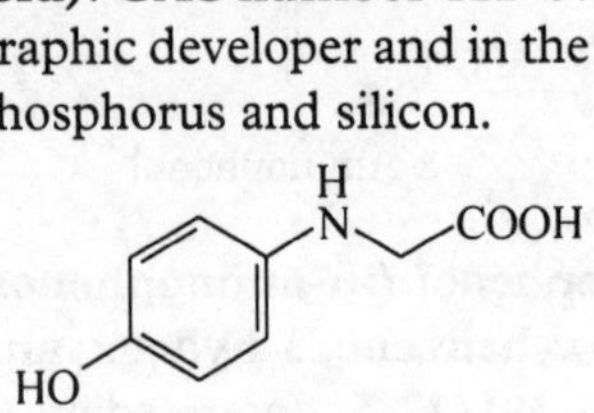

4-Hydroxyplenylglycine

4-methylaminophenol sulfate (monomethyl-*p*-aminophenol sulfate; *p*-hydroxymethylaniline sulfate). CAS number 55-55-0. Used as a photographic developer and fur dye.

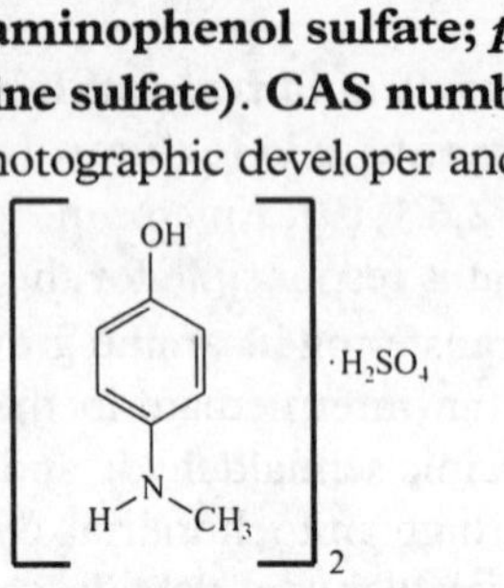

4-Methylaminophenol sulfate

See also DATABASES, TOXICOLOGY.

aminophylline. *See* THEOPHYLLINE.

β-aminoproprionitrile. *See* LATHYRISM.

aminopterin (*N*-[*p*-[(2,4-diamino-6-pteridyl methyl)amino]benzoyl]glutamic acid; 4-amino-folic acid; 4-aminopteroylglutamic acid; 4-amino-PGA). CAS number 54-62-6. A rodenticide; it is also used therapeutically as an antineoplastic agent since it is a folic acid antagonist and therefore serves as an antimetabolite, inhibiting the pathway for purine synthesis. Aminopterin has been used as an abortifacient and has proven to be teratogenic to surviving fetuses, that display hydrocephalus, micrognathia, defective skulls and palates, low-set ears, hypertelorism and abnormalities of the extremities.

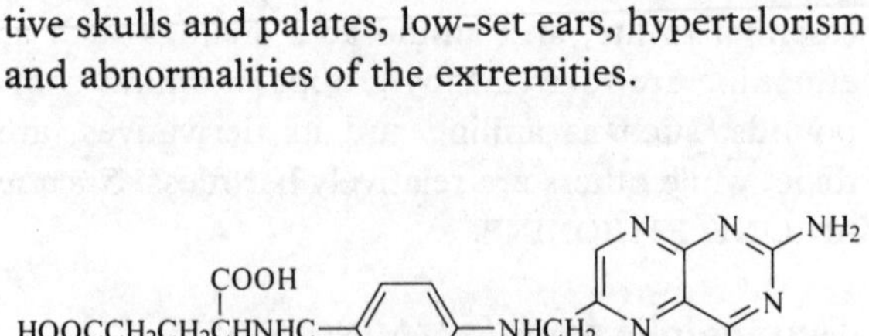

Aminopterin

2-aminopurine-6-thiol. *See* ABNORMAL BASE ANALOGS; THIOGUANINE.

4-aminopyridine. CAS number 504-24-5. A bird repellant used to repel nuisance birds by causing them to signal vocal and physical distress. It is very toxic, with an acute rat oral LD50 of 20 mg/kg.

aminopyrine. *See* ANTIPYRINE; PYRAZOLON DERIVATIVES.

aminotoluenes (*o*-, *m*- and *p*-toluidines). **CAS number 95-53-4.** 2-Aminotoluene (liquid, b.p. 200 °C) and 4-aminotoluene (solid, m.p. 45 °C), CAS number 106-49-0, are prepared by the reduction (e.g., Fe + HCl) of the respective nitrotoluene. They are basic and form salts with mineral acids. They are often used to prepare azo dyes. *See also* *O*-TOLUIDINE, *M*-TOLUIDINE, *P*-TOLUIDINE.

aminotriazole (amitrole; 1,2,4-triazol-3-ylamine; 1H-1,2,4-triazol-3-amine). **CAS number 61-82-5.** A non-selective herbicide. The acute oral LD50 in rats is 1100–24,600 mg/kg; the acute dermal LD50 in rats is more than 10,000 mg/kg. In 476-day feeding trials, rats receiving 50 mg/kg diet suffered no effects on growth or food intake, but male rats developed an enlarged thyroid after 90 days. It is an experimental animal carcinogen and suspected human carcinogen.

Aminotriazole

amitriptyline. *See* TRICYCLIC ANTIDEPRESSANTS.

amitrole. *See* AMINOTRIAZOLE.

AMM (Autorisation Mise sur la Marche). *See* MARKETING AUTHORIZATION.

ammonia (NH₃). **CAS number 7664-41-7.** A colorless gas with a pungent odor, detectable by humans down to concentrations of 53 ppm. Solutions in water, forming ammonium hydroxide (NH_4OH), are alkaline and corrosive. It has numerous industrial uses, such as in the manufacture of nitric acid, fertilizers, explosives and synthetic fibers, and also in refrigeration. Ammonia is also used in household cleaners. Inhalation of concentrated vapors causes severe respiratory system distress, including spasm of the glottis, respiratory

tract, edema and asphyxiation. Such exposure can be life-threatening, but if exposures are not acutely toxic, chronic residual effects do not result. It can cause alkali burns to the eye, with subsequent opacification, perforation of the cornea and iritis.

ammonium nitrate (NH₄NO₃). **CAS number 6484-52-2.** A compound commonly used as a fertilizer and as a component of explosives, herbicides and insecticides. It is the main source of the nitrate run-off from agricultural land that results from excessive fertilizer use. In water it can be pollutant and may cause eutrophication.

amniocentesis. Aspiration of amniotic fluid with a needle inserted into the gravid uterus through the abdominal wall. This process allows the examination of fetal cells contained in the amniotic fluid.

amobarbital. *See* BARBITURATES.

Amoco Cadiz. *See* ENVIRONMENTAL DISASTERS.

AMP. *See* ADENOSINE MONOPHOSPHATE.

amphetamine ((phenylisopropyl)amine; 1-phenyl-2-aminopropane; Dexedrine (D-isomer)). **CAS number 1407-85-8.** Originally found as the most active compound of a synthetic series based on the natural alkaloid ephedrine, the active principle of a Chinese folk medicine used to treat asthma. Amphetamine is one of a group of (phenylisopropyl)amines that has sympathomimetic activity in the periphery, as well as profound actions in the CNS. Amphetamine is believed to act primarily as an indirect-acting agonist, causing the release of monoamine neurotransmitters from existing nerve terminals. The actions of amphetamine in the periphery are at adrenergic nerve terminals, whereas in the CNS many of the important effects of amphetamine result from its actions on dopamine-containing nerve terminals. It also is a weak inhibitor of the uptake of catecholamines into their presynaptic terminals. The central effects of overdoses of amphetamine are countered by antipsychotic drugs, whereas the peripheral actions (a consequence of effects on the autonomic nervous system) can be countered by β-adrenergic antagonists. It also stimulates the medullary respiratory center and lessens depression of this area caused by other drugs, such as barbiturates. Amphetamine can alleviate fatigue, cause wakefulness, alertness, an elevation of mood and increased ability to concentrate. Appropriate clinical uses include the treatment of children with attention deficit disorder ("hyperkinesis") and therapy of narcolepsy. Although amphetamine has been used as an appetite suppressant (anorectic agent), it has little or no long-term effects, especially in persons whose overeating is impelled by psychological factors. The anorexic effects are insufficient to cause significant weight loss without dietary control, and tolerance to anorexic effects develops rapidly. Its widespread use for this purpose probably has contributed more to substance abuse problems than to weight control. One of the consequences of chronic abuse is a condition called "amphetamine psychosis", treatable with antipsychotic drugs and psychological intervention. *See also* AMPHETAMINES; HALLUCINOGENS.

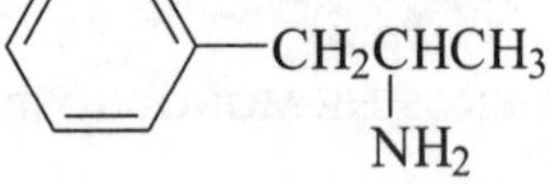

CH₂CHCH₃ structure

Amphetamine

amphetamines. Any molecule possessing a 1-phenyl-2-aminopropane skeleton. Aromatic ring substituents such as methoxy, or methoxy combined with alkyl, halogen or alkylthio lead to potent hallucinogenic substances known as "hallucinogenic amphetamines." The term "amphetamines" is sometimes used in a generic sense, particularly in the context of law enforcement, to denote any of a variety of structures that have stimulant effects similar to amphetamine, such as diethylpropion or phenmetrazine. As a group, these compounds tend to have actions on one or more of the synaptic mechanisms of biogenic amines, including release, uptake or degradation. For this reason, they often have effects on both the sympathetic nervous system and on central monoamine function. *See also* AMPHETAMINE; BIOGENIC AMINES; EPHEDRINE; HALLUCINOGENS; MESCALINE; METHAMPHETAMINE; STIMULANTS.

amphotericin B. *See* ANTIBIOTICS.

amygdalin (laetrile; amygdaloside; [(6-*O*-β-D-glucopyranosyl-β-D-glucopyranosyl)oxy] benzenacetonitrile). CAS number 29883-15-6. A cyanogenic glycoside occurring in seeds of Rosaceae, principally in bitter almonds and peach and apricot pits. It has been touted as being effective in the treatment of cancer, but controlled clinical trials have repeatedly failed to confirm such claims. Its toxic actions are those that can be ascribed to cyanide. It inhibits cellular respiration by binding to the trivalent iron of cytochrome oxidase in mitochondria, blocking oxygen utilization and resulting in cytotoxic hypoxia. Intoxicated individuals often exhibit the characteristic odor of bitter almonds. The therapy for acute poisoning is similar to that for cyanide. Amyl nitrate by inhalation oxidizes hemoglobin to methemoglobin, that provides a large pool of ferric iron to compete for cyanide. *See also* CYANIDE POISONING, THERAPY.

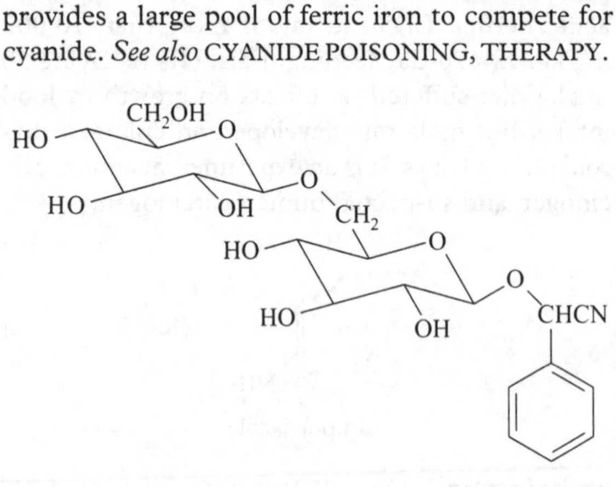

Amygdalin

amygdaloside. *See* AMYGDALIN.

α-amylase, in chronic toxicity testing. An enzyme that hydrolyzes 1,4-glucoside linkages of starch to form a mixture of dextrins, tri- and disaccharides, and glucose. This enzyme can be depressed following hepatobilary toxicity and elevated during renal failure.

amyl nitrite. Amyl nitrate is a mixture of isomers but consists primarily of isoamyl nitrite (isopentyl nitrite, CAS number 110-46-3). A vasodilator used by inhalation in angina episodes. Also used, by inhalation, in the initial treatment of cyanide intoxication because of its ability to bring about the oxidation of hemoglobin to methemoglobin, the latter being an avid binding agent for cyanide ion. Treatment is subsequently followed by intravenous sodium nitrite since the latter is much more effective in the oxidation of hemoglobin.

amyotrophic lateral sclerosis (ALS; Lou Gehrig disease). A rare degenerative neurological condition with an incidence of two per 100,000 for which no known etiology has been demonstrated for the majority of cases. Symptoms result from destruction of innervation of musculature, with death occurring due to respiratory paralysis or secondary respiratory effects. While at least one rare form has been ascribed to a genetic defect in superoxide dismutase, several neurotoxicological hypotheses have been proposed. These are usually based on specific case clusters, including the island of Guam, where both consumption of the cycad nut and exposure to cadmium have been implicated. Exposure to fertilizer containing high concentrations of cadmium has also been suggested as a factor in the USA. Although these hypotheses are either unproven or of local concern, it raises the issue that chemical factors in the environment may be involved. Both cause and effective therapy are, however, unknown at present. *See also* ALUMINUM; CADMIUM.

anabolic steroids. Testosterone is the naturally occurring androgenic steroid, produced by the Leydig cells of the testes, under the stimulation of luteinizing hormone from the adenohypophysis. It is 98% bound by sex hormone-binding protein. The free testosterone binds to an intracellular binding site, that stimulates production of mRNA with resultant protein synthesis (anabolism). Because of a short half-life and rapid hepatic degradation, testosterone is not suitable for therapeutic use. Esterification of testosterone is used to retard degradation; oral synthetic androgens are alkylated in the 17α-position, but the injectable anabolic steroids are not substituted at this position. Studies suggesting an increase in muscle mass are equivocal. It is also unclear if they improve performance beyond levels attained by intensive training alone. Numerous side effects, including hepatic neoplasia, glucose intolerance, decreased HDL-C levels, hypertension, testicular atrophy, oligospermia, virilization, amenorrhea, acne and alopecia have been reported. *See also* ANABOLISM; ANDROGENS; TESTOSTERONE.

anabolism. Metabolism leading to increased structural complexity, such as the synthesis of proteins from amino acids. A preponderence of anabolism over catabolism leads to increased mass or growth. Anabolism can be stimulated by such compounds as the androgens (the anabolic steroids) that promote protein synthesis and, therefore, muscle growth. *Compare* CATABOLISM.

anaerobic. Without oxygen. Anaerobic cells or organisms may be either facultative or obligate anaerobes. A facultative anaerobe normally exists in aerobic conditions, but can live and metabolize in anaerobic conditions when necessary; examples would be oysters and vertebrate skeletal muscle fibers. An obligate anaerobe requires anaerobic conditions to grow and metabolize. From a toxicological standpoint, the bacterial genus *Clostridium* is an extremely important example, with *C. botulinum*, which produces botulinum toxin, and *C. tetani*, which produces tetanus toxin, two extremely dangerous species. *See also* BOTULINUM TOXIN; TETANUS TOXIN.

analeptics. The archaic designation of a class of drugs that are purported to block the effects of depressant drugs (e.g., ethanol, sedative hypnotics or anesthetics). Because of the numerous mechanisms involved in "depressant" drug action and because many "depressants" do not act at a single, competitive site, no truly effective analeptic drug has been available clinically. In fact, many of the compounds that have been so used are probably more dangerous than helpful in reversing the effects of depressants. *See also* PICROTOXIN; STIMULANTS; STRYCHNINE.

analgesics. A group of drugs used to alleviate pain. The earliest narcotic analgesics were alkaloids isolated from the opium poppy. There are also a number of synthetic narcotic analgesics, including meperidine and methadone. The effects of morphine, the prototypical narcotic, can be divided into effects on the gastrointestinal tract and the CNS. The principal CNS effects include analgesia, euphoria and/or sedation, respiratory depression, antitussive action, emetic and/or antiemetic action, miosis, tolerance and dependence with chronic usage. It is now believed that morphine interacts with receptor sites for endogenous opioid peptides. The most important side effect of morphine is depression of the respiratory centers in the medulla and pons. The resulting respiratory depression seriously limits the therapeutic use of morphine. Other narcotic analgesics include codeine, heroin (diacetylmorphine), meperidine and methadone. Non-narcotic analgesics and non-steroidal anti-inflammatory drugs (NSAID) are also used in the control of pain. Aspirin and other salicylates are the most widely used drugs in this class. The major therapeutic and side effects of aspirin-like drugs are related to inhibition of the synthesis of prostaglandins and related autocoids. Aspirin can produce various forms of gastric distress, particularly in patients suffering from peptic ulcers, including gastric hemorrhaging. A more common danger with aspirin is overdosage. The problem is particularly serious in children and not unexpectedly involves flavored aspirin tablets. Salicylate poisoning is initially characterized by respiratory stimulation followed by alkalosis and, occasionally, respiratory acidosis. The 4-aminophenol derivatives such as phenacetin and acetaminophen are also important analgesics. These drugs may be less dangerous than salicylates and have a lower incidence of hypersensitivity. Pyrazolon derivatives, such as phenylbutazone, aminopyrine, antipyrine and apazone, are weaker antipyretics or analgesics than the salicylates, but they do have strong anti-inflammatory properties. The main disadvantage of the pyrazolon derivatives is that they may produce serious blood disorders. Miscellaneous NSAIDs such as indomethacin are also used as analgesics, although there is a high incidence of severe side reactions including gastrointestinal distress, CNS depression, visual disturbances and psychotic reactions, especially upon chronic administration. Propionic acid derivatives, including ibuprofen, naproxen, fenoprofen, flubiprofen and ketoprofen are now the most widely used NSAIDS, and have potent anti-inflammatory, antipyretic and analgesic properties. New NSAIDS with selectivity for only one form of cyclooxygenase have been developed and may soon be used widely. *See also* ACETAMINOPHEN; ANTI-INFLAMMATORY AGENTS; ANTIPYRETIC; ASPIRIN; CYCLOOXYGENASE; PHENACETIN.

Analgesine. *See* ANTIPYRINE.

analysis of variance (ANOVA). A method for testing the significance of mean differences based on partitioning the total variation in a set of scores into additive parts; a parametric statistical procedure for evaluating hypotheses about mean differences. In the case of a single-factor experiment, the variation in the dependent measure can be explained by the variation resulting from the effects of the treatment or independent variable (i.e., differences between mean scores associated with groups receiving different treatments) plus that due to random error (i.e., the summed within group variation). The effect of the independent variable is tested by forming an F-ratio, that is an estimate of the variability (mean square) divided by the appropriate error term. In toxicology, the typical application of this method is to test for mean differences when more than two experimental conditions are being compared. *See also* F TEST; STATISTICS, FUNCTION IN TOXICOLOGY; VARIANCE.

analyte. A molecule that is targeted by a particular quantification method. Quantification techniques may involve detection not only, but also include sample preparation and analytical separation. *See also* ABSORBANCE; ANALYTICAL TOXICOLOGY; CHROMATOGRAPHY; MASS SPECTROSCOPY.

analytical toxicology. The application of qualitative and quantitative chemical and physical techniques to the field of toxicology. Analytical toxicology involves the separation of a substance into constituents and/or the identification and quantification of individual constituents. Analytical techniques include sample preparation, separation, detection and assay calibration. Because of the complex nature of many environmental and tissue samples, as well as the frequently low concentrations of toxicants and/or their derivatives present, many specialized and sophisticated techniques for separation, identification and quantitation are required. *See also* ABSORBANCE; BEER'S LAW; BIOASSAY; CHROMATOGRAPHY; CHROMATOGRAPHY, GAS; CHROMATOGRAPHY, HIGH-PERFORMANCE LIQUID; EXTRACTION; IMMUNOASSAY; SPECTROMETRY, MASS; SAMPLING; SOLVENT PARTITIONING; SPECTROMETRY.

anaphase. *See* MITOSIS.

anaphylactic reaction. *See* ALLERGIC RESPONSE; IMMEDIATE HYPERSENSITIVITY; MAST CELLS/BASOPHILS.

anaphylactic shock. *See* ALLERGIC RESPONSE; IMMEDIATE HYPERSENSITIVITY; MAST CELLS/BASOPHILS.

anaphylaxis. *See* ALLERGIC RESPONSE; IMMEDIATE HYPERSENSITIVITY; MAST CELLS/BASOPHILS.

anaplasia. A characteristic of tumor tissue in which cells become dedifferentiated and lose their orientation within the tissue and with respect to adjacent tissue.

androgen-binding protein (ABP). A protein produced by the Sertoli cells of the testis, secreted into the lumina of seminiferous tubules and transported via efferent ducts to the epididymis. It is a glycoprotein (25% carbohydrate) composed of two subunits (Mr = 47,000 and 41,000). Its function is to bind androgens produced by the Leydig (interstitial) cells of the testis, thus maintaining sufficient local concentrations of testosterone within the testis and epididymis.

androgens (androgenic hormones). Substances, primarily steroids, that confer masculine properties on an individual. Common androgens include testosterone, androstenedione, androsterone and dihydrotestosterone. Androgens are responsible for the development of secondary sex characteristics, the function of sexual accessory glands, the maintenance of spermatogenesis and male sexual behavior. They are produced primarily by the testis, with small amounts being produced by the adrenal gland and ovary as well as by chemical synthesis. Androgens affect a variety of target tissues by binding to a specific cytoplasmic hormone receptor. This hormone-receptor complex binds to DNA and affects transcription, resulting in synthesis of tissue-specific proteins (anabolism). Symptoms of inappropriate production or administration in humans include masculinization, menstrual irregularities, acne, disturbance of bone growth in children, edema,

jaundice, hepatic carcinoma, impotence and azoospermia. *See also* ANABOLIC STEROIDS; TESTOSTERONE.

andromedotoxin. *See* GRAYANOTOXIN.

androsterone. **CAS number 53-41-8**. Typical urinary 17-oxosteroid, formed by the metabolic reduction of testosterone. Less potent than testosterone. *See also* TESTOSTERONE.

Androsterone

anemia. A condition in which the blood hemoglobin concentration is below normal. Causes may include blood loss, increased intravascular destruction of blood cells or decreased production of blood cells. Injury to the gastrointestinal mucosa, with subsequent blood loss, is the most common cause of anemia. This may be drug-induced, stress-induced or congenital in origin. There are two types of drug-induced hemolysis: (1) drug-induced oxidation of hemoglobin in intrinsically defective red blood cells (i.e., pyruvate kinase or glucose-6-phosphate dehydrogenase defects); (2) drug-induced immune hemolysis. Marrow toxicity is manifest either by a direct toxicity on red cell mitosis or by interference with metabolism of essential red cell nutrients (i.e., folate or iron). *See also* HEMOLYSIS.

anemic hypoxia. *See* HYPOXIA.

anesthesia. A condition in which loss of consciousness, usually coupled with loss of response to pain and muscle contraction, permits medical or surgical procedures to proceed without response or discomfort to the patient. The four stages of general anesthesia with diethyl ether, outlined in 1920 by Guedel, are still of general relevance, although newer anesthetics have different properties. Stage I (analgesia) begins with ether administration and lasts until consciousness is lost. Stage II (delirium) lasts from loss of consciousness until surgical anesthesia begins. Excitement and involuntary activity (laughing, shouting, thrashing, incontinence, irregular breathing, hypertension, etc.) may occur, and the intensity and duration of this stage are minimized to prevent injury to patients. Stage III (surgical anesthesia) lasts from the end of the second stage until spontaneous respiration ceases and has been arbitrarily divided into four planes relating to changes in muscle tone, eye reflexes and respiration. This is the stage in which most surgery is done. The final stage (medullary depression) begins when spontaneous respiration ceases and ends when circulatory collapse and death occur. Anesthetics can be administered both by injection and/or inhalation. Sometimes an intravenous drug is used to induce, and a volatile drug to maintain, anesthesia. The uptake, distribution and elimination of the gaseous agents are greatly influenced by the physical laws of gases (e.g., Dalton's or Henry's laws). The mechanism of action of most anesthetics is still unknown. Some (like the barbiturates) act at specific sites on receptors, whereas others may have more generalized actions on cellular membranes. Anesthetics can be toxic due to direct effects on respiration and cardiovascular function, but also through mechanisms that affect temperature regulation (malignant hyperthermia) or as a consequence of anesthetic metabolism (halothane hepatitis). *See also* ANESTHETICS; HALOTHANES; MALIGNANT HYPERTHERMIA.

anesthetics. Compounds that induce loss of sensation either in a specific part of the body (local anesthetics) or the body in general (general anesthetics), the latter generally involving loss of consciousness. Local anesthetics include compounds such as procaine and lidocaine, the actions of which involve neuronal sodium channels, and chlorethane, that acts by reducing the temperature of the skin and underlying tissue. General anesthetics include desflurane, enflurane, halothane, isoflurane, sevoflurane and propofol. Diethyl ether, formally used as an anesthetic, is no longer recommended. *See also* BARBITURATES; CYCLOPROPANE; ETHYL ETHER; HALOTHANE; KETAMINE; NITROUS OXIDE; THIOPENTAL SODIUM.

aneuploidy. *See* CHROMOSOME ABERRATIONS.

"angel dust." *See* PHENCYCLIDINE.

angioma. A benign (non-malignant) tumor consisting of blood vessels (hemangioma) or lymph vessels (lymphangioma). These tumors may occur in any part of the body where these types of vessels are found.

angiosarcoma (hemangiosarcoma; malignant hemangioendothelioma). A malignant tumor of cells of the vascular endothelium. These tumors are designated sarcomas, because the embryonal origin of the cells is considered to be mesenchymal (the progenitor cells of the supporting tissues of the body such as muscle, bone, cartilage, etc.). *See also* SARCOMA.

aniline (aminobenzene). CAS number 62-53-3. A designated hazardous substance (EPA) and hazardous waste (EPA). It is a colorless liquid with a characteristic odor. Aniline is used as an intermediate in the synthesis of dyes, as well as in the manufacture of rubber accelerators and antioxidants, pharmaceuticals, photographic developers, resins, varnishes, shoe polishes and many other organic chemicals. The principal routes of entry are inhalation of the vapor and either percutaneous absorption or ingestion of the liquid. Uptake from the lungs, skin or gastrointestinal tract causes anoxia due to methemoglobin formation, with moderate exposure causing cyanosis.

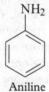

Aniline

Animal and Plant Health Inspection Service (APHIS). A program of the US Department of Agriculture that deals in part with matters of toxicological interest, including residues of pesticides in foods.

animal care. Watchful and concerned attention, heed and caution for the biological (and psychological) needs of animals and for the concerns of people who work with or are aware of those animals. Specific components of animal care are described in the US government's

Principles for the Utilization and Care of Vertebrate Animals Used in Testing, Research and Training. Topics of concern included in these principles are: transportation; ultimate benefit of animal use to humans and other animals; appropriateness of the species for a study and availability of alternatives; nature of the experimental procedures and steps to avoid discomfort, stress and pain; euthanasia; husbandry, including housing, food, environment and social interaction; veterinary care; qualifications of and safety precautions for animal care and research personnel. *Compare* ANIMALS (SCIENTIFIC PROCEDURES) ACT. *See also* GUIDE FOR THE CARE AND USE OF LABORATORY ANIMALS.

animal environment. There are three levels: (1) the microenvironment or cage; (2) the macroenvironment or room; (3) the megaenvironment or building. Factors within these environments that may alter the animal, and therefore its responses, include: ambient temperature; humidity; ventilation; light (intensity, wavelength and on/off cycle); sound (intensity, frequency and pattern); chemical contaminant (properties, interactions, exposure duration and frequency, and route of exposure); recent changes in environment; human interaction (routine or irregular, familiar or unfamiliar, proficient or stressful); vermin; water and food; bedding composition; olfactants; microbial contaminants; social interactions with the same or different species; cage or housing (composition, size, arrangement, comfort, security, ease of seeing into or out of, cleanliness and appropriateness for biological needs). *See also* CHRONIC TOXICITY TESTING.

animal factors. Factors or characteristics of an animal that may alter the response of that animal to its environment. The factors include: species, variety or breed; sex; age; source or previous environment; breeding status; biological cycle and physiological status; surgical alterations; behavior patterns; previous illness; current illness, infections and immune status; history; previous exposure to xenobiotics; genetic constitution; sensory receptor specificity; normal microbial flora and fauna; nutritional status.

animal model selection. The most important factor influencing the selection of an animal model is similarity in mechanism of toxic action and/or expression of toxicity between the proposed model species and the species of primary interest (usually human). The ease with which the actual toxicant exposure to the species of primary interest can be simulated using the proposed model is also critical. Other factors of importance include: ease and cost of producing the model for many investigators; previous experience with the model and existing baseline data; ease of transport and export; size (optimally large enough to permit sequential and/or multiple sampling and small enough to be accommodated easily in laboratories and animal facilities); ease of handling and experimental manipulations; fecundity, longevity, general health and pattern of spontaneous disease. The endangered or threatened status of the species, public concern for the species and the availability of alternatives are also relevant.

Animals (Scientific Procedures) Act. A UK law of 1986 that controls the use of animals in procedures that involve pain, suffering, distress or lasting harm. The Act requires that anyone performing a procedure must hold a license that is granted by the Home Office. In addition, a project license is required and is only granted for a specified program of work carried out at specified places. This Act replaces the Cruelty to Animals Act of 1976.

animal toxins. All phyla of animals include organisms that produce toxins. Some are passively venomous (i.e., from chance ingestion) whereas others are actively venomous, injecting poisons through specially adapted stings or mouth parts. Many toxinologists consider it more appropriate to refer only to the latter group as venomous, the former being considered simply as poisonous. The chemistry of animal toxins includes enzymes, neurotoxic and cardiotoxic peptides, proteins and small molecules such as biogenic amines, alkaloids, glycosides and terpenes. The venoms may be complex mixtures including both proteins and small molecules and depend upon the interaction of the various components for the full expression of their toxic effect. For example, bee venom contains a biogenic amine, histamine, three peptides and two enzymes. Snake venoms frequently contain toxins that are peptides with 60–70 amino acids. The cardiotoxic or neurotoxic effects of these toxins are enhanced by enzymes such as phospholipases, peptidases or proteases that are often present.

anise. *See* ESSENTIAL OILS.

ANOVA. *See* ANALYSIS OF VARIANCE.

anoxia. A lack of oxygen. It also indicates a decrease in the oxygen content of tissues to below physiological levels and is therefore similar to hypoxia. Anoxia may result from low atmospheric oxygen pressure, anemia, interference with blood flow or the inability of tissues to utilize oxygen normally.

anoxic hypoxia. *See* HYPOXIA.

Antabuse. *See* DISULFIRAM.

antagonism. In toxicology, that situation in which the toxicity of two or more compounds administered together, or sequentially, is less than that expected from consideration of their toxicities when administered alone. Although this definition includes lowered toxicity resulting from induction of detoxifying enzymes, such cases are frequently considered separately because of the time that must elapse between treatment with the inducer and subsequent treatment with the toxicant. Reduction of hexobarbital sleeping time and reduction of zoxazolamine paralysis time by prior treatment with phenobarbital are examples of antagonism resulting from induction, as is protection by phenobarbital treatment from the carcinogenic action of benzo[*a*]pyrene or aflatoxin B1. Antagonism not involving induction is often seen at a marginal level of detection and consequently is both difficult to explain and of marginal significance. Such antagonism may involve competition for receptor sites or situations, as in the chelation of metal ions, in which one toxicant combines non-enzymatically with another to reduce their toxic effects. *See also* ANTAGONISTS.

antagonism, pharmacological. *See* ANTAGONISTS.

antagonism, physiological. *See* ANTAGONISTS.

antagonists. Compounds that have actions opposing those of an endogenous molecule, toxicant or administered drug (the agonist). Antagonists are usually divided into two classes—pharmacological and physiological. Pharmacological antagonism occurs when one compound blocks the effects of a second compound by actions at the same molecular locus. An example is atropine blocking muscarinic acetylcholine receptors, preventing the toxicity of excess acetylcholine caused by organophosphate intoxication. Physiological antagonists reverse or attenuate the actions of the agonist, but by mechanisms unrelated to the primary mode of action of the agonist. Pharmacological antagonists can be either competitive or non-competitive. The action of a competitive antagonist is reversible and can be overcome by increasing the concentration of the agonist. Non-competitive antagonists block agonist effects by irreversibly binding to a receptor protein or by acting at a different site on the protein. The potency of a pharmacological antagonist *in vitro* is typically expressed as the K_i or inhibitory constant, that can be derived from the IC50. *In vivo*, the affinity (a predictor of potency) of an antagonist can be expressed as the ID50 or dose at which inhibition of agonist effects are seen in one-half the subjects tested. *See also* AGONISTS; ANTAGONISM; ENZYME KINETICS; INHIBITORY CONCENTRATION; K_i; RECEPTOR; RADIORECEPTOR ASSAYS.

anterior pituitary. *See* ADENOHYPOPHYSIS.

anthelminthics. Agents that kill worms. The worms of greatest concern are roundworms (nematodes) and flatworms (platyhelminthes) that are of both agricultural and medical/veterinary importance.

anthracene. **CAS number 120-12-7**. A polycyclic aromatic hydrocarbon. It is among the chemicals displaying cutaneous phototoxicity

Anthracene

and it is a skin irritant and allergen. It can cause hyperpigmentation. It is a questionable carcinogen.

antianxiety drugs (anxiolytic drugs). A chemically heterogeneous group of agents that produce a reduction of the manifestations of anxiety, where anxiety is a physiological reaction to situations perceived as potentially threatening, but only becomes abnormal when it occurs without sufficient objective reasons or when its manifestations are excessive in intensity or duration. Both barbiturates and propanediol carbamates have been used in the successful treatment of anxiety, but have been largely supplanted by the use of benzodiazepine derivatives. The molecular site of action of antianxiety drugs is thought to consist of specific binding sites coupled to a polymeric cell membrane chloride channel that constitutes the receptor for the neurotransmitter γ-aminobutyric acid (GABA). *See also* BENZODIAZEPINES; DIAZEPAM; GABA.

antibacterials. Physical and chemical agents that either kill or inhibit the proliferation of bacteria. They may be considered bacteriocidal if a lethal effect is exerted or bacteriostatic if growth is inhibited in a non-lethal manner. In the latter case, inhibition is reversible in that growth is resumed upon removal of the agent from the growth medium. The most common antibacterial agents are classified as disinfectants, antiseptics, synthetic drugs or antibiotics. In order to be of value with regard to chemotherapeutic considerations, an antibacterial must exhibit selective toxicity. *See also* ANTIBIOTICS; ANTIMICROBIALS; BACTERIOSTATS.

antibiotics. Biochemicals, originally of microbial origin, that are capable, at low concentrations, of inhibiting the growth of microorganisms. Modern usage of the term includes synthetic and semisynthetic compounds that exhibit antimicrobial activity. Their mechanisms of action result in either cidal or static effects, most often mediated by inhibition of cell wall biosynthesis (e.g., peptidoglycan in bacteria), protein biosynthesis, nucleic acid biosynthesis, intermediary metabolism, and/or cytoplasmic membrane physiology. Selective toxicity must be exhibited in order for a given

antibiotic to be of value chemotherapeutically. Resistance to anti-biotics may be due to one or more of the following: modification of the target in the cell or reduction of the physiological importance of the target; prevention of access to the target; production by the bacteria of inactivating enzymes (e.g., beta-lactamase). Many of the chemically modified antibiotics were produced in order to overcome or bypass resistance to the parent compound. The following are the most important classes of antibiotics.

Penicillins. Compounds produced by *Penicillium chrysogenum* that are bacteriocidal due to inhibition of cell wall biosynthesis. Chemical modifications have yielded compounds, such as benzylpenicillin, carbenicillin and methicillin, with improved properties. Resistance may be due to penicillinase (beta-lactamase) that opens the lactam ring giving rise to penicilloic acid. Toxic side effects in humans include immune reactions, sometimes life threatening.

General structure of penicillins

Cephalosporins. Cephalosporins (e.g., cephalosporin C. CAS number 61-24-5) are produced by *Cephalosporium sp*. They are broad spectrum antibiotics that act by inhibition of cell wall biosynthesis and are active against penicillinase producing organisms. Principal toxic side effects are allergic hypersensitivity reactions, including anaphylactic shock and nephrotoxicity. There is frequently cross-sensitivity with penicillin and penicillin-sensitive patients should not be given cephalosporins.

Cephalosporin C

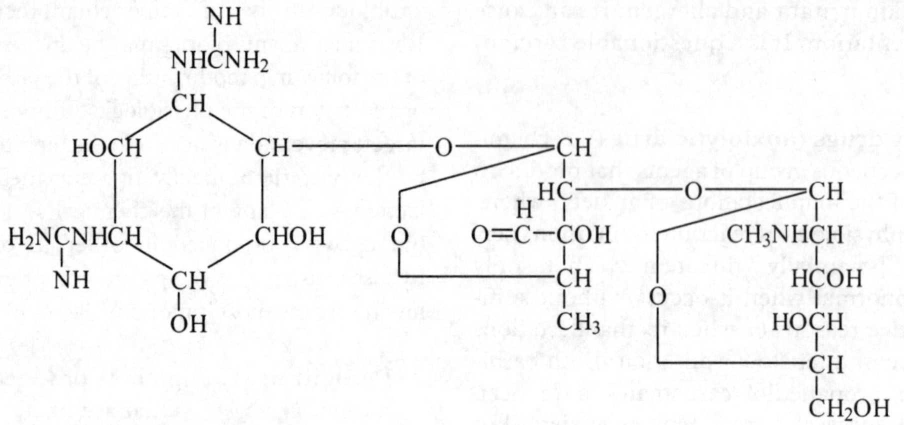

Streptomycin

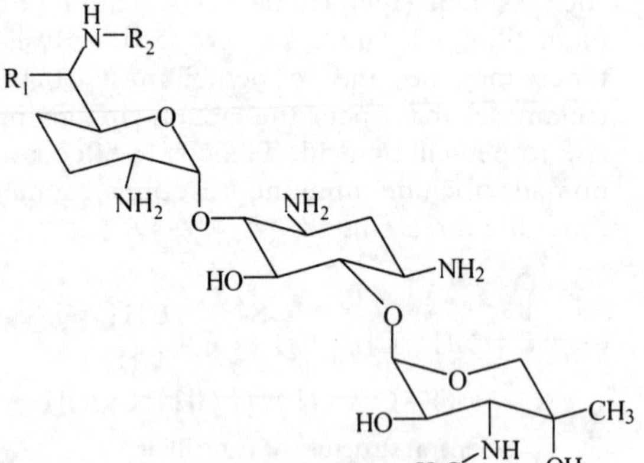

Gentamycin C₁ R₁ = R₂ = CH₃
Gentamycin C₂ R₁ = CH₃, R₂ = H
Gentamycin C₁ₐ R₁ = R₂ = H

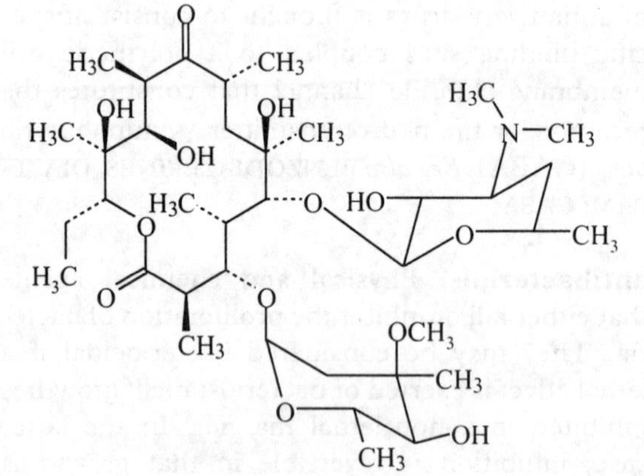

Erythromycin

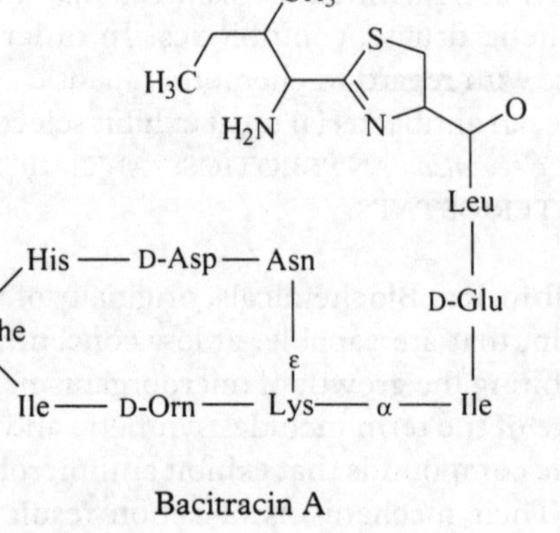

Tetracycline

Bacitracin A

Val—Orn—Leu—D-Phe—Pro
Pro—D-Phe—Leu—Orn—Val

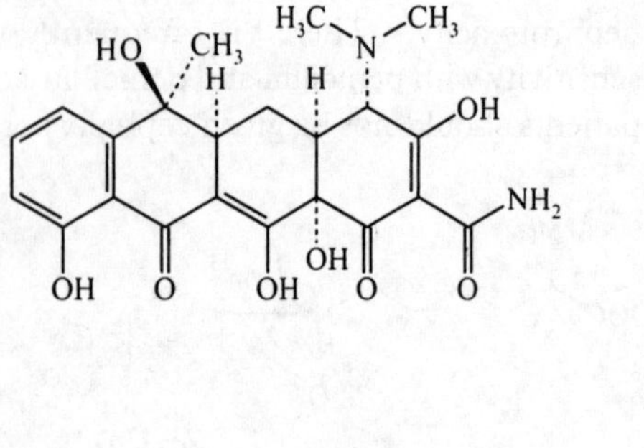

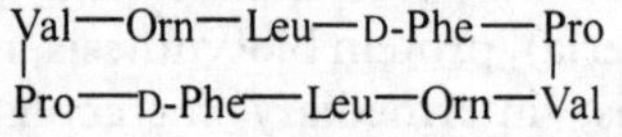

Gramicidin S

Aminoglycosides. A class of antibiotics, all consisting of two or more amino sugars joined in a glycosidic linkage to a hexose nucleus, inositol. Representative members of this group are streptomycin and gentamycin, both produced by soil actinomycetes. Semisynthetic aminoglycosides such as kanomycin also are produced. Aminoglycosides are active against many gram-negative and a few gram-positive bacteria due, apparently, to their ability to inhibit the first step of ribosomal protein synthesis and also, perhaps, from their ability to induce mistranslation of mRNA. Major toxic side effects are renal failure and hearing loss due to cochlear damage.

Tetracyclines. A family of antibiotics effective against gram-positive bacteria. Side effects from continued use in humans include photosensitivity, fatty liver and renal failure. Tetracyclines are deposited at sites of active calcification of teeth and bones and effects after birth on teeth exposed to tetracyclines *in utero* may be severe.

Macrolides. A group of compounds that possess a macrocyclic lactone ring with sugar substituents. Includes the erythromycins produced by *Streptomyces erythreus*. They are broad spectrum, acting by inhibition of protein synthesis.

Peptides. A large group of compounds, either cyclic and/or including one or more D-amino acids. Includes bacitracin and the gramicidins, the mode of action involving effects on the cytoplasmic membrane.

Polyenes. Cyclic compounds containing long chain polyunsaturated moieties. These include antifungal agents such as nystatin, produced by *Streptomyces noursei* and amphotericin B, produced by *Streptomyces nodosus*.

Other miscellaneous antibiotics include chloramphenicol and griseofulvin. Chloramphenicol, an antibiotic produced by *Streptmyces venezulae*, is effective against gram-positive and gram-negative spirochaetes, psittacosis group, and rickettsiae that cause typhus. It blocks the ribosomal site for the attachment of the 3'-terminus of amino acyl-tRNA, thereby inhibiting protein synthesis. Toxic side effects include blood dyscrasias in humans, including aplastic anemia and granulocytopenia. High dosage in the neonate can be fatal. Griseofulvin is produced be *Pennicillium griseofulvum* concentrates in keratin and is effective against fungal infection of nails and hair.

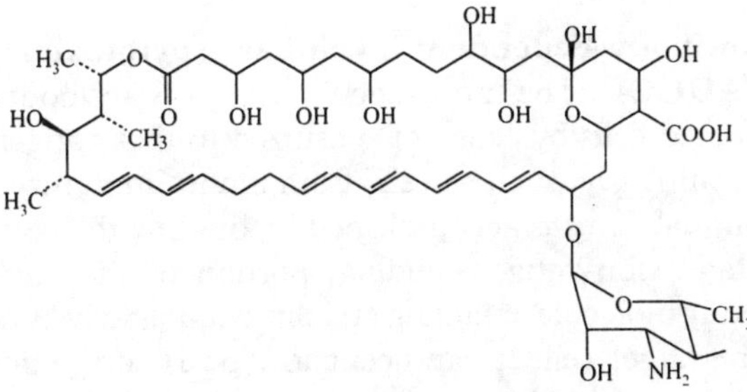

Nystatin

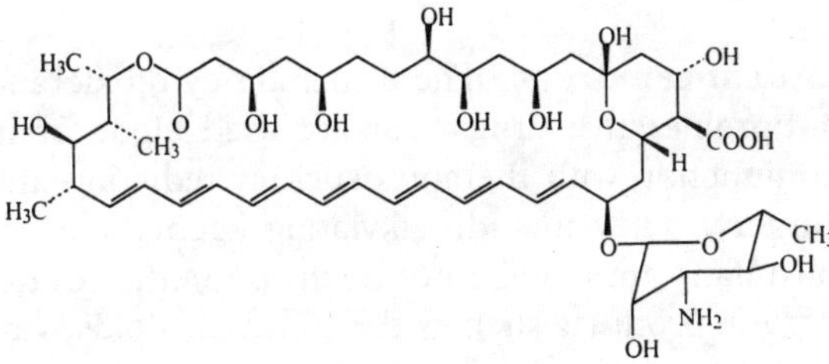

Amphotericin B

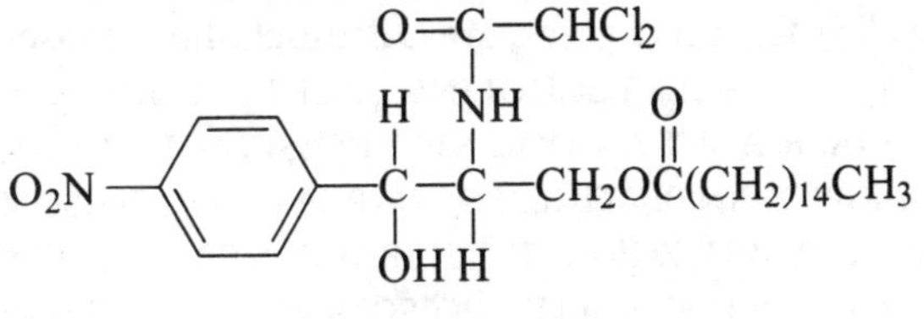

Chloramphenicol

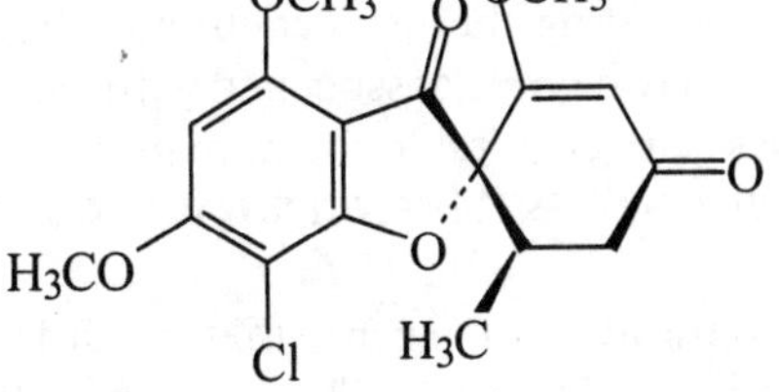

Griseofulvin

antibody. A large protein molecule expressed first on the surface of B cells. Stimulation of an immune response by a substance (antigen) that is complementary to and binds with a particular antibody results in proliferation and differentiation of the B cells bearing that antibody. The end product of this response is one or more clones of plasma cells that secrete the antibody molecules into body fluids. Antibodies bind specifically with the substance that stimulated their production, but may cross-react with other substances. The natural function of antibodies is to bind foreign substances (e.g., microbes or microbial products) and eliminate them by a variety of subsequent mechanisms. Because of their specificity, antibodies are used in a variety of research, diagnostic and therapeutic procedures. See also IMMUNOGLOBULIN.

antibody-dependent cellular cytotoxicity (ADCC). The non-specific lysis of antibody-coated cells by cells not sensitized to that antigen or antibody, such as cells from a non-immunized animal. This is accomplished by binding the constant, non-antigen-binding, portion of the antibody molecule, enabling attachment to and lysis of the target cell. It can occur in type II (cytolytic) allergic responses, as well as in tumor defense and foreign tissue graft rejection. It is believed to be mediated by killer (K) cells and, possibly, natural killer (NK) cells. See also ALLERGIC RESPONSE; NATURAL KILLER CELLS.

anticancer drugs. These include cytotoxic and antiproliferative drugs that are used alone or in conjunction with therapies such as radiation and surgery. They include alkylating agents such as busulfan, antimetabolites such as methotrexate, natural products such as the Vinca alkaloids, vinblastin and vincristine as well as hormones and related steroids and non-steroids. All current anticancer drugs are toxic and sometimes carcinogenic themselves, the risk of deleterious side effects is high. Considering the risk/benefit paradigm, only the extremely high risk associated with cancer renders these drugs suitable for human use. See also ALKYLATING AGENTS; CANCER; CARCINOGENESIS.

anticoagulant. An agent that retards blood coagulation (clotting). These chemicals have medical utility as "blood thinners" to prevent blood clots that could result in heart attacks, strokes or embolisms; coumarin derivatives are examples of therapeutic anticoagulants. Toxicologically, one of the most important uses of anticoagulants is as a rodenticide; warfarin is an example. Both groups act as vitamin K antagonists; vitamin K is a vitamin produced by the gut microflora in vertebrates that is necessary for the hepatic synthesis of thrombin, one of the clotting factors. Internal hemorrhage is the usual cause of death from these rodenticides. See also BLOOD; DICUMEROL.

anticodon. The three adjacent nucleotides in a transfer-RNA molecule that are complementary to, and base pair with, the three complementary nucleotides of a codon in a messenger-RNA molecule during protein synthesis.

anticholinesterases (acetylcholinesterase inhibitors). A number of carbamate or organophosphorus (OP) esters can carbamylate or phosphorylate, respectively, the serine hydroxyl at the esteratic site of acetylcholinesterase (AChE), inhibiting the action of the enzyme. During the reaction, the original ester is cleaved; the leaving group refers to the portion of the toxicant not remaining bound to the enzyme. The carbamylated AChE is spontaneously hydrolyzed quite readily, leading to rapid recovery of enzyme activity; symptoms of poisoning persist for only a few hours. The phosphorylated AChE, however, is spontaneously hydrolyzed much more slowly, and the inhibitory action of OP anticholinesterases and the resultant symptomology are much more persistent, with inhibition by some compounds lasting several days or even weeks. "Aging" of the enzyme occurs with some compounds, after which spontaneous reactivation is impossible. A number of carbamate anticholinesterases are used as insecticides; others (e.g., neostigmine, eserine) are used therapeutically. A large number of insecticides, as well as the nerve gases, are OP anticholinesterases. See also ACETYLCHOLINE; ACETYLCHOLINESTERASE; ACETYLCHOLINESTERASE, AGING; CARBAMATE INSECTICIDES; CARBAMATE POISONING, SYMPTOMS AND THERAPY; NERVE GASES; ORGANOPHOSPHATE POISONING, SYMPTOMS AND THERAPY; ORGANOPHOSPHORUS INSECTICIDES.

anticonvulsants (antiepileptics). Compounds used in the control of seizure disorders. Phenytoin, formerly known as diphenylhydantoin, is one of the most widely used anticonvulsants. Like phenobarbital and primidone, phenytoin is effective in treating grand mal epilepsy and cortical focal (psychomotor) epilepsy, but is not used to treat petit mal seizures. Side effects include visual disturbances, slurred speech, gastrointestinal distress and drug sensitivity reactions. Carbamazepine is useful in patients with temporal lobe epilepsy when the condition occurs alone or in combination with generalized tonic-clonic seizures. Valproic acid (*n*-dipropylacetic acid), the latest antiepileptic agent to be approved for use in the USA, is active against a wide variety of seizures, while causing minimal sedation and CNS side effects. Compared with other agents, valproic acid also has a very low incidence of other side effects. Clonazepam, a benzodiazepine, is used in the therapy of absence seizures, as well as myoclonic seizures in children, but diazepam is particularly useful in treating status epilepticus, a continuing epileptic seizure that may result in death if not treated. Anticonvulsant agents are frequently used to treat symptoms caused by intoxication with seizure-inducing chemicals or by generalized insult of the CNS. *See also* BARBITURATES; BENZODIAZEPINES; CONVULSIONS; DIAZEPAM; PHENOBARBITAL; PHENYTOIN; SEIZURES.

antidepressants. Drugs that are used to treat depression, a very common (c.a. 10% of the population) psychiatric mood disorder. The three classes of drugs that are most commonly used are the selective serotonin reuptake inhibitors (SSRIs), tricyclic antidepressants, and the monoamine oxidase inhibitors (MAOIs). These MAOIs may cause toxicity because of their common property of potentiating the action of endogenous and, when ingested, exogenous monoamines. The tricyclic antidepressants, while very effective, have an extremely low therapeutic index because of cardiovascular effects caused by an increase in synaptic norepinephrine concentration and blockade of muscarinic cholinergic receptors (both actions being cardiostimulatory). Lithium, a drug primarily used to treat mania, may also be used prophylactically against depression. *See also* LITHIUM; MONOAMINE OXIDASE INHIBITORS; SSRIS; TRICYCLIC ANTIDEPRESSANTS.

antidiuretic hormone. *See* VASOPRESSIN.

antidote. A compound that is administered in order to reverse the deleterious effects of a toxicant. Antidotes may be specific, exerting their effect through a mechanism related to the mechanism of action of the toxicant, or non-specific, counteracting the symptoms of toxicity in a manner not clearly related to the mechanism of action. An example of the former is 2-PAM (*N*-methylpyridinium-2-aldoxime), that reverses the effect of organophosphate acetylcholinesterase inhibition by dephosphorylating the phosphorylated enzyme. Syrup of ipecac is an example of a non-specific antidote since its mode of action is to eliminate toxicants from the stomach by induction of vomiting (emesis). *See also* THERAPY.

antiemetics. Drugs that suppress vomiting. The chief antiemetics are the phenothiazines, such as chlorpromazine, perphenazine, prochlorperazine or promethazine. Induction of emesis by apomorphine or certain ergot alkaloids can be blocked by most neuroleptics due to their actions on dopamine receptors in the chemoreceptor trigger zone of the area postrema. Thioridazine is an exception, having no antiemetic effects in humans. Emesis induced by local effects on the gastrointestinal tract are not blocked by neuroleptics, although vestibular stimulation-induced nausea can be blocked by the more potent neuroleptics. In addition, phenothiazines such as chlorpromazine can be used to block the vomiting associated with radiation sickness, carcinomas, gastroenteritis, uremia or emesis induced by opioid analgesics, disulfiram, drugs used in the chemotherapy of carcinomas and tetracyclines. Although not recommended for this use, chlorpromazine will also suppress vomiting associated with pregnancy. Chlorpromazine is not useful in controlling motion sickness. Certain H1 histamine receptor blockers including dimenhydrinate (Dramamine), diphenhydramine, promethazine and other piperazine derivatives are useful in treating or preventing motion sickness. Many of the H1 receptor blockers have antimuscarinic properties, that may contribute to their antiemetic effect. The antimuscarinic agent scopolamine, for example, is a potent anti-motion sickness agent. Also, promethazine, which is one of the most effective anti-motion sickness drugs, has potent antimuscarinic effects. Because morphine and its derivatives frequently result in nausea and vomiting, opiate antagonists, such as naloxone, will exert antiemetic effects like the neuroleptics. *See also* AREA POSTREMA; EMESIS; PHENOTHIAZINES.

antiepileptics. *See* ANTICONVULSANTS.

antigen. A substance that elicits an immune response. In general a molecule must be foreign to the host, have a molecular mass in excess of 5000 daltons and have some degree of molecular complexity in order to be antigenic. Smaller molecules (haptens), including a number of xenobiotics, can be rendered antigenic by covalently coupling them to larger, more complex molecules (carriers). The antibodies elicited by the hapten–carrier conjugate will generally react with that conjugate and with the free hapten as well. *See also* ANTIBODY.

Antigestil. *See* DIETHYLSTILBESTROL.

antihistamines. Drugs, such as diphenhydramine or chlorpheniramine, that exert their pharmacodynamic effect by blocking H_1 and/or H_2 histamine receptors. Antihistamines are used to treat allergic symptoms (H_1), motion sickness (H_1) and stomach ulcers (H_2). They are usually rapidly absorbed from the gastrointestinal tract, showing peak blood levels one to two hours after oral administration. Side effects of non-selective agents include sedation, nausea and vomiting, as well as atropine-like effects such as dry mouth, dysuria, hypotension and weakness. Selective H_2 histamine antagonists (e.g., cimetidine, ranitidine, famotidine, nizatidine) have been widely used recently for treatment of stomach ulcers by suppressing gastric acid secretion. There are new H_1 antagonists that do not cross the blood–brain barrier, such as terfenidine. *See also* CIMETIDINE; DIPHENHYDRAMINE; HISTAMINE; PROMETHAZINE; TERFENIDINE.

antihyperlipidemics. Drugs that reduce the concentration of lipids in the blood. Hyperlipidemia, an excess of lipid (usually either cholesterol or triglycerides) in the blood, has been associated with a variety of disease states, but particularly with premature vascular disease. Hyperlipidemia is, however, usually hyperlipoproteinemia since of the various lipids only free fatty acids are not characteristically associated with lipoproteins in the blood. Such drugs are therefore antihyperlipoproteinemics. They include clofibrate, nicotinic acid and cholestyramine, all of which may have adverse effects in some individuals. *See also* CHOLESTYRAMINE; CLOFIBRATE.

antihyperlipoproteinemics. *See* ANTIHYPERLIPIDEMICS.

anti-inflammatory agents. A large and diverse class of pharmaceuticals that interfere with the inflammatory response, including adrenal corticosteroids, non-steroidal anti-inflammatory drugs (NSAID), gold salts and colchicine. There are six classes of NSAID: salicylates, indenes, propionates, fenamates, pyrazolones and oxicams. The mechanism of action is inhibition of prostaglandin synthesis, with concomitant disruption of inflammatory intercellular communication. All are nonionizable weak acids, that are highly protein-bound. Prostaglandin inhibition accounts for most of the side effects, including nausea, gastritis, peptic ulcer, nephritic syndrome, platelet dysfunction, headaches, confusion, allergic rhinosinusitis, exacerbation of asthma and allergic skin rashes. Competition for the protein-binding sites accounts for many of the drug interactions. Metabolism is hepatic, whereas excretion is primarily renal and secondarily fecal. Drug Evaluations, 6th edn (American Medical Association, Chicago, 1986). *See also* ANALGESICS; ANTIPYRINE; CORTICOSTEROIDS; NSAIDS.

antimetabolites. Chemicals that resemble a normal substrate (metabolite) in a metabolic pathway. An antimetabolite inhibits the enzyme that metabolizes that substrate and therefore blocks the metabolic pathway. If the product of this enzyme reaction is essential for growth, then cellular growth is suppressed. Examples of antimetabolites include sulfanilamide, an antimetabolite of the folic acid precursor *p*-aminobenzoic acid, and 6-mercaptopurine, an antimetabolite of purine. *See also* 6-MERCAPTOPURINE.

antimicrobials. Physical and chemical agents that kill or inhibit the proliferation of microorganisms. Antimicrobials that exert lethal effects are considered to function in a cidal manner, whereas those that merely inhibit growth in a reversible manner are considered to function in a static manner. They are referred to as germicides (e.g., bacteriocides, fungicides, etc.) and microstatic agents (e.g., bacteriostatic agents, fungistatic agents, etc.), respectively. Physical antimicrobial agents include temperature, radiation, ultrasonication and filtration. Chemical antimicrobial agents having non-selective toxicity that are used to kill or inhibit pathogenic (i.e., disease-causing) microorganisms are classified as disinfectants if employed for inanimate objects or antiseptics if they are applied topically to biological tissues. This latter group includes surface-active compounds, dyes, heavy metals, phenols, alcohols, aldehydes, acids, halogens, oxidants, etc. Chemical antimicrobial agents suitable for chemotherapeutic use (i.e., drugs) exhibit selective toxicity in that they inhibit the proliferation of microorganisms at concentrations that do not harm the host. This group includes certain antibiotics and synthetic drugs. In addition to the specific nature of the microorganism being inhibited, the efficacy of an antimicrobial is critically dependent upon concentration, time of exposure, temperature and pH. *See also* ANTIBACTERIALS; ANTIBIOTICS; BACTERIOSTATS.

antimitotic agents. *See* SPINDLE POISONS.

antimony (Sb). A non-essential element. Acute or chronic toxicity results almost exclusively from industrial atmospheric exposure and involves pulmonary, dermal or cardiovascular (altered electrocardiogram) effects. Its oxidation states of +3 and +5 lead to many polyvalent compounds, some of which, like stilbene (SbH_3), are gaseous. Antimony has been used in human medicine for control of parasites. Although in the same group of the Periodic Table as arsenic, antimony is much less toxic. *Compare* ARSENIC.

antineoplastic agents. Drugs used in the chemotherapy of neoplastic diseases. They include many different types of drugs that have many different modes of action. All function, however, by killing neoplastic cells, but their toxicity to normal cells may also be high. Moreover, some of them, particularly the alkylating agents, are themselves carcinogens. Only the life-threatening nature of the disease and the lack of alternate therapies justify the clinical use of such hazardous drugs. They include: alkylating agents, such as nitrogen mustards (e.g., cyclophosphamide), ethylenimines (e.g., thiotepa), alkylsulfonates (e.g., busulfan) and nitrosoureas (e.g., carmustine); antimetabolites, such as the folic acid antagonist methotrexate; natural products such as the Vinca alkaloids vincristine and vinblastine; and hormones and hormone antagonists, such as estrogens (e.g., ethinylestradiol) and antiestrogens (e.g., tamoxifen). *See also* ALKYLATING AGENTS; ANTIMETABOLITES; ESTROGENS; ETHYLENEIMINE; NEOPLASM; NITROGEN MUSTARD; TAMOXIFEN; THERAPEUTIC INDEX; VINBLASTINE; VINCRISTINE.

antioxidants. Chemicals that hinder oxidation, frequently serving as free radical scavengers. Important examples include vitamins C and E, butylated hydroxyanisole (BHA) and butylated hydroxytoluene (BHT). These are frequently used as food preservatives and dietary supplements.

antiproliferative agents. Chemicals that can suppress cell proliferation, such as occurs during tumorigenesis. *See also* CYTOTOXICITY.

antipsychotic drugs. Drugs that are used to treat the most severe mental illnesses—the psychoses. They are widely used and have been given to as many as 300 million people world-wide. They have beneficial effects on mood and thought and are used in all psychoses, not just schizophrenia. The types of symptoms they are used for include delusions, hallucinations, mania and severe paranoia. The primary common mechanism of action of present antipsychotic drugs is as dopamine receptor antagonists. This class of drugs generally has a very high therapeutic index when used alone, and fatal overdoses (even deliberate) are not usually a problem. Many of the side effects are due to the fact that these compounds may also have anticholinergic or antiadrenergic properties. Because of their antihistaminic properties, they may interact with other depressant drugs. The most prevalent toxic effects are neurological in nature and fall into two general categories. There are various extrapyramidal side effects (e.g., pseudoparkinsonism or acute dystonia) that may be controlled by adding an anticholinergic drug or decreasing the antipsychotic dose. A major long-term toxic effect is tardive dyskinesia, a series of bizarre buccolingual or choreoathetoid movements, that usually occurs after long-term administration, more frequently in older patients. These latter movement disorders are usually permanent and are refractory to pharmacotherapy; the underlying mechanisms are not well understood. Many of the biochemical, neurochemical and behavioral effects of antipsychotic drugs occur acutely, yet clinical antipsychotic effects generally have a delayed onset over several weeks. Since these drugs generally achieve fairly rapid brain concentrations, blockade of dopamine receptors must initiate changes in the brain that ultimately causes amelioration of symptoms and possibly toxic side effects. *See also* BUTYROPHENONES; DOPAMINE; DOPAMINE RECEPTORS; EXTRAPYRAMIDAL SIDE EFFECTS; PHENOTHIAZINES; THERAPEUTIC INDEX; THIOXANTHENES.

antipyretics. Drugs that reduce fever, any or all of which may have adverse effects in some individuals. *See also* ANALGESICS; ANTI-INFLAMMATORY AGENTS; ASPIRIN; NONSTEROIDAL ANTI-INFLAMMATORY DRUGS.

antipyrine (1,2-dihydro-1,5-dimethyl-2-phenyl-3H-pyrazol-3-one; 2,3-dimethyl-1-phenyl-3-pyrazolin-5-one; phenazone; Analgesine; Sedatine). CAS number 60-80-0. One of the pyrazolon derivatives, that also include phenylbutazone, aminopyrine and apazone. These drugs tend to be weaker antipyretics or analgesics than the salicylates, but they do have strong anti-inflammatory properties. The main disadvantage of the pyrazolon derivatives is that they also may produce serious blood disorders. Agranulocytosis (i.e., a sudden decrease in white blood cells) may be fatal and can occur in hypersensitive individuals receiving aminopyrine. Skin eruptions occasionally occur with antipyrine. Although the oral LD50

is about 1.8 g/kg in rats, these pyrazolon derivatives seem to be more toxic than the other mild analgesics. They may be useful in patients who are hypersensitive to salicylates. If pyrazolon derivatives are used, it is important to monitor the blood frequently for the possible development of low white blood cell counts. *Compare* SALICYLATES. *See also* ANALGESICS; ANTI-INFLAMMATORY AGENTS; APAZONE; PYRAZOLON DERIVATIVES.

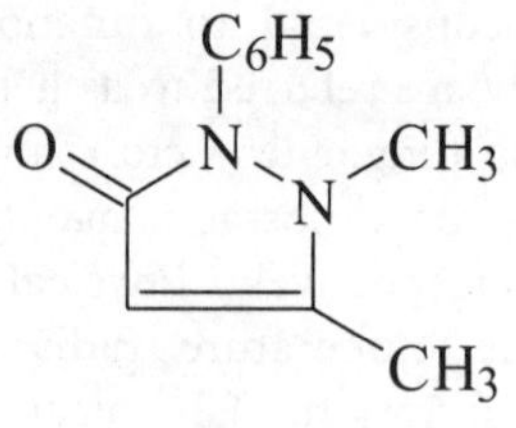

Antipyrine

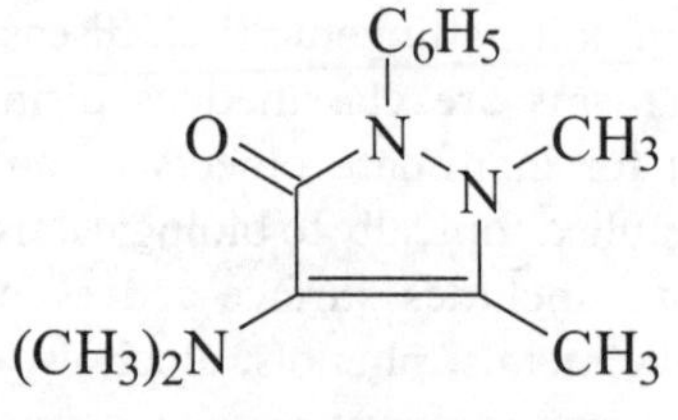

Aminopyrine

antiseptics. *See* ANTIMICROBIALS.

antitoxin. Therapeutic antibodies that have been raised against a microbial, plant or animal toxin, and that can be used in the therapy of poisoned individuals to neutralize the toxin. The antitoxin can also be used prophylactically. *See also* ANTIVENIN.

antitumor agent. *See* ANTINEOPLASTIC AGENTS.

antivenin. A therapeutic agent produced against a venom, such as from snakes or black widow spiders, by animals, frequently horses, that have been immunized against the venom. If delivered soon enough after envenomation, the antivenin can prevent or attenuate signs of poisoning and/or death. Such therapy may cause its own toxicological consequences from immune response to the foreign protein that constitutes the antivenin. *See also* ANTITOXIN.

antivenom. *See* ANTIVENIN.

ANTU. *See* α-NAPHTHOTHIOUREA.

anuria. A condition in which no urine is produced. This condition can be life-threatening because of the accumulation of toxic metabolic wastes in the body.

anxiolytic drugs. *See* ANTIANXIETY DRUGS.

apazone   (5-(dimethylamino)-9-methyl-2-propyl-1H-pyrazolo[1,2-*a*][1,2,4]benzotriazine-1,3(2H)-dione; azapropazone). CAS number 13539-59-8. An anti-inflammatory, analgesic and antipyretic. It is also useful in the treatment of gout due to its uricosuric actions. It is similar in activity to phenylbutazone, although considerably less toxic. Gastrointestinal effects such as nausea, epigastric pain, dyspepsia and heartburn have been reported in only a small percentage of patients. Similarly, few report skin rashes, whereas CNS effects such as headache and dizziness occur even less frequently. Apazone inhibits prostaglandin synthetase and has ulcerogenic properties. *See also* ANALGESICS; ANTI-INFLAMMATORY AGENTS; ANTIPYRETICS; PYRAZOLON DERIVATIVES.

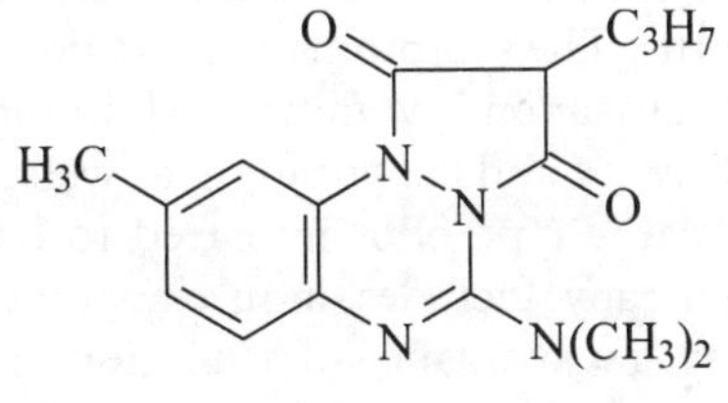

Apazone

APHIS. *See* ANIMAL AND PLANT HEALTH INSPECTION SERVICE.

aplastic anemia. Anemia resulting from the destruction of the ability of the bone marrow to generate all blood cells. This results in loss of erythrocyte concentrations in the blood and, consequently, reduced oxygen transport. This can result from bone marrow damage due to radiation or chemicals. *See also* CHLORAMPHENICOL; CLOZAPINE.

apnea. A condition characterized by lapses in breathing.

apoptosis. The process of programmed cell death. This is a normal part of such processes as embryonic development, metamorphosis, and immune cell differentiation. It is characterized by high levels of energy consumption, condensation of nuclear chromatin, internucleosomal cleavage of DNA, and activation of highly conserved signal transduction pathways. Molecular biological techniques now permit rapid assessment of toxicant-induced apoptosis.

Aquacide. *See* DIQUAT.

aquatic bioassay. A procedure in which aquatic organisms are used to detect or measure biological responses to one or more substances, wastes or environmental factors, alone or in combination. Experimental procedures may vary considerably; therefore, it is important that biological, chemical and physical parameters be defined (e.g., test organism, type of exposure system, length of exposure, water quality). Common test organisms include bluegill sunfish (*Lepomis macrochirus*), fathead minnow (*Pimephales promelas*), rainbow trout (*Oncorhychus mykiss*), sheepshead minnow (*Cyprinodon variegatus*), daphnids (*Daphnia species*) and mysid shrimp (*Mysidopsis species*).

aquatic ecosystem. An ecosystem involving strictly water, sediments and aquatic organisms, but not terrestrial elements. Model aquatic ecosystems have been developed to study the fate of chemicals in the environment. *See also* ECOSYSTEMS; MODEL ECOSYSTEMS.

aquatic toxicology. A branch of toxicology that deals with adverse effects of toxicants on aquatic organisms (marine, estuarine or freshwater) and on aquatic ecosystems; largely a study of water pollution and its ecological effects. *See also* WATER POLLUTION.

ARBD (alcohol-related birth defects). *See* FETAL ALCOHOL SYNDROME.

area postrema. A narrow strip of neural tissue located in the caudal part of the floor of the fourth ventricle (cisterna magna), dorsal to the nucleus tractus solitarius and dorsal efferent nucleus of the vagus. The "blood–brain barrier" is lacking in this area and so circulating compounds can penetrate nervous tissue from capillary blood. The area postrema is thought to be a chemoreceptor trigger zone for emetics such as apomorphine. Additionally, the area postrema is important in mediating the pressor effects of angiotensin II. *See also* ANTIEMETICS; EMESIS.

arene oxides. *See* EPOXIDES.

ARIMA. *See* AUTOREGRESSIVE INTEGRATED MOVING AVERAGE.

Aroclors. Commercial mixtures of polychlorinated biphenyls (PCBs), each containing a large number of isomers and being identified by numbers reflecting the average degree of chlorination of the mixture (e.g., Aroclor 1254). Aroclors and other commercial PCB mixtures have been used for over 50 years as heat exchangers in electrical equipment. Because they have a variety of adverse effects on the immune system and skin, and may be either carcinogenic or promote tumors, their use has been greatly restricted. *See also* POLYCHLORINATED BIPHENYLS.

aromatase. The name given to an enzyme catalyzing the aromatization of the A-ring of the steroid nucleus during the conversion of androgens to estrogens. It is now known to be identical to CYP19, a cytochrome P450 isoform. *See also* AROMATIZATION; CYTOCHROME P450.

aromatic amines. A number of aromatic amines have proven to be carcinogenic in animal tests. Among these are substituted anilines (e.g., *o*-toluidine), biphenyls (e.g., benzidine or 4-biphenylamine), 2-naphthylamine and polycyclic arylamines (e.g., 2-phenanthrylamine and 2-aminofluorene). Many of these aromatic amines cause liver cancer, urinary bladder cancer (primarily in males) and breast cancer in females. Humans developing cancer as a result of occupational exposure to arylamines usually display urinary bladder cancer. Some nitro derivatives of aromatic amines are also carcinogenic. *See also* BENZIDINE; β-NAPHTHYLAMINE; *o*-TOLUIDINE.

aromatic hydrocarbons. *See* POLYCYCLIC AROMATIC HYDROCARBONS.

aromatic hydroxylation. *See* EPOXIDATION AND AROMATIC HYDROXYLATION.

aromatization. A reaction in which a saturated ring structure is converted to an aromatic ring. In addition to the aromatization of steroids by CYP19 there are mitochondrial enzymes in rabbit and guinea pig liver that can aromatize cyclohexane derivatives. This reaction requires oxygen, CoA and ATP. These mitochondrial enzymes are not widely distributed, mitochondria from rodent and primate liver being relatively to completely inactive. *See also* AROMATASE.

arrhythmia. Any variation from the normal cardiac rhythm. Arrhythmias may result from many disease states, but can also be the result of poisoning, or as a drug toxic side effect, usually acute.

arsenate. Pentavalent arsenic; it is used in insecticides, herbicides, fungicides and algicides, and is widely distributed in nature, being a contaminant of metal ores and coal. It is a carcinogen, but is less toxic than arsenite. Arsenate uncouples oxidative phosphorylation by substituting for inorganic phosphorus. The symptoms of acute poisoning are violent nausea and vomiting, abdominal pain, severe diarrhea and dehydration, as well as a sweet metallic garlic-type odor imparted to breath and feces. Therapy includes induction of emesis or gastric lavage, avoidance of aspiration of vomitus, correction of dehydration and electrolyte imbalance and chelation therapy with 3–5 mg/kg, i.m., 2,3-dimercapto-1-propanol. *See also* ARSENIC.

arsenic (As). **CAS number 7440-38-2**. A metalloid element that is used in metallurgy, glassmaking, agriculture and medicine. Human exposure occurs occupationally and via food, tobacco smoke, ambient air and water. Three major groups of arsenic compounds have been defined on the basis of biological considerations: inorganic arsenicals; organic arsenicals; and arsine (gas). The comparative toxicity of these groups are dependent upon the route of exposure and their solubilities; the more quickly absorbed compounds have lower LD50s. Arsenic is readily absorbed by the respiratory and gastrointestinal systems and is concentrated in the skin, hair and nails (Aldrich–Mee's lines). The cellular toxicity of arsenic is related to reactions with SH-containing mitochondrial enzymes that result in impaired respiration. Arsenic may also compete with phosphate during oxidative phosphorylation. Detoxication is via reductive methylation. Methylarsinic and dimethylarsinic acids are excreted into the urine. The acute signs of poisoning include fever, anorexia, hepatomegaly, cardiac arrhythmia, transient encephalopathy and irritation of the gastrointestinal tract. Additional signs may include upper respiratory tract involvement and peripheral neuropathy. Chronic symptoms are exfoliation and pigmentation of skin, symmetrical distal neuropathy, altered hematopoiesis and liver and kidney degeneration. Epidemiological data indicate that arsenic is a human carcinogen. In humans, the fatal dose for arsenic has been reported to range from 1 to 2.5 mg/kg body weight. Biological indicators of poisoning are urine, blood and hair levels. 2,3-Dimercapto-1-propanol is the treatment for acute intoxication, but it is less effective in treating chronic exposures. *See also* ARSENATE; ARSENITE; ARSINE; 2,3-DIMERCAPTO-1-PROPANOL; LEAD ARSENATE.

arsenicals. The general class of compounds containing arsenic in one of its valency forms. *See also* ARSENATE; ARSENIC; ARSENITE.

arsenic reduction. Organic arsenicals in which the arsenic is in pentavalent state may be reduced to trivalent arsenic compounds. In many cases (e.g., Tryparsamide), these compounds are antiparasitic or antiprotozoan compounds, and the reaction is an activation reaction since the reduced compounds are more effective.

arsenite. Trivalent arsenic; it is used in insecticides, herbicides, fungicides and algicides, and is widely distributed in nature and as a contaminant of metal ores and coal. It is a carcinogen, but is also corrosive to epithelial cells and other tissues. Trivalent arsenic binds avidly to sulfhydryl groups of critical enzymes and impairs cellular metabolism. After acute poisoning, there is violent nausea and vomiting, abdominal pain, severe diarrhea and dehydration, with a sweet metallic garlic-type

odor imparted to breath and feces. Therapy includes induction of emesis or gastric lavage, avoiding aspiration of vomitus, correction of dehydration and electrolyte imbalance. In severe cases, chelation therapy with 3–5 mg/kg, i.m., 2,3-dimercapto-1-propanol is used. *Compare* ARSENATE. *See also* ARSENIC; 2,3-DIMERCAPTO-1-PROPANOL.

arsine (hydrogen arsenide; AsH_3). A colorless flammable gas with a slight odor of garlic. It is sometimes formed as a by-product of the metal industries. Arsine poisoning is characterized by nausea, abdominal colic, vomiting, backache and shortness of breath, followed by dark bloody urine and jaundice. Symptomatic measures, but not chelation, are usually effective. *See also* ARSENIC.

arterial hypoxia. *See* HYPOXIA.

Arthus reaction. *See* IMMEDIATE HYPERSENSITIVITY.

Arum family. The family Araceae, containing *Philodendron* species. *P. scandens* is a common houseplant. Plants in this family contain resorcinol and cause contact dermatitis.

arylamidases. *See* HYDROLYSIS.

arylation. The chemical addition of an aryl group to another molecule. In toxicology, covalent binding of aryl groups to macromolecules is important in the mode of toxic action of many toxicants. It usually occurs as a result of the formation of a reactive electrophilic intermediate, such as an epoxide, by the cytochrome P450-dependent monooxygenase system and the subsequent reaction of this intermediate with nucleophilic substituents on macromolecules to give rise to a covalently bound aryl group. For example, the hepatotoxicant bromobenzene is believed to be metabolized to the 3,4-epoxide, that then reacts with liver proteins. Similarly, benzo[a]pyrene-7,8-epoxide reacts with DNA molecules. *See also* REACTIVE INTERMEDIATES.

arylesterases. *See* HYDROLYSIS.

aryl hydrocarbon hydroxylase (AHH). Although the term is often used as if AHH were an enzyme, it is more properly used in the form AHH activity since the ability to hydroxylate polycyclic aromatic hydrocarbons is a reaction catalyzed by one or more isozymes of cytochrome P450. These isozymes also oxidize substrates that are not polycyclic aromatic hydrocarbons. The importance of the reaction in toxicology is the fact that many polycyclic aromatic hydrocarbons are carcinogenic, and AHH activity is involved in the sequence of reactions leading to the formation of the proximal carcinogens. Hepatic cytochrome P450 isozymes that carry out this reaction are also induced by aromatic hydrocarbons such as 3-methylcholanthrene and benzo[a]pyrene, as well as by TCDD and β-naphthoflavone, this induction being mediated by the Ah receptor. *See also* AH RECEPTOR; BENZO[*A*]PYRENE; BENZO[*A*]-PYRENE-7,8-DIOL-9,10-EPOXIDE; CYTOCHROME P450.

aryl sulfotransferase. *See* SULFATE CONJUGATION.

asbestos. CAS number 1332-21-4. Fibrous hydrated mineral silicates that are resistant to thermal and chemical degradation and have, therefore, been widely used as insulating materials. Asbestos has also been used in textiles, paints, plastics, paper, gaskets, brake linings, tiles, cement and filters. The most widely used is chrysotile, a fibrous form of serpentine; other types include crocidolite, amosite and anthophyllite. Asbestos is poorly absorbed from the gastrointestinal tract and therefore displays low acute oral toxicity. Respiratory exposure, however, leads to a pulmonary fibrosis called asbestosis, whose signs include breathlessness, chest pain, cough, decreased lung function and cyanosis. Occupational exposures to asbestos have resulted in higher incidences of lung cancer (especially mesotheliomas), especially in combination with cigarette smoking; the latent period is 15–30 years. This synergism may be the result of the inhibitory effect of trace elements in asbestosis, such as chromium, nickel or beryllium, on the detoxication of smoke carcinogens. Cancers can also occur in the pleurae, peritoneum, bronchi or oropharynx. Mesothelioma, a cancer of the thin membrane that surrounds the lung, is invariably fatal, often within a few months of diagnosis. Although the mechanism of carcinogenesis is unknown, asbestos does not appear to be metabolized, and thus remains permanently within the body. An additional effect of asbestos exposure is the development of pleural or peritoneal mesotheliomas; the latent period is 3.5–30 years. Fibers can eventually become coated with mucopolysaccharides and hemosiderin to form "asbestos bodies." No safe level of asbestos exposure to humans has been observed. Asbestos in the air occurs around asbestos mines and factories, but it also occurs in urban areas because of wear to brake linings and the flaking of insulation materials. Removal of asbestos from existing buildings during renovation or removal has become a major public health and toxicological concern. *See also* ASBESTOSIS; FIBROSIS; PNEUMOCONIOSIS.

asbestosis. A respiratory disorder resulting from inhalation exposure to asbestos, characterized by fibrosis, calcification, bronchogenic carcinoma and mesothelial tumors. The asbestos fibers are not metabolized and are retained within the lungs for the life span of the animal. The mechanism of carcinogenesis is unknown, but resembles solid-state carcinogenesis. The latent period is long. Asbestosis is synergistic to the carcinogenesis caused by smoking. Asbestosis was recognized as long ago as 1907; however, the magnitude of the risk has become apparent only recently, primarily because of the increased incidence of lung cancer among asbestosis sufferers, especially those who are also cigarette smokers. *See also* DUST, PROLIFERATIVE; FIBROSIS; PULMONARY TOXICITY.

ascorbic acid (vitamin C). CAS number 50-81-7. A water-soluble vitamin that has several known biochemical roles including acting as a cofactor in tyrosine metabolism. Ascorbic acid is necessary for formation of bone, cartilage and dentine. Lack of the vitamin leads to scurvy in humans. The principal sources of ascorbic acid in the diet are fruits and vegetables. Dependence on nutritional sources is rare in mammals, being seen in humans and some other primates and the guinea pig; most mammals are able to synthesize enough to supply their metabolic needs. Various roles in the prevention of disease, such as the common cold, cancer, etc., have been claimed for ascorbic acid, but are largely unproven. Nonetheless, ascorbic acid is often taken in large and frequent doses, although symptoms of overdose are rare.

$$CH_2OH$$
$$HC{-}OH$$

Ascorbic acid

aspartame (L-aspartyl-L-phenylalanine methyl ester; Nutrasweet). CAS number 22389-47-0. A dipeptide food additive sweetener; approximately 200 times sweeter than sugar. Although its sweetness properties were discovered in 1965, and FDA approval was obtained in 1974, doubts about the toxicological studies led to a stay of approval until 1981 in the USA. In 1983, the FDA approved aspartame for use in carbonated beverages. It is also an approved additive in the UK. Aspartame is used in more than 200 food products, with an estimated 100 million people ingesting 10 million pounds of aspartame annually. Its intense sweetness makes it unlikely that most individuals will consume more than 500 mg/day, although higher doses may be possible in some people. The acceptable daily intake (ADI) is set at 50 mg/kg/day. Some toxicological concerns are still debated. A very small number of urticarial reactions have been reported, some of which have been demonstrated in double-blind challenge studies. Although it is generally agreed that the methanol and aspartic acid derived from the metabolism of aspartame are safe, the effects of the phenylalanine moiety upon brain function are unclear. It has been suggested that elevated phenylalanine levels may compete for the transport of other amino acids into the brain and result in diminished neurotransmitter levels, leading possibly to headaches, behavioral disturbances,

$$COOCH_3$$
$$H_2NCHCONHCHCH_2{-}$$
$$CH_2COOH$$

Aspartame

diminution of IQ and epileptic fits. Such adverse effects, however, have not been convincingly demonstrated. The phenylalanine derived from aspartame is a clear hazard for homozygous phenylketonuriacs, although its effect on heterozygous patients with phenylketonuria is still under debate. *See also* FOOD ADDITIVES; SWEETENING AGENTS.

l-aspartyl-l-phenylalanine methyl ester. *See* ASPARTAME.

asphyxiants. Toxicants that exert their toxic effects by depriving the tissues of oxygen. They have been divided into the simple asphyxiants and the chemical asphyxiants. The simple asphyxiants act by diluting the oxygen in the inhaled air, thereby reducing its partial pressure in the alveoli and, consequently, its transfer into venous blood. As the partial pressure approaches that of the venous blood, the rate of transfer approaches zero. Such chemicals as nitrogen, nitrous oxide, hydrogen and helium are classified as simple asphyxiants. Chemical asphyxiants, on the other hand, act by chemical interactions, either to prevent oxygen transport to the tissues or to prevent oxygen utilization by the tissues. Carbon monoxide, for example, combines with hemoglobin to form carboxyhemoglobin and thus blocks oxygen transport, whereas cyanide reacts with the cytochrome oxidase complex to prevent oxygen utilization by mitochondria. Chemicals that inflame or irritate the respiratory tract, giving rise to pulmonary edema, may also cause death by asphyxiation, but are usually classified as primary lung irritants. *See also* CARBON MONOXIDE; CYANIDES; IRRITANTS; NITROUS OXIDE.

aspirin (2-(acetyloxy)benzoic acid; salicylic acid acetate; acetylsalicylic acid). CAS number 50-78-2. A member of the class of drugs known as salicylates. The principal therapeutic actions of aspirin include analgesic, antipyretic and anti-inflammatory activity. It is believed that the aspirin-like drugs work by inhibiting the synthesis of prostaglandins and related autocoids by inhibiting the enzymes (e.g., cyclooxygenases) that form them from arachidonic acid. This biochemical locus is inhibited by all of the aspirin-like drugs, thus resulting in both the most important therapeutic and toxic actions of this class of agents.

Aspirin inhibits the cyclooxygenases by an irreversible mechanism, whereas salicylic acid (also a major aspirin metabolite) inhibits the enzyme reversibly. The analgesic activity of aspirin is much less than that of the narcotic analgesics, but aspirin is more widely used than the narcotic analgesics because it does not induce euphoria, and the repeated use of aspirin does not result in tolerance nor lead to physical dependence. Some of the toxic effects of aspirin include gastric distress, particularly in patients suffering from peptic ulcer. Some people are hypersensitive to aspirin, even at very low doses, and these patients may have anaphylactic reactions to the drug. Gastric hemorrhaging, caused by platelet clumping mediated by prostaglandins and related compounds, is sometimes a problem. The LD50 in mice or rats is of the order of 1.1–1.5 mg/kg, with alteration of physiological acid/base balance being a primary danger. A common danger with aspirin is overdosage; it has been estimated that 40% of all drug poisonings result from aspirin. The problem is particularly serious in children and, not unexpectedly, involves flavored aspirin tablets. *See also* ACETAMINOPHEN; ANALGESICS; ANTI-INFLAMMATORY AGENTS; CYCLOOXYGENASES; FOOD COLORS; NSAIDS.

$$\text{COOH}$$
$$\text{OOCCH}_3$$

Aspirin

association constant (K_A, equilibrium association constant, affinity constant, binding constant). A quantitative measure of the likelihood of the interaction of a ligand with its target protein. The affinity constant can be derived from the equilibrium equation

$$K_A = \frac{[TP]}{[T] \cdot [P]} = \frac{1}{K_D}$$

where [TP] is the concentration of the toxicant-protein (or other macromolecule) complex at equilibrium, [T] is the concentration of free toxicant and [P] is the concentration of free protein at equilibrium. Traditionally, values of K_D (or K_A) can also be determined from the Scatchard

equation. *Compare* DISSOCIATION CONSTANT. *See also* BINDING; BINDING AFFINITY; DISSOCIATION CONSTANT; SCATCHARD PLOT.

Association of the British Pharmaceutical Industry (ABPI). A UK trade association that aims to ensure that medicinal and related products are of the highest quality and are readily available for the treatment of human and animal disease. ABPI publishes the Data Sheet Compendium, that contains details, in the form of data sheets, of drugs commercially available in the UK, listing their uses, dosage and administration, contraindications, warnings, etc. Under the Medicines Act of 1968, data sheets have to be supplied to all medical practitioners.

Association for the Assessment and Accreditation of Laboratory Animal Care (AAALAC). *See* AMERICAN ASSOCIATION FOR ACCREDITATION OF LABORATORY ANIMAL CARE.

asthma. Single (rare) or recurrent (common) episodes of labored or difficult breathing involving spasmodic contraction and hypersecretion of the bronchi. Asthma attacks, in the susceptible individual, may result from exposure to naturally occurring allergens (such as pollens or dusts), to chemicals (including drugs, industrial chemicals and environmental pollutants) or may be idiopathic.

ASTM. *See* AMERICAN SOCIETY FOR TESTING AND MATERIALS.

astrocyte. A type of glial cell found in the vertebrate central nervous system, the name being derived from the star-like appearance. Astrocytes provide metabolic and mechanical support to the neurons, synthesize some metabolites used by the neurons and are involved in regulation of the ionic balance of the fluid around the neurons. Astrocytes have been maintained in culture and cultured astrocytes have been used as models in toxicological research.

astroglia. *See* ASTROCYTE.

astrogliosis. *See* GLIOSIS.

ataxia. Inability to control motor coordination.

Athens Treaty on Land-Based Sources of Pollution. An international treaty drawn up in 1980, that came into force in 1983 when six of its 16 signatory governments ratified it. It was designed to reduce pollution in the Mediterranean.

atheroma. The thickening of the wall or the fatty degeneration occurring in the walls of the larger arteries in atherosclerosis.

atherosclerosis. An accumulation of lipid deposits within or beneath the intimal surfaces of blood vessels that partially occludes the lumen of the vessel and roughens its interior surface. This reduces blood flow to tissues, increases the chance of platelet aggregation and blood coagulation by increasing the turbulence within the blood, and increases the chances of occlusion by trapping a circulating blood clot. If calcium becomes deposited in the atherosclerotic plaques, then arteriosclerosis ("hardening of the arteries") results. Certain diets may contribute to atherosclerosis, as may chromium deficiency or excess copper.

atmosphere generation, in inhalation toxicology. Generation of accurate mixtures is essential for accurate toxicity testing of airborne toxicants. Gases can be added to an air flow by any of several measuring devices (flowmeters, syringes, etc.). Vapors of solids and liquids can be generated by heating in a chamber, and the vapor is passed into the air flow to the exposure chamber. Other methods include spraying onto a heated surface or, in the case of liquids, bubbling with a stream of carrier gas such as air or nitrogen. Generation of particulate or aerosol suspensions is more difficult since it is necessary to regulate particle size as well as total toxicant concentration. Powders may be dispersed by air turbulence and aerosols generated by fluidized bed generators. *See also* ADMINISTRATION OF TOXICANTS, INHALATION.

atmospheric analysis, in inhalation toxicology. Due to the difficulties of generating toxicant mixtures for inhalation studies, analysis of the atmosphere within the test chamber is important. This is necessary to estimate actual dose and distribution within the chamber, particularly in the case of particulate test materials. In this case, the distribution of particle sizes relative to the test organism must be determined as well as toxicant concentration since the extent of penetration into the respiratory system is highly dependent upon particle size. Samples can be collected by sedimentation, centrifugation, impaction or electrostatic precipitation, and particle size is determined by any of several methods including direct measurement by light or electron microscopy, or light scattering. *See also* ADMINISTRATION OF TOXICANTS, INHALATION.

atmospheric half-life. The time required for a 50% reduction of the concentration of an air pollutant present in the ambient atmosphere.

atmospheric residence time. The time required for reduction of the concentration of an air pollutant in the ambient atmosphere to a level equal to $1/e$ (c. 37%) of the original concentration.

atomic absorption spectrophotometry. *See* SPECTROMETRY, ATOMIC ABSORPTION.

ATP (adenosine 5′-triphosphate). **CAS number 56-65-5**. A high-energy intermediate essential for normal metabolic processes that require energy (e.g., muscle contraction, active transport, etc.). In toxicology, ATP is important as a precursor of the conjugating group in such phase II reactions as sulfate formation and methylation. Toxicants that block ATP formation either by uncoupling mitochondrial oxidative phosphorylation (e.g., dinitrophenol) or by inhibiting mitochondrial electron transport (e.g., cyanide) are important in toxicology. *See also* S-ADENOSYLMETHIONINE; OXIDATIVE PHOSPHORYLATION; PAPS.

Adenosine triphosphate

ATPase (adenosine triphosphatase). An enzyme that hydrolyzes ATP to release energy to drive endergonic processes. It may be part of a transport pump, such as the ouabain-sensitive Na^+/K^+-ATPase (Na^+ pump), that assists in establishing the cell membrane's electrochemical gradient, or the Ca^{2+}-ATPase (Ca^{2+} pump), that pumps Ca^{2+} out of the cytosol. The term may also be used as the name for the reverse direction of a reaction that normally forms ATP, such as the mitochondrial Mg^{2+}-dependent ATPase, that functions to form ATP using the energy of the proton gradient established across the inner mitochondrial membrane. The term may also refer to an activity of a protein with additional functions, such as the ATPase activity of myosin molecules, that releases the energy used for the mechanical motion of muscle contraction.

ATP-dependent acid:CoA ligase (AMP). *See* AMINO ACID CONJUGATION.

ATP sulfurylase. *See* SULFATE CONJUGATION.

atrazine (2-chloro-4-ethylamino-6-isopropyl-amino-1,3,5-triazine; 6-chloro-*N*-ethyl-*N*′-(1-methylethyl)-1,3,5-triazine-2,4-diamine). **CAS number 1912-24-9**. A selective pre- and post-emergence herbicide. The acute oral LD50 in rats ranges from 1850 to about 3000 mg/kg; the acute dermal LD50 in rabbits is 7500 mg/kg. It is slightly toxic to fish. Experimentally it has been shown to act as a mutagen, carcinogen and teratogen.

Atrazine

Atropa belladonna. Deadly nightshade, a toxic plant containing 1-hyoscamine and scopolamine. *See also* ACETYLCHOLINE RECEPTORS, MUSCARINIC AND NICOTINIC; ATROPINE; SCOPOLAMINE.

atrophy. Reduction in size of a structure or organ. Atrophy can result from lack of nourishment or functional activity, cell death and subsequent reabsorption, or diminished cell proliferation. These effects may result from ischemia, hormone changes or chemical toxicity.

atropine (*dl*-hyoscamine; tropine tropate; tropic acid ester with tropine; *dl*-tropyl tropate; α-(hydroxymethyl)benzeneacetic acid 8-methyl-8-azabicyclo[3.2.1]oct-3-yl ester; 1αH,5αH-tropan-3αol (+)-tropate). **CAS number 51-55-8**. One of the belladonna alkaloids (from *Atropa belladonna*) that crosses the blood–brain barrier. The oral LD50 in rats is 750 mg/kg. Atropine exerts its pharmacodynamic effects by competitively blocking muscarinic acetylcholine receptor sites. Atropine or atropinic drugs result in pupil dilation, dry mouth, inhibition of activity of sweat glands and, at toxic doses, tachycardia, palpitation, speech disturbance, blurred vision, restlessness, irritability, disorientation, hallucinations or delirium. A major cause of poisonings is the ingestion of drugs with atropinic properties, including antihistamines, phenothiazines and tricyclic antidepressants. Infants and young children are particularly susceptible to atropine intoxication, that may result from application of ophthamological treatments. Atropine has potent antispasmodic and antisecretory properties. *See also* ACETYLCHOLINE RECEPTORS, MUSCARINIC AND NICOTINIC; SCOPOLAMINE.

Atropine

ATSDR. *See* AGENCY FOR TOXIC SUBSTANCE AND DISEASE REGISTRY.

attention deficit disorder. *See* ATTENTION HYPERACTIVITY DEFICIENT DISORDER.

attention hyperactivity deficient disorder. The defining attributes of this disorder are developmentally inappropriate lack of attention, impulsivity and hyperactivity. Distractability, failure to listen, inability to concentrate or pay attention to a task, excessive movement, constant fidgeting and excessive shifting from task to task are all common symptoms of this disorder. The etiology of this disorder is unknown; the diagnosis is most often made after the child starts school, and the treatment of choice appears to be stimulant medication (i.e., methylphenidate). Exposure to chemicals or toxic agents may play an etiological role at least in some cases. Hyperactivity in animals following toxic insult usually refers to a significantly increased latency to habituate to a test apparatus. *See also* FEINGOLD'S HYPOTHESIS; LOCOMOTOR BEHAVIOR; MAINTENANCE THERAPY; MENTAL RETARDATION; NEUROBEHAVIORAL TERATOLOGY; NEUROBEHAVIORAL TOXICOLOGY; POSTNATAL BEHAVIORAL TESTS.

atypia. *See* DYSPLASIA.

AUC (area under curve). *See* BIOAVAILABILITY.

auditory startle. An unconditioned or reflexive behavior that involves a whole-body startle response following presentation of an auditory stimulus greater than 90 dB. Presentation of a low-intensity auditory stimulus prior to presentation of the reflex-eliciting stimulus has been shown to inhibit the startle response. Such "pre-pulse inhibition" provides a useful screen for the effects of a drug or toxicant on sensory processing and habituation. This test is particularly useful as the neural circuitry of this reflexive response has been worked out in detail. *See also* NEUROBEHAVIORAL TERATOLOGY; NEUROBEHAVIORAL TOXICOLOGY; POSTNATAL BEHAVIORAL TESTS.

Authorisation Mise sur la Marche. *See* MARKETING AUTHORIZATION.

autocoids. Compounds endogenous to an organism that, although structurally dissimilar and exerting different physiological effects, participate in inter- and intracellular signaling. The derivation of the term, that can be loosely defined as "self-remedy," is from the Greek autos meaning self and akos meaning remedy. Autocoids have historically been thought to play important physiological roles in the body's response to disease and maintenance of health. Compounds classified as autocoids include prostaglandins, prostacyclins, and thromboxanes, as well as the endogenous amines, histamine and 5-hydroxytryptamine (serotonin), polypeptides (e.g., angiotensin, bradykinin and kallidin).

autoimmunity. Any inappropriate immune system response to self components. The immune system, in order to protect the host normally distinguishes effectively between "self" and "nonself." Many different cell types must cooperate in any immune response and must therefore recognize each other as self. Additionally there must be tolerance to all normal host proteins. If normal autologous host proteins are not recognized as self (i.e., they are recognized as foreign or non-self), damage to the host frequently ensues. Autoimmune responses can be humoral (antibodies) or cell-mediated immunity (T cells). Autoimmunity can be a component of any of the four types of allergic response. There are a number of autoimmune diseases where such inappropriate responses are made against tissue antigens and/or antigens not normally accessible to the immune system, such as intracellular contents, brain tissue, sperm, etc. Antibodies to cell surface antigens can cause cell death by lysis or can interfere with cell function (*see* ALLERGIC RESPONSE; ANTIBODY-DEPENDENT CELLULAR CYTOTOXICITY; COMPLEMENT). If the antigens are inaccessible to the antibody, such as nuclear proteins, no harm is done to the intact cell, but soluble immune complexes form in the serum and can lodge in vessel walls, kidneys or lung tissue, producing an immune complex response (*see* ALLERGIC RESPONSE table). These reactions are usually transitory unless the antigens are chronically presented to the immune system, for instance, by continuous cell damage from toxicants or drugs. Many environmental agents can induce an allergic autoimmune reaction. One of the most common ways for a compound to become allergenic is for it, or one of its metabolites, to become conjugated to a protein, either autologous or environmental (e.g., in gastrointestinal contents or a manufacturing contaminant). This process is called haptenization, with the protein called the carrier and the smaller compound the hapten. The hapten–carrier combination is the actual immunogen and is recognized as "altered-self" (i.e., foreign) by the immune system so that antibodies and/or cytotoxic T cells are generated against the entire molecule. It is unclear whether this breakdown of self-tolerance is due to the induction of new helper T cells or the inhibition of suppressor T cells (*see* T CELL). The haptenization of these low-molecular-weight (500–1000) compounds accounts for the allergenicity of poison ivy, toluene diisocyanate and the β-lactam antibiotics such as penicillin. Many drugs can produce autoimmune hemolytic anemia by adsorbing to erythrocytes. Alternatively, some compounds can substantially alter normal antigens without haptenization, so that they are seen as foreign. α-Methyldopa, a drug used in the treatment of essential hypertension, works in this way to modify erythrocyte surface antigens. Heavy metals are implicated in many autoimmune reactions although the mechanisms for this are not well understood. *See also* B CELLS.

automotive gasoline. *See* GASOLINE.

autonomic nervous system. The portion of the efferent nervous system concerned with the regulation of the activity of cardiac muscle, smooth muscle and glands.

autopsy. *See* NECROPSY.

autoradiography. A technique useful for identifying the location of a radioactive chemical in gels, cells, tissue slices or even sometimes in whole organisms. The source containing the radioactive material is placed in close proximity to a photographic film or a photographic emulsion is placed on the sample until an image of the radioactive pattern emerges on development of the film or emulsion. This technique can be qualitative, or with appropriate standards and computerized image digitization, quantitative.

autoregressive integrated moving average (ARIMA). Statistical models for analyzing time series quasi-experiments. Testing the effect of an intervention on a time series can be confounded by the high degree of autocorrelation or serial dependency often found in such data. ARIMA procedures are designed to model and statistically control for serial dependency. ARIMA models identify three major sources of variance: trend, cyclicity and random error. An ARIMA model is conceptualized as a series of random shocks that are normally, independently and identically distributed and that have a zero mean and a constant average. The model is built on three structural parameters: autoregression, or the number of previous observations used to predict the current observation; integration, or the extent to which the series should be differenced to meet the assumptions (e.g., stationarity); and the number of moving averages or preceding random shocks. Once an adequate model has been constructed (i.e., the residuals are white noise and the smallest number of parameters has been used) the effect of an intervention can be validly assessed. *See also* STATISTICS, FUNCTION IN TOXICOLOGY.

avermectins. Microbially derived insecticides and miticides of complex chemical structure that interact as agonists at the GABA receptor/chloride ionophore leading to sedation, anesthesia, coma and depression of vital centers. They may also act as agonists at the glycine receptor leading to paralysis. The avermectins display low acute mammalian toxicity. *See also* IVERMECTINS.

avoidance conditioning. *See* BEHAVIORAL TOXICITY TESTING.

axon. Long extension of a neuron, normally conducting impulses away from the nerve cell body (perikaryon). Axons vary greatly in length from less than 1 mm to more than 1 m. A steady movement of molecules from the neuron cell body along the axon towards the terminal branches and, to a lesser extent, a slower returning passage of molecules are termed anterograde and retrograde, axoplasmic transport, respectively. Axon transport is greatly facilitated by the cytoskeleton of neurofilaments and microtubules. *See also* PERIPHERAL NEUROPATHY; AXONOPATHY.

axonopathy. A form of axonal degeneration where the primary focus of injury is the axon itself. The axon is an extension of neuronal cytoplasm that may have a volume many times that of the neuronal cell body or perikaryon. Since the axon is dependent upon a continuous transport of substrate and macromolecules from the perikaryon, an axon will degenerate whenever the neuronal cell body dies, but this is not an axonopathy. Primary examples of toxicants that directly injure the axon are some organophosphorus compounds, such as tri-o-cresyl phosphate (TOCP), and the γ-diketones. An alternative mechanism for axonal degeneration in toxic, nutritional or metabolic injury has been termed the "dying back" phenomenon in which it is envisioned that the primary focus of injury is in the cell body, and the unsupported distal axon "dies back." This concept arose from the observation that in toxic neuropathies long axons are more vulnerable than short axons to degeneration, apparently reflecting the greater metabolic vulnerability of the cell body. The concept of axonopathy, on the other hand, would suggest that longer axons simply present more target for injury. *See also* γ-DIKETONE NEUROPATHY; PERIPHERAL NEUROPATHY.

azathioprine. CAS number 446-86-6. A carcinogenic immunosuppressive drug that is an antimetabolite drug, and thereby inhibits cell replication. It can cause bladder tumors, leukemia, lymphoma, reticulum cell sarcoma, skin cancer, and possibly Kaposi's sarcoma. Other toxic effects are anemia, bone marrow abnormalities, hair effects, and metabolic effects. Experimentally it has shown teratogenic and reproductive effects, and human mutation data have been reported.

azapropazone. *See* APAZONE.

azides. Inhibitors of cytochrome oxidase with toxicity similar to cyanide as a result of cytotoxic anoxia. The toxicity may be the result of actions in addition to cytochrome oxidase inhibition. Catalase and peroxidase are also inhibited. A variety of CNS parts may be damaged, resulting in hyperactivity. Acute poisonings in humans have resulted in hypotension, breathlessness, tachycardia, nausea, headache, diarrhea and leukocytosis. Occupational exposures have resulted in episodic rises and falls in blood pressure along with headaches, as well as irritation of mucous membranes, bronchitis and pulmonary edema.

azinphosmethyl. CAS number 86-50-0. An organophosphorus insecticide activated by cytochrome P450 to azinphosmethyl oxon, an acetylcholinesterase (AChE) inhibitor. Toxic to mammals, including humans. Inhibition of AChE is the mode of toxic action in both target and nontarget species. *See also* DATABASES, TOXICOLOGY; ORGANOPHOSPHORUS INSECTICIDES.

Azinphosmethyl

aziridine. *See* ETHYLENEIMINE.

azo compounds. A general class of compounds that contain the aminoazo dyes. Azo compounds have been known since the 1930s to be associated with tumors, particularly of the bladder and liver, in animals. Some well-known experimental carcinogens are 4-dimethylaminoazobenzene and o-aminoazotoluene. The azo bond, or even an aminoazo structure, is not necessarily a determinant of carcinogenicity since changes in structure can cause loss of carcinogenic potential, although reductive splitting of the azo bond is usually a detoxication reaction. In some cases, however, such scission produces a carcinogenic aromatic amine. Except for this latter circumstance, carcinogenicity requires an intact azo link and a substituted amino group in the 4-position of one of the rings. *See also* AMINOAZO DYES.

azo dyes. Synthetic compounds containing an azo linkage originally derived, in part, from coal tar. These compounds are often brightly colored, leading to their use as dyestuffs and as food colors. As a group, they are subject to a variety of interesting metabolic events, some of which (e.g., azo reduction) may lead to toxic metabolites. *See also* FOOD COLORS.

azo reduction. *In vitro*, a process, like nitro reduction, that requires anaerobic conditions and NADPH. It is also inhibited by carbon monoxide and presumably involves cytochrome P450, although the ability of mammalian cells to reduce azo bonds is rather poor. Intestinal microflora may also play a role. *See also* REDUCTION.

B

Bacillus cereus. A gram-positive, anaerobic bacillus that produces toxins that cause food-poisoning. They include a thermolabile toxin causing diarrhea and a thermostable toxin causing emesis.

Bacillus subtilis. A bacterial species, deficient in recombinant abilities, that is useful in prokaryote mutagenicity tests to identify mutagens. *See also* PROKARYOTE MUTAGENICITY TESTS.

bacitracin. *See* ANTIBIOTICS.

bacterial mutagenesis. A number of strains of bacteria, typically with aberrations in normal biochemical pathways or deficiencies in DNA repair capability, are useful in short-term *in vitro* tests to detect the mutagenic potential of chemicals. Because of the action of these mutagens on the bacterial DNA, mutagenic activity in these systems implicates the compounds as potential carcinogens. *See also* AMES TEST; PROKARYOTE MUTAGENICITY TESTS.

bacteriostats (bacteriostatic agents). Antimicrobial agents that inhibit the multiplication of bacteria in a non-lethal manner. The inhibition is reversible in that cultural growth is resumed upon removal of the agent from the medium. Chemotherapeutically useful bacteriostats rely primarily on immunological defense mechanisms of the host for the final elimination of active infections. Bacteriostats include dyes, low-temperature, weak antiseptics and certain antibiotics. Bacteriostatic compounds employed to preclude the deterioration of biological products are specifically referred to as preservatives. *See also* ANTIBACTERIALS; ANTIBIOTICS; ANTIMICROBIALS.

BAL (British Anti-Lewisite). *See* 2,3-DIMER-CAPTO-1-PROPANOL.

BALB/3T3. A type of cultured mouse cell used *in vitro* to test the ability of chemicals to induce the transformation of mammalian cells. *See also* MAMMALIAN CELL TRANSFORMATION TESTS.

barbiturates. Derivatives of barbituric acid. They reversibly depress the activity of most excitable cells, especially in the CNS, and are used for their hypnotic and anticonvulsant activity. They act by binding to a specific recognition site (i.e., a receptor) that is part of the $GABA_A$ receptor complex. Caution must be used with administration of any of these drugs since they have a low therapeutic index and may cause respiratory depression. In addition, these compounds are potentially addictive, and abrupt withdrawal may be life-threatening because of the lowering of the seizure threshold. This is a problem not only in barbiturate abuse, but also when barbiturates are administered chronically as anticonvulsant drugs. Long-acting barbiturates (e.g., phenobarbital, mephobarbital) are used mainly for seizure disorders; short-acting barbiturates (e.g., amobarbital, pentobarbital, secobarbital) are used as hypnotics, and ultra-short-acting barbiturates (e.g., thiopental, methohexital, thiamylal) are used i.v. to induce general anesthesia. The barbiturates cause relatively little analgesia, and thus are seldom used alone unless for a medical or surgical procedure in which little pain is involved. Despite the fact that they have low analgesic potency, they are extremely useful in combination with inhalational anesthetics. The short-acting barbiturates cause a rapid pleasant induction of anesthesia and fast recovery upon cessation of administration. Barbiturates with an intermediate duration of action are deactivated in large part by metabolism to polar inactive compounds that are excreted. Various enzymes (e.g., cytochrome P450; glucuronosyltransferases) are responsible for the degradation of many xenobiotics. Because barbiturates may induce these hepatic drug-metabolizing enzymes, they may cause their own metabolism to be markedly increased. Of equal importance, clinical problems may be caused by the induction of the hepatic enzymes, altering the metabolism of other drugs or compounds. As weak acids, barbiturates tend to ionize in a basic solution, but remain non-ionized in an acid solution. Since only the non-ionized drug can cross cell membranes easily, both intracellular and extracellular pH are important. This principle is important in the case of barbiturate poisoning, since only the non-ionized barbiturate can be reabsorbed from alkaline urine. This will increase the proportion of ionized barbiturate, which is then excreted instead of reabsorbed. The generalized CNS depression associated with barbiturates may cause accidental or deliberate overdosage. Clinically used sedative-hypnotic barbiturates include amobarbital, phenobarbital and secobarbital. *See also* BARBITURIC ACID; METHOHEXITAL; PHENOBARBITAL; SECOBARBITAL; SEDATIVE-HYPNOTICS; THIOBARBITURATES.

Amobarbital

barbituric acid (2,4,6(1H,3H,5H)-pyrimidinetrione). The parent compound from which all of the clinically used barbiturates are derived. Barbituric acid itself does not have sedative-hypnotic activity. If both hydrogen atoms at position 5 are replaced with alkyl or acyl groups, sedative-hypnotic activity results. Most of the interesting structure–activity relationships among barbiturates involve position 5. Sedative-hypnotic activity is not very marked until two ethyl groups are placed at position 5 in the barbiturate ring (to form barbital). In general, increasing the chain length has three effects: (1) it increases potency; (2) it increases the speed of the onset of action; (3) it decreases the duration of action. Thus, barbiturates with a fast onset of action tend to have a short duration of action, and they are more potent than short-chain barbiturates. There is an upper limit to which the chain length can be increased. After the total number of carbon atoms reaches eight, the drugs become very toxic. Substitution of the phenyl ring at position 5 confers antiepileptic activity on this drug. Groups larger than seven carbons also have anticonvulsive potency. Another important structure–activity relationship is when the oxygen at position 2 is replaced with sulfur, giving rise to the thiobarbiturates. Thiobarbiturates are more lipid-soluble than the corresponding oxybarbiturates, and disposition rather than metabolism is important in termination of their action. *See also* BARBITURATES; THIOBARBITURATES.

Barbituric acid

barium (Ba). CAS number 7440-39-3. An element; the heaviest of the stable alkaline earths. Barium sulfate is used as a diagnostic aid in radiology due to its radio-opaqueness and, because of its insolubility and lack of absorption, it is safe barring iatrogenic episodes. Poisoning usually results from deliberate or accidental ingestion of soluble barium compounds. The Ba^{2+} ion is a muscle poison due to the blocking of the K^+ channels of the Na^+/K^+ pump in cell membranes. Because cases of barium poisoning are accompanied by severe hypokalemia, potassium infusion is an effective antidote. The toxicity of barium compounds depends on their solubility, with the free ion being readily absorbed from gastrointestinal tract or lung, whereas the sulfate is essentially unabsorbed. Thus, administration of soluble sulfates immediately after ingestion is another effective antidote.

Bartlett's test. One basic assumption underlying parametric statistics is that within-group error variances are homogeneous. Bartlett's statistic is used to test for departures from homogeneity of variance. In the case of homogeneous error variances, the sampling distribution of the Bartlett's statistic is approximated by the χ^2 distribution with $k-1$ degrees of freedom, where k equals the number of groups. It is important to point out, however, that the F test is quite robust to departures from homogeneity of variance. *See also* COCHRAN'S TEST; STATISTICS, FUNCTION IN TOXICOLOGY.

base pair. The Watson–Crick model for DNA requires that the two helical chains be held together by hydrogen bonds between pairs of bases, a purine and a pyrimidine always being paired together. Because of steric and hydrogen-bonding factors, adenine must always pair with thymine and guanine with cytosine. Changes in the bases give rise to mutations, since they can affect duplication (each chain serves as a template for the other) or the reading of the genetic code. *See also* FRAMESHIFT MUTATION; MUTATION; POINT MUTATION.

base-pair substitution. *See* POINT MUTATION.

base-pair transformation. *See* POINT MUTATION.

base-pair transition. *See* POINT MUTATION.

base-pair transversion. *See* POINT MUTATION.

basophils. *See* MAST CELLS/BASOPHILS.

batrachotoxin (BTX; 3′,9′-epoxy-14α,18α-(epoxyethano-*N*-methylimino)-5β-pregna-7,16-diene-3β,11α,20α (2,4-dimethyl-1H-pyrrole-3-carboxylate). One of the most toxic (LD50 in mice is 2 μg/kg, i.v.) of the four steroidal alkaloids extracted from the skin of the Columbian arrow poison frog *Phyllobates aurotaenia*. Three other steroidal alkaloids are present: iso-BTX, pseudo-BTX and BTX-A. BTX is one of the most potent and specific activators of sodium channels. BTX modifies the activation and inactivation of sodium channels, causing them to remain open at the resting membrane potential thereby increasing the resting sodium permeability. BTX binds to the same receptor site as several other lipid-soluble neurotoxins (i.e., veratridine, aconitine and grayanotoxin), but the BTX site is distinct from that of tetrodotoxin. The increase in membrane sodium permeability is irreversible. BTX has no effect on intact skin, but causes long-lasting pungent pain, not unlike a bee sting, when in contact with broken

skin. Consumption of material exposed to BTX is dangerous only if in contact with an abrasion of the digestive tract. BTX blocks neuromuscular transmission and evokes muscular contracture. Death results from respiratory paralysis. BTX also causes arrhythmias, ventricular tachycardia and fibrillation. Treatment of acute poisoning involves general supportive therapy and artificial respiration. Khodorov, B.I. Prog. Biophys. Molec. Biol. 45, 57–148 (1985). *Compare* TETRODOTOXIN. *See also* ACONITINE; GRAYANOTOXIN.

Batrachotoxin

Bay. *See* ESSENTIAL OILS

B cells (B lymphocytes; bone marrow-derived lymphocytes). A major class of cells responsible for the humoral response of the immune system. They are derived from the bursa of Fabricius in birds and the bone marrow in mammals. B cells arise from the pluripotent stem cells in the bone marrow, differentiate into mature B cells in an antigen-independent fashion and migrate to the lymphoid follicles of the lymph nodes and spleen. The mature B cells can then be stimulated in an antigen-dependent manner to differentiate terminally into antibody-forming cells called plasma cells. Plasma cells secrete antibody with antigen-binding specificity identical to that of the membrane-bound immunoglobin expressed by the mature B cell. B cells generally require interaction with helper T cells to differentiate into plasma cells. The end result of B cell activation is a high serum concentration of specific antibody and the generation of immunological memory. Although antibodies generally bind to foreign proteins and facilitate their removal, they can participate in reactions detrimental to the host, such as type I allergic reaction (anaphalaxis) and autoimmune diseases. *See also* ALLERGIC RESPONSE; ALLERGY; ANTIBODY; AUTOIMMUNITY; IMMUNOGLOBULIN.

BCNU. *See* BIS(2-CHLOROETHYL)NITROSOUREA.

bearded lizard. *Heloderma horridum*, a venomous lizard occurring in the southwestern United States and Mexico.

Beer's Law. This equation is the basis for much analytical toxicology that uses the absorbance of electromagnetic radiation as a method of quantifying an analyte. The equation is:

$$A = abc$$

where A is the absorbance (formerly called optical density), a is the absorptivity, b is the pathlength of the sample container (e.g., spectrophotometer cuvette), and c is the concentration of the analyte. The absorptivity a (formerly called ε) has units of concentration^{-1}pathlength^{-1} (e.g., mM^{-1}cm^{-1}) and is an intrinsic property of the analyte under the experimental conditions that are used. *See also* ABSORBANCE; ANALYTICAL TOXICOLOGY; CHROMATOGRAPHY.

bee sting. Honey bee stings can cause IgE-mediated sensitivity. The bees that cause these reactions are from European varieties (primarily *Apis mellifera mellifera* and *A. m. ligustica*), although the so-called Africanized honey bees (*A. m. scutellata*) present a particular threat because these bees are sensitive to slight disturbance of their colony and frequently mount massive attacks, occasionally delivering hundreds of stings in an individual attack. In non-sensitized individuals, systemic toxic reactions from bee stings may require 50 simultaneous stings. The toxic reactions include vomiting, diarrhea, hemoglobinuria, acute renal failure with elevated serum levels of BUN, creatinine and creatine phosphokinase, rhabdomyolysis and thrombocytopenia. Stings in airway regions tend to increase the risk of fatality. Whole venom from European and Africanized bees is biochemically similar, although some chromatographic differences have been found. The content of hyaluronidase has been reported to be less in Af venom than in Eu venom. Individual components of honey bee venom are known to act synergistically. For example, melittin from bee venom acts synergistically with bee venom phospholipase A$_2$ on phospholipid structures. Hyaluronidase is thought to facilitate distribution of other venom components through tissues surrounding the sting site, and melittin may facilitate entry of other more toxic components into the bloodstream. Since anaphylactoid manifestations comprise only a part of the symptom complex that results from massive envenomation, specific treatment for anaphylaxis may be inadequate in the management of these patients, and antivenom treatment may sometimes be appropriate.

behavior. *See* NEUROBEHAVIORAL TERATOLOGY; NEUROBEHAVIORAL TOXICOLOGY.

behavior, in chronic toxicity testing. *See* TOXIC ENDPOINTS.

behavior, in subchronic toxicity testing. *See* TOXIC ENDPOINTS.

behavioral teratology. *See* NEUROBEHAVIORAL TERATOLOGY.

behavioral toxicity testing. For a number of years tests of the effects of chemicals on behavior have been part of the regulatory process in the USSR, but not in the USA or Western Europe. Although the claim that behavioral tests are more sensitive than pathological tests is difficult to document, it is clear that behavior is the functional integration of all of the various activities of the nervous system and, in part, of some other systems, such as the endocrine glands, whose activity affects the nervous system. For this reason behavioral tests are necessary to fully evaluate toxicity. Many behavioral tests have been described, but no particular set or sequence has been prescribed for regulatory purposes. However, the categories of methods fall into two principal classes: stimulus-oriented behavior and internally generated behavior. The former includes two types of conditioned behavior: operant, in which animals are trained to perform a task in order to obtain a reward or to avoid a punishment; and classical (Pavlovian) conditioning, in which an animal learns to associate a conditioning stimulus with a reflex action. Stimulus-oriented behavior also involves unconditioned responses in which the animal's response to a particular stimulus is recorded. Internally generated behavior includes exploratory behavior, circadian activity, social behavior, etc., and tests involve observation of animal behavior in response to various experimental situations. The performance of animals treated with a particular chemical is compared with untreated controls. As with other types of toxicity testing, sex, age, species, strain, environment, diet and animal husbandry must all be controlled, since behavior may vary with any of these. Norton has described a series of four tests that may form an appropriate series, inasmuch as they represent four different types of behavior and should, therefore, reflect different types of nervous system activity. They are as follows: (1) Passive avoidance. This test involves the use of a shuttle box in which animals can move between a light and dark side. After an acclimatization period in which the animal can move freely between the two sides, it receives an electric shock while in the dark side. During subsequent trials the time spent in the "safe side" is recorded. (2) Auditory startle. This involves the response (movement) to a sound stimulus either without or preceded by a light flash stimulus. (3) Residential maze. Movements of animals in a residential maze are automatically recorded during both light and dark photoperiods. (4) Walking patterns. Characteristics of gait such as the length and width of stride and the angles formed by the placement of the feet are measured in walking animals. Problems associated with behavioral toxicology testing include the functional reserve and adaptablity of the nervous system. Frequently behavior is maintained despite clearly observable injury. Other problems are the statistical ones associated with multiple tests, multiple measurements and the inherently large variability in behavior. The use in behavioral tests of human subjects occupationally exposed to chemicals is often attempted, but such tests are complicated by the subjective nature of the endpoints (dizziness, incoordination, etc.). *See also* AUDITORY STARTLE; PASSIVE AVOIDANCE; PAVLOVIAN CONDITIONING; POSTNATAL BEHAVIORAL TESTS.

behavioral toxicology. *See* NEUROBEHAVIORAL TOXICOLOGY.

belladonna (*Atropa belladonna*; deadly nightshade). A toxic plant associated with the production of the so-called belladonna alkaloids, most of which are quite toxic and some of which

have clinical utility at lower doses. Deadly nightshade produces mostly atropine. Serious intoxication can result from ingestion of berries of this or other solanaceous plants that produce these alkaloids. *See also* ATROPINE; BELLADONNA ALKALOIDS; SCOPOLAMINE.

belladonna alkaloids. Organic esters formed from tropic acid and an organic base such as tropine or scopine. Atropine and scopolamine are the two most important belladonna alkaloids. These alkaloids are associated not only with *Atropa belladonna*, which produces mostly atropine, but also with other solanceous plants such as *Datura stramonium* (Jimson weed), *Hyoscyamus niger* (henbane) and *Scopolia carniolica* . The latter two plants produce scopolamine. Poisoning is not uncommon from ingestion of pharmacological preparations or, particularly in children, from ingestion of berries or plants. Typically the patient has a dry mouth, blurred vision and increased temperature. Memory and orientation are disturbed, and hallucinations are common. In severe cases depression and circulatory collapse may occur, followed by death from respiratory failure. Atropine and related belladonna alkaloids exert their toxic action by binding to muscarinic cholinergic receptors in the nervous system. Treatment of poisoning is both non-specific (gastric lavage, artificial respiration, temperature reduction, etc.) or specific (physostigmine). In severe cases diazepam may be given to control convulsions, but problems can occur if the central depressant action coincides with the respiratory depression characteristic of severe belladonna poisoning. *See also* ACETYLCHOLINE RECEPTORS, MUSCARINIC AND NICOTINIC; ATROPINE; SCOPOLAMINE; TROPAN ALKALOIDS.

Tropic acid   Tropine

Belladonna alkaloids

belmark. *See* FENVALERATE.

Benadryl. *See* DIPHENHYDRAMINE.

Benedictin. *See* DOXYLAMINE.

benign. A benign neoplasm, as compared with a malignant neoplasm, may increase in size but remains localized and has limited potential to metastasize or invade other tissues. The morphological and functional characteristics of a benign neoplasm tend to vary less from the tissue of origin than would those of a malignant neoplasm.

benzene (benzol). **CAS number 71-43-2**. A designated carcinogen (IARC), hazardous substance (EPA), hazardous waste (EPA) and priority toxic pollutant (EPA). It is a flammable, volatile, colorless liquid with a characteristic odor. Benzene is a constituent of motor fuels and is used as an intermediate in many chemical syntheses, as well as a solvent in many industrial processes. The principal route of entry is via inhalation of the vapor. Local exposure to benzene causes irritation to the skin, eyes and upper respiratory tract. Defatting of the skin may cause erythema, blisters or dermatitis. Acute systemic exposure to benzene causes CNS depression, headache, dizziness, etc. Nausea, convulsions, coma and death may result. Epidemiological studies and case histories of benzene-related blood dyscrasias have led to the conclusion that benzene is leukemogenic, with depression of the bone marrow leading ultimately to aplastic anemia. Benzene also causes chromosome abnormalities indicative of genetic damage, both in bone marrow and other tissues. Subsequent experimental studies have confirmed these findings, and benzene is currently being phased out of many of its former uses. *See also* ATSDR DOCUMENT, AUGUST 1995; DATABASES, TOXICOLOGY.

Benzene

benzidine (4,4-diaminobiphenyl; 4,4′-diphenylenediamine). **CAS number 92-87-5**. A designated human carcinogen (IARC), hazardous waste (EPA) and priority toxic pollutant (EPA). It is a crystalline solid with significant vapor pressure. Benzidine is used primarily in the manu-

facture of azo dyes. Other uses in the rubber industry, in the manufacture of plastic films and as a laboratory reagent have largely been discontinued. The principal routes of entry are inhalation of the vapor or by percutaneous absorption. Benzidine is a known urinary tract carcinogen in humans with a relatively long latent period. Dyes synthesized from benzidine, including Direct Blue 6, Direct Black 38 and Direct Brown 95 have all been shown to be carcinogenic in experimental animals and there is some evidence that the first two are associated with bladder cancer in humans. *See also* ATSDR DOCUMENT, AUGUST 1995; DATABASES, TOXICOLOGY.

$$H_2N - \text{---} - \text{---} - NH_2$$
Benzidine

benzodiazepine receptors. High-affinity, specific recognition sites for which the presently available benzodiazepines (e.g., diazepam, chlordiazepoxide, oxazepam) compete. These binding sites, as well as those for barbiturates, picrotoxin and other toxicants, are located on the $GABA_A$ receptor-chloride ionophore complex. The interaction of the clinically important benzodiazepines with this receptor facilitates GABA-ergic transmission by facilitating the binding and function of GABA. Recently, drugs have been found that bind to benzodiazepine receptors, but cause opposite physiological effects, or bind with no functional consequences. *See also* BENZODIAZEPINES; CHLORIDE CHANNEL; GABA.

benzodiazepines. Formerly called minor tranquilizers, they are a class of drugs used largely for their anxiolytic, sedative-hypnotic, muscle relaxant and/or anticonvulsant properties. They have largely superseded the barbiturates as sedative-hypnotic agents because of their much higher therapeutic index. The benzodiazepines (e.g., diazepam, chlordiazepoxide, oxazepam) are clinically indicated for the treatment of a variety of disorders, including anxiety, insomnia, acute alcoholic withdrawal syndrome, seizures and muscle spasms. Different benzodiazepine derivatives differ in the potency or efficacy with which they produce these effects. In general, the clinical toxicity of the benzodiazepines is low. A behavioral dependence may result in some patients, although the frank physical withdrawal seen with alcohol or the barbiturates is usually not seen. Side effects of benzodiazepines are usually extensions of the pharmacological actions of these drugs. Teratogenic effects of benzodiazepines are minimal, although a small increase in the incidence of cleft deformities of the lip or palate has been reported. The actions of these compounds probably involve their binding to specific CNS receptors associated with the $GABA_A$ receptor complex. Although the clinically used benzodiazepines have antiepileptic properties, only clonazepam has received approval in the USA for chronic treatment of certain types of seizures. Clonazepam is used in the therapy of absence seizures, as well as myoclonic seizures in children. Diazepam, another benzodiazepine, is particularly useful in treating status epilepticus, a continuing epileptic seizure of any type. Diazepam is frequently used as part of the treatment of toxicant-induced seizures. The benzodiazepines bind to a specific nervous system receptor, thereby facilitating GABA transmission in the CNS. Their binding site, as well as those of barbiturates and picrotoxinin, is located on the GABA receptor-chloride ionophore complex. *See also* ANTIANXIETY DRUGS; BENZODIAZEPINE RECEPTORS; DIAZEPAM; GABA; SEDATIVE-HYPNOTICS.

benzodioxole ring cleavage. *See* METHYLENEDIOXYPHENYL RING CLEAVAGE.

benzofuran **(2,3-benzofuran, cumaron, cumarone, benzo(b)furan, 1-oxindene). CAS number 271-89-6**. Isolated from coal oil and used in the manufacture of coumarone-indene resin. This resin is used in paints, glue, etc. and is allowed on food packaging. Little is known about the toxicity of benzofuran to humans but acute toxicity in experimental animals involves liver and kidney failure. Chronic toxicity to animals involves damage to the liver, kidneys, lungs and stomach. Lifetime administration (oral administration) caused cancer in both rats and mice.

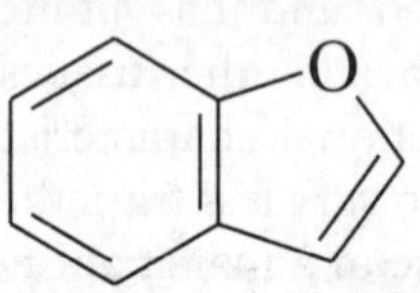

Benzofuran

benzol. *See* BENZENE.

benzo[*a*]pyrene **(3,4-benzpyrene; B[*a*]P). CAS number 50-32-8**. A polycyclic aromatic hydrocarbon (PAH) that is a by-product of combustion. It was isolated by Cook in 1932 from coal tar and has been shown to be highly carcinogenic. It is estimated that 1.8 million pounds per year are released from stationary sources such as coal mines and combustion of coal. The general population is exposed to B[*a*]P from air pollution, cigarette smoke and food sources. B[a]P is metabolically activated by the cytochrome P450-dependent monooxygenase system to the ultimate mutagen and carcinogen as indicated below. B[*a*]P has both local and systemic carcinogenic effects and has produced tumors in nine tested species by oral, skin and intratracheal routes. The cytochrome P450 monooxygenase system forms arene oxides with B[*a*]P at the 2,3-, 4,5-, 7,8- and 9,10-positions, all of which are further hydrolyzed to the diols and/or conjugated. However, only the 7,8-*trans*-dihydrodiol-9,10-epoxide is a potent mutagen and ultimate carcinogen. *See also* BENZO[*A*]PYRENE-7,8-DIOL-9,10-EPOXIDE; POLYCYCLIC AROMATIC HYDROCARBONS.

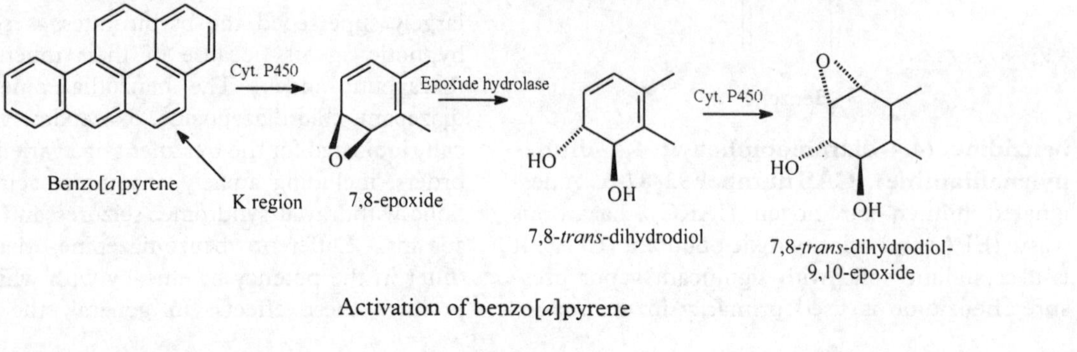

Activation of benzo[*a*]pyrene

benzo[*a*]pyrene-7,8-diol-9,10-epoxide. A group of stereoisomers resulting from the metabolism of benzo[*a*]pyrene. These metabolites arise by prior formation of the 7,8-epoxide by the cytochrome P450-dependent monooxygenase system, subsequently giving rise to the 7,8-dihydrodiol through the action of epoxide hydrolase. This is further metabolized by the cytochrome P450 system to the 7,8-diol-9,10-epoxides, which are potent mutagens and are unsuitable for further epoxide hydration. Of the four isomers of the diol epoxide, the (+)-benzo[*a*]pyrene-7,8-diol-2-epoxide is much more toxic than the others. *See also* BENZO[*A*]-PYRENE.

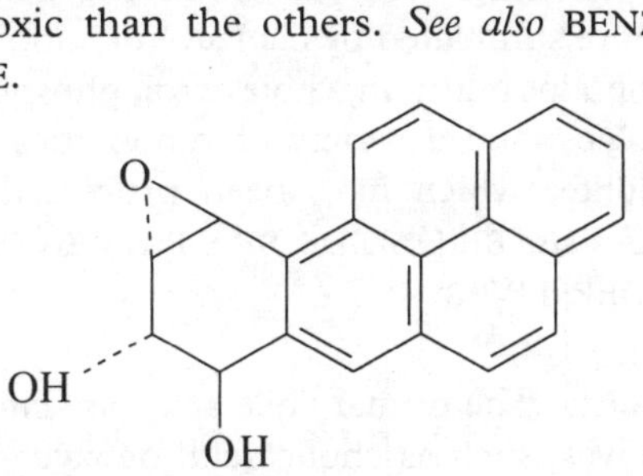

7,8-Diol-9,10-epoxides of benzo[*a*]pyrene

benzo[*a*]pyrene hydroxylase. *See* ARYL HYDROCARBON HYDROXYLASE.

benzotrichloride (trichlorotoluene). A designated hazardous waste (EPA). It is a colorless, oily, fuming liquid boiling at 221 °C. Benzotrichloride is used in the production of dyes such as Malachite Green, Rosamine and Alizarin Yellow, as well as an intermediate in the synthesis of ethyl benzoate. In animal studies benzotrichloride is irritating to the skin and eyes of rabbits and gives rise to carcinomas, leukemia and papillomas in mice.

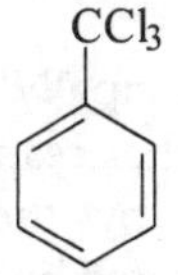

Benzotrichloride

benzphetamine (*N*,α-dimethyl-*N*-(phenylmethyl)-benzeneethanamine; *N*-benzyl-*N*,α-dimethylphenethylamine). Developed as an anorectic; a compound that has proven invaluable for the assay of certain isozymes of cytochrome P450. *See also* BENZPHETAMINE *N*-DEMETHYLATION.

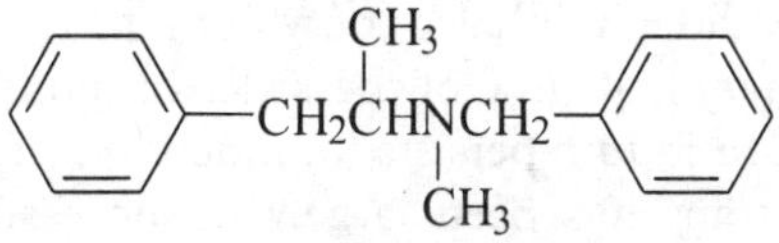

Benzphetamine

benzphetamine *N*-demethylation. An important reaction for the estimation of certain isozymes of cytochrome P450, particularly those induced by phenobarbital and phenobarbital-like inducers. The *N*-methyl group is oxidized, probably initially to an *N*-methylol group and is released as formaldehyde. The formaldehyde is measured colorimetrically or radiometrically if [*N*-14C-methyl]benzphetamine is used. *See also* CYTOCHROME P450.

3,4-benzpyrene. *See* BENZO[*A*]PYRENE.

benzyl alcohol (benzenemethanol, phenylmethanol, alpha hydroxytoluene, phenyl carbinol). CAS number 100-51-6. Simplest aromatic monohydric alcohol. Esters are naturally occurring constituents of plants, such as jasmine and hyacinth, and of many essential oils. It is prepared synthetically for use in the synthesis of other benzyl compounds, as a solvent, in perfumary and as an antimicrobial in pharmaceuticals. Its use in neonatal intravenous solutions discontinued after fatalities characterized by metabolic acidosis, bradycardia, hepatorenal failure and cardiovascular collapse. It is relatively non-toxic to adults although benzyl alcohol can cause skin and eye irritation.

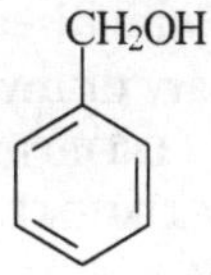

Benzyl alcohol

benzylisoquinolines. *See* TETRAHYDROISOQUINOLINES.

Bergamot. *See* ESSENTIAL OILS

berylliosis. *See* BERYLLIUM.

beryllium (Be). An element that differs from other alkaline earths in that its oxide is amphoteric. Compounds of beryllium are not readily absorbed from the skin or gastrointestinal tract because they tend to form insoluble precipitates at physiological pHs. Although inhaled beryllium has an initial pulmonary half-time of the order of months, particulate residuum persists for much longer. Chelation therapy has been largely unsuccessful. The primary results of inhalation are acute pneumonitis and chronic pulmonary granulomatosis ("berylliosis"), the latter an insidious disease with great mortality. Although beryllium is sometimes associated with carcinogenicity, the epidemiological evidence is controversial. Beryllium metal has been designated an animal carcinogen (IARC), hazardous waste (EPA) and priority toxic pollutant (EPA). A number of beryllium compounds, including the chloride, fluoride and nitrate, have been designated hazardous substances and hazardous wastes (EPA). Beryllium metal is important in atomic energy as a fission moderator or, mixed with uranium, as a neutron source. Various alloys of beryllium are in commercial use (e.g., beryllium-copper, beryllium-nickel, etc.). These alloys have a wide variety of engineering applications. The uptake of beryllium and beryllium compounds into the body is almost entirely by inhalation of dusts or fumes in the workplace. Local exposure to beryllium compounds can cause a variety of skin lesions or eye and mucous membrane irritation. Chronic beryllium disease can vary from a mild non-disabling form with respiratory distress, joint pains and weakness to a serious disabling disease in which death is caused by pulmonary insufficiency or cardiac failure. Beryllium is a highly toxic element, since even in the mild form of chronic beryllium disease the patient eventually shows pulmonary or myocardial failure. *See also* CARCINOGEN, INORGANIC; CHELATING AGENTS; ATSDR DOCUMENT, APRIL 1993; DATABASES, TOXICOLOGY.

B-esterases. *See* HYDROLYSIS.

beta-blockers. *See* β-ADRENERGIC ANTAGONISTS.

Beta-Chlor. *See* CHLORAL DERIVATIVES.

γ-BHC. *See* γ-HCH.

Bhopal. A town in India where, on 3 December 1984, an accident at a pesticide factory owned by Union Carbide India released a cloud of methyl isocyanate, killing about 2500 people and injuring about 200,000. *See also* ENVIRONMENTAL DISASTERS; METHYL ISOCYANATE.

BIBRA. *See* BRITISH INDUSTRIAL BIOLOGICAL RESEARCH ASSOCIATION.

bile. The secretion of the liver that contains bile acids for the emulsification of dietary lipids. Bile is typically stored in the gallbladder until needed and is delivered to the small intestine through the bile duct, following contractions of the gallbladder which are stimulated by cholecystokinin. The bile also contains bilirubin, cholesterol, phospholipids, electrolytes and a variety of xenobiotics or their metabolites which have been processed by the liver. *See also* BILE ACIDS; BILE PIGMENTS; GALL-BLADDER; LIVER.

bile acids. The primary bile acids are cholesterol derivatives, such as cholic acid, deoxycholic acid and chenodeoxycholic acid, which are synthesized by the liver, secreted in the bile (choleresis) and stored in the gallbladder. When needed to assist in the emulsification of dietary fats, bile is delivered into the duodenum by contraction of the gallbladder. A large percentage of the bile acids is recycled by enterohepatic circulation. The bile acids can be metabolized by the gut microflora into secondary bile acids, such as lithocholic acid, which are effective promoters of colon carcinogenesis. Some of the bile salts can cause cholestasis or hepatic necrosis.

bile duct. *See* BILE ACIDS; BILE PIGMENTS; GALLBLADDER; LIVER.

bile pigments. Principally bilirubin and biliverdin, the pigments that result from the degradation of hemoglobin by the reticuloendothelial system. They are excreted by the liver into the bile. The presence of excess bilirubin in the blood gives rise to the condition known as jaundice. *See also* HEME OXIGENASE; JAUNDICE.

bile salts. *See* BILE ACIDS.

bile salt sulfotransferase. *See* SULFATE CONJUGATION.

bile sampling. Continuous sampling of bile secreted by the liver in the intact animal is important in toxicokinetic studies, as well as in studies of xenobiotic excretion by the liver. This is particularly true because bile is normally mixed with the gut contents, because some components are reabsorbed, and thus subjected to enterohepatic circulation, and because all are subjected to the bacterial action of the gut microflora. Normally the abdominal cavity is surgically opened, the bile duct cannulated, the cannula exteriorized, and the incision closed. The animal may be restrained, and samples collected from the cannula or a suitable collection container may be attached to the animal so that restraint is unnecessary. In long-term studies, a modified technique must be adopted since removal of bile would prevent recirculation of bile salts, cause changes in bile composition and affect lipid processing. A second cannula returns to the duodenum all of the bile not removed during sampling. *See also* BILE; LIVER; TOXICOKINETICS.

bilirubin. *See* BILE PIGMENTS; HEME OXYGENASE.

bilirubin, in chronic toxicity testing. *See* TOXIC ENDPOINTS.

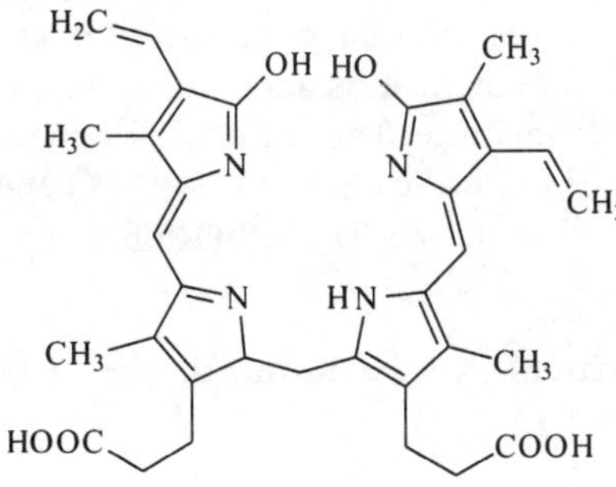

Bilirubin

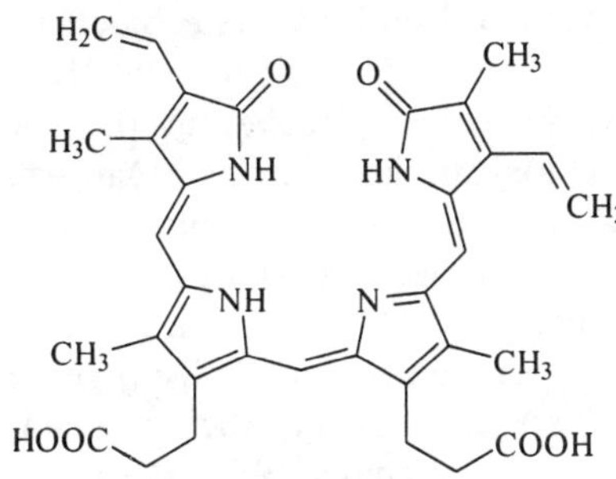

Biliverdin

biliverdin. *See* BILE PIGMENTS.

binary agent. A military toxic agent ("war gas") formed by reaction between two primary agents during delivery. Is used either to allow storage and transport of less toxic primary agents, or to allow battlefield synthesis of an agent with limited stability.

binding. The thermodynamically favorable association of one molecule with another to form a molecular complex of varying stability. This may or may not lead to the formation of additional products resulting from a chemical reaction initiated by the association. In toxicology the most important binding reactions are between small molecules (ligands), usually of toxicants or potential toxicants, and target macromolecules such as proteins or nucleic acids. Such binding is also important in the transport and distribution of toxicants and their metabolites and may be either covalent or non-covalent. *See also* COVALENT BINDING; EQUILIBRIUM DIALYSIS; HYDROGEN BONDING; HYDROPHILIC BINDING; LIGAND; PROTEIN BINDING; RADIORECEPTOR ASSAYS; VAN DER WAALS' FORCES.

binding, covalent. *See* COVALENT BINDING.

binding, to cellular macromolecules. The binding of xenobiotics to cellular macromolecules is of considerable importance in many areas of toxicology. Covalent binding is a feature of many types of toxic action leading to long-term effects such as carcinogenicity or immune responses. Various types of reversible binding to macromolecules are involved in transport of xenobiotics by lipoproteins and albumins and in receptor binding. The latter may be involved in toxic action as, for example, when xenobiotics bind to receptor sites in the nervous system, perturbing the normal function of neurotransmitters or when xenobiotics function as inducers, as in the binding of TCDD and polycyclic aromatic hydrocarbons to the Ah receptor. *See also* AH RECEPTOR; BINDING AFFINITY; BINDING SITES AND TRANSPORT; COVALENT BINDING; HYDROGEN BONDING; PROTEIN BINDING; VAN DER WAALS FORCES.

binding affinity. The strength of the interaction in ligand binding. It is described quantitatively by the affinity constant, which is determined by Scatchard analysis of data derived from equilibrium dialysis or ultrafiltration determinations. There are two principal types of toxicant–protein interactions: (1) non-specific, low-affinity and high-capacity; (2) specific, high-affinity and low-capacity. High-affinity implies an affinity constant of 10^8 M^{-1} or greater, low-affinity being 10^4 M^{-1} or less. Low-affinity binding is characteristic of the binding of lipophilic toxicants to lipoproteins. *See also* ASSOCIATION CONSTANT; BINDING; DISSOCIATION CONSTANT; EQUILIBRIUM DIALYSIS; K_D; PROTEIN BINDING; SCATCHARD PLOT.

binding constant. *See* AFFINITY CONSTANT.

binding sites and transport. The nature and number of binding sites on blood proteins is a critical parameter in determining the rate and efficiency of transport and, therefore, distribution of toxicants and their metabolites in the body. A number of binding possibilities exist for the attachment of toxicants to blood or other proteins. Although highly specific (high-affinity, low-capacity) binding is common with drugs, examples of specific binding for other toxicants seem less common. It seems probable that low-affinity, high-capacity binding is more common with toxicants in general and is a function of their lipophilicity. Because of the non-specific nature of these interactions, the actual number of binding sites can only be estimated. *See also* ALBUMINS; BINDING; COMPETITIVE BINDING AND TRANSPORT; DISTRIBUTION OF TOXICANTS; LIPOPROTEINS; PROTEIN BINDING; SCATCHARD PLOT.

bioaccumulation. The accumulation of a chemical by organisms from water directly or through consumption of food containing the chemical. Efficient transfer of chemical from food to consumer, through two or more trophic levels, results in a systematic increase in tissue residue concentrations from one trophic level to another. *See also* FOOD CHAINS.

bioactivation. *See* ACTIVATION.

bioassay. (1) The use of a living organism to measure the amount of a toxicant present in a sample or the toxicity of a sample. This is done by comparing the toxic effect of the sample with that of a graded series of concentrations of a known standard. (2) The use of animals to investigate the toxic effects of chemicals, as in chronic toxicity tests. This is the less appropriate meaning.

bioavailability. From an environmental toxicology standpoint, the term refers to the extent to which a chemical is available for absorption by an organism. For example, if a chemical is strongly adsorbed to clays in sediments and has little tendency to partition into the interstitial water, then it will not be highly bioavailable and will have little tendency to be absorbed by organisms. In pharmacokinetics bioavailability is a dual mathematical function describing the rate and extent of absorption of a drug or a drug-like substance. The rate function is a measure of the rate at which a substance passes from the site of administration into the systemic circulation. The extent of absorption may be characterized by application of the Wagner–Nelson method or the Loo–Riegelman methods. Bioavailability is most often characterized by calculation of the area under the curve (AUC) of the plasma concentration versus the time profile of a substance measured over the interval from time 0 to infinity. Wagner, J.G. & Nelson, E.J. Pharm. Sci. 53, 1392 (1964). Loo, J.C.K.J. Pharm. Sci. 57, 918 (1968).

biochemical oxygen demand. *See* BIOLOGICAL OXYGEN DEMAND.

biochemical toxicology. The biochemical and molecular aspects of any phase of the complex series of events that make up the interaction between a toxicant and a living organism. Thus it may deal with the role of membrane structure in toxicant absorption, with transport mechanisms in body fluids, with the nature and function of the enzymes of xenobiotic metabolism, generation of reactive intermediates and their interaction with cellular macromolecules, etc. Because it deals largely with mechanism, it is central to most aspects of toxicology.

biocide. Any substance that kills or inhibits the growth of a living organism. It is generally used more specifically to refer to chemicals synthesized and used for the purpose of killing or inhibiting the growth of living organisms, e.g., pesticides and antibiotics.

bioconcentration. Accumulation of a chemical in an organism to levels greater than in the surrounding medium. Most often used for accumulation in aquatic organisms of chemicals found in the water in which they exist. *See also* BIOACCUMULATION.

biodegradation. The environmental destruction of toxicants as a result of microbial and/or fungal action. This is an extremely important mechanism for the detoxication of environmental pollutants in soil and water, such as pesticides, organometallics, plasticizers and petroleum products, as well as other industrial and municipal wastes.

biogenic amines. Neurotransmitters that contain an essential primary amine group. This designation usually refers to the catecholamines dopamine, norepinephrine and epinephrine, and the indoleamine serotonin. However, histamine and acetylcholine have sometimes been included in such a description. *See also* CATECHOLAMINES; DOPAMINE; EPINEPHRINE; NOREPINEPHRINE; SEROTONIN.

biological factors, in toxicity testing. *See* TESTING VARIABLES, BIOLOGICAL.

biological half-life. The time required for a 50% reduction in the concentration of a particular chemical in the body.

biological marker. *See* BIOMARKER.

biological monitoring. Monitoring current exposure or internal load by measurement of a biological parameter in the exposed individuals. This may be by measuring either the chemical and/or its metabolites in blood or urine or by determining some related enzyme activity in the blood. For example, xylene exposure can be estimated from the methylhippurate concentration in the urine, the xylene concentration in the blood or the xylene concentration in the expired air. Nitrobenzene exposure can be estimated from *p*-nitrophenol concentration in the urine or methemoglobin levels in the blood. Exposure to organophosphorus insecticides can be estimated from measurements of plasma or erythrocyte cholinesterase activity.

biological oxygen demand (BOD; biochemical oxygen demand). The amount of oxygen required by aerobic bacteria to oxidize organic matter in a volume of water. BOD is calculated by measuring the decline in oxygen tension from an oxygen-saturated volume of raw water at 20 °C for five days, expressed as units of oxygen per liter of water. BOD is a function of nutrient load and, hence, is a useful indicator of organic pollution. BOD, together with concentration of oxygen, helps determine the quality and quantity of biota that a body of water is capable of supporting.

biological TLV. *See* THRESHOLD LIMIT VALUE, BIOLOGICAL.

biomagnification. *See* BIOACCUMULATION.

biomarker. A parameter (pharmacokinetic, physiological or pharmacological) that can be used to predict a toxic event in an individual animal and also can be used to extrapolate to a similar toxic endpoint across species.

biomarker, of effect. Any biochemical or physiological change that is quantifiable and related to an actual or potential health impairment. Many, such as the release of liver enzymes into the blood, are not toxicant specific, while others, such as DNA adduct formation, may indicate only a potential for harmful effect. DNA adduct formation may also be considered a biomarker of exposure.

biomarker, of exposure. A xenobiotic, one or more of its metabolites, or a product of its interaction with a target molecule that can be measured within some compartment of an organism. The preferred biomarkers of exposure to toxicants are usually the concentration of the toxicant itself or one of its metabolites in a readily available body fluid.

biomarker, of susceptibility. Any indicator of an organism's reduced capacity to respond to a toxicant challenge, for example the identification of a polymorphism in a cytochrome P450 isoform may be a marker for increased susceptibility to drug toxicity in those cases where the drug is a substrate for the particular isoform.

biomass. Total weight of living matter in a defined system such as a population, ecosystem, etc. Biomass is usually expressed as dry weight per unit volume or area

biomathematics. The branch of mathematics that deals with quantitative relationships in biological systems and their formulation into mathematical models that define and describe the interrelationships in mathematical terms. Ideally such models have predictive value. In toxicology, biomathematics has played an important role in toxicodynamics (toxicokinetics) and risk analysis, but not, as yet, in other areas. Important roles may be predicted with some confidence in such areas as environmental toxicology and epidemiology. Biomathematics is not to be confused with statistics. *Compare* STATISTICS.

biomethylation, of elements. The addition of methyl groups to toxic elements, such as mercury and lead, is an important reaction in environmental toxicology. Primarily bacterial, and in many cases favored by anaerobic environments, such methylations may greatly increase the toxicity of the metal in question. For example, the formation of methyl- and dimethyl-mercury in bottom sediments is held to be responsible for the severity of the Minamata Bay poisoning episode. Such methyl derivatives penetrate biological membranes more readily than inorganic forms of the elements in question and thus are absorbed more effectively. *See also* METHYLMERCURY; MINAMATA DISEASE; ORGANOMETALS.

Biomet TBTO. *See* TRIBUTYLTIN.

biotic index. A rating used in assessing the quality of the environment in ecological terms. Rivers can be classified according to the type of invertebrate community present in the water using a biotic index which is largely an indication of the amount of dissolved oxygen present, this in turn being a measure of the level of organic pollution. Very clean water, holding a wide variety of species including pollution-sensitive animals (e.g., stonefly and mayfly nymphs), has a high biotic score. As pollution increases, oxygen levels decrease, and the more sensitive species disappear. Badly polluted water, in which only a few tolerant species (e.g., red midge larvae and annelid worms) can survive, together with a few animals that breathe air at the surface, has a very low biotic score.

biotransformation. *See* METABOLISM.

biotransformation of xenobiotics. *See* XENOBIOTIC METABOLISM.

biphasic effects on metabolism: inhibition and induction. Inhibitors of monooxygenase activity can also act as inducers. Inhibition of activity is fairly rapid and involves a direct interaction with the enzyme; induction is a slower process, involving gene expression and protein synthesis. Therefore, after a single dose of a suitable compound, an initial decrease due to inhibition is followed by induction, and then as the compound and its metabolites are eliminated the levels return to normal. Examples of compounds acting in this way include methylenedioxyphenyl synergists, such as piperonyl butoxide. *See also* INDUCTION; INHIBITION.

bipyridyl herbicides. There are two important herbicides, paraquat and diquat, based on bipyridylium ions. They are both toxic to mammals and appear to exert their toxicity to animals, as well as their herbicidal action, via free radical mechanisms. *See also* DIQUAT; PARAQUAT.

BIRA. *See* BRITISH INSTITUTE OF REGULATORY AFFAIRS.

birth defects. Anatomical, physiological or behavioral abnormalities present in the offspring at parturition. They can be due to chemical effects *in utero*, genetic effects on the parents or disease. *See also* TERATOGENESIS; TERATOGENIC FACTORS; TERATOGENIC MECHANISMS; TERATOLOGY; TERATOLOGY TESTING; TOXIC ENDPOINTS.

4-[bis(2-chloroethyl)amino]-l-phenylalanine. *See* MELPHALAN.

5-[bis(2-chloroethyl)amino]uracil. *See* URACIL MUSTARD.

N,N-bis(chloroethyl)-2-naphthylamine (chlornaphazine). A nitrogen mustard developed as an antineoplastic agent. This compound is an alkylating agent and a known human bladder carcinogen.

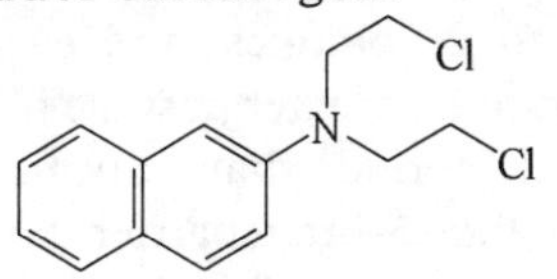

N,N-bis(chloroethyl)-2-naphthylamine
(chlornaphazine)

bis(2-chloroethyl)nitrosourea (BCNU; carmustine). CAS number 154-93-8. A nitrosourea; an alkylating agent used in the treatment of Hodgkin's disease and other lymphomas, as well as in the treatment of meningeal leukemia and metastatic brain tumors. Toxic effects include CNS toxicity, pulmonary fibrosis and renal and hepatic toxicity. It is cytotoxic, immunosuppressive and is probably a carcinogen itself since it alkylates DNA and RNA.

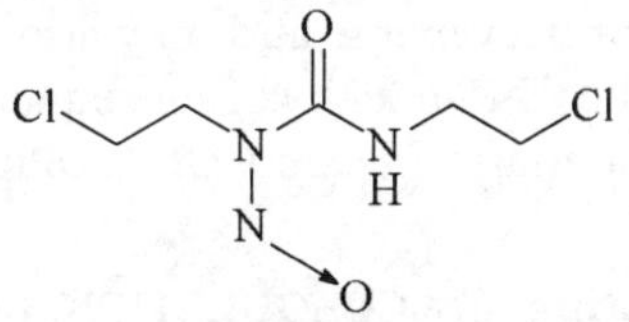

Carmustine

bis(2-chloroethyl)sulfide. *See* MUSTARD GAS.

bis(chloromethyl) ether (dichloromethyl ether). A designated human carcinogen (IARC), hazardous waste (EPA) and priority toxic pollutant (EPA). It is a colorless volatile liquid that has been used in the manufacture of polymers and ion exchange resins and as a chemical intermediate. It is also known to be formed spontaneously from formaldehyde and hydrogen chloride. The most important route of entry into the body is inhalation with possible percutaneous absorption. Locally the vapor is irritating to the skin and mucous membranes. Systemically it is a carcinogen with a latent period of 10–15 years.

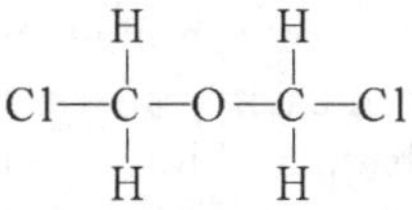

Bis(chloromethyl)ether

bis-dithiocarbamates. *See* CARBAMATE AND THIOCARBAMATE HERBICIDES.

bismuth (Bi). An element that has no known essential function for life. It has been widely used in various therapeutic agents and is still commonly found in cosmetics. Although not extremely toxic, occasional episodes of toxicity have been observed for several bismuth compounds (but not for the metal itself). Toxicity is likely to involve the CNS, liver and/or kidney. Therapy includes the chelating agent *d*-penicillamine or, less effectively, 2,3-dimercapto-1-propanol. *See also* CHELATING AGENTS.

bis(tributyltin) oxide. *See* TRIBUTYLTIN.

Black Leaf 40. *See* NICOTINE.

black widow spider venom (latrotoxin). The toxic fraction of the venom from spiders of the genus *Latrodectus*; a protein with a molecular weight of 5000 containing predominantly basic residues. Its LD50 in mice is 0.55 mg/kg. It is a neurotoxin that appears to be preferentially accumulated in central and peripheral nervous systems. It causes explosive, non-specific release of vesicle-bound neurotransmitters, followed by destruction of prejunctional nerve endings. Common symptoms include intense pain, restlessness, irritability, tremors, superficial breathing, tachycardia and hypertension. Black widow spider bites are more serious and life-threatening to children than adults. There is no effective first aid treatment. Intravenous calcium gluconate, muscle relaxants and meperidine may be useful in relieving muscle pain. The use of antivenin is normally restricted to children. *Compare* SNAKE VENOMS. *See also* NEUROTRANSMITTERS.

blastocyst. An early stage of development, occurring during the preimplantation period in mammals, after cleavage and before gastrulation. The blastocyst consists of a hollow ball of cells surrounding a central cavity, the blastocoel. It corresponds to the blastula of lower vertebrates.

blastocyte. An undifferentiated embryonic cell. *See also* BLASTOCYST.

blastomogen. *See* CARCINOGEN.

blastula. *See* BLASTOCYST.

BLAVA. *See* BRITISH LABORATORY ANIMAL VETERINARY ASSOCIATION.

bleaches. Solutions which can remove stains or pigments, and also which can have a disinfectant action. They frequently act through chlorine-containing compounds, such as hypochlorite, or through oxygen-containing compounds such as peroxide.

blood. The circulating fluid of the circulatory system that is responsible for the transport of oxygen and carbon dioxide, as well as of nutrients and hormones. About 55% of the blood in mammals is plasma, the liquid matrix, whereas 45% is cellular, primarily erythrocytes (red blood cells), but also leukocytes (white blood cells) and platelets. In toxicology the blood is important for many reasons. (1) Toxicants that affect hemoglobin may exert their deleterious effects by blocking oxygen transport (e.g., carbon monoxide, nitrites). (2) Toxicants are distributed from the portal of entry via the blood, involving primarily transport by plasma proteins, either albumin or lipoproteins. (3) Metabolites of toxicants are distributed to the organs of excretion to permit their elimination from the body. (4) Leukocytes play an important role in the immune system. (5) Toxicants may exert their effects by interfering with the coagulation mechanism. *See also* CIRCULATORY SYSTEM; DIAGNOSTIC FEATURES, BLOOD; ERYTHROCYTES.

blood–brain barrier. A permeability barrier that limits the influx of circulating substances into the immediate brain interstitial space. This barrier is due to tight junctions between the endothelial cells and their lack of fenestrations. Brain sites are protected from most toxicants as passage of large molecules does not usually occur or is severely hindered, and polar molecules are generally physically excluded due to the highly lipophilic nature of the blood–brain barrier. However, specific transport systems may facilitate the passage of certain toxicants into the brain, and supraependymal sites (extra blood–brain barrier structures) may also be particularly vulnerable to toxicants. Finally, many factors can influence blood–brain permeability. The most important of these is the age of the target animal. It is generally accepted that embryonic or fetal forms have higher central accessibility to xenobiotics, and even after birth there appears to be greater passage in the immediate postnatal period than during adulthood. Alterations in blood–brain barrier function may be caused by many types of toxicant exposure. For example, substances that alter membrane function directly—such as the bile salt sodium deoxycholate or high concentrations of various organic solvents, including alcohols—disrupt the blood–brain barrier. Increases in blood–brain barrier permeability are also seen after exposure to cobra venom, presumably because the phospholipases in these venoms hydrolyze membrane lipids. Heavy metals (e.g., lead) are also believed to alter blood-barrier function, although the specific biochemical site of action is not known. It should be noted that changes caused by these and other agents may be reversible or irreversible and may also profoundly influence the CNS toxicity of subsequent exposure to other materials. *See also* P-GLYCOPROTEIN.

blood clotting. *See* COAGULATION, BLOOD.

blood coagulation. *See* COAGULATION, BLOOD.

blood urea nitrogen (BUN). The concentration of urea in blood; a measure of kidney function, more specifically of glomerular function. As filtration diminishes or stops, BUN rises. Changes in BUN are normally paralleled by changes in blood creatinine, although conditions that cause mobilization and breakdown of protein may give rise to an increase in BUN unrelated to kidney failure and to a BUN/creatinine ratio that is higher than usual. *See also* NEPHROTOXICITY.

bluegill sunfish (*Lepomis macrochirus*). A standard warm water fish species for aquatic toxicology tests.

B lymphocytes. *See* B CELLS.

B_{max}. The term representing the theoretical number of binding sites in a radioreceptor assay. It is usually determined experimentally from a saturation assay using nonlinear regression or graphical analyses (e.g., Scatchard, Eadie–Hofstee or Woolf plot). The B_{max} is used to quantify the number of toxicant-binding sites (e.g., receptors), as well as to characterize how intoxication may change the number of endogenous binding sites. *See also* EADIE–HOFSTEE PLOT; ENZYME KINETICS; K_D; RADIO RECEPTOR ASSAYS; SCATCHARD PLOT; WOOLF PLOT; XENOBIOTIC METABOLISM, REVERSIBLE INHIBITION.

Board on Environmental Studies and Toxicology. *See* NATIONAL RESEARCH COUNCIL.

bob white quail. A standard avian test species for wildlife toxicology tests.

BOD. *See* BIOLOGICAL OXYGEN DEMAND.

body burden. The total amount of a chemical present in the whole body of the organism at a particular time. The body burden is determined by exposure, rate of uptake and rate of elimination or biotransformation. It may be distributed more or less evenly between tissues or may be localized primarily in one or a few locations in the body. The study of the rates of change of the body burden and the rates of change of its distribution, as well as the development of predictive mathematical models of them, is the province of toxicokinetics (toxicodynamics) and pharmacokinetics. *See also* PHARMACOKINETICS; TOXICOKINETICS.

body fluids. All of the internal fluids of the body: blood, including subfractions such as serum or plasma; lymph; cerebrospinal fluid; etc. It is an ill-defined term of little utility that is used most often in clinical chemistry to refer to groups of tests that may be carried out on such fluids.

body fluids, in chronic toxicity testing. *See* TOXIC ENDPOINTS.

body fluids, in subchronic toxicity testing. *See* TOXIC ENDPOINTS.

body weight, in chronic toxicity testing. *See* TOXIC ENDPOINTS.

bone. The connective tissue of the skeleton, comprising osteocytes, a collagen matrix and calcified ground substance (hydroxyapatite). This is the target for the deleterious effects of excessive fluoride (fluorosis), for the accumulation of a number of toxicants (e.g., strontium, lead) and for the damaging effects of lathyrogens which inhibit collagen synthesis.

bone marrow. The hematopoietic tissue that has stem cells capable of differentiating into erythrocytes, leukocytes or platelets (thrombocytes). Cobalt toxicity results in polycythemia from stimulation of erythropoiesis. Vitamin B_{12} or folic acid deficiencies, folic acid antagonists such as some cancer chemotherapeutic agents (e.g., methotrexate) or antimalarials (e.g., pyrimethamine) can induce the premature release of blast cells from the bone marrow because of excessive stimulation of production, a condition called megaloblastic anemia. A number of chemicals are toxic to the bone marrow, including benzene, antimetabolites, gold, arsenic, mustards and chloramphenicol, as is ionizing radiation. If damage is extreme, aplastic anemia results. Most of this damage is the result of damage to DNA structure or function. Thrombocytopenia also results when bone marrow function is depressed by chemicals or radiation, and appears to result specifically following exposure to cytosine arabinoside. Granulocytopenia can result from exposure to ionizing radiation, alkylating agents, antimetabolites, phenothiazines, non-steroidal anti-inflammatory drugs, antithyroid drugs and some anticonvulsants. Acute myelogenous leukemia may be caused by benzene, chloramphenicol and phenylbutazone.

bone marrow-derived lymphocytes. *See* B CELLS.

bone marrow evaluation. Bone marrow is the site of formation of the blood cells. Not only is the pluripotent stem cell particularly sensitive to chemical damage, but also overall evaluation of stem cell proliferation may be a sensitive indicator of effects on the immune system. Thus differential staining and examination of cell types may be carried out as part of either acute or chronic toxicity tests or as part of an evaluation of immunotoxic effects. Specific tests for *in vivo* genetic toxicity involve examination of bone marrow cells recovered from treated animals (for chromosome rearrangements, breaks, etc.). *See also* BONE MARROW.

botanical insecticides. Insecticides which have been extracted from plants. Some of the main botanical insecticides are pyrethrum from *Chrysanthemum* and rotenone from *Derris eliptica*.

botulinum toxin. A generic term referring to at least eight biological substances produced during anaerobic growth of the bacterium *Clostridium botulinum*. These bacterial toxins comprise a family of structurally homologous proteins, designated A–G, indicating that they derive from a common ancestor. Botulinum toxin is highly potent, with an LD50 in mice of 2 ng/kg, i.p. Botulinum toxin acts to block release of acetylcholine from cholinergic nerve endings. Interaction between the toxin and cholinergic nerve endings involves binding of the toxin to a receptor. Binding is essential to paralysis, but is not toxic in itself. After binding, translocation of the receptor-toxin complex or some portion thereof occurs. The internalized toxin evokes a lytic effect, resulting in the blockade of transmitter release. It appears that the heavy chain of the toxin provides the mechanism of intracellular delivery, and the light chain is the actual inhibitor of the release of neurotransmitters. β-Bungarotoxin, another presynaptic blocker of acetylcholine release, does not antagonize the effects of the botulinum toxin. Symptoms in humans include nausea, vomiting, diarrhea, abdominal distress, double vision and muscular paralysis eight hours to eight days after ingestion. Marked muscular fatigability, ptosis and dysarthia lead to death due to respiratory paralysis. Treatment involves emesis using sodium bicarbonate or activated charcoal, gastric lavage, ABE botulinum antitoxin, artificial respiration and oral guanidine hydrochloride (15–40 mg/kg/day) for neuromuscular block. *See also* ACETYLCHOLINE; β-BUNGAROTOXIN; CLOSTRIDIUM.

botulism. The poisoning caused by consumption of food in which there has been growth of one or more strains of the anaerobic bacterium *Clostridium botulinum*. Such growth results in production of the proteinaceous botulinum exotoxin, often occurring as a result of home canning where insufficient heat processing or inadequate sealing is at fault. There are occasional commercial episodes, and there has been some speculation that growth of this bacterium *in vivo* (e.g., in infants) may sometimes causes toxicity. The toxin interferes with cholinergic neurotransmission and ultimately causes death by peripheral mechanisms (respiratory failure and cardiac arrest), although there are also profound CNS effects. Botulinum antiserum may prevent further damage when poisoning is confirmed, but the only other therapy is supportive. In survivors, there are often significant permanent sequelae. Although the toxin is heat-labile, all suspected food should be discarded due to the extreme toxicity of the toxins. *See also* BOTULINUM TOXIN.

bradycardia. Slow heart rate, can result from excess parasympathetic stimulation.

brain. *See* NERVOUS SYSTEM.

brain, perfusion. *See* PERFUSION STUDIES, BRAIN.

breaks. *See* CHROMOSOME ABERRATIONS.

Brevital. *See* METHOHEXITAL.

Bright's disease. *See* RENAL FAILURE.

British Agrochemicals Association. A UK trade association for the agrochemical industry, based in Peterborough, England

British Anti-Lewisite (BAL). *See* 2,3-DIMERCAPTO-1-PROPANOL.

British Industrial Biological Research Association (BIBRA). A non-commercial organization that undertakes sponsored research into the safety evaluation of cosmetics and other environmental chemicals. BIBRA also performs toxicological testing of intentional food additives and of residues in foods derived from packaging materials, processing aids, pesticides and herbicides.

British Institute of Regulatory Affairs (BIRA). A body of professionals engaged in the registration (licensing) of pharmaceuticals and other compounds.

British Laboratory Animal Veterinary Association (BLAVA). A division of the British Veterinary Association (BVA) for members working in laboratory animal science.

British Standards Institution (BSI). The recognized authority in the UK for the preparation and publication of national standards for industrial and consumer products. It publishes British Standards (about 600 new or revised standards per annum) covering quality, performance or safety, methods of testing and analysis, glossaries of terms and codes of practice.

bromobenzene. A synthetic intermediate, a solvent and a motor oil additive. It is known to be a hepatotoxicant, the toxicity of which is mediated by the 3,4-epoxide formed by the action of the cytochrome P450-dependent monooxygenase system. This intermediate can either be detoxified by a glutathione S-transferase-mediated reaction or it can exert its toxic effect by forming covalent adducts with nucleophilic substituents on proteins. Formation of the 2,3-epoxide, a pathway stimulated by 3-methylcholanthrene induction, has less serious consequences. *See also* ARYLATION; CYTOCHROME P450.

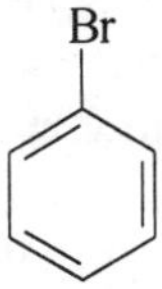

Bromobenzene

bromocriptine (2-bromo-12′-hydroxy-2′-(1-methylethyl)5′-(2-methylpropyl)ergotaman-3′,6′,18-trione; 2-bromoergocryptine; Parlodel). An ergot alkaloid derivative that exhibits potent dopamine agonist properties, particularly at D_2 dopamine receptors. Bromocriptine, like dopamine, inhibits prolactin release from the pituitary and so is used in endocrine disorders, such as hyperprolactinemia. It is also used in the treatment of Parkinson's disease. A large "first-pass" effect is seen with bromocriptine, and peak concentrations occur about 1.5–3 hours after ingestion, with a half-life of about three hours. Nausea, vomiting and orthostatic hypotension are among the acute adverse effects. Long-term use has been associated with dyskinesias, constipation, psychoses, digital spasm and erythromelalgia. The LD50 in rabbits exceeds 1 g/kg, p.o., and 12 mg/kg, i.v. *See also* DOPAMINE; ERGOT ALKALOIDS.

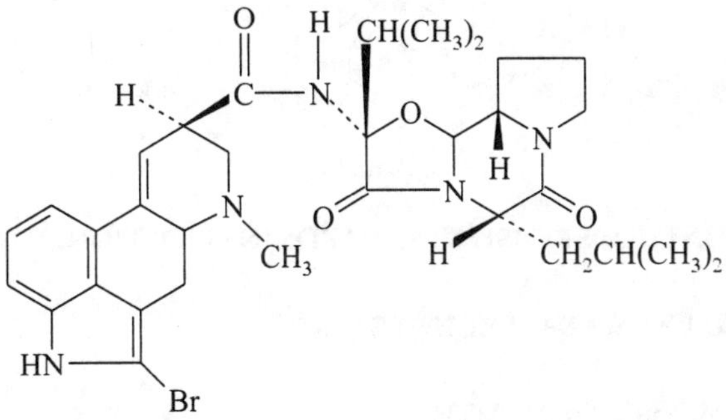

Bromocriptine

bromo-DMA. *See* DOB.

2-bromoergocryptine. *See* BROMOCRIPTINE.

bromomethane. *See* METHYL BROMIDE.

5-bromouracil. *See* ABNORMAL BASE ANALOGS.

bronchiectasis. Pathological dilation of the bronchus.

bronchiole. A subdivision (branch) of the bronchus. Terminal bronchioles lead to respiratory bronchioles that, in turn, lead into the alveolar ducts.

bronchitis. Inflammation of the lining of the bronchus.

bronchogenic. Originating in the bronchus (e.g., bronchogenic carcinoma).

bronchus. One of the two large branches of the trachea in the mammalian respiratory system.

brown recluse spider. *See* SPIDER, BROWN RECLUSE.

brucine. Occurs with strychnine, extracted from *Strychnos nux-vomica* seeds; m.p. 178 °C. Used to denature alcohols and oil, and as a lubricant additive.

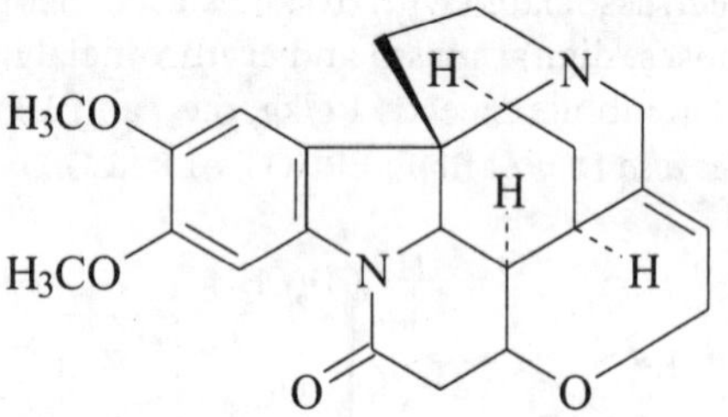

Brucine

BSI. *See* BRITISH STANDARDS INSTITUTION.

BTX. *See* BATRACHOTOXIN.

buccal. *See* MOUTH.

buckthorn toxins (Coytillo, Tullidora). Toxins found in the fruit of the spineless shrub *Karwinskia humboldtiana*, a desert species found in northern Mexico and southwest Texas, USA. The four principal *K. humboldtiana* toxins are 7-[3′,4′-di-hydro-7′,9′-dimethoxy-1′,3′-dimethyl--10′-hydroxy-1′H-naphtho(2′,3′-*c*′)pyran-5′-yl]-3,4-dihydro-3-methyl-3,8,9-trihydroxy-1(2H)-an-thracenone (T-544); 3,4-dihydro-3,di-3′-methyl-1′,3,8,8′,9-pentahydroxy (7,10′-bianthracene)-1,9′ (2H,10′H)-dione (T-496); 7-(2′-aceto-6′,8′-dimethoxy-3′-methyl-1′-hydroxynaphth-4′yl)-3,4-dihydro-3-methyl-3,8,9-trihydroxy-1(2H)-anthracenone (T-516); 3,3′-dimethyl-3,3′,8,8′,9,9′-hexahydroxy-3,3′,4,4′-tetrahydro-(7,10′-bi-anthracene)-1,1′ (2H,2′H)-dione (T-514). Buckthorn toxins produce segmental demyelination of peripheral nerves in man and animals. Clinical manifestations of the demyelinating neuropathy in humans begin five to 20 days after ingestion of the fruit and include malaise, quadriparesis and paralysis of bulbar and respiratory muscles. Recovery requires three to 12 months.

Therapy consists of general supportive care. It has been suggested that daily administration of thiamine may be of therapeutic value. Spencer, P.S. et al. Experimental and Clinical Neurotoxicology (Williams & Wilkins, Baltimore, 1980).

Buehler test. A dermal sensitization test involving repeated application of the test chemical under occlusive patches followed two weeks later by a challenge dose under the same conditions. *See also* DERMAL IRRITATION TESTS.

BUN. *See* BLOOD UREA NITROGEN.

α-bungarotoxin. A neurotoxin isolated from the venom of the elapid snakes *Bungarus multicinctus* and *B. caerulus* (Indian Krait). The LD50 of the venom in mice is 0.09 mg/kg. Electrophoresis of crude venom yields at least three fractions, α-, β- and γ-bungarotoxin, with α-bungarotoxin being the main fraction. The structure consists of a single polypeptide chain containing 74 amino acids (molecular weight about 8000) cross-linked by five disulfide bridges. α-Bungarotoxin is a highly specific blocker of the junctional postsynaptic acetylcholine receptor. When labeled with ^{125}I, it is used to quantify acetylcholine receptors. α-Bungarotoxin suppresses the sensitivity of the endplate membrane to acetylcholine. There is no effect on resting or action potentials of muscle, and there is no presynaptic effect. The neuromuscular block can be reversed by neostigmine and prevented by pretreatment with *d*-tubocurarine. Symptoms in humans include headache, dizziness, unconsciousness, visual and speech disorders, and sometimes convulsions. Also abdominal pain and muscular paralysis that is particularly severe occur within 10 hours and may last for 4 days. Death is from respiratory paralysis. Treatment involves supportive therapy and administration of antivenom (300–350 ml, i.v.) as soon as possible. Although anaphylaxis from the latter is observed in 3% of cases, the risk of dying from the venom is greater. Narahashi, T. Physiol. Rev. 54, 813–889 (1974).

β-bungarotoxin. A neurotoxin isolated from the venom of the elapid snakes *Bungarus multicinctus* and *B. caeruleus* (Indian Krait). The LD50 of the venom in mice is 0.09 mg/kg. The toxin exists in the form of two polypeptide chains: the A chain of 71 amino acids and the B chain of 60 amino acids. The A and B chains appear to differ with respect to enzymatic activity. β-Bungarotoxin acts presynaptically to block neuromuscular transmission through a specific increase in transmitter release. Spontaneous miniature endplate potentials (MEPPs) disappear completely after an initial period of increased frequency. Endplate potentials evoked by nerve stimulation are also blocked. It has no effect on endplate sensitivity to acetylcholine, and blockade is not prevented by pretreatment with *d*-tubocurarine. Synaptic vesicles disappear after exposure to β-bungarotoxin, but not α-bungarotoxin, in contrast to botulinum toxin which causes no ultrastructural changes despite presynaptic action. Symptoms include headache, dizziness, visual and speech disorders, unconsciousness, convulsions, abdominal pain and muscular paralysis that may last four days, with death resulting from respiratory paralysis. Treatment involves general supportive therapy and administration of antivenom (300–350 ml, i.v.) as soon as possible. Although anaphylaxis is observed in 3% of the latter cases, the risk of dying from venom is greater. Narahashi, T. Physiol. Rev. 54, 813–889 (1974).

Busulfan (1,4-butanediol dimethane sulfonate; myleran). An alkylating agent that has been used as an antineoplastic agent for the treatment of chronic myeloid leukemia and as an insect chemosterilant. Since it is an alkylating agent, it is also a primary carcinogen, a clastogen and a teratogen. It has also been shown to produce cataracts and is immunosuppressive.

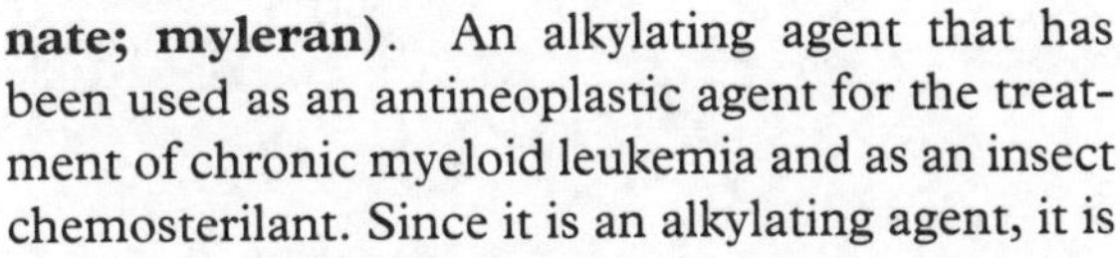

Busulfan

1,3-butadiene. CAS number 106-99-0. A colorless, flammable gas with a sharp aromatic odor. It may be more important as a fire and explosion hazard than as a chemical toxicant because its flash point is low. 1,3-Butadiene is used in the manufacture of synthetic rubber and in rocket fuels, plastics and resin manufacture. The principal route of entry into the body is via inhalation of gas or by contact with the skin. Butadiene gas is somewhat irritating to mucous membranes, and dermatitis may result from exposure to the liquid. High concentrations of the gas can act as an irritant and as a narcotic, causing fatigue, drowsiness, loss of consciousness, respiratory paralysis and possibly death. Chronic exposure may affect the CNS and liver, and may cause a decreased hemoglobin level. Butadiene is carcinogenic in rats and mice with mice being the more sensitive, but it is not known if butadiene presents a cancer risk for humans. The DNA-reactive metabolites appear to be the monoepoxide and the diepoxide both formed by the cytochrome P450-dependent monooxygenase system.

$$CH_2=CHCH=CH_2$$

Butadiene

1,4-butanediol dimethyl sulfonate. *See* BUSULFAN.

Butazolidin. *See* PHENYLBUTAZONE.

Butinox. *See* TRIBUTYLTIN.

butter yellow (*p*-dimethylaminoazobenzene). A food color that has been banned from use because of its demonstrated carcinogenicity. *See also* FOOD COLORS.

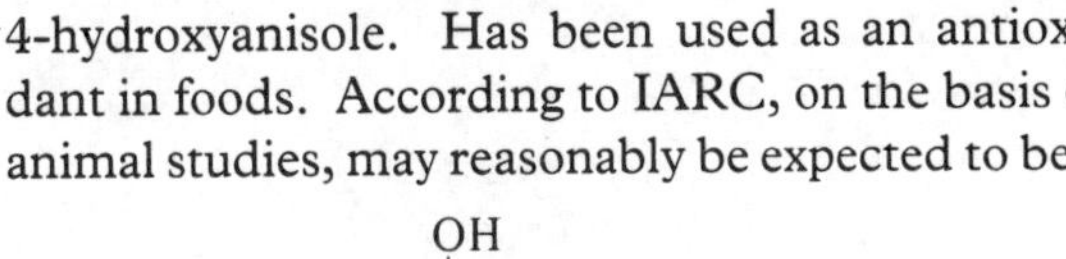

Butter yellow

butylated hydroxyanisole ((1,1-dimethylethyl)-4-methoxyphenol, BHA). **CAS number 25013-16-5.** A mixture of 2-*tert*- and 3-*tert*-butyl-4-hydroxyanisole. Has been used as an antioxidant in foods. According to IARC, on the basis of animal studies, may reasonably be expected to be a

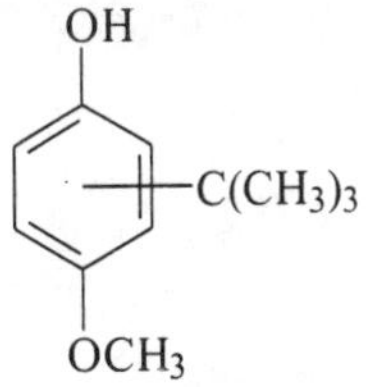

Butylated hydroxyanisole

carcinogen (category 2B). *See also* DATABASES, TOXICOLOGY; MERCK INDEX, 12TH EDN, NUMBER 1582.

butylated hydroxytoluene (2,6-bis (1,1-dimethylethyl)-4-methylphenol, BHT). CAS number 128-37-0. Used as an antioxidant in foods. No evidence of carcinogenicity. *See also* DATABASES, TOXICOLOGY; MERCK INDEX, 12TH EDN, NUMBER 1583.

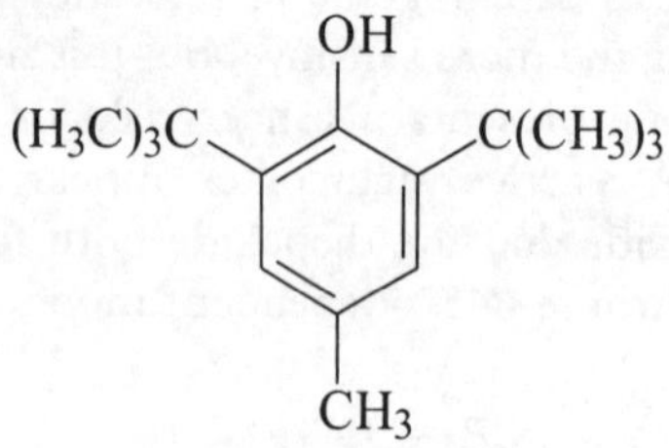

Butylated hydroxytoluene

butyrophenones. One of the classes of antipsychotic drugs, whose most well-known member is haloperidol. Haloperidol is believed to act by being a selective antagonist of the D_2 class of dopamine receptors. Such compounds are usually of high potency and tend to cause a relatively high incidence of extrapyramidal side effects. *See also* ANTIPSYCHOTIC DRUGS; DOPAMINE; DOPAMINE RECEPTORS.

byssinosis. *See* DUST, PROLIFERATIVE.

BZ. Code designation for a glycollate psychotomimetic agent with potential use as an antipersonnel smoke.

C

C3H10T1/2 cells. A cell line derived from mouse embryo fibroblasts that can be cultured indefinitely and is useful in cell transformation tests for carcinogenicity or promotion. C3H10T1/2 cells are somewhat limited by their lack of activating capacity and their aneuploidy in the untransformed state. *See also* MAMMALIAN CELL TRANSFORMATION TESTS.

CAA. *See* CLEAN AIR ACT.

CAC. *See* CODEX ALIMENTARIUS COMMISSION.

cacodylic acid (dimethylarsinic acid, hydroxydimethyl arsine oxide). CAS number 75-60-5. Has been used as a herbicide; use currently restricted by USEPA. Although there is clear evidence that inorganic arsenic is a human carcinogenic, the evidence for organic arsenic compounds is more equivocal. There is evidence, based on studies on experimental animals, for cancer promotion by cacodylic acid. *See also* ATSDR DOCUMENT; DATABASES, TOXICOLOGY.

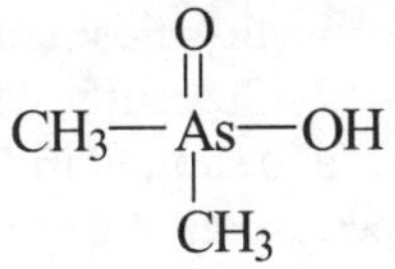

$$CH_3 \overset{\overset{\displaystyle O}{\|}}{\underset{\underset{\displaystyle CH_3}{|}}{As}} OH$$

Cacodylic acid

cadmium (Cd). A metal that is used for electroplating and in batteries, as a color pigment for paints and as a stabilizer in plastics. The oral LD50 in rats is about 0.88 mg/kg and the LC50 in fathead minnows is about 3.06 mg/1. Cadmium is a nephrotoxicant and hepatotoxicant, probably acting by displacement and substitution of essential metals in proteins and enzymes. In humans acute poisoning can cause nausea and vomiting, diarrhea, headache, muscular aches, salivation, abdominal pain and shock. In acute poisoning

unabsorbed cadmium is removed by catharsis. Cadmium contamination of the environment from industrial processes is well known. Perhaps the most dramatic illustration is the outbreak of itai-itai disease in Japan caused by contamination of rice paddies. Another cause of concern is the accumulation of cadmium in sewage sludges. Since cadmium is readily taken up by plants the utilization of such sludges has been opposed due to the potential for cadmium toxicity. *See also* ATSDR DOCUMENT, APRIL 1993.

caffeine (3,7-dihydro-1,3,7-trimethyl-1H-purine-2,6-dione; 1,3,7-trimethylxanthine). CAS number 58-08-2. One of the methylxanthine central stimulants. It is consumed as part of the diet and is found in high concentrations in coffee, cocoa, chocolate, cola and other soft drinks. In addition, caffeine is found in several over-the-counter and prescription drugs. Caffeine has effects on the periphery and also causes significant CNS stimulation. Its effects include elimination of fatigue and drowsiness, promotion of a clearer flow of thought and, at higher doses, diuresis and increased gastrointestinal motility, nervousness, restlessness, insomnia and tremors. Still higher doses may cause focal and generalized seizures. The oral LD50 in various rodent species ranges from 127 to 355 mg/kg. The nature of the urinary metabolites excreted by humans after ingestion of caffeine may be used as a biomarker for certain polymorphisms in xenobiotic-meta-

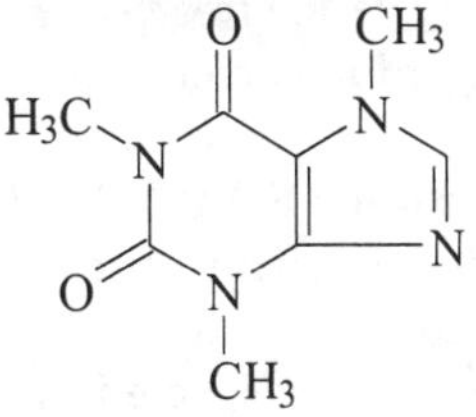

Caffeine

bolizing enzymes, in particular cytochrome P450 1A2 and *N*-acetyl transferase. *See also* METHYL-XANTHINES; PURINES.

C-Agents (CN, CS, CR). Code designations for sensory irritant smokes. CS (*ortho*-chlorobenzylid-ene malanonitrile) has been widely used as a riot control agent. All have been considered for mili-tary use. *See also* CN; CR; CS; D-AGENTS; TEAR GASES.

calcitonin (thyrocalcitonin). Straight-chain polypeptide containing 32 amino acid residues, produced by mammalian thyroid gland. It lowers blood calcium (and phosphate) levels and operates in opposition to parathyroid hormone.

calcium channel blockers. A chemically diverse group of drugs that affect sinoatrial and atrioven-tricular properties of both smooth and cardiac muscle. Primarily used as antiarrhythmic and anti-anginal agents, the group includes such drugs as diltiazem, verapamil and nifedipine. They appear to act at several Ca^{++} channels, including the voltage-dependent Ca^{++}-ion channel, but probably act at different sites, either between channels or even within the same channel. Toxic effects at high doses often involve moderate to severe hypoten-sion and there is some anecdotal evidence that children may be particularly sensitive.

California. *See* PROPOSITION 65.

cAMP. *See* CYCLIC AMP.

camphor. *See* ESSENTIAL OILS.

Canadian Health Protection Branch. An agency of the Canadian Federal Government responsible for the regulation of drugs and other hazardous chemicals and the promulgation of rules and protocols for toxicity testing, including carcinogenicity, mutagenicity and teratogenicity.

cancellation, under FIFRA. Under the US Fed-eral Insecticide, Fungicide and Rodenticide Act (FIFRA), a cancellation order is used to initiate review of a pesticide suspected of causing unrea-sonable adverse effects on humans or the envi-ronment. The cancellation proceedings usually involve a scientific review and public hearings, which may extend over several years. During the proceedings, manufacture and marketing of the pesticide are permitted. *See also* FEDERAL INSEC-TICIDE, FUNGICIDE AND RODENTICIDE ACT; SUSPENSION, UNDER FIFRA.

cancer. Malignant cellular growth consisting of genetically and functionally modified cells capable of invading other tissues. *See also* CARCINOGENE-SIS; CARCINOMA; SARCOMA.

cancer potency factor. A concept used in cancer risk assessment related to the slope of the dose response curve. Cancer potency, or Q, is the slope of the dose response curve and its upper 95% con-fidence is known as Q^*. For genotoxic carcinogens it is assumed that there is no threshold dose below which carcinogenesis does not occur.

Cannabiaceae (Cannabidaceae). A family of dicotyledoneae that contains only two genera *Humulus* and *Cannabis*. *Humulus lupulus* (hop) is a perennial climbing herb widely cultivated for its inflorescences, used to flavor beer. *Cannabis sativa* (hemp) is cultivated in temperate and tropical regions for its fiber, and for the drug (known vari-ously as ganja, marijuana, charas, bhang, pot, etc.) contained in its resin. *See also* CANNABINOIDS.

cannabinoids. The group of C21 compounds typical of and present in *Cannabis sativa*. It includes their carboxylic acids, analogs and trans-formation products. Currently 61 different can-nabinoids have been identified in *Cannabis* and, as yet, none have been isolated from any other plant or animal species. The nomenclature of these compounds is confusing because in North Amer-ica the dibenzopyran numbering system is used (i.e., Δ-9-THC), whereas in Europe the monoter-pene numbering system is used (i.e., Δ-1-THC). The development of a pharmaceutical preparation to administer cannabinoids i.v. to man made it possible to conduct safely comparative studies of the pharmacological activity and potency of these compounds. Currently information about the psy-choactive potency of only the most abundant can-nabinoids (cannabinol and cannabidiol) is available. The results of these investigations indicate that cannabinol has approximately 5% of the potency of Δ-9-THC and that cannabidiol is inactive. The active cannibinoids work by binding to specific high affinity receptors in the brain, whose endogenous function is not known. *See also* CANNABIS SATIVA; MARIHUANA; Δ⁹-*TRANS*-TETRAHYDROCANNABINOL.

***Cannabis sativa* (bhang; charas; dagga; ganja; hashish; hemp plant; marihuana).** A plant that was named and described by Linnaeus in 1753. The psychoactivity of *Cannabis* has been known since antiquity. The plant has been used for its drug effects in India for about 3500 years, and Moslems have used the drug for centuries. Various preparations of this plant are smoked or ingested by 200–300 million people throughout the world. Accordingly, these preparations undoubtedly constitute the most widely used group of illicit drugs. *Cannabis* has been cultivated for at least 5000 years, spreading originally from central Asia to all temperate and tropical areas of the world. *Cannabis* has been a valued agricultural crop for many reasons. The durable fibers of the woody trunk are known as hemp and have been used to produce rope and twine, as well as fine or rough cloth. The *Cannabis* plant is possibly the most efficient source of paper pulp, producing up to five times as much cellulose per acre per year as trees. *Cannabis* seeds are used as food by man, poultry and other birds, as well as furnishing hemp seed oil for paint and soap. The plant produces as many as 61 specific C21 compounds known as cannabinoids, of which Δ-9-*trans*-tetrahydrocannabinol (THC) is the major source of psychoactivity. The concentration of THC in the plant is highest in the bracts, flowers and leaves, and practically non-existent in the stems, roots or seeds. The THC content of the plant and the proportion of other cannabinoids vary greatly and are probably controlled more by the type of seed than by the soil or climatic conditions. According to their THC content *Cannabis sativa* plants are subdivided into fiber-type (less than 0.5% THC) or drug-type (more than 1% THC). In 1987, the average THC content found in samples of confiscated marihuana was approximately 3.0%. Due to seed selection and improved methods of cultivation, however, some samples of confiscated plant material

(Sinsemilla) have been found to contain as much as 15% THC. *See also* CANNABINOIDS; CANNABIACEAE; MARIHUANA; Δ⁹-*TRANS*-TETRAHYDROCANNABINOL.

cannulation. The insertion of any type of tube into the lumen of a blood vessel or duct or into a body cavity for the purpose of withdrawing or infusing fluids. Cannulation of blood vessels is essential in toxicokinetic studies for continuous sampling and cannulation of the bile duct for studies of liver function. Blood vessels are also cannulated for toxicological studies of isolated perfused organs. Cannulae from vessels and ducts are frequently exteriorized through the body wall to allow for continuous sampling for an extended period.

capsaicin. *See* CAPSICUM.

capsicum. The generic name of the red peppers, also a mixture of closely related vanillyl acids (*N*-[(4-hydroxy-3-methoxyphenyl)-methyl]8-methyl-6-noneamide; *trans*-8-methyl-*N*-vanillyl-6-nonenamide). The most active hot component is capsaicin. The red pepper is a member of the Solanaceae family which also includes tomatoes, potatoes and tobacco. The genus *Capsicum* encompasses five species, including *C. annuum*, *C. frutescens*, *C. pendulum*, *C. pubescens* and *C. chinense*, and some other varieties, of which *C. annuum* (milder) and *C. frutescens* (hotter) are commercially most important. Most capsicums have some capsaicin, but in such varieties the amount has been minimized through cultivation. In consumer terms, the capsicums include: paprika, red pepper ("cayenne"), chili pepper, chili powder and sweet pepper flakes. Generally speaking the hottest types of peppers are grown and consumed in the hot tropical areas of Africa, America and Asia. Large amounts of hot pepper consumption are known in India, certain parts of China, Malaysia, Japan, Mexico, Korea, Spain, Hungary, Turkey, Pakistan, Morocco, etc. Capsicum contains a mixture of at least seven closely related vanillyl acids, with approximate composition being: capsaicin (69%), dihydrocapsaicin (22%), nor-dihydrocapsaicin (7%), homocapsaicin (1%), homodihydrocapsaicin (1%), and nor-capsaicin (<0.1%). Capsaicin causes severe pain in humans and experimental animals upon administration. Capsaicin appears to act selectively on primary afferent neurons, depleting these processes of the peptide substance P. As a result, chronic administration causes an insensitivity to some types of nociceptive stimuli. Neonatal rodents are particularly sensitive to capsaicin, which causes a selective, profound and permanent degeneration of C and A fibers. The sensory deficits induced by capsaicin appear to be due to plasma membranes that are in a chronic depolarized state. It thus has use as a neurobiological research tool, as well as a condiment.

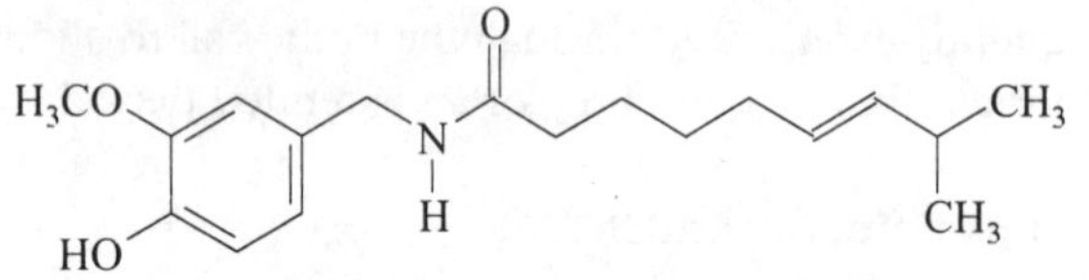

Capsaicin

captan (1,2,3,6-tetrahydro-*N*-(trichloromethylthio)phthalimide; *N*-(trichloromethyl-thio)cyclohex-4-ene-1,2-dicarboximide; 3*a*,4,7,7*a*-tetrahydro-2-[(trichloromethyl)thio]-*H*-isoindole-1,3(2*H*)-dione). CAS number 133-06-02. A fungicide with an acute oral LD50 in rats of 9000 mg/kg. It may cause skin irritation. In two-year feeding trials the no "effect" level for rats was 1000 mg/kg diet. Experimentally it has been shown to cause carcinogenic and teratogenic effects.

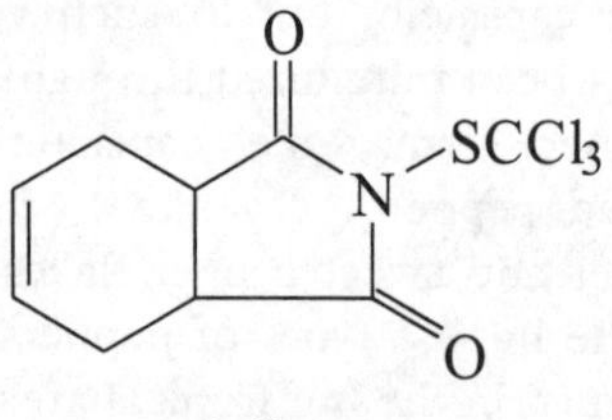

Captan

carbachol (2-[(aminocarbonyl)oxy]-*N*,*N*,*N*-trimethylethanaminium chloride; (2-hydroxyethyl)trimethyl ammonium chloride carbamate). CAS number 51-83-2. The carbamyl ester of acetylcholine. It has actions at both muscarinic and nicotinic cholinergic receptors. Its nicotinic actions occur particularly at autonomic ganglia. Carbachol has relatively little effect on cardiovascular function, but greater effects on the gastrointestinal and urinary tract, and also produces miosis. Carbachol is also a potent dipsogen. The LD50 in mice is 15mg/kg, p.o., and 0.3 mg/kg, i.v. *See also* ACETYLCHOLINE; ACETYLCHOLINE RECEPTORS, MUSCARINIC AND NICOTINIC.

$$(CH_3)_3NCH_2CH_2OCNH_2$$

Carbachol

carbamate. Substituted carbamic acids. The best known are anticholinesterases and serve as insecticides (e.g., carbaryl, propoxur), drugs for such disorders as myasthenia gravis (e.g., physostigmine) or prophylactic agents when anticholinesterase chemical warfare agents (i.e., nerve agents, nerve gases) are anticipated (e.g., pyridostigmine). *See also* ANTICHOLINESTERASES.

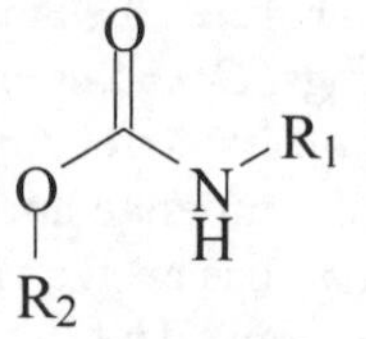

Carbamate

carbamate and thiocarbamate herbicides. A class of herbicides comprising esters of carbamic or thiocarbamic acid: for example, isopropyl carbanilate (propham). In general, both acute and chronic mammalian toxicity is low and, unlike the insecticidal carbamates, they are not inhibitors of cholinesterase.

carbamate insecticides. *N*-Methyl or *N*,*N*-dimethyl derivatives of esters of carbamic acid. They exert their insecticidal activity, as well as their toxicity to other animals, by virtue of their ability to act as potent cholinesterase inhibitors. Symptoms are typically cholinergic with lachrymation, salivation, miosis and, in extreme cases, death from respiratory failure. Atropine is an effective antidote, but 2-PAM is not useful. *See also* ALDICARB; CARBAMATE POISONING, SYMPTOMS AND THERAPY; CARBARYL.

carbamate poisoning, symptoms and therapy. Although the mode of action is similar to that of organophosphorus cholinesterase inhibitors, the carbamylated cholinesterase is less stable than the phosphorylated enzyme, and its regeneration cannot be accelerated by 2-PAM. Thus the non-specific therapy is the same as that for organophosphate compounds, but only atropine is used as a specific antidote. *See also* ORGANOSPHOSPHATE POISONING, SYMPTOMS AND THERAPY.

carbamazepine (5*H*-dibenz[*b*,*f*]azepine-5-carboxamide; Tegretol). An anticonvulsant drug and a specific analgesic for trigeminal neuralgia, also used in certain neuropsychiatric disorders. Its use must be carefully monitored, however, because it may cause significant effects on the hemopoetic system, including aplastic anemia. These latter effects can be minimized by careful monitoring of patients, with the discontinuation of the drug at the first sign of changes in the blood count. The oral LD50 in rodents ranges from 920 to 3750 mg/kg. *See also* ANTICONVULSANTS.

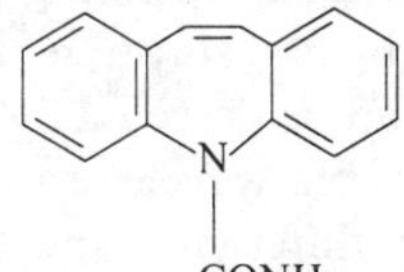

CONH$_2$

Carbamazepine

carbamylated. The chemical entity resulting from the covalent addition of a carbamyl moiety (e.g., from a carbamate insecticide) to a macromolecule, such as the enzyme acetylcholinesterase.

carbaryl (1-naphthalenyl methyl carbamate; Sevin). CAS number 63-25-2. A broad-spectrum contact insecticide with an acute oral LD50 in male rats of 850 mg/kg and an acute dermal LD50 in rats of 4000 mg/kg and in rabbits of 2000 mg/kg. It is a neurotoxicant by virtue of its ability to inhibit acetylcholinesterase. *See also* CARBAMATE INSECTICIDES; CARBAMATE POISONING, SYMPTOMS AND THERAPY.

OCONHCH$_3$

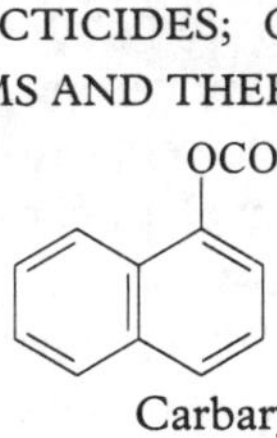

Carbaryl

carbazole (9H-carbazole; 9-azafluorene; dibenzopyrrole; diphenylenimine). CAS number 86-74-8. Intermediate in production of dyes and UV-sensitive photographic plates. *See also* LEWIS, HCDR, NUMBER CBN000; DATABASES, TOXICOLOGY.

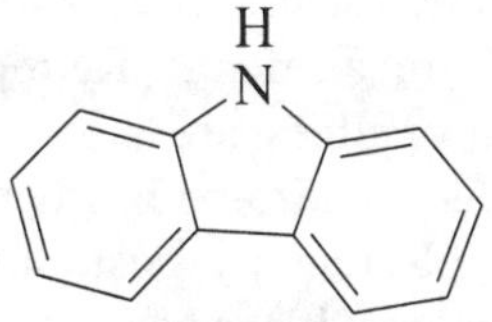

Carbazole

β-carbolines. Derivatives of tryptoline or 1,2,3,4-tetrahydro-β-carboline. The β-carbolines are formed by the non-enzymatic Pictet–Spengler condensation of aldehydes (like acetaldehyde) and arylethylamines, such as serotonin, its precursors or metabolites. Some of these compounds have potent activity on the nervous system (e.g., as serotonin agonists), and some are found to occur endogenously in the nervous system where it has been hypothesized that they serve a role as neurotransmitters or neuromodulators. Several of the β-carbolines are found in sufficient concentrations in some foods (e.g., fermented soy sauce) that they may cause toxicological effects under unusual circumstances. *See also* TETRAHYDROISOQUINOLINES.

carbon dioxide (CO$_2$). CAS number 124-38-9. As a gas, at high levels, it can be an eye irritant and an asphyxiant by replacing oxygen in air, and it causes headache, shortness of breath, dizziness, muscular weakness, drowsiness and a ringing in the ears. As a solid (dry ice) it can cause frostbite. It has many uses, including (as a gas) carbonation of beverages, in the textile, leather and chemical industries, in water treatment, in food preservation, as a fire extinguisher, as a pressure medium, as a propellant in aerosols, as a respiratory stimulant medically, as an inert atmosphere when a fire hazard exists and (as a solid or liquid) as a refrigerant. Carbon dioxide can produce teratogenic effects by causing hypoxia. Increased atmospheric levels of carbon dioxide resulting from the increased burning of fossil fuels is believed to contribute to the greenhouse effect. *See also* GREENHOUSE EFFECT.

carbon disulfide (CS$_2$). CAS number 75-15-0. A flammable and volatile liquid with a boiling point of 46 °C that is used as a fumigant and as an industrial solvent in the rayon and rubber industries. Prolonged exposure can cause severe intoxication marked by severe encephalopathies, toxic psychoses, agitated delirium, seizures and permanent mental impairment. Retinopathies and peripheral neuropathies are also marked, and a Parkinsonian-like syndrome has been reported in young people. No therapy exists for any of these toxic manifestations. It has been hypothesized that the mechanism of toxicity of carbon disulfide involves chelation of copper and zinc by the metabolite-amino acid condensation product diethyldithiocarbamate, thus causing secondary enzyme inhibition. The observation that carbon disulfide-induced peripheral neuropathies are marked by neurofilament-filled axonal swellings similar to those induced by γ-diketones, however, suggests that the degeneration of distal axons may be due to covalent cross-linking of neurofilaments. Carbon disulfide is metabolized to carbonyl sulfide by the cytochrome P450-dependent monooxygenase system, the carbonyl disulfide being further metabolized to yield inorganic sulfur. The reactive sulfur initially released may inhibit cytochrome P450 by interaction with the heme iron or may ultimately be excreted as sulfate ion, although the excretion of inorganic sulfate appears to be low in humans. Carbon disulfide may also be conjugated with amino acids to form dithiocarbamates or with cysteine or glutathione. *See also* γ-DIKETONE NEUROPATHY; PERIPHERAL NEUROPATHY.

carbonic anhydrase. The enzyme that catalyzes the reversible reaction between water, carbon dioxide and carbonic acid. Its presence in erythrocytes is very important for the transport of carbon dioxide by the blood and in the buffering capacity of the blood. Interference with the activity of carbonic anhydrase by the organochlorine insecticides has been implicated in the eggshell thinning phenomenon. *See also* DDT; ORGANOCHLORINE INSECTICIDES.

carbon monoxide (CO). CAS number 630-08-0. An odorless, colorless and tasteless, but highly reactive gas that burns in air. It is formed by incomplete combustion of carbon or organic compounds and is used as an intermediate in certain industrial processes. It is produced for these purposes by partial oxidation of natural gas or by coal gasification. Carbon monoxide is produced in large quantities from combustion of fossil fuels, and atmospheric levels due to automobiles may rise as high as 20 ppm in the air of large cities. Its importance in toxicology lies in its ability to bind, with high affinity, to hemoglobin, forming carboxyhemoglobin. Since the latter cannot transport oxygen, anoxia, often leading to death, occurs. *See also* CARBON MONOXIDE POISONING, THERAPY; CARBOXYHEMOGLOBIN; CARBOXYHEMOGLOBINEMIA.

carbon monoxide binding spectra. Carbon monoxide binds to the heme iron of hemoproteins that normally bind oxygen. Such complexes are frequently of importance in toxicology, either due to their role in poisoning by carbon monoxide or in experimental techniques for the investigation of hemoproteins. Since the binding of carbon monoxide affects the light absorption of the heme chromophore, they can be detected by spectroscopy in the ultraviolet/visible wavelength, either as absolute spectra or difference spectra. Spectra of importance include those of the carbon monoxide complexes of cytochrome oxidase and reduced cytochrome P450, as well as that of carboxyhemoglobin. *See also* CARBOXYHEMOGLOBIN; CYTOCHROME P450, OPTICAL DIFFERENCE SPECTRA; OPTICAL DIFFERENCE SPECTRA.

carbon monoxide poisoning, therapy. Carbon monoxide is a common cause of both deliberate and accidental poisoning. Carbon monoxide is produced by the incomplete combustion of fossil fuels, in automobiles, industrial machinery, home furnaces, etc., and binds reversibly with high-affinity to hemoglobin forming carboxy hemoglobin. The affinity of carbon monoxide is 250 times that of oxygen, and thus it is imperative to remove the victim from the source of carbon monoxide. The patient is kept at rest to reduce oxygen demand. The specific therapy involves competition for the receptor, hemoglobin, by the physiological ligand, oxygen. Respiration is maintained artificially and either oxygen or a mixture of 95% oxygen and 5% carbon dioxide is administered. Since the affinity of carbon monoxide is high, the use of high oxygen concentration is critical. The use of a compression chamber at about 2 atmospheres is extremely helpful, permitting more oxygen to be available to compete for the hemoglobin and increasing the solubility of oxygen in the blood plasma. *See also* CARBON MONOXIDE.

carbon tetrachloride (CCl₄). CAS number 56-23-5. A designated animal carcinogen (IARC), hazardous substance (EPA), hazardous waste (EPA) and priority toxic pollutant (EPA). It is a colorless liquid with a high vapor pressure and a characteristic odor. It forms phosgene and hydrogen chloride on combustion. Carbon tetrachloride has been used as a solvent for oils, fats, waxes and resins, and as a solvent in dry cleaning. It has also been used as a pesticidal fumigant and as an intermediate in fluorocarbon synthesis. Although the use of carbon tetrachloride was formerly widespread, substitution of less toxic compounds is now recommended. Carbon tetrachloride may cause dermatitis on repeated skin contact, and acute systemic effects include CNS depression and gastrointestinal effects, and liver and kidney damage accompanied by nausea, abdominal pain and jaundice. These effects are aggravated when ethanol has also been ingested, and in serious cases coma and death may result from renal failure. Hepatotoxicity is caused by the generation of the trichloromethyl radical $\left(CCl_3^{\bullet}\right)$ by the action of cytochrome P450, an electrophilic radical that binds to nucleophilic substituents on proteins. *See also* ATSDR DOCUMENT, MAY 1994.

$$
\begin{array}{c}
Cl \\
| \\
Cl-C-Cl \\
| \\
Cl
\end{array}
$$

Carbon tetrachloride

carboxyhemoglobin (COHb). Hemoglobin (Hb) in combination with carbon monoxide is incapable of transporting oxygen. Since the affinity of Hb for carbon monoxide is about 250 times greater than its affinity for oxygen, carboxyhemoglobin can be formed at relatively low concentrations of carbon monoxide. *See also* CARBON MONOXIDE; CARBON MONOXIDE POISONING, THERAPY; CARBOXYHEMOGLOBINEMIA; HEMOGLOBIN.

carboxyhemoglobinemia. The condition in which a significant part of the circulating hemoglobin (Hb) is in the form of its carbon monoxide derivative, carboxyhemoglobin. Poisoning by carbon monoxide occurs because of its ability to combine effectively with hemoglobin to form carboxyhemoglobin. Carboxyhemoglobin cannot bind oxygen. Symptoms of poisoning include headaches, dizziness, nausea, breathing difficulty and finally death. Since hemoglobin binds carbon monoxide so much more effectively than it binds oxygen, victims of high-level carbon monoxide exposure can only achieve sufficient oxygen transport by increasing the dissolved oxygen content of the plasma. *See also* CARBON MONOXIDE; CARBON MONOXIDE POISONING, THERAPY; CARBOXYHEMOGLOBIN; HEMOGLOBIN.

carboxylesterases (aliesterases; carboxylic ester hydrolase; E.C. 3.1.1.1). Hydrolases that are found in liver, erythrocytes, muscle, kidney, intestinal mucosa, etc., and that hydrolyze aliphatic and aromatic esters. These enzymes are inhibited by 10^{-7} M paraoxon, as well as other organophosphorus inhibitors. Carboxylesterases hydrolyze *p*-nitrophenyl butyrate faster than *p*-nitrophenyl acetate. A carboxylesterase capable of hydrolyzing the ethyl ester group of the insecticide malathion is largely responsible for the selectivity of this insecticide, since it is common in mammals and unusual in insects. Aldridge, W.N. Biochem. J. 53, 110 (1953). Dauterman, W.C. Toxicol. Clin. Toxicol. 19, 623 (1982–3). *See also* HYDROLYSIS.

carboxylic acid. One of the organic acids in which a carbon atom is attached to a carboxyl (-COOH) group. The carboxylic acids include aliphatic acids, such as formic acid (HCOOH), acetic acid (CH₃COOH) and stearic acid (CH₃(CH₂)₁₆COOH) and aromatic acids, such as benzoic acid.

carcinogen (blastomogen; oncogen; tumorigen). A chemical that induces neoplasms that are not usually observed, the earlier induction of neoplasms that are commonly observed and/or the induction of more neoplasms than are usually found; fundamentally different mechanisms may be involved in these three situations. Chemical carcinogens share many common biological properties, that includes metabolism of some precarcinogens to reactive electrophilic intermediates capable of interacting with DNA. They may differ widely, however, in the dose required to produce a given level of tumor induction. Although the term carcinogen literally means giving rise to carcinomas (such as epithelial malignancies), in general usage it also includes agents producing sarcomas of mesenchymal origin. Carcinogens are a highly diverse collection of chemical substances including organic and inorganic chemicals, hormones, immunosuppressants and solid-state materials.

carcinogen, chemical. Chemicals that can induce tumors without prior or subsequent exposure to other chemical or physical agents.

carcinogen classification systems. Various national and international agencies, frequently those charged with the regulation of carcinogens, have developed systems for carcinogen classification. These systems reflect the risk associated with exposure to a particular chemical, chemical mixture, or occupation, or the potential for risk based on hazard determination in experimental animals. The most accepted system for the classification of carcinogens is that of IARC, the International Agency for Research on Cancer. The system consists of three groups of chemicals, with group 2 being further divided into groups 2A and 2B. They are defined as follows.

Group 1. The chemical, group of chemicals, industrial process or occupational exposure is carcinogenic to humans. This category is used when there is sufficient epidemiological evidence to support a causal association between the exposure and human cancer. This group contains approximately 30 chemicals or processes including benzene, benzidine, vinyl chloride, nickel refining, etc.

Group 2. The chemical, group of chemicals, industrial process or occupational exposure is probably carcinogenic to humans. To reflect the wide range of probabilities within the group it is further subdivided into 2A in which there is at least limited evidence of cancer causation in humans but adequate evidence from animal studies and 2B in which there is inadequate data on humans but sufficient evidence for cancer causation in animals. Group 2A contains

such compounds as acrylonitrile, beryllium and beryllium compounds, phenacetin, etc., while 2B, a much larger group, contains compounds such as DDT, ethylene oxide, phenytoin, uracil mustard, etc.

Group 3. The chemical, group of chemicals, industrial process or occupational exposure cannot be classified as to its carcinogenicity in humans.

The US Environmental Protection Agency uses a similar system in which group A corresponds approximately to IARC group 1, group B to IARC group 2A, group C to IARC group 2B and group D to IARC group 3. An additional group, E, includes chemicals for which there is evidence of non-carcinogenicity. The US National Toxicology Program and OSHA use similar, but simplified systems. *See also* DATABASES, TOXICOLOGY.

carcinogen, complete. Chemicals that can induce tumors without prior or subsequent exposure to other chemical or physical agents.

carcinogen, direct-acting. *See* CARCINOGEN, PRIMARY.

carcinogen, epigenetic (non-genotoxic carcinogen). An agent causing an increase in malignant tumors that does not directly interact with DNA, but may cause changes in methylation patterns or the tertiary structure of DNA. Carcinogens that do not produce responses in assays for mutation, cell transformation, chromosome aberration or DNA binding or damage are described as producing their carcinogenic effect by epigenetic mechanisms. There are no direct methods for identifying epigenetic carcinogens except for those agents that are active in promoter assays. Epigenetic carcinogens are identified only indirectly by their apparent failure to produce a response in short-term carcinogenicity assays. Examples of epigenetic carcinogens include hormones (estrogens, androgens, thyroid hormone), solid-state carcinogens, immunosuppressants, cytotoxic agents and promoters.

carcinogen, genotoxic. A chemical that acts through genetic mechanisms by interacting with DNA, causing gene mutation or duplication, or a change in the chromosome structure or number. Carcinogens that produce a consistent response in short-term tests for mutagenicity are defined as acting by genetic mechanisms. They are frequently called initiators or early-stage carcinogens, indicating that they affect an early stage of the multistep process of carcinogenesis. Genotoxic carcinogens, probably because of their effects on DNA, usually produce neoplasms in more than one target organ, have a short latent period, are occasionally effective after a single exposure and frequently are carcinogenic at doses that are physiologically subtoxic.

carcinogen, inorganic. A carcinogen that induces neoplasms by an ambiguously defined mechanism such as by altering the fidelity of DNA polymerases and replication to yield cells with altered DNA. Inorganic carcinogenesis is associated with a wide range of metals and their compounds (e.g., arsenic, beryllium, chromium, nickel, cadmium, lead), as well as fibrous mineral asbestos.

carcinogen, known human. *See* CARCINOGEN CLASSIFICATION SYSTEMS.

carcinogen, primary (direct-acting carcinogen). An agent that is reactive or toxic enough to act directly to cause cancer in its parent, unmetabolized form. Examples of primary carcinogens include alkylating agents, nitrogen or sulfur mustards, sulfonic esters, sulfones, epoxides, bis(chloromethyl) ether, peroxides, dimethyl sulfate, and radiation. Such a carcinogen is a chemically and biologically reactive entity by virtue of its specific structure. These agents can interact specifically with certain elements of tissues, cells, and cellular component macromolecules to yield modified cellular macromolecules that are typical of the neoplastic state.

carcinogen, probable human. *See* CARCINOGEN CLASSIFICATION SYSTEMS.

carcinogen, proximate (procarcinogen). A chemical that must undergo metabolism to another chemical form before the carcinogenic action can be expressed. Examples include nitrosamines, nitrosoureas, polyaromatic hydrocarbons, aromatic and heterocyclic amines, azo dyes, chlorinated hydrocarbons, aflatoxin and mycotoxins. Some proximate carcinogens are often chemically or spontaneously converted to the ultimate carcinogens by hydrolytic reactions. These are specific, spontaneous or biochemical (e.g., host-mediated and controlled) activation reactions that can convert proximate carcinogens to the corresponding reactive ultimate carcinogens.

carcinogen, solid-state. A carcinogen whose solid physical form is crucial to the carcinogenesis process, although acting by an as yet unknown mechanism. Examples of solid-state carcinogens include asbestos, metal foils and plastics.

carcinogen, ultimate. The form of a carcinogen that directly interacts with a cell constituent (presumably DNA) to initiate carcinogenesis. Many, if not most, chemical carcinogens are not intrinsically carcinogenic, but require metabolic activation to express their carcinogenic potential. The terms precarcinogen, proximate carcinogen and ultimate carcinogen are used to describe the initial compound, its more active products and the compound that is actually responsible for carcinogenesis by its interaction with DNA, respectively. *See also* CARCINOGEN, PROXIMATE; PRECARCINOGEN.

carcinogenesis. The process encompassing the conversion of normal cells to neoplastic cells and the further development of neoplastic cells into a tumor. It can be the result of the action of specific chemicals, certain viruses, or radiation from ultraviolet light, X- or gamma-rays, or α- and β-particles. Chemical carcinogens have been classified into those that are genotoxic and those that are not, but are epigenetic. Genotoxic carcinogens can be shown to be reactive with DNA, to be mutagenic in prokaryotic and eukaryotic cells, and to induce DNA repair in mammalian cells. *See also* CO-CARCINOGENESIS; INITIATION; NEOPLASTIC TRANSFORMATION; PROGRESSION; PROMOTION; TRANSPLACENTAL CARCINOGENESIS.

carcinogenesis, extrapolation to humans. Carcinogenesis testing is carried out at high doses in species other than man. Extrapolation to humans is necessary to estimate the risk of carcinogenesis that might be attendant upon continued use and/or manufacture and dissemination of the chemical. It involves extrapolation from one species, usually a rodent, to humans, and also from the high doses used in the tests to the low doses typical of human exposure. Although the presence or absence of threshold concentrations for chemical carcinogens is still a matter of controversy for regulatory purposes, there are assumed to be no threshold concentrations for the purpose of extrapolation to humans. *See also* EXTRAPOLATION; EXTRAPOLATION TO HUMANS; LOW-DOSE EXTRAPOLATION; SPECIES EXTRAPOLATION.

carcinogenesis, occupational. A high risk of cancer resulting from engagement in a particular occupation. Occupations are classified in the IARC system in the same way as specific chemicals or groups of chemicals, being placed in the same groups using the same weight and type of evidence. For example, nickel mining is associated with excess incidence of cancers of the nasal cavity, lung, and larynx. *See also* DATABASES, TOXICOLOGY.

carcinogenesis, radiation. *See* RADIATION CARCINOGENESIS.

carcinogenesis, transplacental. *See* TRANS-PLACENTAL CARCINOGENESIS.

carcinogenic potency database. A tabulation and analysis of all chemicals tested for carcinogenicity that meet certain criteria designed to permit the estimation of carcinogenic potency. The database has been developed by Gold, Ames and numerous co-workers. As of 1995, it contained 1230 chemicals.

carcinogenicity testing. Carcinogenicity tests have most requirements in common (physical facilities, diets, etc.) with chronic and subchronic toxicity tests. Most tests are carried out using rats and/or mice, but in some cases an additional, non-rodent, species may also be used. The test chemical may be administered in the food, the drinking water, by gavage, by dermal application or by inhalation, the first and third being most common. Since the oncogenic potency of chemicals varies through extreme limits, the purity of the test chemical is of great concern. Dosing is carried

out over the major part of the lifespan (1.5–2.0 years for mice and 2.0 years or more for rats), starting at weaning. The highest dose used is the maximum tolerated dose (MTD), together with one lower dose, usually 0.5 MTD. The principal endpoint is tumor incidence, as determined by histological examination. The statistical problem of distinguishing between spontaneous tumor occurrence in the controls and chemical-related tumor incidence in the treated animals is great and, for that reason, large numbers of animals are used. A typical test involves 50 rats or mice of each sex per treatment group. Some animals are necropsied at intermediate stages of the test (e.g., at 12 months), as are any animals that are found dead or moribund, and all surviving animals are necropsied at the end of the test. *See also* CHRONIC TOXICITY TESTING; SUBCHRONIC TOXICITY TESTING; TOXIC ENDPOINTS.

carcinoma. A malignant neoplasm of a tissue derived from the embryonic ectoderm and endoderm. Cancers that arise in the epithelial cells are called carcinomas. Pitot, H.C. Fundamentals of Oncology 3rd edn (Marcel Dekker, New York & Basel, 1986).

carcinostatic. Tending to check the growth of a carcinoma. *See also* CHEMOTHERAPY.

cardiac arrest. A sudden cessation of functional circulation. Cardiac arrest may occur as a result of drugs that interfere with cellular ion transport, general anesthesia, carbon monoxide poisoning, following asphyxia resulting from pulmonary edema, and other causes. *See also* MAINTENANCE THERAPY, CIRCULATORY SYSTEM.

cardiac glycosides. A series of alkaloids that have been used clinically as cardiotonic agents and diuretics. These compounds generally work by inhibiting Na^+/K^+-ATPases. *See also* DIGITALIS; DIGITOXIN; NA^+/K^+-ATPASES; OUABAIN.

cardiovascular system. The anatomical/physiological system consisting of the heart and blood vessels.

carmustine. *See* BIS(2-CHLOROETHYL)NITRO-SOUREA.

case-control studies. *See* EPIDEMIOLOGY STUDIES.

CAS number. A number assigned by the Chemical Abstracts Service to provide an unambiguous identification of a chemical. *See also* CHEMICAL ABSTRACTS SERVICE.

CAST. *See* COUNCIL FOR AGRICULTURAL SCIENCE AND TECHNOLOGY.

Castillo de Belmer. *See* ENVIRONMENTAL DISASTERS.

castor beans (*Ricinus communis*). A toxic plant of the family Euphorbiaceae. The beans contain ricin, a toxic lectin, and hemagglutinin, ricinine, and a triglyceride of ricinoleic acid. This fatty acid comprises 90% of the triglyceride fraction of castor oil, which is used medicinally as a cathartic. *See also* RICIN; RICININE; RICINOLEIC ACID.

catabolism. Metabolism involving the breakdown of large molecules to smaller units, usually to transduce energy into a form that can be utilized for cellular functions.

catalepsy. The inhibition of the ability of an animal to initiate motor movement, such that the animal will remain in an externally imposed posture for some duration of time. Antipsychotic drugs and some other centrally active agents can induce catalepsy in a dose-dependent fashion. Although several variations are used, the most common method of testing for catalepsy involves placing the rat's forepaws on a horizontal bar that is elevated 10–12 cm above the floor of the test chamber. The descent latency, or time it takes for the animal to return to the test chamber floor, is then measured. *See also* ANTIPSYCHOTIC DRUGS; CATATONIA.

catalytic converter. A device fitted to the exhaust system of a gasoline-driven motor vehicle to reduce emissions of pollutants, especially of unburned hydrocarbons, carbon monoxide and nitrogen oxides, by catalyzing chemical reactions to trap the pollutants. The device is very efficient, and can be fitted only to engines burning lead-free gasoline.

catatonia. The state associated with marked psychomotor disturbance, including stupor, negativism, rigidity, excitement and abnormal posturing. It is often seen with some schizophrenic patients who are mute, exhibit stereotypies and mannerisms, and remain in an externally imposed posture. It may be related to perturbation of dopamine neurotransmission. *See also* CATALEPSY.

catechol. (1) Pyrocatechol, *o*-dihydroxybenzene; an organic compound used as an antiseptic, in photography, in electroplating and in dyestuffs, specialty inks, antioxidants and light stabilizers. Its oral LD50 in rats is 3.89 g/kg. Skin contact can lead to eczematous dermatitis. Absorption leads to phenol-like symptoms, but with more pronounced convulsions. It increases blood pressure, probably from peripheral vasoconstriction, and it can cause death from respiratory failure. Catechol is also a co-carcinogen or a promoter of carcinogenesis. (2) Catechin; a bioflavonoid found in some higher woody plants. It is used in dyeing and tanning, and as an astringent.

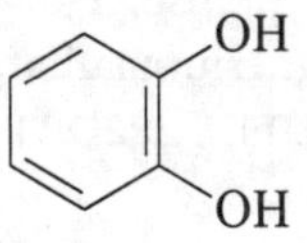

Catechol 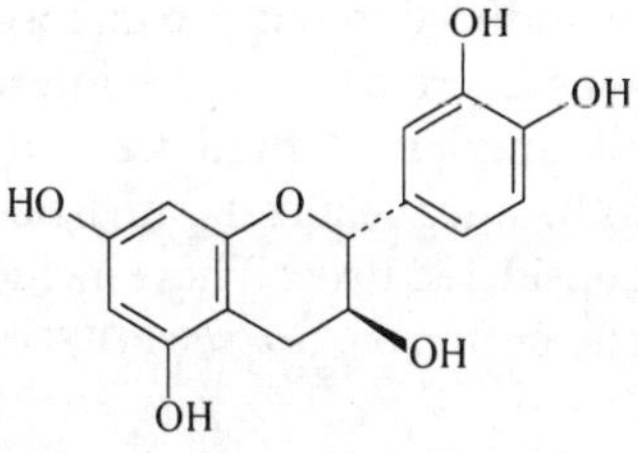   D-Catechin

catecholamines. A class of compounds containing the 3,4-dihydroxyphenylethylamine nucleus. This group includes the mammalian neurotransmitters dopamine, norepinephrine and epinephrine, and non-mammalian compounds such as octopamine. They subserve a variety of important functions including sensory-motor integration, movement and memory. In addition to their widespread importance in many CNS functions, their study was aided by early development of sensitive assay methods for their quantification. The catecholamine biosynthetic pathway begins with the hydroxylation of tyrosine by tyrosine hydroxylase to form 1,3,4-dihydroxyphenylalanine (L-dopa), which is decarboxylated by aromatic amino acid decarboxylase to form dopamine. Norepinephrine is formed from dopamine by the enzyme dopamine β-hydroxylase, and epinephrine is formed from norepinephrine by the enzyme phenylethanolamine *N*-methyltransferase. Catecholamines have been implicated in major psychiatric disturbances such as schizophrenia and depression. Symptoms seen after intoxication with such agents as manganese or MPTP are believed to be primarily due to effects on catecholamine systems. Chemicals that affect catechol systems in the brain can induce depression or psychoses. In the periphery, changes can affect blood pressure and cardiac function. *See also* DOPAMINE RECEPTORS; MPTP; MANGANESE.

catechol *O*-methyltransferase. *See* O-METHYLATION.

catharsis. The stimulation of defecation. Compounds causing such an effect are known as cathartics. Although cathartic and laxative are sometimes held to be synonymous, in many cases the term cathartic is used to mean a compound with a more potent effect than a laxative. Catharsis may be induced to remove unabsorbed poisons or poisons excreted into the intestine. Since excessive elimination of fluid feces may cause electrolyte imbalance, clinical cathartics may themselves be considered toxic. These include magnesium sulfate and croton oil. *See also* POISONING, LIFE SUPPORT.

cathepsins. Proteolytic enzymes active at acid pH that are characteristic of lysosomes. Cathepsins A and C are exopeptidases, whereas cathepsins B and D are endopeptidases. These enzymes are frequently used as marker enzymes for lysosomes during isolation of the lysosomal fraction from cell homogenates. *See also* LYSOSOME.

Caxtat. *See* ENVIRONMENTAL DISASTERS.

CCNU. *See* 1-(2-CHLOROETHYL)-3-CYCLOHEXYL-1-NITROSOUREA.

CCPR. *See* CODEX COMMISSION ON PESTICIDE RESIDUES.

CDC. *See* CENTERS FOR DISEASE CONTROL.

cecum. A blind pouch comprising the cephalic region of the large intestine and having the vermiform appendix attached.

ceiling limit. A concentration of a chemical in the work place that should not be exceeded, even transiently. *See also* THRESHOLD LIMIT VALUE, CEILING.

celiac sprue. *See* GLUTEN, WHEAT.

cell. The basic structural and functional biological unit. Although morphology and composition vary greatly with function, the typical cell has a nucleus containing the chromatin bounded by the nuclear envelope, the endoplasmic reticulum, mitochondria, ribosomes, Golgi apparatus, lysosomes, cytoskeleton, cell membrane and cytosol. Cells in multicellular organisms are differentiated for specialized functions. Cells are the basic components of tissues.

cell–cell interaction. The interaction of cells by physical connections or by chemical communication. Physical connections (junctions) include: tight junctions, which fuse cell membranes of adjacent cells and form impermeable barriers around cells; gap junctions, which allow small cytoplasmic channels to exist between adjacent cells that allow for communication of small chemicals (an example is an electrotonic synapse); and desmosomes, points of very strong attachment between cells for adhesion. Cells may communicate chemically via neurotransmitters and neuromodulators at chemical synapses, by hormones and by autocoids. *See also* AUTOCOIDS; NEUROTRANSMITTERS.

cell culture. General term used to indicate the growing of cells *in vitro*, either in tissue culture or as single cells. Cells in culture are not normally organized into tissues. Cells may be established in culture by making an explant of cells from the living organism under sterile conditions and placing the explant in a suitable sterile tissue culture medium. Many cells will grow only for a few generations and then die out and there is evidence to suggest that many or most vertebrate cells that become established in culture are virally transformed cells. Cells established in culture are referred to as a cell line (e.g., HeLa cell). Cells may be cultured either in a stirred suspension, on a glass or plastic surface of a roller tube or petri dish, or, in a recently developed technique, on the surface of inert minispheres which are themselves maintained in suspension. In recent years cell culture has become an invaluable tool for the investigation of mechanisms of toxicity, of xenobiotic metabolizing enzymes and for toxicity testing.

cell cycle. Sequence of phases (see figure) in cell activity between successive cell divisions. While in interphase the cell grows; it is difficult to delineate stages in this growth, but DNA is replicated during a discrete phase called the S (synthesis) phase. The cell division phase (which includes nuclear division—mitosis—and cytoplasmic division—cytokinesis) in called the M (mitotic) phase. The phase between the M phase and the start of the S phase is the G1 (gap or growth) phase; that between the end of DNA synthesis and the next M phase is the G2 phase. Consequently, cells in G1 have only one-half of each chromosome (one chromatid) present, and chromatid replication takes place during the S phase. Interphase, comprising the G1, S and G2 phases, usually comprises about 90% of the cell cycle time. Rates of cell division are very variable, mainly reflecting variations in the G1 phase from a few hours to several years. The length of time taken to progress from the start of the S phase to the end of the M phase tends to be relatively constant. The cell cycle can be arrested in the G1 phase by adverse conditions such as deprivation of essential nutrients. Once a restriction point (R point) late in G1 has been reached, however, cells complete their cycles at the normal rate notwithstanding any unfavorable environmental

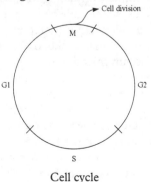

Cell cycle

conditions. It is suggested that cells need to accumulate by the R point a threshold amount of a trigger (or U) protein which then "triggers" the cell to go beyond the R point to commence a new cycle of division.

cell death. Normal cells die after a limited number of divisions (e.g., cultured mammalian lung fibroblasts die after 20–50 divisions), depending upon the age of the source animal. Aging cultures of cells take longer and longer to go through their cell cycles until division eventually ceases, the cellular contents become disorganized and obstructed with waste materials, and the cells die. The reason why such cell strains die is not known. It has been suggested that as cells differentiate they become programmed to die after a specified, finite number of divisions. This number of divisions is sometimes called the Hayflick limit, after its discoverer, and the phenomenon has been called programmed cell death. Cancerous cell lines (e.g., HeLa cells) will go on dividing indefinitely, as will some apparently normal, non-cancerous cell strains which are described as immortalized. *In vivo*, cell death after a fixed number of divisions may ensure that "rogue" cells that have escaped normal cell division control processes do not grow in an unbridled fashion. *See also* APOTOSIS.

cell division. Process by which a single cell divides to yield two daughter cells. Nuclear division (mitosis in somatic cells and meiosis in germ cells), is followed by division of the cytoplasm (cytokinesis) to yield the two daughter cells. Following division of animal cells a new membrane is synthesized to permit the growth that follows, whereas in plant cells, cell walls and middle lamellae are also laid down.

cell injury. Any process that harms or wounds a cell. Toxicants may cause cell injury directly or secondarily via disruption of normal physiological mechanisms. *See also* CELL TOXICITY.

cell junction. Connection between cells. Plant cells often have substantial cytoplasmic connections—plasmodesmata—and many embryonic cells are connected by cytoplasmic bridges. Other cell junctions function as communicating connections (e.g. gap junctions, synapses), as impermeable junctions controlling chemical communication and providing tissue integrity (e.g. tight junctions, septate junctions), and adhering junctions to provide tissue strength and elastic adhesion (e.g. belt desmosomes, spot desmosomes, hemidesmosomes). *See also* GAP JUNCTION.

cell-mediated immunity. An immunological response or reaction performed by cells, not by antibodies. It is usually initiated by T cells which may directly kill infected cells or may secrete soluble mediators which contribute to inflammation and subsequent elimination of the foreign material (antigen) that stimulated the response. Cell-mediated immune responses are specific for the antigen that elicited them, and a second encounter with that antigen produces a faster and more vigorous response. Cell-mediated immunity is especially important in resistance to infections caused by viruses, fungi and bacteria that can survive within phagocytic cells. It is also involved in immunity to immunogenic tumors and rejection of tissue grafts. Non-adaptive immunity to tumors probably involves non-T, non-B cells termed natural killer (NK) cells. *See also* CYTOTOXICITY; IMMUNE SYSTEM.

cell proliferation. The rapid growth of cells accompanied by assimilation of nutrients, high metabolic activity and an elevated mitotic index. This process is accompanied by an increase in tissue mass. Normal cells undergo division until contact with other cells inhibits their growth, whereas transformed cells lack this control mechanism.

cell toxicity. Any detrimental change in cellular physiology, biochemistry or morphology. Toxicants may cause cell toxicity directly by acting on specific biochemical loci or on many intracellular sites. Toxicants may also cause cell toxicity indirectly via disruption of normal physiological mechanisms, that secondarily cause poisoning of a cell. *See also* POISON; TOXIC ENDPOINTS.

cell transformation. The acquisition by a cell of the capacity for uncontrolled growth. It is one step in the series of events known as carcinogenesis that starts with initiation and ends with the formation of a tumor. *See also* MAMMALIAN CELL TRANSFORMATION TESTS.

cellular macromolecules. The large polymers within animal cells. They include proteins, nucleic acids and glycogen. Targets for toxicants among these are proteins and DNA. The protein targets may be enzymes, channel proteins, transport proteins or receptors, whose activities or functions can be inhibited or enhanced by interaction with toxicants. Covalent binding of toxicants to DNA leads to mutagenicity with subsequent alteration of genic expression and, therefore, of cellular function. This may lead to carcinogenesis.

Centers for Disease Control. Formerly the Communicable Disease Center, housed in Atlanta, Georgia, USA. An agency of the Department of Health and Human Services, formed to investigate the etiology of human diseases caused by either pathogens or chemicals.

centipedes. Venomous arthropods of the family *Myriopoda*. In the United States, bites are very painful but rarely fatal to humans. In some tropical regions, some centipedes are dangerous to humans.

central nervous system (CNS). The vertebrate brain and spinal cord. The nerves to the tissues comprise the peripheral nervous system. The peripheral nervous system consists of the somatic system and the autonomic (sympathetic and parasympathetic) system. The nervous system provides rapid communication between sensory and motor systems, as well as integrating sensory input to activate complex physiological and behavioral responses. This is accomplished by the conduction of waves of depolarization (nerve impulses) along specialized membranes in the axons of nerve cells (neurons). Communication between nerve cells is accomplished by a system of chemical messengers (neurotransmitters) and specialized receptors. The nervous system is a critically important site of toxic action. Due to the enormous complexity of the nervous system, neurotoxicology is a highly diverse and specialized branch of toxicology. The effects of neurotoxicants may be reflected in behavioral deficits and/or physiological deficits.

See also BLOOD–BRAIN BARRIER; DIAGNOSTIC FEATURES, CENTRAL NERVOUS SYSTEM; NEUROTOXICITY; NEUROTOXICOLOGY.

Centre National d'Information Toxicologiques Veterinaire (CNITV). Based at the Lyon veterinary school (France), providing advice on clinical poisoning cases as well as carrying out pharmacovigilance and toxicovigilance work.

centromere. The point of attachment of the two sister chromatids during the early events of mitosis. This may also be synonymous with kinetochore, the point of attachment of the chromosome to the spindle.

cephalosporins. Principal toxic side effects are allergic hypersensitivity reactions, including anaphylactic shock, and nephrotoxicity. There is frequently cross-sensitivity with penicillin, and penicillin-sensitive patients should not be given cephalosporins. *See also* ANTIBIOTICS.

CEQ. *See* COUNCIL ON ENVIRONMENTAL QUALITY.

CERCLA. *See* COMPREHENSIVE ENVIRONMENTAL RESPONSE, COMPENSATION AND LIABILITY ACT.

cervical. Pertaining to the cervix or the neck of an organ. *See also* CERVIX.

cervix. The neck of an organ. The term usually refers to the posterior-most region of the uterus, which extends slightly into the vagina and contains the opening for menstrual flow and for the birth of the fetus. The cervix is a frequent site of cancer.

cGMP. *See* CYCLIC GMP.

chambers, inhalation. *See* ADMINISTRATION OF TOXICANTS, INHALATION; EXPOSURE CHAMBERS.

charcoal. *See* ACTIVATED CHARCOAL.

chelating agents. Polydentate ligands capable of forming multiple coordinate covalent bonds with a metal. Chelating agents may have broad specificity or may be relatively selective for one or several metals. Chelation therapy is the use of chelating agents therapeutically to bind free metal ions, preventing their toxicity until the metal-chelate complex can be excreted. To a lesser extent, chelation therapy may assist in the removal of some metals from physiological stores, permitting their excretion and decreasing the body burden. Chelating agents may be toxic because they decrease the availability of essential trace minerals. For example, EDTA can form a complex with inorganic lead, but it also causes a rapid and harmful loss of calcium. Thus, the calcium chelate of EDTA is used in therapy, the lead chelate being formed by exchange of the calcium for lead. There is also some evidence that the mobilization of toxic metals by chelators may actually result in more delivery to the nervous system. *See also* DEFEROXAMINE; 2,3-DIMERCAPTO-1-PROPANOL; EDTA; PENICILLAMINE; TRIENTINE.

chelation therapy. *See* CHELATING AGENTS.

Chemical Abstracts Service (CAS). A service of the American Chemical Society which publishes abstracts of numerous journals, books and conference proceedings which are broadly related to the chemical sciences. Many toxicology works are represented. The abstracts are published biweekly and also contain indices and authors' addresses.

chemical effects on metabolism, induction. *See* XENOBIOTIC METABOLISM, CHEMICAL EFFECTS.

chemical effects on metabolism, inhibition. *See* XENOBIOTIC METABOLISM, CHEMICAL EFFECTS.

chemical oxygen demand (COD). The weight of oxygen taken up by the organic matter in a sample of water, assessed as the oxygen taken up from a solution of boiling potassium dichromate in two hours. The test is used to assess the strength of sewage and trade wastes. *Compare* BIOLOGICAL OXYGEN DEMAND.

Chemical Manufacturers Association (CMA). An association representing the US chemical industry. Includes groups that consider such toxicology-related aspects of chemical use as chemical safety, risk analysis, occupational health and environmental effects and management. The National Chemical Response and Information Center (NCRIC), established by CMA, consists of three services: the Chemical Transportation Emergency Center (CHEMTREC) provides information in the event of chemical emergencies; the Chemical Referral Center (CRC) provides safety and health information about chemicals through referrals to contacts within member companies; and CHEMNET is a network of shippers and contractors that provides advice and assistance in the event of chemical transportation emergencies.

Chemical Referral Center (CRC). *See* CHEMICAL MANUFACTURERS ASSOCIATION.

chemical sensitivity. An immunological reaction to chemical exposure in which an individual might react to the exposure by an allergic reaction or by a delayed hypersensitivity reaction.

Chemical Transportation Emergency Center (CHEMTREC). *See* CHEMICAL MANUFACTURERS ASSOCIATION.

CHEMNET. *See* CHEMICAL MANUFACTURERS ASSOCIATION.

chemoreceptor trigger zone. *See* ANTIEMETICS; AREA POSTREMA; EMESIS.

chemotherapy. The use of chemicals, singly or in combination, to reduce the rate of proliferation and to kill a population of cells causing a tumor, and in which the tumorigenic phenotype is heritable. The objective of chemotherapy is the selective destruction of the aberrant cells that in most aspects are identical to normal cells.

CHEMTREC. *See* CHEMICAL MANUFACTURERS ASSOCIATION.

Chernobyl. The site in the Ukraine of a large complex of nuclear power plants where, on 26 April 1986, one of four operational RMBK reactors failed catastrophically as a result of experiments conducted on it during a routine maintenance shut-down. The reactor building, partly destroyed by explosions and fire, released large clouds of radioactivity, amounting to an estimated total of 10^{16} becquerels. The fallout affected principally what was then the western part of the USSR, Poland and, to a lesser extent, parts of northwestern Europe. One worker was killed by falling debris, a second by steam burns and a further 29 from injuries or radiation sickness. Estimates of long-term cancer deaths have varied from less than 1000 to about 75,000 over 50 years. *See also* ENVIRONMENTAL DISASTERS.

chiasma. The visible result of crossing-over (breakage and reunion) between homologous chromatids of paired homologs during prophase of meiosis. The chiasma is manifested at late prophase and metaphase of meiosis as a cross-shaped region of the bivalent (pair of homologs) because of the fact that two sets of homologous chromatids are physically joined at the site of crossing-over. In order to avoid meiotic non-disjunction and resulting aneuploidy, every pair of homologs must acquire at least one chiasma during meiotic prophase. Therefore, the distribution of chiasmata among the linkage groups cannot be assumed to be uniform. White, M.J.D. Animal Cytology and Evolution, 3rd edn (Cambridge University Press, Cambridge, 1973).

Chimie et Ecologie. French association, with offices in Paris, formed to enhance developments of knowledge of effects of chemical and biological products on man and the environment.

Chinese hamster ovary cells (CHO cells). A cell line originally from a Chinese hamster ovary. These cells are used for *in vitro* mutagenicity testing to detect clastogenic agents and agents causing sister chromatid exchange (SCE). Following culture with the test chemical, either non-activated or activated with the S-9 fraction, the stained cells are scored for chromosomal aberrations, such as gaps, deletions, breaks and fragments, or for SCEs, for comparison with negative and positive controls. Two agents that can be employed in the non-activated and activated positive controls are ethylmethane sulfonate (EMS) and *N*-dimethylnitrosamine (DMN), respectively. Mitotic indices and the frequencies of M1, M2 and M3 cells (cells in first, second and third divisions, respectively) can also be recorded as signs of toxicity. *See also IN VIVO* TOXICITY TESTS; MAMMALIAN CELL MUTATION TESTS.

Chinese restaurant syndrome (CRS syndrome). A syndrome described in 1968 by Kwok et al. as a classic triad of symptoms that commences shortly after eating Chinese food and includes "numbness at the back of the neck, gradually radiating to both arms and the back, general weakness and palpitations". Single- and double-blind studies in humans provide little or no support for the theory that monosodium glutamate (MSG) is the sole causative agent in CRS. A dose of 12 g of MSG was required to produce at least one of the CRS symptoms in a study performed by Schaumburg. In clinical studies, only very large doses of MSG (doses that are much higher than those consumed in a Chinese meal) have mimicked CRS, making the causal link of MSG to CRS uncertain at best. Perhaps other ingredients, or combinations of ingredients, in a Chinese meal are responsible for CRS. Alternatively, only a very small fraction of the population may be sensitive to the CRS-producing effects of MSG. *See also* GLUTAMATE.

chi-square test (χ-square test). A statistical test typically used for testing hypotheses about the variance of a normally distributed population of scores. This test provides an estimate of the deviation of a sample ratio from a hypothetical population ratio. The test statistic is the ratio of the variance estimate for a sample of n observations multiplied by $(n-1)$ to the hypothesized value of the population variance. If the data are categorical, the χ-square statistic is obtained by summing the squared differences between observed and expected frequencies with each squared difference being divided by the expected frequency. In this instance, if the sample frequencies are the same as the hypothetical or expected frequencies, the value of χ-square would be zero. *See also* STATISTICS, FUNCTION IN TOXICOLOGY.

chloracne. A disfiguring skin rash caused by excessive exposure to chlorinated chemicals, especially noteworthy for TCDD. It is difficult to treat and has been known to persist for 15 years,

although workers exposed to TCDD at the Bolsover, Derbyshire, UK, factory of Coalite and Chemical Products Ltd in 1968 were free from chloracne after four years. Many cases of chloracne occurred as a result of the accident at Seveso, Italy. *See also* ENVIRONMENTAL DISASTERS; SEVESO; SEVESO DIRECTIVE; TCDD.

chloral betaine. *See* CHLORAL DERIVATIVES.

chloral derivatives. Any of the pharmaceutical formulations (e.g., chloral hydrate (Noctec); trichlofos (Triclos); chloral betaine (Beta-Chlor), β-chloralose, dichloral phenazone, chloral alcoholate) that have chloral as a basis, including the hemiacetals. These compounds are presumed all to be converted rapidly *in vivo* to 2,2,2-trichloroethanol, the apparent active species. There are many similarities between chloral derivatives and barbiturates. Both are used widely as sedative hypnotics, both induce xenobiotic metabolizing enzymes, both produce tolerance and physical dependence, and both produce a withdrawal syndrome marked by convulsions and delirium. *See also* MICKEY FINN.

chloral hydrate (2,2,2-trichloro-1,1-ethanediol; Noctec). CAS number 302-17-0. An oral sedative-hypnotic. Its oral LD50 in rats is 479 mg/kg. In overdose, its effects on the nervous system resemble those of the barbiturates. It causes slow, rapid and shallow breathing, pinpoint pupils, hypothermia, hypotension, coma and death. Therapy includes emptying the stomach with gastric lavage or induction of vomiting and symptomatic support. *See also* CHLORAL DERIVATIVES; MICKEY FINN.

$$Cl_3C-\underset{\underset{\textstyle OH}{|}}{C}HOH$$

Chloral hydrate

chlorambucil. CAS number 305-03-3. A nitrogen mustard used in the treatment of chronic lymphocytic leukemia. It is an alkylating agent, is itself a primary carcinogen and is cytotoxic and immunosuppressive. It is also known to affect reproductive function. *See also* NITROGEN MUSTARD.

$(ClCH_2CH_2)_2N$—⟨benzene ring⟩—$CH_2CH_2CH_2COOH$

Chlorambucil

chloramphenicol (D(-)-threo-2,2-dichloro-
N-[β-hydroxy-α-(hydroxymethyl)-p-nitro-
phenethyl]acetamide; chloromycetin; sinto-
mycetin; synthomycin). CAS number
56-75-7. An antibiotic produced by *Streptomyces*
venezulae (see structure in antibiotics entry). It is
effective against gram-positive bacteria and gram-
negative pathogenic spirochetes, psittacosis group
and rickettsiae that cause typhus. It blocks the site
on ribosomes where the 3′-terminus of amino
acyl-tRNA attaches, thus inhibiting protein synthesis. The oral LD50 in rats is 279 mg/kg. Chloramphenicol can cause blood dyscrasias in
humans, including aplastic anemia and granulocytopenia. High dosage in the neonate can cause
death. The therapy is discontinuance of the drug
and the employment of an alternate therapy. *See*
also ANTIBIOTICS; APLASTIC ANEMIA.

$$O=C—CHCl_2$$

$$O_2N—\text{⟨benzene ring⟩}—\underset{\underset{OH}{|}}{\overset{\overset{H}{|}}{C}}-\underset{\underset{H}{|}}{\overset{\overset{NH}{|}}{C}}-CH_2O\overset{\overset{O}{\|}}{C}(CH_2)_{14}CH_3$$

Chloramphenicol

chlordane. *See* CYCLODIENE INSECTICIDES.

chlordecone (decachlorooctahydro-1,3,4-meth-
eno-2H-cyclobuta[*cd*]pentalen-2-one; Kepone).
CAS number 143-50-0. An insecticide developed for
the control of ants and roaches, it also possesses activity as a fungicide. Its use was largely terminated following contamination of the James River estuary (Virginia, USA) as a result of improper production
practices. The oral LD50 in rats is 125 mg/kg. It is a
neurotoxicant, hepatotoxicant, and xenoestrogen. It has
been found to cause hepatocellular carcinoma in rats
and mice. In humans, it causes tremors, chest pain,
weight loss, mental changes, arthralgia, skin rash,
muscle weakness, incoordination and slurred speech.
Therapy is initially symptomatic, but administering

cholestyramine, a non-absorbable anion exchange
resin, increases the rate at which chlordecone is eliminated from the body.

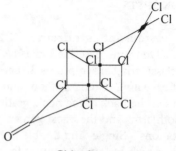

Chlordecone

chlordimeform (N′-(4-chloro-o-tolyl)-N,N-
dimethylformamidine; chlorophedine; chlo-
rophenamidine; bermat; C 8514; ENT 27567;
EP-333; Fundal; Galecron; SN 36268). CAS
number 6164-98-3. A formamidine acaricide and
ovicide effective against a variety of lepidopteran
species. The oral LD50 in male rats is 120–300
mg/kg and in female rats is 250–650 mg/kg. Chlordimeform is a neurotoxicant. The proposed mechanisms of action are reversible inhibition of
monoamine oxidase, as an octopaminergic agonist
in insects, and as an adrenergic agonist/antagonist
(low/high doses) in mammals. Symptoms and signs
in humans include hemorrhagic cystitis, dysuria,
nocturia, hematuria, proteinuria, abdominal pain,
respiratory failure and dermatitis. There is no specific antidote; treatment is symptomatic.

$$Cl—\text{⟨benzene ring with } CH_3\text{⟩}—N=CHN\overset{\diagup CH_3}{\diagdown CH_3}$$

Chlordimeform

chlorfenvinphos (organophorus insecticide).
CAS number 470-90-6. Cholinesterase inhibitor. Not known to cause cancer in animals or
humans. *See also* ATSDR DOCUMENT, AUGUST
1995; DATABASES, TOXICOLOGY; ORGANOPHOS-
PHORUS INSECTICIDES; ORGANOPHOSPHORUS
POISONING, SYMPTOMS AND THERAPY.

chloride channel. Chloride ions are distributed
almost at equilibrium in many animal cells so that
the equilibrium potential for chloride is near the

resting potential. For this reason chloride channels provide a stabilizing influence by opposing normal excitability and repolarizing cells after depolarization. Three broad categories exist: steeply voltage-dependent channels; weakly voltage-dependent "background" channels; and transmitter-activated synaptic channels. Steeply voltage-dependent channels in reconstituted membranes are permeable to Cl⁻ and Br⁻ only. A significant stabilizing action by "background" channels exists in some excitable membranes. These channels are permeable to Cl⁻ and are blocked by Zn^{2+}. Transmitter-activated synaptic channels are specialized for mediating chemical synaptic transmission or for transducing sensory stimuli. Although these channels gate ion movement and generate electrical signals, they do so in response to non-electrical stimuli. The acetylcholine-activated channels of the neuromuscular junction are activated by acetylcholine to open and subsequently initiate depolarization. The GABA receptor complex, like the acetylcholine receptor complex, includes an ion channel permeable to Cl⁻.

chlorinated alicyclic insecticides. *See* CYCLODIENE INSECTICIDES.

chlorinated hydrocarbon insecticides. *See* ORGANOCHLORINE INSECTICIDES.

chlorination of water. A process used to make water supplies safe from contamination by microorganisms. It has resulted, however, in the presence of several potentially carcinogenic halogenated hydrocarbons in the treated water, including chloroform, carbon tetrachloride, 1,2-dichloroethane, bromodichloromethane, dibromochloromethane and bromoform.

chlorine (Cl). CAS number 7782-50-5. A nonflammable gas, with a pungent odor. Chlorine is used as a bleaching agent for paper, pulp and textiles, as a disinfectant, in detinning and dezincing iron, and in the manufacture of chlorinated lime, inorganic and organic compounds, such as metallic chlorides, chlorinated solvents, pesticides and polymers. Fires and explosions can result from its reaction with some substances. Chlorine is extremely irritating to the eyes and skin, but it is usually considered to be a respiratory toxicant.

Chlorine forms acids when in contact with body water, so causes irritation of eyes, skin and respiratory membranes, as well as corrosion of teeth and chloracne. Systemically, it causes choking, swelling of mucous membranes, nausea, vomiting, anxiety, and syncope. Respiratory tract symptoms can include cough, chest pain, dyspnea, cyanosis, pulmonary edema, rales and pneumonia. The one-hour LC50 by inhalation is 293 ppm (by volume) for rats and 137 ppm for mice.

chlornaphazine. *See* N,N-BIS(CHLOROETHYL)-2-NAPHTHYLAMINE.

chlorodibenzofurans. A family of chemicals (135 congeners) with from one to eight chlorine substituents on the parent compound, dibenzofuran. Produced primarily by thermal degradation of polychlorinated biphenyls (PCBs) or fires involving electrical equipment containing PCBs. Acute and chronic effects similar to the chlorinated benzodioxins. *See also* ATSDR DOCUMENT, MAY 1994.

1-(2-chloroethyl)-3-cyclohexyl-1-nitrosourea (CCNU; Lomustine). CAS number 13010-47-4. CCNU and its methyl analog semustine (methyl-CCNU) are alkylating agents used in the treatment of Hodgkin's disease and other lymphomas. Clinical toxicity includes delayed bone marrow suppression, nausea and vomiting.

$$ClCH_2CH_2-\underset{\underset{N=O}{|}}{N}-\overset{\overset{O}{\|}}{C}-NH-\bigcirc$$

CCNU

chloroethyl phosphate, tris. *See* TRIS (2-CHLOROETHYL) PHOSPHATE.

chlorofluorocarbons. *See* FLUOROCARBONS.

chloroform (trichloromethane; $CHCl_3$). CAS number 67-66-3. A colorless liquid with a high vapor pressure and a characteristic odor. It has been used as an anesthetic, but its use has been discontinued because it is hepatotoxic and nephrotoxic, and may cause cardiac arrhythmias leading to death. The liver and kidney damage, accompanied by nausea, abdominal pain and jaundice, often occurred within days of surgery. It is still used as an industrial solvent. Like carbon tetrachloride, hepatotoxicity probably is mediated via cytochrome P450, with the resulting trichloromethyl radical $\left(\text{CCl}_3^{\bullet}\right)$ electrophilically attacking nucleophilic substituents of cells. Animal carcinogen. Classified as a possible human carcinogen by IARC and as a probable human carcinogen by the US EPA. *See also* CARBON TETRACHLORIDE; DRY-CLEANING SOLVENTS; ATSDR DOCUMENT, AUGUST 1995; DATABASES, TOXICOLOGY.

chloromethane. *See* METHYL CHLORIDE.

chloromethyl methyl ether. A designated suspected human carcinogen (IARC), hazardous waste (EPA) and priority toxic pollutant (EPA). It is a volatile liquid that is often contaminated with bis(chloromethyl) ether, which is a known human carcinogen. It is used as an intermediate in the synthesis of organic chemicals. Entry into the body is primarily by inhalation. It is irritating to the skin and mucous membranes, and systemically appears to be carcinogenic. It is not clear, however, whether this is due to its intrinsic activity or to the contaminant, bis(chloromethyl) ether. Animal studies with the pure compound show very low, if any, carcinogenicity. *See also* BIS(CHLOROMETHYL) ETHER.

$$CH_3OCH_2Cl$$

Chloromethyl methyl ether

chloroquine (7-chloro-4-(4-diethylamino-1-methylbutylamino)quinoline). CAS number 54-05-7. An effective antimalarial drug that causes especially high incidences of injuries to the visual system. Dose-related retinopathies have been reported, as well as damage to the hearing. Because of concentration in the liver, it is also contraindicated in patients with liver damage. *See also* RETINOPATHY.

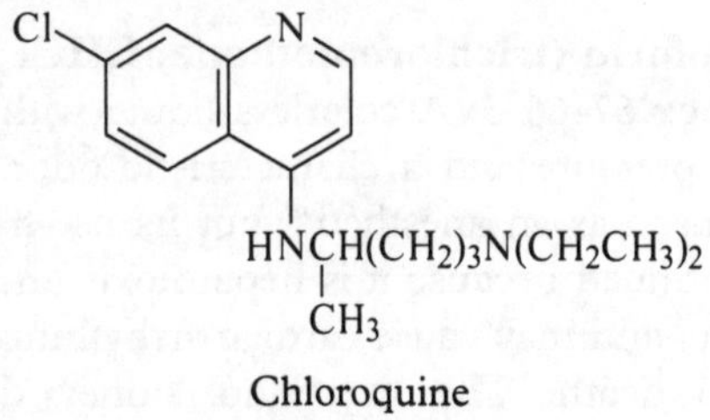

Chloroquine

chloroquinol (Enterovioform). An antidiarrhea drug used extensively in Japan. It has been shown to be the cause of subacute myelooptic neuropathy, a syndrome in which stiffness of the joints is accompanied by damage to the optic nerve.

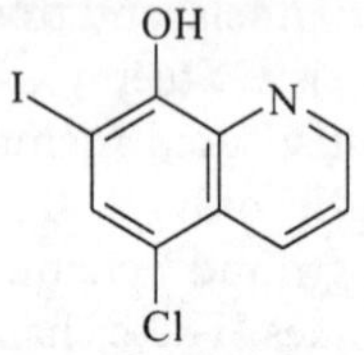

Chloroquinol

chlorpheniramine. Antihistaminic drug that blocks H_1 histamine receptors. Causes drowsiness and sedation that can be addictive with other central nervous system depressants. *See also* ANTIHISTAMINES; DATABASES, TOXICOLOGY.

chlorpromazine (2-chloro-10-(3-dimethylaminopropyl)phenothiazine; Thorazine). CAS number 50-53-3. The prototypical phenothiazine antipsychotic drug. Derivatives were used as dyestuffs in the late 19th century, and Ehrlich suggested that the resulting aniline dyes might be used to treat psychoses. It was first synthesized while searching for better anesthetic-potentiating agents. It was found to cause more than symptomatic relief of agitation or anxiety and was ameliorative of various symptomatologies. The introduction of chlorpromazine in the early 1950s led to the development of numerous phenothiazine analogs and also resulted in the structurally related tricyclic antidepressants. Although relatively safe in terms of acute toxicity, chlorpromazine causes some acute neurological effects (extrapyramidal side effects) and, like other antipsychotic drugs, may increase the incidence of tardive dyskinesia. Drug metabolism may markedly alter clinical response for chlorpromazine, and it has been proposed that it may have nearly 200 metabolites, although there are significant circulating

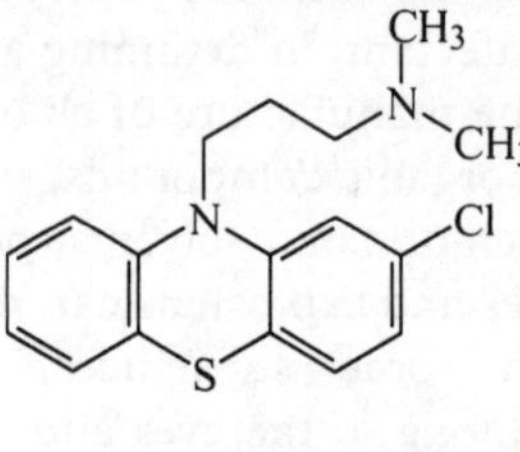

Chlorpromazine

concentrations of only six or eight of these. Chlorpromazine is a relatively potent dopamine receptor blocker and has slight antihistaminic and antiadrenergic properties. *See also* ANTIPSYCHOTIC DRUGS; DOPAMINE; DOPAMINE RECEPTORS; TARDIVE DYSKINESIA; TRICYLIC ANTIDEPRESSANTS.

chlorpyrifos. CAS number 2921-89-2. Organophosphorus insecticide. Cholinesterase inhibitor. Not known to cause cancer in animals or humans. *See also* ATSDR DOCUMENT, AUGUST 1995; DATABASES, TOXICOLOGY; ORGANOPHOSPHORUS INSECTICIDES; ORGANOPHOSPHORUS POISONING, SYMPTOMS AND THERAPY.

CHO. *See* CHINESE HAMSTER OVARY CELLS.

cholera toxin (choleragen). An 87,000-dalton protein, A1 peptide linked to an A2 peptide and five B peptides. It is secreted by the gram-negative bacterium *Vibrio cholerae*. It is a gastrointestinal toxin that increases adenylate cyclase activity of mucosa of the small intestine, thereby increasing cyclic AMP within these cells. Cyclic AMP stimulates active transport of ions by these epithelial cells, resulting in a large efflux of Na^+ and water into the gut. The toxin enters cells by interacting with a GM1 ganglioside on the cell surface. After entry, the A1 subunit catalyzes the transfer of an ADP-ribose unit from NAD^+ to an arginine side chain of the adenylate cyclase regulatory G protein, blocking its GTPase activity. Thus the adenylate cyclase deactivation mechanism is destroyed, and cyclic AMP is continually produced. The major sign of cholera poisoning is severe diarrhea; several liters of body water may be lost within a few hours, leading to shock and death if fluid is not replaced. Treatment involves physiological support (including i.v. fluids) and antibiotics. *See also* ADENYLATE CYCLASE; CYCLIC AMP.

cholestasis. An arrest or decrease in the flow of bile, resulting in hyperbilirubinemia and retention of sulfobromophthalein, a dye excreted almost exclusively in bile. Cholestasis can be induced by a wide variety of compounds (e.g., α-naphthylisothiocyanate, lithocholate, steroid D-ring glucuronides, manganese) by, as yet, ill-defined mechanisms.

cholesterol (5-cholesten-3β-ol, $C_{27}H_{46}O$). CAS number 57-88-5. Present in all parts of the animal body; concentrated in spinal cord, brain, skin secretions and gallstones. An unsaturated, unsaponifiable alcohol (m.p. 149 °C). It is synthesized in the body from ethanoate units; its metabolism is regulated by a specific set of enzymes. It is the parent compound of many other steroids and its presence in high concentrations in the blood is suspected as being a contributory factor in cardiovascular disease.

Cholesterol

cholestyramine. An anion exchange resin (main component: polystyrene trimethylammonium as Cl^- anion) that can be administered orally to bind the insecticide chlordecone. It enhances the excretion of chlordecone several fold, reduced the half-life of chlordecone in the body and enhances the rate of recovery from toxic signs. It has also been used to minimize absorption of cardiac glycosides, and to disrupt their enterohepatic circulation. It binds bile salts very effectively, and by this action it indirectly lowers serum low-density lipoproteins. It can cause digestive tract distress, such as constipation, and can retard fat absorption.

choline acetyltransferase (ChAT). The mitochondrial enzyme that synthesizes the neurotransmitter acetylcholine from its precursors acetyl CoA and choline. The rate-limiting step in acetylcholine formation is high-affinity choline uptake into nerve terminals, not choline acetyltransferase activity. *See also* ACETYLCHOLINE.

cholinergic crisis. The excessive accumulation of acetylcholine with resultant symptomology characteristic of hyperactivity of cholinergic pathways. The term is used to describe the overtreatment of myasthenics with an anticholinesterase, such as neostigmine. The same effects occur in poisoning with organophosphate or carbamate anticholinesterases. *See also* CARBAMATE POISON-ING, SYMPTOMS AND THERAPY; ORGANOPHOS-PHATE POISONING, SYMPTOMS AND THERAPY.

cholinesterase. *See* ACETYLCHOLINESTERASE.

cholinesterase, in chronic toxicity testing. *See* ACETYLCHOLINESTERASE; TOXIC ENDPOINTS.

cholinesterase, in subchronic toxicity testing. *See* ACETYLCHOLINESTERASE; TOXIC END-POINTS.

cholinesterase inhibitors. *See* ANTICHOLINES-TERASES.

choline uptake, high-affinity, sodium-dependent. A specific sodium-dependent process for choline entry into cholinergic nerve terminals, whereby choline can be used for synthesis of acetylcholine by the enzyme choline acetyltransferase. The process proceeds at low concentrations of choline, and demonstrates typical saturation kinetics. It is a marker for cholinergic neurons and is distinguishable from the widespread low-affinity choline uptake process, which requires higher choline concentrations. Unlike the situation with most other neurotransmitters, choline uptake is often the rate-limiting step in acetylcholine formation. The process is inhibited specifically by hemicholinium-3. *See also* HEMICHOLINIUM-3.

cholinoreceptors. *See* ACETYLCHOLINE RECEP-TORS, MUSCARINIC AND NICOTINIC.

chorionic gonadotropins. Gonadotropins (i.e., hormones that stimulate the gonads) are produced by the chorionic villi of the placenta. They are found in the blood of pregnant women (human chorionic gonadotropin, hCG) and mares (pregnant mare serum, PMG). hCG has an action like luteinizing hormone (LH), stimulating the ovarian corpus luteum to produce progesterone and estrogen to maintain the pregnancy and to prevent menstruation. The presence of hCG in the urine is the basis for many pregnancy tests. It is produced for about the first 10 weeks of pregnancy. hCG is produced in high levels by a hydatiform (hydatid) mole during a molar pregnancy.

chromatid. One of the DNA molecules in the replicated DNA into which the chromosome will separate during mitosis. It is connected to its sister chromatid in the early stages of mitosis at the centromere and, later, by the interaction of its kinetochore with the spindle, it is moved to one of the poles and the sister moves to the other pole.

chromatid exchange assay. *See* SISTER CHRO-MATID EXCHANGE.

chromatin. The diffuse, thread-like DNA with its associated nucleoproteins in the interphase (non-dividing) nucleus. The chromatin will condense during mitosis into chromosomes.

chromatogram. A trace indicating the zones to which a chemical (i.e., an analyte) has migrated during chromatography. Detector output is recorded in the form of a continuous trace in gas–liquid chromatography and high-performance liquid chromatography. In paper chromatography and thin-layer chromatography, it is the developed surface on which the separate zones have been revealed; if the surface is scanned with a densitometer (or other suitable device) a similar trace can be obtained (*see* figure). t_1, t_2, and V_1, V_2 are the retention times and volumes, respectively, for components 1 and 2. The resolution (R_s) is given by

$$R_s = \frac{2(t_2 - t_1)}{V_1 + V_2}$$

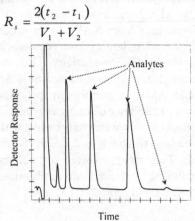

Example of a chromatogram

chromatography. Physical methods of separation in which the components or solute compounds to be separated are distributed between two phases, one of which is stationary and the other mobile. The chromatographic process occurs as a result of repeated sorption/desorption acts during the movement of the solute compounds through the stationary phase. Separations are based on differences in the extent to which solutes are partitioned between the mobile and stationary phase; described quantitatively by the temperature-dependent partition coefficient (K)

$$K = \frac{c_s}{c_m}$$

where c_s and c_m are the total analytical concentrations of the solute in the stationary and mobile phases, respectively. The assumption that K is constant is generally satisfied provided the concentrations are low. This process results in a differential migration of the solute compounds and hence their separation. Chromatography takes many forms depending upon the nature of the stationary and mobile phase comprising the system. See also CHROMATOGRAPHY, COLUMN; CHROMATOGRAPHY, GAS–LIQUID; CHROMATOGRAPHY, HIGH-PERFORMANCE LIQUID; CHROMATOGRAPHY, PAPER; CHROMATOGRAPHY, THIN-LAYER.

chromatography, affinity. Technique that depends on the highly biospecific interaction between an immobilized ligand and the macromolecule of interest. The ligand (e.g., enzyme, nucleic acid, hormone, antigen, dye) is bound by a hydrophilic spacer arm to a matrix. Molecules that bind with the immobilized ligand are retarded by the column matrix to be eluted later under conditions in which the binding affinity is reduced. Immobilized boronic acid has an extremely broad specificity for the separation of nucleosides, nucleotides, glycoproteins, catecholamines, carbohydrates and tRNA. Anti-immunoglobulin ligands are used for antibody purification, triazine dyes for enzymes and lectins (e.g., concanavalin A) for specific sugars, carbohydrate residues or sequences in glycoproteins. See also CHROMATOGRAM; CHROMATOGRAPH.

chromatography, column. A chromatographic separation technique in which the stationary phase is confined to a tube and the solute compounds are gradually eluted as the mobile phase percolates through the column of the stationary bed. The composition and dimensions of the tube depend upon the particular type of column chromatography used. For instance, high-performance liquid chromatography utilizes special stainless steel columns to furnish sufficient mechanical strength to withstand the column operating pressure associated with the delivery of the mobile phase at relatively high positive pressure. Column chromatography permits the controlled elution of solute compounds and provides a means of concentrating the stationary phase and performing chromatographic separations at pressures other than atmospheric. See also CHROMATOGRAPHY; CHROMATOGRAPHY, HIGH-PERFORMANCE LIQUID; CHROMATOGRAM.

chromatography, gas–liquid (GLC; GC). A chromatographic technique for separating volatile solute compounds in which the mobile phase is an inert gas and the stationary phase is a liquid distributed over the surface of a porous, inert support. The compounds to be separated are carried through the column by a carrier gas, partitioned between the carrier gas and a non-volatile solvent (the stationary phase) supported on an inert size-graded solid (the solid support). The stationary phase selectively retards the solute compounds, according to their differences in solubility in the stationary phase, until they form separate bonds in the carrier gas. The versatility and selectivity of gas–liquid chromatography are due to the wide variety of stationary phases available. The formation of less polar, more volatile derivatives permits the assay of solute compounds that are not amenable to gas–liquid chromatographic separation in the underivatized form. Elution time can be modified as a function of column temperature, with chromatograms obtained under isothermal conditions or by the increase of column temperature during an analysis (temperature programming) to permit the separation of compounds of widely varying retention in a single chromatographic run. See also CHROMATOGRAPHY; CHROMATOGRAPHY, COLUMN; CHROMATOGRAM.

chromatography, gel filtration. Separation technique dependent on the shape and size of the solute molecules. The mixture applied at the top of a column of gel is washed through the gel with water, buffer solution or organic solvent. Solutes with molecules larger than the largest pores of the swollen gel beads (above the exclusion limit) cannot penetrate the particles and pass through the bed in the liquid phase outside the gel and emerge from the bottom first. Smaller molecules can penetrate the particles to varying extents resulting in a partition between the liquid inside the gel and that outside. The gels are based on cross-linked dextrans, polyacrylamides, high-molecular-mass polysaccharides (e.g., agarose), etc. The technique can be used not only for the separation of macromolecules, but also for an approximate determination of relative molecular mass (M_r). *See also* CHROMATOGRAPHY.

chromatography, high-performance liquid. (HPLC; high-pressure liquid chromatography; liquid chromatography). A chromatographic technique for separating solute compounds in which the mobile phase is a liquid and the stationary phase is typically a polar absorbent (e.g., microparticulate silica) to which an array of functional groups may be bonded. As with other forms of chromatography, retention is dependent upon the relative affinity of the solute compounds for the mobile phase and the stationary phase, the functionalities of the stationary phase and the physical and chemical properties of the solute compounds. Unlike gas–liquid chromatography, the mobile phase is not inert, but instead contributes greatly to solute retention. Two major forms of HPLC are generally recognized: normal-phase (adsorption) and bonded-phase chromatography. In adsorption chromatography, the retention of the solute is a consequence of the interaction with the surface of the polar absorbent using non-polar organic mobile phases, in which acyl carbon chains of varying length are chemically bonded to the polar absorbent. Reversed-phase chromatography represents the most popular form of bonded-phase chromatography. Typically, reversed-phase chromatography utilizes polar mobile phases and non-polar stationary phases. The stationary phase in ion exchange chromatography consists of absorbents to which anionic or cationic groups have been bonded. *See also* CHROMATOGRAPHY; CHROMATOGRAPHY, COLUMN; CHROMATOGRAM.

chromatography, high-performance liquid affinity (HPLAC). Technique combining affinity chromatography for selectivity with high-performance chromatography for high resolution, speed of analysis and sensitive detection. Typical HPLAC columns, based on 10 μm spherical silica for high-dimensional stability are boronate for the separation of nucleotides, nucleosides, carbohydrates, etc. and concanavalin A for the separation of closely related carbohydrates and glycoproteins.

chromatography, paper. A planar chromatographic system in which solute compounds are separated using a mobile phase composed of varying proportions of polar and non-polar solvents and a stationary phase consisting of purified cellulose paper of varying fiber coarseness and packing density. Solutes are "spotted" as solutions in volatile solvents on the paper and developed by capillary action in an ascending or descending mode using an appropriate solvent system. The separation mechanism involves adsorption (e.g., hydrogen bonding, van der Waals forces) on the cellulose fibers, ion exchange with the carboxy groups on the cellulose and partition between the mobile phase and the water content of the cellulose. As with thin-layer chromatography, relative migration of solutes is expressed as R_f values, defined by the ratio between the distance that the solute has travelled from the origin and the distance that the solvent front has travelled from the origin. *See also* CHROMATOGRAPHY; CHROMATOGRAPHY, THIN-LAYER.

chromatography, reversed phase. Technique in which the mobile phase is hydrophilic and the stationary phase hydrophobic. The mobile phase (commonly a mixture of aqueous buffer with methanol, ethanol or acetonitrile) is the more polar phase, and polar solutes will move with this phase rather than remain with the less polar stationary phase. Reversed-phase chromatography is now widely used in toxicology research and with thin-layer chromatography.

chromatography, reversed phase high-performance liquid (RP-HPLC). Powerful method of separation of peptides and proteins, using a stationary hydrophobic phase and a polar mobile phase (*see* REVERSED-PHASE CHROMATOGRAPHY). The extent of retention of a molecule depends on the number, size and stereochemistry of its hydrophobic and hydrophilic groups, and is manifested by the combined interactions of each group with the stationary and mobile phases and even with each other. Reversed phases such as octadecylsilyl (ODS), octylsilyl, butylsilyl and propylsilyl functions bonded to silica supports, and mobile phases consisting of aqueous solutions of various acids with ethanenitrile, methanol or propanol have been used with success in the separation of a range of proteins.

chromatography, thin-layer (TLC). A chromatographic separation technique using a liquid mobile phase that moves by capillary action through a thin layer of sorbent (the stationary phase) coated on an inert, rigid backing material or plate. The mobile phase or solvent system consists of a single solvent or a mixture of solvents of varying polarity, and common stationary phases include silica, alumina, cellulose, polyamides and ion exchangers. The separation mechanisms vary with the sorbent used and the physiochemical properties of the solute compounds and include hydrogen bonding, phase partitioning and ion exchange. Typically, the sample to be separated is applied to the edge of the sorbent layer as a spot, and the plate is developed in an enclosed chamber by contacting the solvent system. Additional separation power can be obtained by two-dimensional development in which a developed plate is rotated through $90°$ and redeveloped using a different solvent system. Relative migration of a solute compound is expressed as an R_f value, defined by the ratio between the distance travelled by the solute from the origin and the distance travelled by the solvent front from the origin. *See also* CHROMATOGRAPHY; CHROMATOGRAPHY, PAPER.

chromium (Cr). Elemental chromium and certain chromium compounds have been designated as carcinogens, hazardous substances, hazardous waste constituents and priority toxic pollutants. Some of those compounds designated as hazardous are chromic acetate, chromic acid, chromic sulfate and chromous chloride. The chromium atom in chromium compounds is in one of three valence states (2^+, 3^+ or 6^+). Chromium trioxide is the most commonly used chromium compound, being employed in chrome plating, aluminum anodizing, as a catalyst in organic syntheses and in

other industrial processes. It is clear that a number of chromium compounds are human carcinogens, and they are regulated as such. The structure–activity relationships, however, are less clear. Although chromium in the 6^+ state is regarded as being the most carcinogenic, there are 6^+ compounds that appear to be non-carcinogenic. In addition to their possible carcinogenicity, chromium compounds may have local allergic effects leading to dermatitis. Systemically, 6^+ chromium compounds are irritants to the respiratory system and may give rise to pulmonary edema. *See also* ATSDR DOCUMENT, APRIL 1993; DATABASES, TOXICOLOGY.

chromosome. The condensed form of chromatin (DNA plus nucleoproteins) visible during mitosis. *See also* CHROMATID; CHROMATIN.

chromosome aberrations. All chromosomal changes that are detectable by light microscopy. Gaps are achromatic lesions in a chromosome that vary in length and are thought to be due to loss of DNA. Breaks are broken ends of chromatids that are seen to be dislocated, but are still contained within the metaphase. Several genetic diseases (e.g., Bloom's syndrome and Fanconi's anemia) are correlated with chromosomal breaks, and many chemicals, as well as ionizing radiation, can cause breakage of chromosomes. Alkylating agents, especially bifunctional alkylating agents, may cause breaks by cross-linking with DNA. Chromosomal mutations are changes in chromosomes arising from incorrect reincorporation of broken parts. The main types of change are deletions, translocation, duplications and inversions. Deletions and translocations are relatively easy to detect using microscopy and are important in mutagenicity testing. Numerical aberrations are a consequence of unequal division of chromosomes and result in a cell with either more or fewer chromosomes than normal (i.e., aneuploidy). Such cells may or may not be viable. Genetic diseases that result from the unequal division (nondisjunction) of chromosomes include Down's syndrome (mongolism), Klinefelter's syndrome, and Turner's syndrome. Several chemicals are known to induce polyploidy, a condition in which each chromosome occurs more than the normal number of times. The best known examples are the metaphase poisons. Colchicine, a specific spindle poison, binds to the spindle protein tubulin and inhibits its polymerization thus blocking mitosis at metaphase, resulting in polyploidy. Other compounds that can cause similar effects are the *Vinca* alkaloids vincristine and vinblastine, and podophyllotoxin, which binds to the same site as colchicine. Polyploidy is well known in plants and is used extensively in plant breeding. In animals, however, polyploidy is not usually viable and is generally a lethal mutation. *See also* FRAMESHIFT MUTATION; MUTATION; PODOPHYLLOTOXIN; POINT MUTATION; VINBLASTINE; VINCRISTINE.

chromosome aberration tests. Tests for chromosomal damage using eukaryotic cultured cells or intact organisms that assess large effects in chromosomes, such as breaks or exchange of DNA between chromosomes. These include sister chromatid exchange tests *in vitro* with Chinese hamster ovary (CHO) cells or cells from animals exposed to the toxicant *in vivo*, the *in vivo* micronucleus test in mice and the *in vivo* dominant lethal test in rodents. In addition, chromosomal aberrations can be observed microscopically in cultured CHO cells treated *in vitro* or in bone marrow cells or lymphocytes obtained from animals treated *in vivo*. Aberrations to be observed include: gaps, breaks or deletions in chromatids or chromosomes; chromosome fragments; translocations; ploidy. The heritability of translocations and other chromosome aberrations can also be observed in the progeny of treated animals. *See also* DOMINANT LETHAL (RODENTS) TEST; MICRONUCLEUS TEST; SISTER CHROMATID EXCHANGE TEST.

chromosome breaking agents. *See* CHROMOSOME ABERRATIONS; CLASTOGEN.

chromosome mutations. *See* CHROMOSOME ABERRATIONS.

chronic exposure. *See* EXPOSURE, CHRONIC.

chronicity index. A numerical expression of cumulative toxicity. It is the ratio between the single-dose LD50 [LD50(1)] and the 90-dose LD50 [LD50(90)], the latter being defined as that dose which, administered daily, will cause 50% mortality in the test population i.e.

$$\frac{LD50(1)}{LD(90)}$$

Considering the number of animals, time, facilities and personnel required to conduct the LD50(90), it is doubtful whether the accurate determination of the chronicity index can be justified. A semi-quantitative expression of cumulative toxicity can be derived from the acute, subchronic, and chronic tests prescribed for other regulatory purposes.

chronic obstructive pulmonary disease (COPD). A lung disease that involves increased resistance to air flow in the bronchial airways and decreased tissue elasticity, leading to decreased ventilation. COPD can be the long-term result of chronic bronchitis, emphysema, asthma or chronic bronchiolitis. Since these health effects may, in some cases, result from exposure to chemicals, COPD can, in those cases, be considered a chronic toxic endpoint.

chronic toxicity. The adverse effects manifested after a long time period of uptake of small quantities of a toxicant. The dose is small enough that no acute effects are manifested, and the time period is frequently a significant part of the expected normal lifetime of the organism. The most serious manifestation of chronic toxicity is carcinogenesis, but other types of chronic toxicity are also known (e.g., reproductive or neural effects). *See also* CARCINOGENICITY TESTING; CHRONIC TOXICITY TESTING.

chronic toxicity testing. Chronic tests are those conducted over the greater part of the lifespan of the test species or, in some cases, in more than one generation. The most important tests of this type are chronic toxicity, carcinogenicity, teratogenicity, and reproduction. Chronic toxicity tests are designed to discover any of numerous toxic effects, and to define safety margins to be used in the regulation of chemicals. As with subchronic tests, usually either a rat or a mouse strain is used, and the tests are run for 2.0–2.5 years or 1.5–2.0 years, respectively. Less commonly a non-rodent species (e.g., dog), a non-human primate or a small carnivore (e.g., ferret) is used. Chronic toxicity tests may involve administration in the food, in the drinking water, by gavage, or by inhalation, the first route being the most common. The doses used are the maximum tolerated dose (MTD) and usually two lower doses of 0.25 MTD and 0.125 MTD. The requirements for animal facilities, housing and environmental conditions are similar to those for subchronic studies (*see* TESTING VARI-ABLES, NON-BIOLOGICAL). Special attention must be paid to the diet formulation since it is impractical to formulate a single batch of each for a two-year study or even longer. Semi-synthetic diets of specified components are formulated regularly, and analyzed before use. The endpoints used in these studies are the same as those for a subchronic study (i.e., appearance, ophthalmology, food consumption, body weight, clinical signs, behavioral signs, hematology, blood chemistry, urinalysis, fecal analysis, organ weights, histology). Some animals may be sacrificed at fixed intervals during the test (e.g., at 6, 12 or 18 months) for histological examination. Particular attention is paid to organs or to animals from dose levels that showed compound-related effects in preliminary subchronic studies. *See also* CARCINOGENICITY TESTING; CHRONIC TOXICITY TESTING, END-POINTS; REPRODUCTIVE TOXICITY TESTING; TERATOLOGY TESTING; TESTING VARIABLES, BIOLOGICAL; TOXIC ENDPOINTS.

chronic toxicity testing, endpoints. The endpoints examined in both chronic and subchronic tests are similar, covering a wide variety of physiological, clinical, biochemical and pathological parameters. *See also* TOXIC ENDPOINTS.

chronic toxicity testing, factors affecting. *See* TESTING VARIABLES, BIOLOGICAL; TESTING VARIABLES, NON-BIOLOGICAL.

chrysotile asbestos. *See* ASBESTOS.

cigarettes. Units for smoking containing tobacco wrapped in paper. When smoked, the smoke releases a variety of carcinogenic and toxic chemicals, most notable of which are the polycyclic aromatic hydrocarbons, that are part of the "tar" and are carcinogenic; metals may also be contained in the smoke. Nicotine is present in the smoke, and makes the use of cigarettes addictive. Various brands of cigarettes differ in their nicotine and tar content. Cigarette smoking is implicated strongly in the etiology of lung cancer, emphysema and cardiovascular disease, as well as some other diseases. In addition to the effects of smoke on the smoker, there is also toxicological concern about the effects of sidestream (second-hand) smoke on non-smokers; this issue is highly controversial. *See also* NICOTINE; POLYCYCLIC AROMATIC HYDROCARBONS; SECONDHAND SMOKE.

ciguatera. Ciguatera refers to intoxication resulting from the ingestion of tropical and subtropical fin fish, distinct either from histaminic poisonings or those associated with the pufferfish. Unlike other dinoflagellate toxins, ciguatoxin is rarely concentrated by filter feeding mollusks (shellfish) because of the sessile existence of the ciguatoxigenic dinoflagellates on macro-algae. The term "ciguatera" is derived from the Spanish word for snail (cigua) based on the belief that a marine turban snail was responsible for poisoning settlers in Cuba. Ciguatera is the most common disease associated with the consumption of fish in the United States and its territories. The illness is characterized initially by gastrointestinal inflammation, leading to severe dehydration and weakness and eventually cardiovascular and neurological distress. The most distinctive features of ciguatera are severe puritus, hot/cold reversal, and tingling and numbness of the extremities. The neurological symptoms can persist for months or even years, occasionally recurring in seemingly healthy individuals long after their recovery. Ciguatera symptoms are highly variable among individuals and among regions. A large dinoflagellate (*Gambierdiscus toxicus*) produces two toxins, ciguatoxin and maitotoxin, with similar chemical and pharmacological properties. Similarly active compounds have been extracted from the *Gymodinium sanguineum*, *Gonyaulax polyhedra*, *Coolia menotes* and *Amphidinium elegans*. Intoxication caused by brevetoxins is similar to ciguatoxin, distinguished only by time of onset. Ciguatoxin is insoluble in water or benzene, but readily partitions with methanol, acetone, ethanol or isopropanol. Ciguatoxin is a white solid lipid with the probable configuration of a highly oxygenated long-chain fatty acid. Proton NMR suggests a molecular weight of 1111 daltons and a polymer formula of

$C_{53}H_{77}NO_{24}$ or $C_{54}H_{78}O_{24}$, and may be structurally related to okadaic acid and brevetoxin c. Two additional toxins have been extracted from ciguatoxic fish; one (scaritoxin) is ether-soluble and the other (maitotoxin) is more water-soluble. Scaritoxin is found predominantly in many species of parrotfish (*Scarus*). Scaritoxin has not been detected in the diet of the parrotfish. Ciguatoxin is the predominant toxin in the gut and liver of the parrot fish. This suggests that scaritoxin is not produced by the dinoflagellate, but is a metabolite of ciguatoxin. Maitotoxin was originally isolated from the surgeonfish *Ctenochaetus striatus* and *G. toxicus* and possibly *P. concavum*. Maitotoxin has been produced in abundance in dinoflagellate cultures; however, it is not well characterized. Purified material yields an amorphous white solid whose molecular weight is around 3300 daltons. Some data support a molecular weight of approximately 50,000 daltons. There are no amino acid and fatty acid moieties in the molecule, and there appear to be no chemical similarities between maitotoxin and ciguatoxin.

ciguatoxin. *See* CIGUATERA.

cilia. Locomotory organelles comprising microtubule bundles with associated motor proteins. The ciliary motion either moves the cell (such as a protozoan) or it moves materials across the surface of cells, such as mucus through the respiratory tract or the ovum through the oviduct. The ciliated tracheobronchial cells are a major means of removing dusts and other accumulated particles from the respiratory tract.

ciliated epithelial cell. *See* EPITHELIAL CELL, CILIATED.

cimetidine (*N*-cyano-*N*'-methyl-*N*''-[2-[[(5-methyl-1*H*-imidazol-4-yl)methyl]thio]ethyl]-guanidine; Tagamet; Eureceptor; Gastromet; Ulcidine). CAS number 51481-61-9. H_2 histamine receptor antagonist used in the treatment of duodenal and gastric ulcers. It reversibly inhibits gastric acid secretion normally stimulated by endogenous histamine. Side effects have been reported in 1–2% of patients and include headache, dizziness, nausea and loss of libido. Less common and more serious effects include CNS dysfunction marked by slurred speech and delirium, most common in older patients.

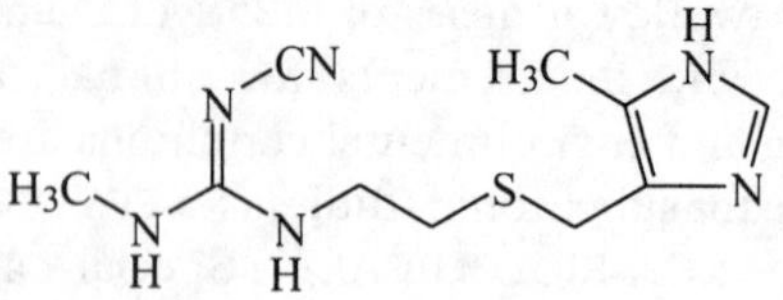

Cimetidine

***Cinchona* alkaloids**. Alkaloids derived from the bark of *Cinchona officinalis* L. They include the antimalarials quinine and cinchonine as well as the antiarrhythmic quinidine. *See also* CINCHONINE; QUINIDINE; QUININE.

Cinchonine ((9*s*)-cinchonan-9ol). CAS number 118-10-5. An alkaloid derived from the bark of *Cinchona officinalis* L. *See also* CINCHONA ALKALOIDS.

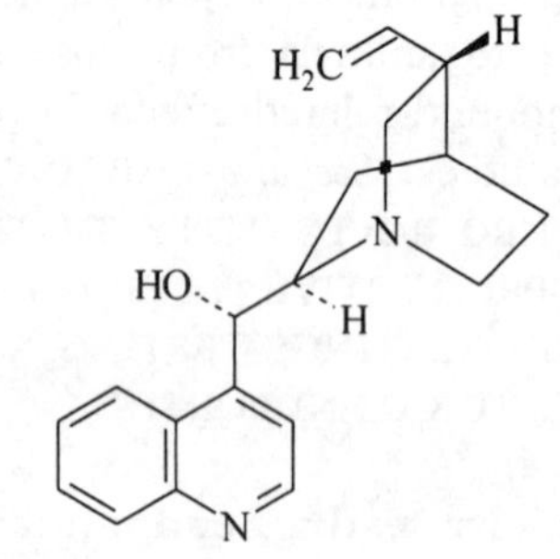

Cinchonine

cinnamene. *See* STYRENE.

cinnamol. *See* STYRENE.

cinnamon. *See* ESSENTIAL OILS.

circulatory system. Each cell in complex organisms carries out many functions in common, such as protein synthesis, ATP synthesis, etc., whereas at the same time different cell types also have specialized functions such as hormone synthesis and impulse transmission. These cells all need a supply of oxygen and nutrients, as well as a mechanism to eliminate carbon dioxide and organic wastes. Although single-cell and very small organisms can do this directly from the medium surrounding the organism, larger animals require a transport system. This system, characteristically closed and high-pressure in vertebrates, is known as the circulatory system, and the circulating fluid is known as blood. The pumping organ is the heart, the number of chambers of which varies with the taxonomic group, being four in mammals. The principal vessel exiting the heart to the organs is the aorta and that to the lungs is the pulmonary artery. The pulmonary veins return blood to the heart from the lungs, whereas the vena cava returns blood from the other organs. Between the arteries and the veins there is a capillary bed consisting of numerous thin-walled capillaries through which exchange of gases, nutrients and waste products with the tissue occurs. Blood pressure, heart beat, etc. are controlled by the nervous system. The circulatory system is important in toxicology as a means of transport and as a site of toxic action. Most invertebrates have a low pressure, open circulatory system involved in the movement of nutrients and waste products but not respiratory gases. *See also* BLOOD; DIAGNOSTIC FEATURES, CIRCULATORY SYSTEM.

cirrhosis. A chronic liver disease characterized by dense perilobular connective tissue, degenerative changes in parenchyma cells, fatty infiltration and single-cell necrosis. The pattern of blood flow is changed with increased resistance and decreased flow. In humans the most common cause is chronic ethanol poisoning, but it can also arise from dietary deficiency of protein, methionine or choline. Cirrhosis can be induced in animals by a number of hepatotoxicants including carbon tetrachloride and aflatoxins. *See also* HEPATOTOXICITY.

cisplatin (*cis*-diammineplatinum II; CDDP; *cis*-DDP; *cis*-platinum; Cisplatyl; diaminodichloro-(SP-4-2)-platinum; Cis-Pt II; Platinol). CAS number 15663-27-1. A cytotoxic antineoplastic with an LD50 in mice of 13.0 mg/kg, i.p. Cisplatin is a carcinogen that inhibits DNA replication by binding to DNA, producing interstrand cross-links (similar to bifunctional alkylating agents). In humans, acute treatment causes nausea and vomiting, with delayed bone marrow depression and renal toxicity, neurotoxicity, ototoxicity and the potential for anaphylaxis.

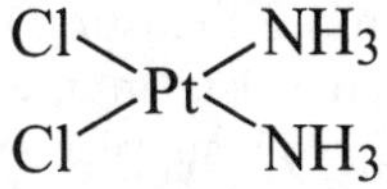

Ciplatin

citrus red (1-[(2,5-dimethoxyphenyl)azo]-2-naphthol). CAS number 6358-53-8. A color used for coloring the skin of mature oranges. This compound has been described as being carcinogenic. *See also* FOOD COLORS.

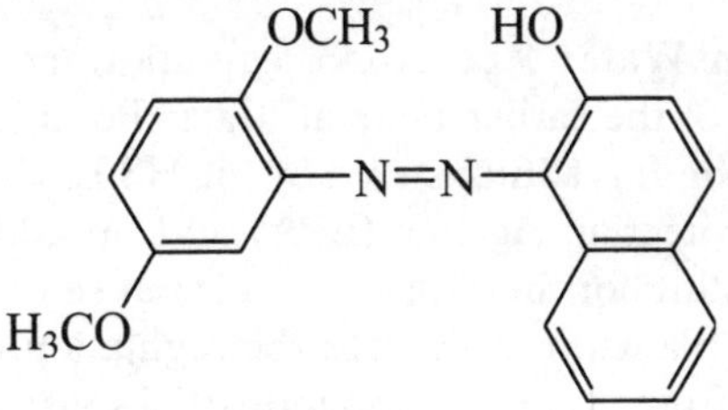

Citrus red 2

Clara cells. Metabolically active, unciliated bronchiolar cells containing a monooxygenase system that may detoxify or activate contaminants entering the lungs. Clara cells are characterized in some animals by basal granular endoplasmic reticulum (ER) and apical smooth ER. Cholesterol and carbohydrates are synthesized in these cells and secreted into the bronchiole lumen.

classical conditioning. *See* PAVLOVIAN CONDITIONING.

clastogen. A chemical that is able to cause structural changes in chromosomes, primarily breaks. Such agents are referred to as clastogenic.

clastogenic. *See* CLASTOGEN.

Clean Air Act. A US law administered by the US Environmental Protection Agency (EPA). Although the principal enforcement provisions are the responsibility of state and local governments, overall administrative responsibility rests with the EPA. This act requires criteria documents for air pollutants and sets both national air quality standards and standards for sources that create air pollutants, such as motor vehicles, power plants, etc. Important actions taken under this law include standards for a phased-out elimination of lead in gasoline and the setting of sulfuric acid air emission guidelines for existing industrial plants. Similar legislation exists in the UK under the Clean Air Act of 1956, supplemented in 1968.

Clean Air Acts. UK legislation, passed in 1956 and 1968, that prohibits the emission of dark smoke from any chimney or trade premises. The Act also enabled local authorities to declare smoke control areas, in which the emission of any smoke is an offense.

Clean Water Act. A US legislation; an amendment of the earlier Federal Water Pollution Control Act. It is administered by the US Environmental Protection Agency (EPA) and, in addition to providing for funding for municipal sewage treatment plants, it authorizes the regulation of emissions from municipal and industrial sources. Some important actions taken under this statute include setting standards for emissions of inorganics from smelter operations and publishing priority lists of toxic pollutants. This act also allows the US government to recover clean-up and other costs as damages from the polluting agency, company or individual.

clearance. A measure of the ability of the body or of an organ to remove a substance by processes of elimination such as metabolism, excretion or exhalation. Clearance does not indicate how much of a substance is removed, but is a measure of the volume of blood or plasma from which the substance is completely removed in a given time period. Clearance is thus expressed in units of volume per unit of time (e.g., ml/min). Clearance relates the concentration to the rate of elimination. Thus when linear kinetics exists, as the concentration increases so the rate of elimination increases proportionately such that the clearance remains constant. Total body clearance represents the sum of all organ clearances. Dividing the rate of elimination at each organ by the concentration gives individual organ clearance estimates. Organ clearances calculated from a more physiological perspective (by multiplying the flow rate of blood through the organ by the extraction ratio of the organ) can give additional insights into effects of physiological or environmental factors on clearance. *See also* KINETIC EQUATIONS; KINETIC EQUATIONS, ELIMINATION; KINETIC EQUATIONS,

HEPATIC CLEARANCE; KINETIC EQUATIONS, RENAL CLEARANCE; PHARMACOKINETICS; TOXICOKINETICS; VOLUME OF DISTRIBUTION.

clearance, from lungs. *See* ALVEOLAR CLEARANCE.

cleft palate. *See* TERATOGENIC EFFECTS, EXTERNAL MALFORMATIONS.

clinical chemistry. The chemical analysis and study of body fluids, excreta and tissues in the diagnosis and treatment of disease. In toxicology, clinical chemistry is important in the diagnosis of poisoning in humans and in the evaluation of toxicity in toxicity tests, including acute, subchronic and chronic tests. *See also* TOXIC ENDPOINTS.

clinical chemistry, in chronic toxicity testing. *See* TOXIC ENDPOINTS.

clinical chemistry, in subchronic toxicity testing. *See* TOXIC ENDPOINTS.

clinical surveillance. The surveillance of workers in industrial settings that involve chemical exposure is important for several reasons: (1) to detect effects not readily detected by studies of experimental animals, particularly hypersensitivity or other immunotoxicologic effects and effects on higher nervous activities such as incoordination; (2) as a continuing test of the appropriateness of the permitted exposure levels established for the particular chemical to which the workers are exposed. They could, eventually, provide the data necessary to establish biological threshold limit values. *See also* THRESHOLD LIMIT VALUES, BIOLOGICAL.

clinical toxicology. The branch of toxicology that deals with the diagnosis and treatment of poisoning in humans. It is primarily a specialty of medical practice rather than an experimental science. *See also* DIAGNOSTIC FEATURES; MAINTENANCE THERAPY; THERAPY.

clofibrate **(2-(4-chlorophenoxy)-2-methyl-propanoic acid ethyl ester)**. **CAS number 637-07-0**. A drug that lowers the concentration of plasma very low-density lipoproteins (and plasma triglycerides). It inhibits cholesterol synthesis and increases excretion of neutral steroids. Side effects include nausea, diarrhea, muscle cramps, stiffness, weakness and muscle tenderness. *See also* CHO-LESTEROL.

Clofibrate

clonal expansion. In any given animal a small percentage of lymphoid cells have receptors specific for a given antigen. Upon exposure to this antigen, these cells bind the antigen and are stimulated to divide (i.e., expand their population) and differentiate into effector cells, which have the same antigen specificity. Lymphocytes with receptors for unrelated antigens are not stimulated to divide and differentiate. Since any antigen of moderate complexity has multiple sites that are immunogenic (epitopes), many cells will respond to the stimulus, generating a polyclonal response. This is in contrast to the response of only one cell, which is monoclonal. *See also* MONOCLONAL ANTIBODY.

clonazepam. *See* BENZODIAZEPINES.

clonic. Describing marked rhythmical involuntary muscle contractions associated with convulsions due to seizure disorders. *See also* CONVULSIONS.

closantel. A veterinary drug for the treatment of fluke and nematode infestations. In 1993 some was included in a batch of donated drugs sent to Lithuania. Attempts to match the product with the names of other medicines on accompanying literature resulted in its misidentification as a treatment for endometriosis. Eleven women lost their eyesight; though this has since returned, they were left with eye pain and are unable to work.

closed segment technique. A technique for the estimation of intestinal absorption in which a section of the exposed intestine is ligated at each end and the test chemical introduced (via a hypodermic needle passed through one of the ligatures). Following a preselected time, the closed segment is removed and analyzed *in toto* for the chemical, the amount absorbed being estimated from the loss of injected material. *See also* PENETRATION ROUTES, GASTROINTESTINAL; PERFUSION STUDIES, INTESTINAL.

Clostridium. Genus of obligate spore-forming anaerobic bacteria of the family Bacilaceae. They are widely distributed in soil and also commonly occur in human and animal intestinal tracts. There are several species, several of which produce very potent toxins. *Cl. botulinum* produces botulinum toxin which can contaminate improperly processed food and is responsible for botulism. *Cl. perfringens* is the most common cause of gas gangrene. *Cl. tetani* produces tetanus toxin which is responsible for tetanus or lockjaw. *See also* BOTULINUM TOXIN; BOTULISM; TETANUS.

clotting, blood. *See* COAGULATION, BLOOD.

cloves. *See* ESSENTIAL OILS.

clozapine (8-chloro-11-(4-methyl-1-piperazinyl)-5H-dibenzo[*b,e*][1,4]diazepine; Clozaril; Leponex). CAS Number 5786-21-0. When first developed, this "atypical" antipsychotic drug produced fewer neurological side effects than did equally effective doses of other available agents like chlorpromazine or haloperidol. There is a lower incidence of tremor, rigidity, and bradykinesia, and it does not produce acute dystonic reactions. Moreover, there are no documented cases of tardive dyskinesia directly attributable to chronic treatment with clozapine. Clozapine has a complex mechanism of action therapeutically, acting at multiple neurotransmitter receptors, including dopamine D_2 and D_4, serotonin $5HT_2$, $5HT_6$, and $5HT_7$, and α_1- and α_2-adrenergic, and muscarinic cholinergic receptors. Unfortunately, treatment with this drug causes agranulocytosis in 1–3% of the patients using it, requiring constant therapeutic monitoring and discontinuation of therapy if blood dyscrasias develop. The mechanism(s) responsible for the agranulocytosis are unknown, although several clozapine-like drugs are in development that do not have this side effect. *See also* ANTIPSYCHOTIC

DRUGS; CHLORPROMAZINE; DOPAMINE; DOPA-MINE RECEPTORS; EXTRAPYRAMIDAL SIDE EFFECTS; HALOPERIDOL; TARDIVE DYSKINESIA.

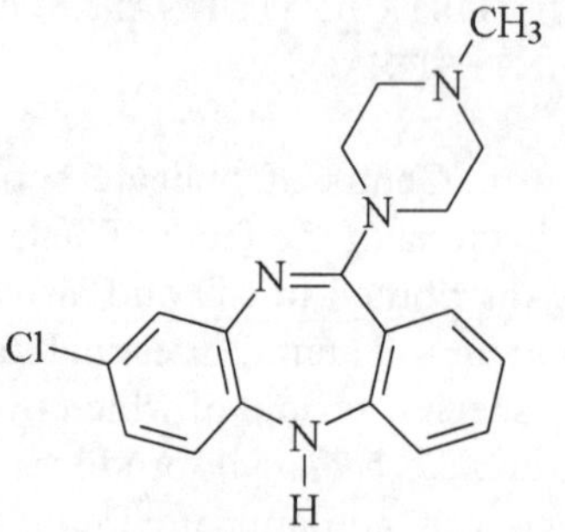

Clozapine

CMA. *See* CHEMICAL MANUFACTURERS ASSOCIATION.

CN (1-chloroacetophenone). A potent lacrimator and alkylating agent that is used in civil disturbances, resulting in stinging and burning of the eyes, nose and throat, salivation, lacrimation, rhinorrhea, irritation of the skin, tightess of the chest, shortness of breath, and gagging. Most of the signs and symptoms are generally transient. CN is of greater potency than the tear gas CS. *See also* C-AGENTS.

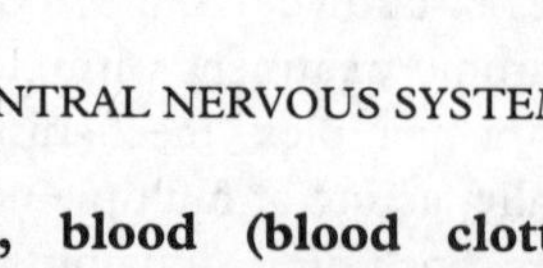

CN

CNITV. *See* CENTRE NATIONALE D'INFORMATION TOXICOLOGIQUES VETERINAIRE.

CNS. *See* CENTRAL NERVOUS SYSTEM.

coagulation, blood (blood clotting). The process of forming an insoluble fibrous network of the protein fibrin, in which blood cells become trapped to seal off a damaged blood vessel. It is the third stage of hemostasis, the process of stopping blood flow from a wound. Formation of the fibrin network is the final step of a multi-step process, involving calcium ions and various protein clotting factors, including prothrombin, the precursor of thrombin, which activates the conversion of fibrinogen into fibrin. The coagulation process can be initiated by injury to the blood vessel walls or by trauma to the blood itself, such as the turbulence resulting from passage of the blood over the roughened vessel walls created by atherosclerotic plaques. A deficient blood coagulation system can result in uncontrolled bleeding from wounds, as well as internal hemorrhage. Vitamin K is required for the hepatic synthesis of some of these clotting factors. Vitamin K antagonists, such as warfarin and other hydroxycoumarins, slowly diminish the ability of an animal to form blood clots and serve as effective rodenticides.

coal tar. The distillate produced by the destructive distillation of coal is condensed and fractionated into a variety of products, some of which are further processed. They include: coal tar; coal tar pitch; coal tar distillate; and creosote. These products are used in a number of industries including constructional (roofing, wood preserving) and electrical. Contact with the body is primarily cutaneous, but volatile components may be inhaled. Coal tar and related fractions should be considered probable human carcinogens, since a number of identified components are known carcinogens (e.g., benzo[*a*]pyrene, benzanthracene, chrysene, phenanthrene and possibly anthracene, carbazole, fluoranthrene and pyrene). Coal tar distillate yields four fractions: light oil that boils below 200 °C and contains benzene, toluene, xylenes, thiophene, phenol, cresol, etc.; middle oil, that boils at 200–250 °C and contains naphthalene, phenols, creosols, pyridine, methylpyridines, etc.; heavy oil, that boils at 250–300 °C and contains naphthalene, cresols, xylenols, quinoline, etc.; and anthracene oil, which boils at 300–350 °C and contains phenanthrene, anthracene, carbazole, etc. *See also* BENZO[*A*]PYRENE.

coal tar dyes. Chemically synthesized compounds for which anthracene is one of the starting materials. The first of these compounds, aniline purple, was synthesized in 1856 and led ultimately to the development of various synthetic food colors. *See also* FOOD COLORS.

cobalt (Co). An element essential for life through its role in vitamin B_{12}. The major problem with cobalt toxicity is industrial. This includes pneumoconiosis from occupational exposure during working of cobalt-containing alloys. In addition, skin contact may cause an erythematous papular-type of dermatitis, especially in workers in the hard metal industries, offset printers and cement handlers. Cobalt toxicity also results in polycythemia due to stimulation of erythropoiesis, and high doses for long periods may even have carcinogenic or mutagenic effects. *See also* BONE MARROW.

cobra venom (cobratoxin). A small basic protein ($Mr = 7000$). It contains 62 amino acids in a single chain, cross-linked by four disulfide bonds. The toxin comprises 10% of the venom by weight. It is a neurotoxin that is secreted by glands of the cobra snake and injected into its prey via immobile, grooved fangs. Cobratoxin may be radiolabeled and used as a specific radioligand in binding studies performed on acetylcholine receptors. Cobratoxin is absorbed from the subcutaneous tissues and is distributed throughout the body. After intoxication, high concentrations are found at the motor endplates of neuromuscular junctions, where it irreversibly binds to acetylcholine receptors. The primary action is similar to that of curare, but the binding process is slower. Symptoms include drooping of the eyelids, accompanied by flaccid paralysis and neck flexor weakness. Respiratory failure may occur due to paralysis of the diaphragm or pharynx. For therapy, the patient should be immobilized in a horizontal position. Cobratoxin antivenom is not commercially marketed in the USA, but may be available at zoos. It should be administered parenterally as soon as possible following exposure. Respiratory assistance may be a necessary and crucial part of treatment. Most deaths due to cobra bites occur in the very young and old. *See also* NEUROTRANSMITTERS; SNAKE VENOMS.

coca (*Erythroxylon coca*; hayo; ipado). A plant originally found in Bolivia, Brazil and Peru (but now cultivated elsewhere) that contains the alkaloid cocaine in its leaves. The leaves were often chewed by South American Indians to eliminate fatigue. *See also* COCAINE.

cocaine (3-(benzoyloxy)-8-methyl-8-azabicyclo-[3.2.1] octane-2-carboxylic acid methyl ester; ethylbenzoylecgonine). CAS number 50-36-2. A natural product isolated from the leaves of the South American coca plant *Erythroxylon coca*. Administration causes feelings of well-being, stimulation and euphoria, although at higher doses dysphoria may result. It may cause elevation of blood pressure, palpitation and tachycardia, as well as various CNS effects, including psychotic effects at higher doses. Chronic use, especially at high doses as often occurs with drug abuse, can cause a condition often indistinguishable from schizophrenia. Abrupt withdrawal may result in fatigue, depression and sleep changes. Several biochemical mechanisms may be involved in the actions of cocaine in the CNS, principally inhibition of monoamine uptake. This resulting increase in the synaptic availability of dopamine, norepinephrine and serotonin is responsible for its central actions, whereas adrenergic effects cause most of its peripheral sympathomimetic effects. Lethality of cocaine is probably due to the local anesthetic properties of cocaine and actions on various CNS neurons, possibly coupled with its effects on monoamine uptake. Although both the free base and salts (principally the hydrochloride) have been used clinically, the recent trend in abuse of cocaine is in the form of the free base. Its i.v. LD50 in rats is 17.5 mg/kg. Many of its actions can be blocked by adrenergic and dopamine antagonists. *See also* ALKALOIDS; CATECHOLAMINES; COCA; HALLUCINOGENS; STIMULANTS.

Cocaine

co-carcinogen. A chemical that enhances the action of a complete carcinogen when given simultaneously with the latter. Although not carcinogenic itself, the agent may act to increase absorption, increase bioactivation, or inhibit detoxication of the carcinogen it is administered with. Examples of co-carcinogens include ethanol, solvents and catechol.

co-carcinogenesis. The enhancement of the conversion of normal cells to neoplastic cells. This process is manifested by the enhancement of carcinogenesis when the agent is administered either before or together with a carcinogen. Co-carcinogenesis should be distinguished from promotion, as, in the latter case, the promoter must be administered after the initiating carcinogen. *Compare* PROMOTION. *See also* CARCINOGENESIS; INITIATION; PROGRESSION.

cocculin. *See* PICROTOXIN.

Cochran's *Q* statistic. A test for mean differences in a single-factor experiment with repeated measures when the dependent variable is dichotomous. The sampling distribution of the Q statistic is approximated by a chi-square distribution with degrees of freedom equal to the number of conditions (n) minus one, unless n is small (e.g., less than 10). *See also* CHI-SQUARE TEST; STATISTICS, FUNCTION IN TOXICOLOGY.

Cochran's test (Cochran's *C* test). A computationally simpler statistic than Bartlett's test for evaluating departures from homogeneity of variance. In this case, C equals the ratio of the largest sample variance to the sum of the within-group variances. The observed value for C can be evaluated by reference to special tables that provide critical values for C based on the number of groups and the degrees of freedom for each of the variances ($n-1$). *See also* BARTLETT'S TEST; STATISTICS, FUNCTION IN TOXICOLOGY.

Code of Federal Regulations (CFR). In the USA the Federal Register is issued daily and includes proposed rules authorized by statute and presented for public comment as well as rules and regulations authorized by statute and issued in their final form. Includes rules governing the regulation of toxic chemicals and authorized under such statutes as the Toxic Substances Control Act (TSCA) the Federal Fungicide, Insecticide and Rodenticide Act (FIFRA), the Federal Clean Air Act and others.

codeine (7,8-didehydro-4,5-epoxy-3-methoxy-17-methylmorphinan-6-ol; methylmorphine). **CAS number 76-57-3.** An alkaloid of the opium poppy present in opium from 0.7 to 2.5%, depending on source; it is also prepared by methylation of morphine. It is almost as effective as morphine as an antitussive agent, yet it is felt to be less likely to cause addiction. Codeine is more effective orally than morphine, increasing its utility as an antitussive agent. Codeine has many of the actions of morphine and also works by being an agonist on opioid receptors. The oral LD50 for codeine phosphate in rabbits is 100 mg/kg, the s.c. LD50 for codeine hydrochloride in mice is 300 mg/kg. *See also* MORPHINE; NARCOTICS; OPIOIDS; OPIUM.

Codeine

Codex Alimentarius. Published with the full title "Recommended International Codes of Hygienic Practice for Fresh Meat, for Anti-Mortem and Post-Mortem Inspection of Slaughter Animals and for Processed Meat Products," this is a data system that provides information on food standards for pesticides, commodities, and pesticide/commodity combinations. Topics covered include: pesticide residues in food; residues of veterinary drugs in foods; foods for special dietary uses, including food for infants and children; processed and quick frozen fruits and vegetables; tropical fresh fruits and vegetables; fruit juices and related products; cereals, pulses, legumes, and derived products and vegetable proteins; fats, oils, and related products; meat and meat products, including soups and broths; sugars, cocoa products, and chocolate and miscellaneous products; and methods of analysis and sampling. It was last updated in 1992 by the Secretariat of the Joint FAO/WHO Food Standards Programme (Codex Alimentarius), Food and Agriculture Organization (FAO) of the United Nations.

Codex Alimentarius Commission (CAC). Commission established by the Codex Alimentarius. The Commission meets biennially.

Codex Commission on Pesticide Residues (CCPR). *See* CODEX ALIMENTARIUS COMMISSION.

Codex Committee on Food Additives and Contaminants. *See* CODEX ALIMENTARIUS COMMISSION.

Codex Committee on Residues of Veterinary Drugs in Food. *See* CODEX ALIMENTARIUS COMMISSION.

codon (coding triplets, triplet codon). Sequence of three nucleotides coding for the incorporation of one specific amino acid into a polypeptide chain or of other specific genetic information. This code is almost universal in nature, identical sets of three nucleotides being used by viruses, bacteria and higher organisms. Recent studies have shown, however, that mitochondria have some minor alterations of the code in their genetic apparatus. Since there are 64 possible combinations of the four nucleotides in sets of three, there is redundancy in the system, which means that most amino acids can be coded for by more than one triplet. Extremes are tryptophan (one codon: UGG) and leucine (six codons). The genetic code is therefore said to be degenerate. The ambiguity exists in only one direction; although there are a number of possible combinations of codons that will produce a given amino acid sequence, any particular set of codons will code for just one particular polypeptide sequence. It has also been found that not all possible codons for any one amino acid are utilized with the same frequency, although the reasons for this variability are not known. Codons exist in the messenger RNA and are thus transcribed from complementary sequences in the DNA template. They are also matched with complementary triplets, known as anticodons, present in the specific transfer RNA molecules which bring the amino acids to the site of protein synthesis on the ribosome. The interaction of codons and anticodons is further complicated by a phenomenon known as wobble, such that only two out of three bases need to be properly matched by the normal base pairing rules. Finally, some triplets are signals to the ribosome either to start protein (usually AUG) or to stop it (e.g., UGA).

coenzymes. Organic, non-protein molecules necessary for the activity of an enzyme which are loosely associated with the enzyme as compared with tightly associated prosthetic groups. Coenzymes participate in the substrate–enzyme interaction by donating or accepting protons or other groups. They may be structurally altered during the reaction, but are usually regenerated in subsequent reactions. The most important coenzymes are those involved in biological oxidation/reduction reactions, (i.e., hydrogen/electron transfer reactions). Adenosine triphosphate, biotin, coenzyme A, and pyridoxal phosphate all act as coenzymes in various group transfer reactions (e.g., transaminations involving amino acids and a-keto acids). NADPH is involved in the reactions of the cytochrome P450-dependent monooxygenase system and the flavin-containing monooxygenase, both important in the oxidation of xenobiotics. NAD is a coenzyme for alcohol dehydrogenase. *See also* ALCOHOL DEHYDROGENASE; ATP; NAD; NADP; CYTOCHROME P450; FLAVIN-CONTAINING MONOOXYGENASE.

cohort epidemiological study. *See* EPIDEMIOLOGICAL STUDIES, COHORT.

colcemid. *See* COLCHICINE.

colchicine (colcemid). CAS number 64-86-8. An alkaloid first isolated from the meadow saffron *Colchicum autumnale* that binds specifically to the β-tubulin dimer and, in so doing, blocks assembly of microtubules. Because the intrinsic dissociation rate is not altered by colchicine binding, the result will be net disassembly of existing microtubules. Because of its relatively slow rate of penetration of the cell membrane, this drug has been superceded by nocodozole.

Colchincine

colchicine-binding protein. *See* TUBULIN.

colon. The large intestine; the site of much water and electrolyte absorption. The colon is the frequent site of cancer from carcinogens.

Colouring Matter in Food Regulations. Regulations for England and Wales, and for Scotland, that were produced in 1973 by the Ministry of Agriculture, Fisheries and Food. These regulations incorporated directives of the European Economic Community (EEC) on the use of permitted colors in food as recommended by the Scientific Committee for Food. All additives with E numbers (e.g., cochineal, E120) have been recognized as safe by the EEC. Numbers without the prefix E are proposals and are yet to be adopted.

Colubridae. The family of venomous rear-fanged snakes, most of which are not a major hazard to humans because the rear-fanged delivery system does not lend itself to effective delivery of venom to larger animals. Exceptions are the highly dangerous boomslang and bird snake of Africa, the rednecked keelback of Asia, and a few others. This family is of lesser concern to humans than the families Elapidae, Viperidae and Crotalidae.

column chromatography. *See* CHROMATOGRAPHY, COLUMN.

COM. *See* COMMITTEE ON MUTAGENICITY OF CHEMICALS AND FOOD.

coma. Unconsciousness from which a patient cannot be aroused. Coma may be caused by primary disease of the CNS or by drugs, toxins, trauma, stroke or asphyxia. *See also* DIAGNOSTIC FEATURES, CENTRAL NERVOUS SYSTEM; MAINTENANCE THERAPY.

combustion products. The chemicals which result from the burning of fuels and other organic materials. If combustion is complete, the main products are carbon dioxide and water. Carbon dioxide generated in high levels from the burning of large amounts of fossil fuels is implicated in contributing to the greenhouse effect, still a controversial topic. Combustion in the presence of limited amounts of oxygen generates carbon monoxide. Incomplete combustion of organic matter, usually occurring at very high temperatures, generates polycyclic aromatic hydrocarbons. Metals and sulfur oxides may also be released by combustion if the material being burned contains metals and sulfur. Burning in air can generate nitrogen oxides.

Residue not released from the combustion as a gas is ash, particulates of various sizes which contribute to smoke. All of these products are a part of air pollution, and are produced largely by fuel combustion for transportation, industrial and municipal needs. *See also* AIR POLLUTION; CARBON DIOXIDE; CARBON MONOXIDE; POLYCYCLIC AROMATIC HYDROCARBONS; GREENHOUSE EFFECT.

Commission of the European Communities. Proposes Directives, which provide a framework for the abatement of pollution, control of additives in food, the use and labeling of pesticides, etc.

Committee 17 report. A report, entitled "Environmental Mutagenic Hazards", prepared by a committee appointed by the Council of the Environmental Mutagen Society. It contains important suggestions concerning species extrapolation of value in risk assessment. Committee 17 Science 187, 503–514 (1975). *See also* MOLECULAR DOSIMETRY; RATE-DOUBLING CONCENTRATION; SPECIES EXTRAPOLATION.

Committee for Environmental Conservation (CoEnCo). A body, formed in 1969, and made up of representatives of all the major UK national, non-governmental conservation bodies, covering such interests in wildlife, archaeology, architecture, outdoor recreation or amenities, with the purpose of facilitating exchange of views and information among them and of coordinating their approach to national issues.

Committee on Mutagenicity of Chemicals in Food, Consumer Products and the Environment (COM). A UK non-statutory expert committee providing advice to government departments, etc. Prepares the "Guidelines for the Testing of Chemicals for Mutagenicity" (published by HMSO, London).

Committee on Safety of Drugs (CSD). *See* COMMITTEE ON SAFETY OF MEDICINES.

Committee on Safety of Medicines (CSM). A committee within the Medicines Division of the UK Department of Health and Social Security established in 1971 as a result of the Medicines Act 1968. The Sub-Committee on Adverse Reactions is responsible for monitoring any suspected adverse reactions reported by medical practitioners to the Medical Assessor. The CSM replaced the Committee on Safety of Drugs (CSD), which had provided a voluntary system of consultation within the UK pharmaceutical industry.

Committee on Toxicity of Chemicals in Food, Consumer Products and the Environment (COT).

A UK expert committee that has reported on the safety of the use of sweeteners, caffeine, nitrosamines, metals (lead, mercury and cadmium) and enzymes. Prepares the "Guidelines for the Evaluation of Chemicals for Carcinogenicity" (published by HMSO, London).

comparative toxicity, indices for.

The comparative toxicity of two different chemicals for the same adverse effect or of the same chemical for two different adverse effects can be expressed numerically in a manner analogous to the therapeutic index for drugs. For example, in the first case, the comparative toxicity index is

$$\frac{\text{LD50 for compound A}}{\text{LD50 for compound B}}$$

in the case of lethality or

$$\frac{\text{ED50(A)}}{\text{ED50(B)}}$$

if the effect is non-lethal. In the second case, the index is

$$\frac{\text{ED50 for effect X}}{\text{ED50 for effect Y}}$$

See also MARGIN OF SAFETY; THERAPEUTIC INDEX.

comparative toxicology.

The study of the variation in the expression of toxicity of exogenous chemicals towards organisms of different taxonomic groups or of different genetic strains. Although any aspect of toxicology can be studied from a comparative point of view, in fact the majority of such studies are either on acute toxicity or on the metabolism of xenobiotics. The most important practical applications of comparative toxicology are in the development of appropriate animal models for toxic phenomena seen in humans, the development of selective toxicants and the study of environmental xenobiotic cycles. *See also* ENVIRONMENTAL XENOBIOTIC CYCLES; SELECTIVITY.

comparative variation in xenobiotic metabolism.

Differences in xenobiotic metabolism specific for large taxonomic groups are rare; formation of glucosides by insects and plants rather than the glucuronides of other animal groups is, perhaps, the best known. Differences between species are common and often of toxicological significance, but they are usually quantitative in nature and occur both within and between taxonomic groups. Such differences can be seen at many levels: *in vivo* toxicity; *in vivo* metabolism; *in vitro* metabolism. *See also* COMPARATIVE VARIATION IN XENOBIOTIC METABOLISM, *IN VITRO* METABOLISM; COMPARATIVE VARIATION IN XENOBIOTIC METABOLISM, *IN VIVO* METABOLISM; COMPARATIVE VARIATION IN XENOBIOTIC METABOLISM, *IN VIVO* TOXICITY.

comparative variation in xenobiotic metabolism, *in vitro* metabolism.

Since many factors alter enzymatic rates *in vitro*, caution must be exercised in interpreting data in terms of species variation. For example, enzymes are often sensitive to the experimental conditions used in their preparation, and this sensitivity may vary from one enzyme to another. Species variation in the oxidation of xenobiotics is usually quantitative; qualitative differences are seldom seen. Since there are multiple forms of microsomal cytochrome P450 in each species, the relative amounts of these forms may differ from one species to another. Reductive reactions, like oxidations, proceed at different rates with enzyme preparations from different species, microsomes from mammalian liver being up to 18 times higher in azo reductase activity and more than 20 times higher in nitro reductase activity than those from fish liver. Several animal species possess hepatic microsomal UDP glucuronyltransferase activity and as with other phase II reactions, species variation is apparent, being as much as 12-fold with *p*-nitrophenol as a substrate. *Compare* COMPARATIVE VARIATION IN XENOBIOTIC METABOLISM, *IN VIVO* METABOLISM.

comparative variation in xenobiotic metabolism, *in vivo* **metabolism**. The biological half-life is governed by the rates of metabolism and excretion, and thus its comparative variation is frequently dependent upon variation in metabolism between species. For example, phenylbutazone is metabolized slowly in humans, with a half-life of about three days, whereas in the monkey, rat, guinea pig, rabbit, dog and horse the half-life varies from three to six hours. The effects of hexobarbital are an example of the interdependence of metabolic rate, half-life and pharmacological action and its variation between species. Mice inactivate hexobarbital rapidly and both biological half-life *in vivo* and sleeping time are short. In dogs, hexobarbital is inactivated slowly, and the reverse is true of both half-life and sleeping time. Xenobiotics, once inside the body, usually undergo a series of biotransformations. Since these biotransformations are catalyzed by a number of enzymes, it is probable that they will vary between species. There may be species differences, however, even in the case of xenobiotics undergoing a single reaction. In humans, rats and guinea pigs, papaverine is metabolized via *O*-demethylation to phenolic products, but these products are not formed to any extent in dogs. A few studies suggest some relationship between the evolutionary position of a species and its conjugation mechanisms. In most mammals the principal mechanisms involve conjugation with glucuronic acid, glycine, glutamine or sulfate, mercapturic acid synthesis, acetylation and methylation. In conjugation, in some birds and reptiles, ornithine replaces glycine, whereas in plants, bacteria and insects, glucose replaces glucuronic acid. Minor conjugative processes are also found in only a few species. These include conjugation with phosphate, taurine, *N*-acetylglucosamine, ribose, glycyltaurine, serine, arginine, formic acid and succinate. Glucuronide synthesis itself, however, varies within taxonomic groups. The cat and closely related species have a defective glucuronide-forming system. They form little or no glucuronide from many phenols, although they form glucuronides from other compounds. This defective glucuronidation is probably related to the absence of the appropriate transferase isozyme. *Compare* COMPARATIVE VARIATION IN XENOBIOTIC METABOLISM, *IN VITRO* METABOLISM.

comparative variation in xenobiotic metabolism, *in vivo* **toxicity**. Variations in both acute and chronic toxicity between species are well known. In general, insecticides are more toxic to mammals than are herbicides and fungicides. Carbon tetrachloride, a potent hepatotoxicant to most mammals, is virtually without effect on chickens. *See also* COMPARATIVE VARIATION IN XENOBIOTIC METABOLISM, *IN VITRO* METABOLISM; COMPARATIVE VARIATION IN XENOBIOTIC METABOLISM, *IN VIVO* METABOLISM.

compartment. A hypothetical volume of an animal system wherein a chemical acts homogeneously in transport and transformation. A single mathematical compartment may be one, two or more physiological tissues or entities. *See also* COMPARTMENTAL MODEL; MULTI-COMPARTMENT MODELS; ONE-COMPARTMENT MODEL; TWO-COMPARTMENT MODEL.

compartmental model. A mathematical depiction of physiological reality. Transport into, out of, or between compartments is described by rate constants which describe movement of the chemical in the animal system. *See also* MULTI-COMPARTMENT MODELS; ONE-COMPARTMENT MODEL; TWO-COMPARTMENT MODEL.

competitive binding and transport. Competition for the same binding sites on a transport or other protein can have an important toxicological significance. If a toxicant competes for sites already occupied by a previously applied compound displacement results. For example, the anticoagulant warfarin is important in treatment of heart disease, but many fatty acids, and some drugs, also bind to the same site on proteins. Concurrently administered phenylbutazone, an anti-inflammatory agent, displaces warfarin, and the resultant increases in free warfarin can appreciably increase anticoagulant effects. *See also* BINDING; PROTEIN BINDING.

complement. The complement system is composed of 20 serum proteins and nine membrane proteins which, when activated, react in a cascade fashion to facilitate clearance of antigen–antibody complexes and destruction of foreign bacteria. The process of activation, which occurs on the target membrane or particle, is called complement fixation. The complement cascade can be initiated via two different pathways: the classical pathway and the alternative pathway. The classical pathway can be activated by immune complexes of IgG and IgM with antigen. The classical pathway was the first described, and the components were named in order of discovery. The alternative pathway is activated by certain bacteria (usually gram-negative) viruses and tumors in the absence of antibody and by aggregated antibody of all classes. The deposition of component C3, via either pathway, faciliates the phagocytosis of the target particle or cell. Additionally, C5b, C6, C7, C8 and C9 can then react to form a membrane attack complex, which leads to colloid osmotic lysis of the cell. Erythrocytes, many phagocytic cells and granulocytes have receptors for various intermediate complement components, many of which have powerful biological effects. C3b is a chemoattractant for phagocytic leukocytes. C3a, C4a and C5a have inflammatory actions, increasing vascular permeability and promoting smooth muscle contractions. C5a is the most potent of these and also promotes granulocyte participation, leading to release of histamines and toxic oxygen metabolites into the tissues. Deficiencies in the complement system lead to increased susceptiblity to bacterial infections and immune complex problems similar to those seen in systemic lupus erythematosis (SLE). Tissue damage in autoimmune processes and some allergic responses is due to complement fixation in and of healthy tissues and their subsequent destruction and inflammation of the surrounding area. Deficiencies in regulatory factors can lead to complete consumption of different components and to chronic inflammatory processes. Individual components can be monitored (usually by RIA) to follow the progress of infection or determine the nature of the causative agent by determining which pathway has been activated. Complement is used in many immunological assays. After specific antibody–antigen reactions occur, complement is added causing lysis of the antibody-coated target cells and release of cellular contents (e.g., hemoglobin from erythrocytes) which can easily be quantitated. Release of hemoglobin from previously sensitized erythrocytes

after the addition of complement also provides a direct quantitative assessment of the complement system. *See also* ALLERGIC RESPONSE.

complete carcinogen. *See* CARCINOGEN, COMPLETE.

complete Freund's adjuvant. *See* FREUND'S ADJUVANT.

compliance. (1) Operating in accordance with rules and regulations set forth by the government, such as the regulations required of industries producing toxicant-containing effluents entering the air or water, or the rules required of federal grantees. (2) In the area of pulmonary physiology, it is the expansibility of the lungs and thorax; in the area of cardiovascular physiology, the distensibility of the blood vessels.

compliance, pulmonary. The change in volume per unit of pressure change for the thorax and/or the lung.

composition. An EC term synonymous with formulation of medicines.

compound 1080. *See* FLUOROACETATE.

compound 1081. *See* FLUOROACETAMIDE.

Comprehensive Environmental Response, Compensation and Liability Act (CERCLA). An act passed in 1980 authorizing the United States Environmental Protection Agency to identify and clean up hazardous waste sites, many of which resulted from industrial dumping. It mandates that the companies responsible for generating the hazardous waste are financially liable for the clean up procedures. The term "Superfund" is usually used for this legislation referring to the funds provided for this clean up which have been accumulated into a large trust fund, the superfund. CERCLA was amended in 1986 by the Superfund Amendments and Reauthorization Act (SARA). Concern exists that a disproportionately large amount of these funds have gone into legal matters and not the clean-up itself.

conantokins. Marine snails produce a variety of peptides that can affect ion channel function. The three major families of paralytic toxins have been categorized according to their biological activities and have provided useful tools for the study of nicotinic acetylcholine receptors (alpha-conotoxins), voltage-gated sodium channels (mu-conotoxins), and voltage-gated calcium channels (omega-conotoxins). These compounds totally block ion flow through the channels to which they bind, and thus induce paralysis and death. A fourth group of snail peptides, the conantokins, were named for antokin, the Philippine word for sleepy, because, when injected into the brains of mice, they cause sleep instead of paralysis. Conantokin-T (ConT) and ConG are found in the venoms of *Conus tulipa* and *C. geographus*, respectively. ConG acts as an antagonist of the NMDA-type glutamate receptor, but is not a typical NMDA antagonist because it inhibits only the polyamine portion of NMDA receptor activation, and it is specific for only one subtype of NMDA receptors. *See also* CONOTOXIN; CONUS.

conditioned avoidance (active avoidance). An operant or instrumental procedure to assess learning and/or retention. The procedure involves the animal making a response to avoid presentation of a noxious stimulus (e.g., shock). Typically, the animal is placed in one chamber of the test area. A conditioned stimulus (e.g., tone) is presented followed by the noxious stimulus. The animal can escape, and later avoid, the noxious stimulus by moving to another chamber or location in the test area. If the animal fails to avoid, but successfully escapes, the noxious stimulus learning deficits are inferred. *See also* NEUROBEHAVIORAL TERATOLOGY; NEUROBEHAVIORAL TOXICOLOGY.

conditioned behavior. Behavior that is acquired by conditioning or learning; an archaic term. *See also* CONDITIONED AVOIDANCE; NEUROBEHAVIORAL TERATOLOGY; NEUROBEHAVIORAL TOXICOLOGY.

confidence interval. *See* CONFIDENCE LIMIT.

confidence limit (upper confidence limit). The confidence limit is the upper value of the confidence interval, the latter being a set of values that has a specified probability (e.g., 90%) of containing a given characteristic.

congenital. Present at birth but not necessarily genetic; applied particularly to structural and functional defects or diseases.

congestive heart failure. A failure of the heart to maintain adequate blood circulation. It is characterized by weakness, lack of breath and edema, resulting from venous stasis and reduced outflow of blood. Congestive heart failure can be caused by poisons that induce myocardial damage.

conjugation reactions. *See* PHASE II REACTIONS.

conjunctiva. The mucous membrane in the eyes, lining the eyelid and covering part of the eyeball. It is subject to irritation and damage by eye irritants, including a number of xenobiotics that are respiratory system poisons.

coniine (2-propylpiperidine). Piperidine alkaloid obtained from poison hemlock, *Conium maculatum*. Alkaline, steam volatile liquid (b.p. 167 °C), mousy odor. Darkens and polymerizes in air. It can be reduced at high temperature with HI to *n*-octane and oxidized to pyridine-1-carboxylic acid. The hydrochloride is used as an antispasmodic. *See also* HEMLOCK.

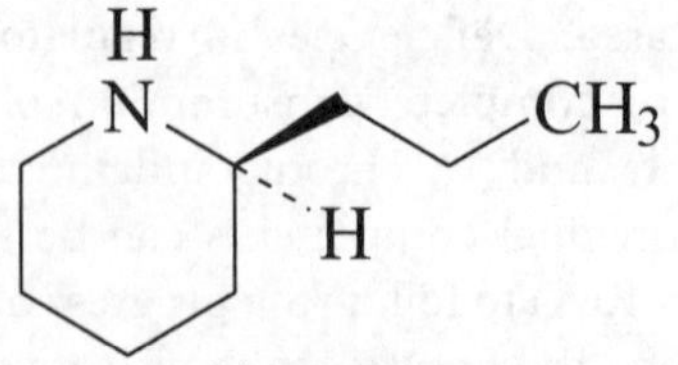

Coniine

connective tissue. A diverse group of tissues characterized by widely spaced cells with extensive interstitial material. Collagen is an important component of the interstitial material, forming the structural matrix. Chemicals inhibiting collagen synthesis, such as lathyrogens, adversely affect connective tissue.

conotoxins (ω-). Neurotoxins isolated from marine snails (*Conus geographus* and *C. magus*). They block N-type calcium channels in neuronal preparations, and can therefore inhibit calcium-mediated release of several neurotransmitters. *See also* CONANTOKINS.

Consumer Products Safety Act (Consumer Products Safety Commission Improvements Act). A US act, administered by a Consumer Products Safety Commission, that is designed to protect the public against risk of injury from consumer products and to set safety standards for such products. Although many of the actions taken under this law relate to non-chemical (primarily mechanical) injury, it is also concerned with chemical safety. *See also* CONSUMER PRODUCTS SAFETY COMMISSION.

Consumer Products Safety Commission. An agency of the US government charged with the protection of the public from unreasonable risk of injury from consumer products. This is done by the evaluation of the comparative safety of different products and by research into the causes and prevention of product-related illness, death and injury. The Consumer Products Safety Commission has been active in the formulation of toxicity-testing protocols and was one of the agencies that established the Interagency Regulatory Liaison Group to reform the various processes and protocols used in the regulation of chemicals.

contaminant. An undesired chemical present in a sample that contains one or more principal components. Contaminants are derived from the synthetic process as by-products, were present in the starting materials or may have entered post-production. In many cases, the purity of the product may not be critical, particularly in industrial chemicals, and it is less expensive to conduct the synthetic process without extensive purification of either the starting materials or the final product. Since such contaminants may be toxic, perhaps more toxic than the parent compound, both regulatory agencies and toxicologists are confronted with a dilemma: whether to test the mixture for toxicity or to test the purified active ingredient. The former may approach actual exposure conditions, but little is learned of the mechanisms

involved; moreover, contaminants often vary from batch to batch and from one synthetic process to another. The latter is more informative from a toxicological mechanism point of view, but says little of the additional toxicity of contaminants or possible interactions. Ideally both the parent compound and the commercial mixture should be tested.

continuous variables. Describing a variable when its values are not limited theoretically, but only by the precision of measuring instruments. Thus, the concentration of a toxicant is a continuous variable, whereas the occurrence of a toxicant-induced behavior, as defined by a rating of 1–6, is a discontinuous variable. *See also* STATISTICS, FUNCTION IN TOXICOLOGY.

Controlled Substances Act. A US law concerned with the controlled use of therapeutic drugs and the control of drugs of abuse. It is administered by the Drug Enforcement Administration. All legitimate manufacturers, dispensers or investigators must be licensed under the act. For the purposes of licensing, controlled substances are divided into five schedules. Schedule I includes drugs with a high potential for abuse and of no current medical use in the USA (e.g., heroin, mescaline, psilocybin). Schedule II includes drugs with great potential for abuse and high potential for psychological or physical dependence, but they may have legitimate clinical uses (e.g., codeine, amphetamines, morphine). Schedule III includes drugs with a lower potential for abuse than those in Schedule I or II. Schedule IV includes drugs or preparations with relatively low potential for abuse of dependence, whereas Schedule V includes drugs with a low enough potential for abuse that they may be dispensed without prescription. Schedule V preparations, however, must be distributed by a pharmacist following regulations concerning amounts, record keeping, etc. This law not only applies to physicians, but also to research workers in both clinical and non-clinical research. The act not only strengthens law enforcement in the field of drug abuse, but also provides for research into methods for the prevention and treatment of drug abuse.

Control of Pollution Act. UK legislation, passed in 1974, that covers the pollution of land, water and the atmosphere. It restricts the depositing of toxic wastes on land. Controlled waste may only be deposited or disposed of using the plant of a license-holder. Licenses are granted by the disposal authority with the agreement of the water authority. The Act also prohibits the discharge of poisonous or polluting matter into a stream.

Control of Substances Hazardous to Health Regulations (COSHH). Regulations (1988) under the UK Health and Safety at Work Act of 1974. *See also* HSC.

controls, in toxicity testing. A test run in parallel to the toxicity assay to ensure the viability and validity of the assay system. Except for the omission of the test chemical, a negative control would have all the same conditions as the test assay, include any vehicle (solvent), thus ensuring accurate comparison. The parameter measured (e.g., survival, tumor incidence, cell growth, enzyme activity, etc.) must be significantly different, as assessed by appropriate statistical methods, from the negative control for the test to be considered positive. Any effect in the negative control, such as the level of mortality or vehicle-induced inhibition, must be used to correct the data before these data are subject to further analysis. Unexpected results in the negative control such as a high level of mortality or excessive vehicle-induced inhibition may invalidate the entire test. A positive control is frequently conducted in which a chemical known to induce the endpoint that the test is designed to measure is tested parallel to the test chemical to ensure that the test system, as set up for the particular test, is functional.

Conus. There are about 400 species within the cone snail genus, and it constitutes the most dangerous group of mollusks. They occur in tropical and subtropical regions, and in the oceans. They produce a very potent potent neurotoxic venom (conotoxin); each species of *Conus* contains in its venom 50–200 different peptides directed at different molecular targets. These include presynaptic Ca^{2+} channel blockers, competitive antagonists of postsynaptic nicotinic receptors, nicotinic receptor channel blockers, Na^+ channel activators, Na^+ channel blockers, selective for channels in skeletal muscle, K^+ channel blockers, and NMDA receptor blockers (conantokins). The conotoxins are small paralytic peptides, 10–30 amino acids in length. *See also* CONOTOXIN; CONANTOKINS.

Convention for the Prevention of Marine Pollution from Land-Based Sources (Paris Convention). An international agreement to augment earlier agreements controlling the dumping of wastes at sea was signed in March 1974 by Denmark, France, Iceland, Luxembourg, the Netherlands, Norway, Spain, Sweden, the UK and West Germany.

Convention to Protect the Ozone Layer. An international convention, drawn up under the auspices of United Nations Environment Program and signed by 49 countries in March 1985, under which nations cooperate to monitor the ozone layer, to note changes in it and to agree upon recommendations for action to mitigate any depletion of it.

convulsions. The motor component of a generalized tonic–clonic seizure. Often a sign seen as a primary or secondary consequence of intoxication of the CNS. Tonic–clonic or grand mal seizures are characterized by sudden onset (sometimes preceded by an aura) and loss of consciousness, followed by body rigidity (tonic) and then marked involuntary muscle contractions (clonic). At the conclusion of a tonic–clonic seizure, the patient is usually lethargic and disoriented, and will often sleep. Other generalized seizures, not associated with convulsions, include myoclonic, atonic (brief loss of postural tone) or akinetic (loss of movement without loss of tone) seizures, and absence (petit mal) seizures which involve very brief losses of consciousness. Convulsions limited to a single limb or muscle group may occur as part of a simple partial or focal seizure. The generalized tonic–clonic convulsions (grand mal) and focal convulsions are usually controlled by such drugs as carbamazepine or phenytoin. The absence seizures generally will respond better to sodium valproate or ethosuximide. *See also* CLONIC; DIAGNOSTIC FEATURES, CENTRAL NERVOUS SYSTEM; MAINTENANCE THERAPY; SEIZURES.

cooxidation. The simultaneous oxidation of two substrates. In toxicology, cooxidations in which at least one of the substrates is a xenobiotic are important. Two such cases are of special interest: cooxidation by microorganisms and, in mammals, cooxidation of xenobiotics during prostaglandin biosynthesis. *See also* COOXIDATION, BY MICROORGANISMS; COOXIDATION, DURING PROSTAGLANDIN BIOSYNTHESIS.

cooxidation, by microorganisms. Organic chemicals not suitable as the sole carbon source or the sole energy source for a microorganism may nevertheless be oxidized in the presence of suitable carbon and/or energy sources. This is important in the oxidation of environmental contaminants otherwise recalcitrant to microbial metabolism. *See also* COOXIDATION.

cooxidation, during prostaglandin biosynthesis. During the biosynthesis of prostaglandins, a polyunsaturated fatty acid (e.g., arachidonic acid) is oxygenated to yield a hydroperoxy endoperoxide, prostaglandin G. This is then further metabolized to prostaglandin H2, both reactions being catalyzed by the same enzyme, prostaglandin synthase. During the second (peroxidase) step of the above sequence many xenobiotics can be cooxidized. Prostaglandin synthase is located in the microsomal membrane and is found in high levels in such tissues as seminal vesicle. It is a glycoprotein with a subunit molecular mass of about 70,000 daltons, containing one heme per subunit. Many of the xenobiotic reactions yield products that are similar or identical to those formed by other peroxidases and also by microsomal monooxygenases. They include both detoxication and activation products, thus this mechanism may be important in xenobiotic metabolism, particularly in tissues low in cytochrome P450 and/or the FAD-containing monooxygenase, but high in prostaglandin synthase. *See also* COOXIDATION.

COPD. *See* CHRONIC OBSTRUCTIVE PULMONARY DISEASE.

copper (Cu). A metal used extensively in electronics and the electric power industry because of its excellent conducting properties. It is also used in a number of important alloys. Dietary copper is an essential nutrient, and not only is copper the prosthetic group for several enzymes, including tyrosinase, superoxide dismutase and amine oxidases, but it is also necessary for the utilization of iron. Entry of toxic concentrations of copper into the body is either by inhalation of dusts or by ingestion. Copper exists in two valence states and can form monovalent (cuprous) and divalent (cupric) compounds. A number of copper compounds are regarded as toxic compounds, including cupric acetate, cupric acetoarsenite, cupric chloride, cupric nitrate, cupric oxalate, cupric sulfate and cupric tartrate. Copper compounds are used as pesticides, pigments, antifouling paints and in electroplating. Copper salts may act as irritants to the skin. Inhalation of dust or fumes may cause irritation of the respiratory tract. Chronic human intoxication is not common except in the case of Wilson's disease. This is a condition characterized by retention of high levels of copper, which can be fatal.

coprine (1-cyclopropanol-1-N5-glutamine). A compound produced by edible mushrooms of the genus *Coprinus* that on ingestion causes a marked ethanol sensitivity. The mechanism appears to be inhibition of the low K_m form of liver acetaldehyde dehydrogenase by the active metabolite cyclopropanone hydrate. Although the overall effect resembles that of disulfiram, coprine does not affect dopamine-β-decarboxylase and is a more potent ethanol sensitizing agent.

$$
\begin{array}{c}
\text{COOH} \\
| \\
\text{H}_2\text{N}-\text{C}-\text{H} \\
| \\
\text{CH}_2\text{CH}_2\text{CONH} \\
\text{HO}
\end{array}
$$

Coprine

Coramine. *See* NIKETHAMIDE.

coriander. *See* ESSENTIAL OILS.

Cornfield and Ryzin model. *See* LOW-DOSE EXTRAPOLATION.

correlation coefficient. A quantitative assessment of the direction and magnitude of the relationship between two variables. The appropriate correlation coefficient to be used depends on the scaling properties of the data (i.e., nominal, ordinal, interval or ratio) and whether the relationship has a linear or nonlinear shape. The most frequently employed correlation coefficient is the Pearson product moment correlation, which specifies the relationship between two variables expressed as standard scores. The product moment correlation is derived by summing the product of pairs of standard scores on the two measures and dividing by N. The ϕ, point biserial and ρ coefficients are all special cases of the product moment coefficient and are used when one or more variables are dichotomous or ranked. In interpreting the correlation between two variables, it is useful to square the r value to obtain the proportion of variance in one measure accounted for by the other. *See also* LINEAR REGRESSION; NONLINEAR REGRESSION; STATISTICS, FUNCTION IN TOXICOLOGY.

corrosives. Materials that cause a surface-destructive effect on contact. In toxicology, a corrosive refers specifically to any substance that causes visible destruction of human skin tissue or the lining of the gastrointestinal tract. Corrosives are usually acids or bases. *See also* POISONING, EMERGENCY TREATMENT.

corticosteroids. The steroids produced from cholesterol by the adrenal cortex. They possess 21 carbon atoms with a double bond at C-4 and ketonic groups at C-3 and C-20 (*see* CORTICOSTERONE). There are several major classes. The glucocorticosteroids which have principal action on carbohydrate, fat and protein metabolism; promoting the deposition of glycogen in the liver and the formation of glucose from tissue protein and mobilization of fat. Hydrocortisone (17-hydroxycorticosterone, cortisol), the main glucocorticosteroid hormone in humans, is used extensively in the treatment of acute inflammation of various tissues. Cortisone (m.p. 215 °C) is manufactured from the saponin, diosgenin. It is used beneficially in the treatment of rheumatoid arthritis; the 9-fluoro derivative (dexamethasone) has a higher activity and fewer side effects than either cortisone or hydrocortisone. The mineralocorticoids have principal action on water and electrolyte metabolism. Aldosterone causes the retention of sodium and is probably the principal hormonal factor in maintaining electrolyte balance in mammals. *See also* CORTICOSTERONE; CORTISOL; CORTISONE.

corticosterone (11β,21-dihydroxypregn-4-ene-3,20-dione). CAS number 50-22-6. An adrenocortical steroid with modest glucocorticoid and mineralocorticoid activity. It is the primary glucocorticoid in the rat. *See also* ADRENAL GLAND TOXICITY; CORTICOSTEROIDS.

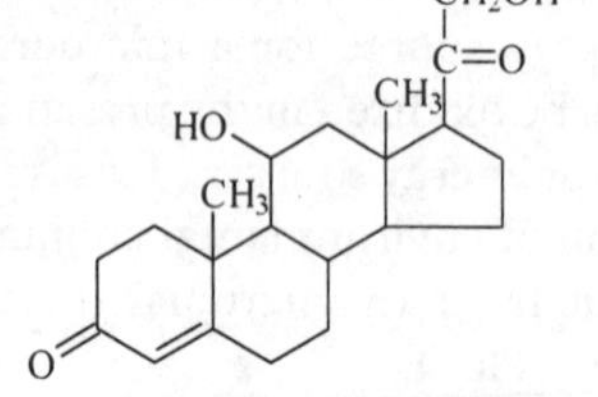

Corticosterone

cortisol (11β,17,21-trihydroxypregn-4-ene-3,20-dione; hydrocortisone). An adrenocortical steroid with glucocorticoid and weak mineralocorticoid activity. It is the primary glucocorticoid in the human, and its presence reflects activation of the HPA axis. *See also* ADRENAL GLAND TOXICITY; CORTICOSTEROIDS.

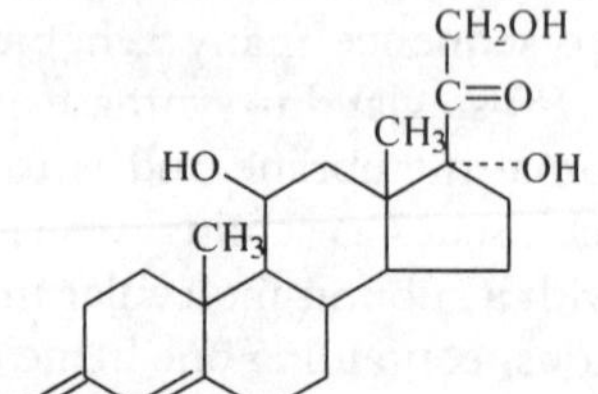

Cortisol

cortisone (17α,21-dihydroxy-4-pregnene-2,11,20-trione). CAS number 53-06-5. A corticosteroid with glucocorticoid and weak mineralocorticoid activity. In rats, it is the primary circulating glucocorticoid. *See also* ADRENAL GLAND TOXICITY; CORTICOSTEROIDS.

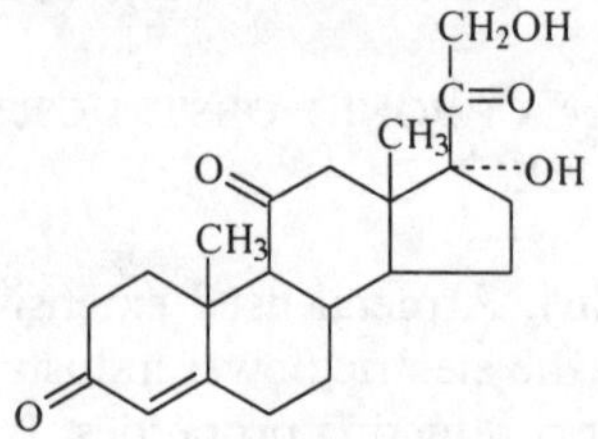

Cortisone

COSHH. *See* CONTROL OF SUBSTANCES HAZARDOUS TO HEALTH REGULATIONS.

Cosmegen. *See* ACTINOMYCIN D.

cosmetics. Chemical formulations intended to enhance appearance or beauty. These preparations require extensive safety testing before approval for marketing is granted.

cost benefit analysis. An analysis of the costs of an action, or a proposed action, relative to the benefits that might accrue from that action. In regulatory toxicology the costs are usually those that might be caused by the regulation of a particular chemical compared with the societal benefits that might accrue from such regulation.

COT. *See* COMMITTEE ON TOXICITY OF CHEMICALS IN FOOD, CONSUMER PRODUCTS AND THE ENVIRONMENT.

coumarin ($C_9H_6O_2$). CAS number 91-64-5. Used as a natural perfume and flavoring material, coumarin is widely distributed in plants as the glycoside. Warfarin is a coumarin derivative. Coumarin is oxidized by cytochrome P4502A6 to 7-hydroxycoumarin. It can also be oxidized to the hepatotoxicant coumarin-3,4-epoxide which subsequently forms 3-hydroxycoumarin. *See also* LEWIS, HCDR, NUMBER CNV000; DATABASES, TOXICOLOGY.

Coumarin

Council for Agricultural Science and Technology (CAST). A US based organization for the rational and safe use of chemicals and modern technology in agriculture. Membership consists of agriculturally oriented scientific societies and individual members. Publishes studies for both scientists and laymen in the above areas.

Council on Environmental Quality (CEQ). The US federal agency, formed under the terms of the National Environmental Policy Act, 1969 (NEPA) for the enforcement of measures for environmental protection. The aim of the Act is to "encourage productive and enjoyable harmony between Man and his environment; to promote efforts which will prevent or eliminate damage to the environment and biosphere and stimulate the health and welfare of Man; to enrich the understanding of the ecological systems and natural resources important to the Nation; and to establish a Council on Environmental Quality."

covalent binding. The formation of a covalent bond or "shared electron pair" bond. Each covalent bond consists of a pair of electrons shared between two atoms and occupying two stable orbitals, one of each atom. Although this is distinguished from the ionic bond or ionic valence, in fact chemical bonds may show both covalent and ionic character. In toxicology, covalent binding is used in a less precise way to refer to the binding of toxicants or their reactive metabolites to endogenous molecules (usually macromolecules) to produce stable adducts resistant to rigorous extraction procedures. A covalent bond between a ligand and macromolecule is generally assumed. Many forms of chronic toxicity involve covalent binding of the toxicant to DNA or protein molecules within the cell.

covalent binding tests. The measurement of DNA adducts provides an indication of genotoxic (carcinogenic) potential, and DNA adducts in the urine are an indication, obtained by a non-invasive technique, of recent exposure. Protein adducts provide an integrated measure of exposure since they accumulate over the lifespan of the protein and may also indicate organ toxicity. Tissue protein adducts are demonstrated in experimental animals by injection of radiolabeled chemicals and, after a period of time, removing the organs, homogenizing and removing all of the non-covalently bound material by rigorous extraction. Extraction methods include lipid solvents, acids and bases, concentrated urea solutions and solubilization and precipitation of the proteins. Newer methods involve dialysis against detergent solutions. Blood proteins, such as hemoglobin, may be used in tests of human exposure, since blood is readily and safely accessible. The exposure of mice to ethylene oxide or dimethylnitrosamine has been estimated by measuring alkylated residues in hemoglobin. The method has subsequently been extended to people occupationally exposed to ethylene oxide by measuring *N*-3-(2-hydroxyethyl)-histamine residues in hemoglobin. Methylcysteine residues in hemoglobin can be used as a measure of methylation. DNA/RNA adducts can also be measured in a variety of ways, including rigorous extraction, separation and precipitation following administration of labeled compounds *in vivo*, or by the use of antibodies raised to chemically modified DNA or RNA. Many compounds of different chemical classes have been shown to bind covalently when activated by microsomal preparations *in vitro* (e.g., aflatoxin, ipomeanol, stilbene, vinyl chloride). Although routine testing procedures based on these observations would be useful in predicting toxic potential, they have not yet been developed. *See also* COVALENT BINDING.

Coytillo. *See* BUCKTHORN TOXINS.

CPSC. *See* CONSUMER PRODUCT SAFETY COMMISSION.

CR (dibenz(b.f.)-1:4-oxazepine). A potent lacrimator which is chemically stable and retains its irritancy in water and so can be used in liquid jets in personnel control. In addition to lacrimation, it causes eye pain, blepharospasm, eyelid swelling, irritation of the conjunctiva, a rise in intraocular pressure, and erythema of the skin. Because it can be used in water, its use is less affected by changes in climatic conditions. It is a more potent lacrimator than CS but it is less potent in lethality than CS. *See also* C-AGENTS.

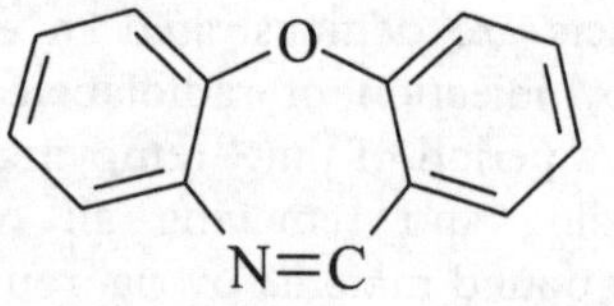

CR

creatine. A compound that is phosphorylated to phosphocreatine, which represents a store of high-energy phosphoryl groups in muscle that can be transferred to ADP, yielding ATP for muscle contraction. The enzyme involved in phosphate transfer between them is creatine phosphokinase, that catalyzes the reaction

$$\text{phosphocreatine} + \text{ADP} \rightarrow \text{ATP} + \text{creatine}$$

An increase in serum creatine phosphokinase may be indicative of damage to non-hepatic tissue, but not to the liver.

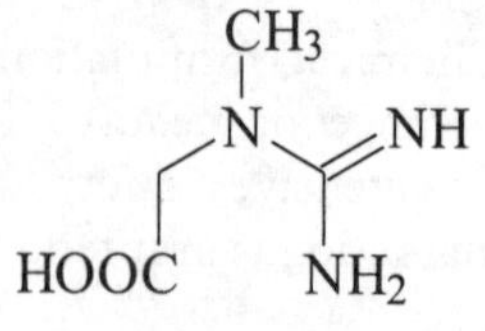

Creatine

creatine phosphokinase. *See* CREATINE.

creatinine. **CAS number 60-27-5**. A degradation product of creatine. Serum creatinine is elevated after eating meat. High serum creatinine may also be indicative of renal failure. *See also* CREATINE.

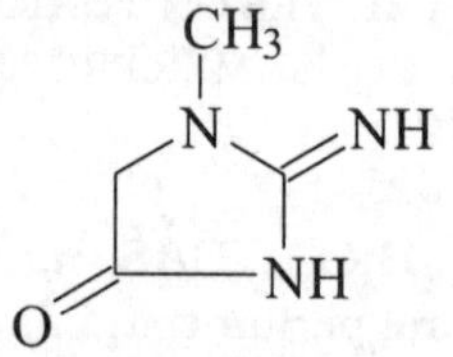

Creatinine

creosote. **CAS number 8001-58-9**. Fractions obtained in the distillation of coal tar are used for preserving timber; a dark liquid mixture of hydrocarbons, phenols, cresols and other aromatic compounds with a characteristic odor. Medical creosote, CAS number 8021-39-4, an almost colorless liquid mixture of phenols, mainly guaiacol and creosol, is obtained by the destructive distillation of wood. It is used as an antiseptic (less toxic than phenol) and as an expectorant. IARC and the US EPA have classified coal tar creosote as a probable human carcinogen. *See also* COAL TAR; ATSDR DOCUMENT, APRIL 1993.

critical endpoint. *See* TOXIC ENDPOINT, CRITICAL.

critical periods. *See* TERATOGENESIS.

crocidolite asbestos. *See* ASBESTOS.

cross-resistance (cross-tolerance). The situation in which either resistance or tolerance is induced by exposure to a different toxicant. This is commonly seen in resistance of insects to insecticides, in which selection with one insecticide brings about a broad spectrum of resistance to insecticides of the same or different chemical classes. Such cross-resistance is usually caused by the inheritance of a high level of non-specific xenobiotic-metabolizing enzymes. *See also* ADAPTATION TO TOXICANTS.

cross-sectional epidemiological study. *See* EPIDEMIOLOGICAL STUDIES, CROSS-SECTIONAL.

cross-tolerance. *See* CROSS-RESISTANCE.

Crotalidae. The family of pit vipers, venomous snakes such as rattlesnakes (*Crotalus*), the copperhead (*Agkistrodon*) and the water moccasin in North America and the bushmaster and fer-de-lances of South America and Asia. The crotalid venoms are high in proteolytic enzymes. *See also* RATTLESNAKE VENOM.

CRS. *See* CHINESE RESTAURANT SYNDROME.

crude oil. Petroleum as it is extracted from its deposits, prior to refining. *See also* PETROLEUM; POLLUTION, FOSSIL FUELS; POLLUTION, PETROLEUM PRODUCTS.

Cruelty to Animals Act. A UK act that placed restrictions on the use of animals in whole-animal experiments. This Act has recently been replaced by the Animals (Scientific Procedures) Act. *See also* ANIMALS (SCIENTIFIC PROCEDURES) ACT.

CS (*o*-chlorobenzylidene malonitrile). A fine powder used in riot control because of its property of inducing acute irritation to the eyes, to any skin abrasion and to the tissues of the respiratory passages, causing coughing and nausea. *See also* C-AGENTS; TEAR GASES.

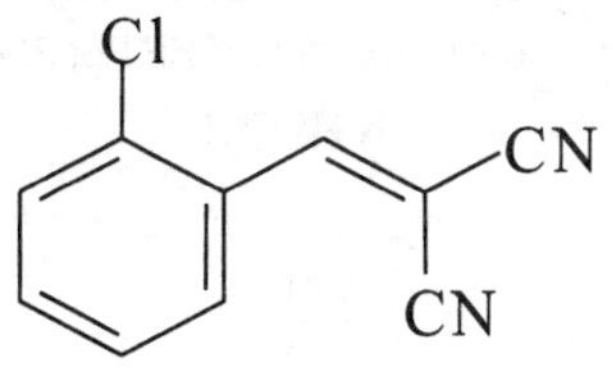

CS

CSA. *See* CONTROLLED SUBSTANCES ACT.

CSD (Committee on Safety of Drugs). *See* COMMITTEE ON SAFETY OF MEDICINES.

CSM. *See* COMMITTEE ON SAFETY OF MEDICINES.

cumulative exposure. The sum of all exposures to an organism over a stated period of time.

Cuprid. *See* TRIENTINE.

curarization. The administration of curare to induce the relaxation of skeletal muscle, usually prior to surgery. The neuromuscular-blocking action allows the patient to receive a lighter level of anesthesia than ordinarily would be required. The technique is also used in orthopedic procedures. *See also* TUBOCURARINE.

CWA. *See* CLEAN WATER ACT.

cyanide poisoning, therapy. The mode of action of cyanide ion is the inhibition of cytochrome oxidase, thus blocking cellular respiration. The toxic dose is very small, and the resultant poisoning is rapid and often fatal. Chronic poisoning due to prolonged exposure to very small amounts is, however, also known to occur. Emergency measures for either inhaled or ingested cyanide include amyl nitrite, artificial respiration and 100% oxygen. In the case of ingestion, gastric lavage may also be used. There are two forms of specific therapy. Sodium nitrite is administered to convert hemoglobin to methemoglobin, the latter combining with cyanide to form cyanomethemoglobin. Although the affinity of cyanide for methemoglobin is lower than its affinity for cytochrome oxidase, the large amount of hemoglobin available makes this a useful therapy. Methemoglobinemia may be hazardous, however, and the nitrite doses must be calculated so as to give 25–40% conversion of hemoglobin. Thiosulfate is also administered to provide a sulfur donor for a reaction catalyzed by the enzyme cyanide-thiosulfate sulfur transferase. This enzyme converts cyanide to thiocyanate (CN^- to CNS^-). In one of these specific therapies, there is removal from the site of action by competition with another binding site, and in the other a detoxication mechanism is stimulated by providing a reactant that is normally rate-limiting *in vivo*. In an experimental setting, these two therapies are synergistic, being much more than additive in their effect. *See also* CYANIDES; AMYL NITRITE.

cyanides. Potassium cyanide (KCN) and sodium cyanide (NaCN) have been designated hazardous substances (EPA), hazardous waste constituents (EPA), and priority toxic pollutants (EPA). Both are white crystalline solids with a faint odor of bitter almonds. Sodium and potassium cyanides are used primarily in the extraction of ores, electroplating and various manufacturing processes. Entry into the body can be via inhalation, ingestion or percutaneous absorption. The cyanides are acutely toxic, their mode of action being the inhibition of cytochrome oxidase with the consequent inhibition of mitochondrial electron transport and oxidative phosphorylation. Symptoms include weakness, headaches, confusion, nausea, vomiting, respiratory failure and death. *See also* CYANIDE POISONING, THERAPY; OXIDATIVE PHOSPHORYLATION; OXIDATIVE PHOSPHORYLATION INHIBITORS.

cyanogenic. Producing cyanide (CN⁻) on metabolism. *See also* AMYGDALIN.

cyanosis. A discoloration of the skin that is slightly blue, purple or grey-blue and that derives from the circulating blood. Due to reduced oxygenation of the blood, cyanosis can be caused by a number of factors, some of which are toxicological in nature. That due to methemoglobin formation is sometimes called enterogenous cyanosis or false cyanosis. Cyanosis is also characteristic of carbon monoxide poisoning. The classical form, that due to reduced oxygenation of normal hemoglobin can be due to non-toxicological causes such as congenital heart disease, but may also result from pulmonary edema, asphyxiant gases, etc. *See also* DIAGNOSTIC FEATURES, SKIN.

cycad. Consumption of flour made from nuts of the cycad plant (e.g., on the island of Guam) has been asssociated with hepatotoxicity, carcinogenicity, teratogenesis, and neurotoxicity. The toxic component is cycasin, a glucoside that is hydrolyzed *in vivo* to the toxic species methylazoxymethanol. Because the nervous system disorders resemble in some ways both amyotropic lateral sclerosis and Parkinsonism, it has been suggested that there may be an environmental link to these diseases. *See also* CYCASIN; METHYLAZOXYMETHANOL.

cycasin   (methylazoxymethanol-β-D-glucoside). CAS number 14901-08-7. A naturally occurring alkylating agent that is produced by the cycad and is found in flour made from the cycad nut. When fed to rats, cycasin causes cancer of the liver, kidney and digestive tract. Ingestion of this plant by animals or humans has been associated with hepatotoxicity, carcinogenicity, teratogenesis, and neurotoxicity that have been linked to its conversion to the active agent methylazoxymethanol. If cycasin is injected i.p. rather than given orally, or if it is fed to germ-free rats, it is not carcinogenic, because glucosidases in the intestinal microflora are necessary for conversion to methylazoxymethanol. *See also* CYCAD; METHYLAZOXYMETHANOL.

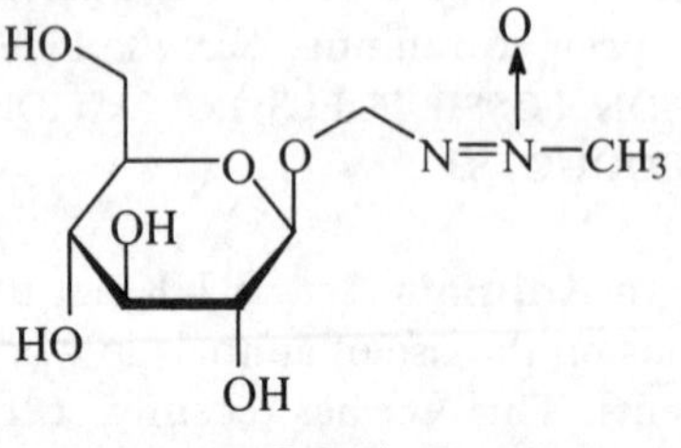

Cycasin

cyclamate. CAS number 100-88-9. Sodium cyclamate is a non-nutritive sweetener that is about 30 times sweeter than cane sugar. The oral LD50s in rats and mice are 15.25 and 17.0 g/kg, respectively. It was banned as a food additive because of findings that it caused bladder cancer in rodents. It appears to act as a promoter. There is also evidence that it causes toxicity in the male reproductive system. *See also* SWEETENING AGENTS.

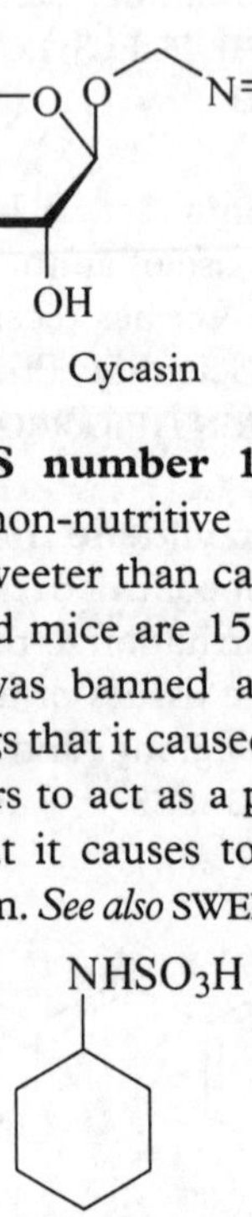

Cyclamate

cyclic adenosine-3′,5′-monophosphate. *See* CYCLIC AMP.

cyclic AMP (cAMP; adenosine-3′,5′-monophosphate; cyclic adenosine-3′,5′-monophosphate). The product formed by the adenylate cyclase enzymes from ATP. It is a cellular "second messenger," participating in the regulation of many intracellular events. Toxicants may cause physiological changes by interfering with aspects of cyclic AMP metabolism. *See also* CHOLERA TOXIN; PERTUSSIS TOXIN; PHOSPHOPROTEINS; RECEPTOR; SECOND MESSENGERS.

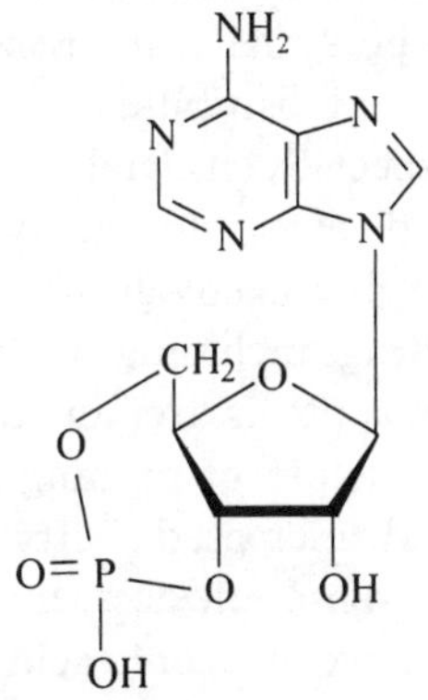

Cyclic AMP

cyclic GMP (cGMP; guanosine-3′-5′-monophosphate; guanosine-3′,5′-cyclic monophosphate; cyclic guanosine-3′,5′-monophosphate). The product formed by the guanylate cyclase enzymes from GTP. It is a cellular "second messenger," participating in the regulation of many

intracellular events. Toxicants (e.g., nitroprusside) may cause physiological changes by interfering with aspects of cyclic GMP metabolism. *See also* CYCLIC AMP; SECOND MESSENGERS.

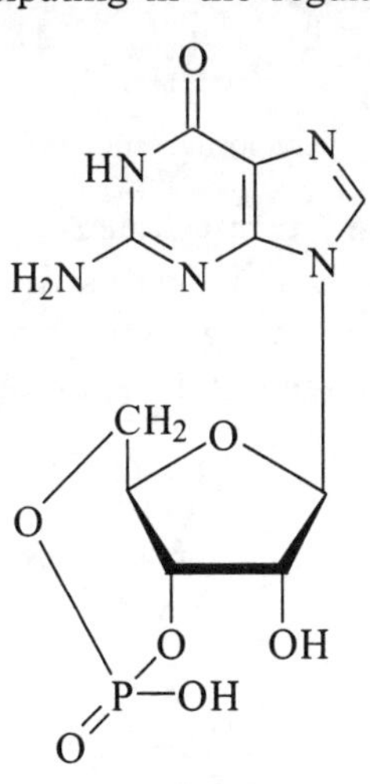

cyclic guanosine-3′,5′-monophosphate. *See* CYCLIC GMP.

cyclic nucleotide cyclases. *See* ADENYLATE CYCLASE; GUANYLATE CYCLASE.

cyclic nucleotide phosphodiesterase. *See* PHOSPHODIESTERASE.

cyclodiene insecticides. Chlorinated insecticides based on the cyclodiene ring structure; formerly widely used for the control of agricultural pests and for structural pest control. All are neurotoxicants, although the signs of poisoning are quite different to those produced by DDT. In humans and animals, seizures are often induced, in addition to the very general symptoms such as nausea, vomiting, headaches, etc. Chronic toxicity is said to include carcinogenicity and/or tumor promotion, and use of cyclodienes has been discontinued in some countries (e.g., aldrin, CAS number 309-00-2, and dieldrin, CAS number 60-57-1, in the USA) as a result. The mode of action (in acute toxicity) is now generally believed to involve effects on GABA$_A$ receptors in the brain. Cyclodienes are metabolized to their epoxides *in vivo*. Since the epoxides are approximately equitoxic and equally persistent with the parent compound, this

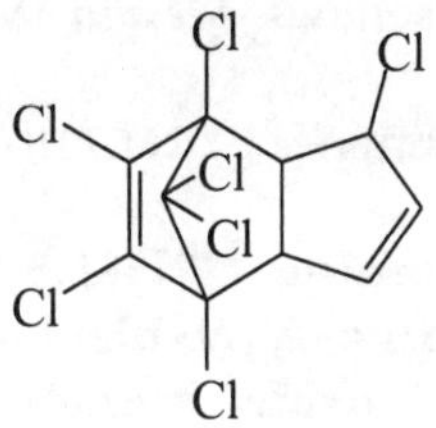

Heptachlor

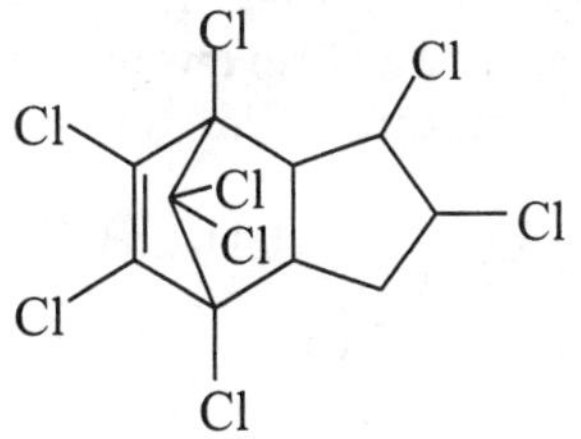

Chlordane

is not a detoxication reaction. Subsequent microsomal cytochrome P450-dependent hydroxylations may occur usually at considerably slower rates, and elimination of aldrin and dieldrin can be accentuated by cytochrome P450 inducers such as phenobarbital. The cyclodiene insecticides are themselves potent inducers of certain cytochrome P450 isozymes. Important representatives of the group include aldrin; dieldrin; endrin, CAS number 72-20-8; heptachlor, CAS number 76-44-8; chlordane, CAS number 57-74-9; and endosulfan, CAS number 115-29-7.

cyclooxygenase. Enzymes that convert arachidonic acid (cleaved from cellular membranes by phospholipase A2) to one of several cyclic endoperoxides known as prostaglandins. The prostaglandins have important cellular actions, but can also be metabolized further to prostacyclins and thromboxanes. Aspirin and related non-steroidal anti-inflammatory drugs (including acetaminophen and ibuprofen) interfere with prostaglandin synthesis by inhibiting cyclooxygenase, thus causing many of their therapeutic effects and side effects. *See also* ACETAMINOPHEN; ANALGESICS; ANTI-INFLAMMATORY AGENTS; ASPIRIN.

cyclopeptides. Amino acids linked by peptide bonds into a variety of cyclic arrangements. Many, including the amatoxins, are highly toxic. They are found particularly in species of two genera of mushrooms, *Amanita* and *Galerina*. One species, *A. phalloides,* is responsible for over 50% of all mushroom poisonings. *See also* AMANITIN.

cyclophospham. *See* CYCLOPHOSPHAMIDE.

cyclophosphamide (2H-1,3,2-oxazaphosphorin-2-amine-N,N-bis(2-chloroethyl)-tetrahydro-1,2-oxide monohydrate; cyclophospham; Cytoxan; Procytox; Endoxan). CAS number 6055-19-2. A cytotoxic antineoplastic with an i.v. LD50 in rats of 160 mg/kg. It is a carcinogen, teratogen and immunosuppressive that strongly inhibits DNA synthesis by being metabolically activated to phosphoramide mustard, a bifunctional alkylating agent. In humans acute exposure causes nausea and vomiting; prolonged exposure causes bone marrow depression, alopecia, hemorrhagic cystitis and cardiotoxicity.

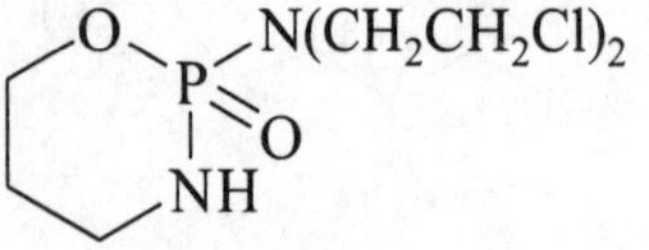

cyclopiazonic acid. A fungal mycotoxin synthesized by several different species of the fungi *Aspergillus* and *Penicillium*. Cyclopiazonic acid is a natural contaminant of cheese, corn and peanuts. Due to the lack of analytical methods for quantifying cyclopiazonic acid, the amount present in the food supply and the potential health risks are uncertain. Cyclopiazonic acid distributes widely in mammalian tissues, especially skeletal muscle, and produces equally diverse cytotoxicity. This toxicant shares many pharmacological properties with antipsychotic drugs including catalepsy, hypothermia, hypokinesia, ptosis, tremor, gait disturbance, sedation without loss of righting reflex, atypical convulsion and increased barbiturate sleeping time. Some of these effects seem to result from direct effects of cyclopiazonic acid on muscle. *See also* MYCOTOXINS.

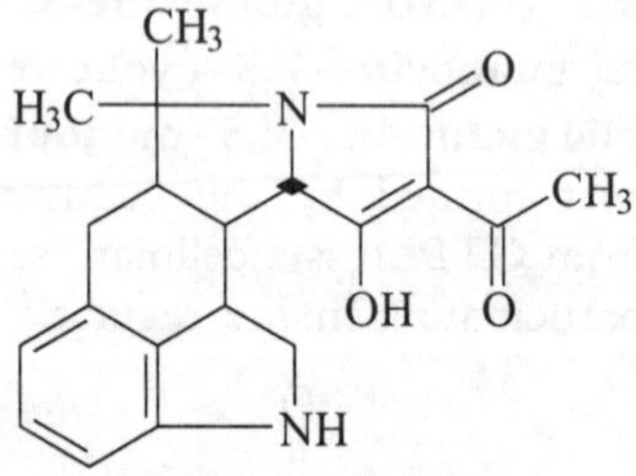

Cyclopiazonic acid

cyclopropane (trimethylene). An inhalation anesthetic that is no longer used due to explosion hazard in the operating room. A mixture of cyclopropane and oxygen or air explodes when ignited.

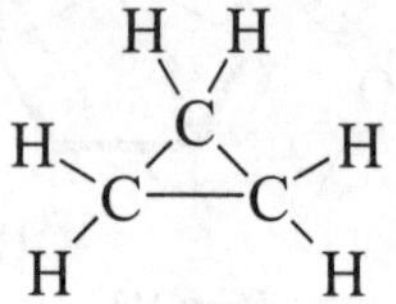

Cyclopropane

Cyclophosphamide

Cygon. *See* DIMETHOATE.

cypermethrin (R,S)-cyano(3-phenoxyphenyl) methyl(R,S)-*cis,trans*-3-(2,2-dichloro-ethenyl)-2,2-dimethylcyclopropane carboxylate). CAS number 52315-07-8. A synthetic analog of the naturally occurring pyrethrins found in pyrethrum extract from certain species of chrysanthemum flower. It is an excellent stomach and contact insecticide, being effective against a variety of insects, especially Lepidoptera, and is widely used in the control of agricultural pests. It exhibits low vertebrate toxicity (acute oral LD50 in rats is 251–4123 mg/kg) and does not accumulate in the environment. It is classified as a type II pyrethroid due to the presence of an α-cyano group, and it acts as a neurotoxicant by increasing nerve membrane sodium permeability by the modification of the sodium channel, leading to depolarization and nerve block. There is evidence that type II pyrethroids may have primarily CNS effects. Signs and symptoms in humans include gastrointestinal irritation, nausea, vomiting, diarrhea, numbness of the tongue and lips, syncope, hyperexcitability, incoordination, convulsions, muscular paralysis, collapse and death due to respiratory paralysis. Treatment involves gastric lavage, use of emetics, demulcents and cathartics, artificial respiration if necessary, and short-acting barbiturates for convulsions.

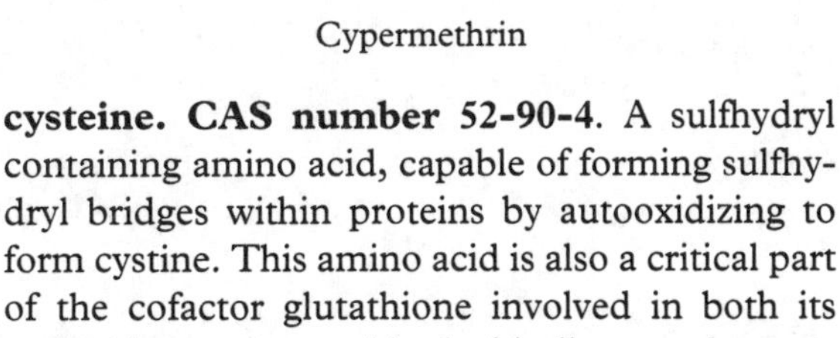

Cypermethrin

cysteine. CAS number 52-90-4. A sulfhydryl containing amino acid, capable of forming sulfhydryl bridges within proteins by autooxidizing to form cystine. This amino acid is also a critical part of the cofactor glutathione involved in both its antioxidant action and in the binding to substrates in glutathione conjugation pathways. Additionally, it is the amino acid catalyzing hydrolysis at the active site of cysteine hydrolases. *See also* ANTI-OXIDANTS; GLUTATHIONE TRANSFERASES; MERCAPTURIC ACIDS.

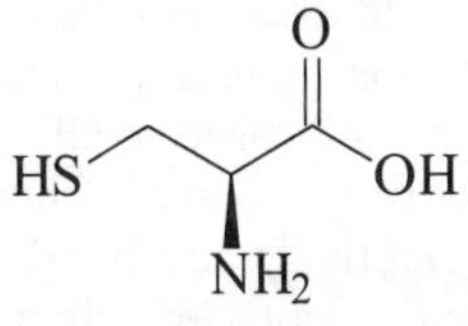

Cysteine

cysteine conjugate β-lyase. An enzyme that metabolizes cysteine conjugates, the products being the thiol derivative of the xenobiotic, pyruvic acid and ammonia. Subsequent methylation of the thiol forms the methylthio derivative. The enzyme from rat liver is a soluble pyridoxal phosphate-requiring protein of about 175 kilodaltons. The best substrates are the cysteine conjugates of aromatic compounds. *See also* METHYLTHIOLATION.

cysteinyl glycinase. The peptidase activity involved in the penultimate step of mercapturic acid formation although a number of aminopeptidases are known that catalyze the hydrolysis of cysteinyl peptides. The membrane-bound glycinases are glycoproteins with molecular weights of around 100,000 daltons. They appear to be metalloproteins, one of the better known being a zinc-containing enzyme. *See also* ACETYLATION; GLUTATHIONE TRANSFERASES; γ-GLUTAMYL TRANS-PEPTIDASE; MERCAPTURIC ACIDS.

Cythion. *See* MALATHION.

cytochrome b$_5$. A microsomal cytochrome involved in such metabolic activities as fatty acid desaturation. It may be involved in the reduction of cytochrome P450. The possibility that the second electron in cytochrome P450 reduction is derived from NADH via cytochrome b$_5$ is still to be resolved. This pathway is not, however, essential for all cytochrome P450-dependent monooxygenations since many occur in systems reconstituted from NADPH, oxygen, phosphatidylcholine and purified NADPH-cytochrome P450 reductase and cytochrome P450. Nevertheless, cytochrome b$_5$ is stimulatory for some monooxygenations and may facilitate oxidative activity in the intact endoplasmic reticulum.

cytochrome oxidase (cytochrome a + a$_3$). The last component of the mitochondrial electron transport system. It receives electrons from cytochrome c and transfers them to oxygen to allow the formation of water; in the process, sufficient free energy is released to allow the formation of ATP. The complex contains heme and copper and can be effectively inhibited by cyanide or carbon monoxide, both of which stop electron transport and prevent ATP formation.

cytochrome P420. A degradation product of cytochrome P450 often seen in microsomal preparations. The carbon monoxide difference spectrum has a prominent absorption peak at 420 nm. Although without oxidative activity, cytochrome P420 binds carbon monoxide and many type II ligands. Its formation, which appears to be irreversible, is believed to be due to rupture of a sulfatide bridge between the heme iron and a protein cysteine residue. *See also* CYTOCHROME P450.

cytochrome P450. The carbon monoxide-binding pigments of microsomes; an enzyme that is a hemoprotein of the b cytochrome type, containing protoporphyrin IX. It was discovered, independently, by Klingenberg and Garfinkel in 1958. Unlike most cytochromes, it is named, not from the absorption maximum of the reduced form in the visible region, but from the unique wavelength of the absorption maximum of the carbon monoxide derivative of the reduced form. The role of cytochrome P450 as the terminal

enzyme in the cytochrome P450-dependent mono-oxygenase system is well documented, and it is the key enzyme in both detoxication and activation reactions of numerous xenobiotics. For example, cytochrome P450, in conjunction with another enzyme, epoxide hydrolase, is responsible for the metabolism of benzo[a]pyrene to its ultimate carcinogenic form, the 7,8-diol-9,10-epoxide. Although the reaction mechanism of cytochrome P450 is not understood, it involves NADPH-cytochrome P450 reductase and may be summarized as shown in the figure. Cytochrome P450 has been studied most in mammalian liver, but is also known to be widely distributed in plants, microorganisms and animals. It occurs in many organs in mammals, including the liver, kidney, lung, skin and placenta, usually as a complex mixture of different isozymes. Many isozymes can be induced by xenobiotics and thus, since xenobiotics can act as substrates, inducers or inhibitors, cytochrome P450 is the focal point for many interactions of profound toxicological significance. In contrast to the microsomal forms of cytochrome P450, the mitochondrial forms are not primarily involved with xenobiotic metabolism, but rather with the metabolism of endogenous steroids. *See also* CYTOCHROME P420; CYTOCHROME P450, ISOZYMES; CYTOCHROME P450, OPTICAL DIFFERENCE SPECTRA; CYTOCHROME P450, PURIFICATION; CYTOCHROME

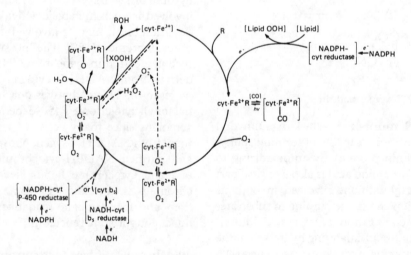

Cytochrome P450
From Hodgson, E.A. & Levi, P.E.A. *Textbook of Modern Toxicology* (New York, Elsevier, 1987)

P450, SUBSTRATE SPECIFICITY; ENDOPLASMIC RETICULUM; INDUCTION; MICROSOMES; MONO-OXYGENASES; PHASE I REACTIONS.

cytochrome P450, classification. A system of nomenclature for cytochrome P450 based on protein sequence as inferred from the cDNA base sequence, was proposed in 1987 and has been updated several times since, most recently in 1996. P450 genes are designated CYP followed by an Arabic numeral designating the gene family, an upper case letter designating the subfamily and finally an Arabic numeral designating the individual gene, for example CYP1A1. The protein sequence of any member of a gene family is 40% or less similar to that of any member of any other gene family. Protein sequences are greater than 55% similar within mammalian subfamilies and 46% within non-mammalian subfamilies. Sequences with less than 3% divergence are considered allelic variants or polymorphisms unless evidence exists to the contrary. The gene products, cytochrome P450 proteins, may still be designated P450 rather than CYP, although the same numbering system is used as described above for the genes.

cytochrome P450, evolution. Cytochrome P450s are found throughout the plant, animal and microbial kingdoms and are evidently of ancient origin. Evolutionary trees have been generated by comparison of derived amino acid sequences. Such trees can be compared with the species divergence time derived from fossil evidence. As a result of such comparisons it has been suggested that the earliest cytochrome P450s are those that metabolize fatty acids and steroids and probably functioned in the maintenance of membrane integrity. Subsequently cytochrome P450s were adapted for the oxidation of lipophilic compounds that, if accumulated, would cause toxicity. The rapid divergence into the large number of xenobiotic-metabolizing isoforms known today may have received its biggest impetus with the emergence of vertebrates onto land.

cytochrome P450, isozymes. The cytochromes P450 that constitute the cytochrome P450-dependent monooxygenase system of the endoplasmic reticulum exist as many distinct cytochrome P450s (e.g., at least ten different cytochrome P450s have been purified to homogenity from rat liver). These proteins represent different gene products and, although the substrate specificity is not identical, the cytochrome P450 forms do exhibit a broad and overlapping substrate specificity for many similar types of compound. Thus, the different cytochrome P450 enzymes are usually referred to as isozymes or isoforms. Many of these isozymes are inducible by drugs and other lipophilic xenobiotics (e.g., phenobarbital will induce certain isozymes, whereas 3-methylcholanthrene will induce others). *See also* CYTOCHROME P450; ISOZYMES.

cytochrome P450, optical difference spectra. Cytochrome P450 has a characteristic absorption spectrum in the visible region that can be perturbed by the addition of many organic, and some inorganic, ligands. These perturbations, measured as optical difference spectra, have been used in characterization of the cytochrome. The most important difference spectra of oxidized cytochrome P450 are: type I, with an absorption maximum at 385–190 nm and a minimum around 420 nm: and type II, with a peak at 420–135 nm and a trough at 390–410 nm. Type I ligands are found in many different chemical classes and include drugs, environmental contaminants, insecticides and industrial chemicals. They appear to bind to a hydrophobic site in the protein that is close enough to the heme to allow both spectral perturbation and interaction with the activated oxygen. Although type I ligands are generally substrates, it has not been possible to demonstrate a quantitative relationship between K_s (the concentration required for half-maximal spectral development) and K_m (the Michaelis constant). Type II ligands interact directly with the heme iron of the cytochrome and are generally organic compounds having nitrogen atoms with sp^2 or sp^3 non-bonded electrons that are sterically accessible. Many type II ligands are inhibitors of cytochrome P450-dependent monooxygenase activity. The two most important optical difference spectra of the reduced cytochrome are the carbon monoxide spectrum, with its maximum at or about 450 nm, and the type III spectrum, with two pH-dependent peaks at approximately 430 and 455 nm. The carbon monoxide spectrum forms the basis for the quantitative estimation of cytochrome P450. The best known type III ligands for cytochrome P450 are ethyl isocyanide and compounds such as the methylenedioxyphenyl synergist piperonyl butoxide, that form stable type III complexes that appear to be related to the mechanism by which they inhibit monooxygenase reactions. *See also* OPTICAL DIFFERENCE SPECTRA.

cytochrome P450, polymorphisms. A true genetic polymorphism is defined as having more than one allele of the same gene in a population. Genetic polymorphisms have been arbitrarily defined as having a frequency of 1% or more, rarer genetic defects being designated as rare traits. Functional polymorphisms result in more than one phenotype within a population when the enzyme is absent due to gene deletions, splice variations or premature stop codons. Other functional polymorphisms may result when the enzyme is expressed at different levels or have altered catalytic activity or substrate specificity. Polymorphisms in cytochrome P450 enzymes result in interindividual variations in the ability to metabolize drugs and are more common in humans than in inbred laboratory animals. Genetic polymorphisms in human CYP2D6 result in differences in the ability to metabolize a variety of drugs including antihypertensive agents such as debrisoquine, the analgesics codeine and dextromethorphan, antiarrhythmic drugs, certain beta blockers and antidepressants. Another polymorphism occurs in the enzyme CYP2C19, responsible for the metabolism of mephenytoin and omeprazole. Allelic variants in CYP2C19 affect its catalytic activity toward substrates such as tolbutamide, warfarin, and various anti-inflammatory drugs. It has been suggested that alterations in the upstream region of CYP2E1 alter its catalytic activity. Base changes in intron and 3'-noncoding regions of various CYP genes have also been reported and their associations with various cancers studied but in these cases the functional significance is more questionable. *See also* POLYMORPHISMS.

cytochrome P450, purification. Considerable progress has been made on the purification of cytochrome P450, although the numerous isozymes have not all been purified. Instability on solubilization, leading to formation of the inactive form, cytochrome P420, is minimized by the use of glycerol and dithiothreitol. Following solubilization, reaggregation due to the hydrophobicity of the protein can be overcome by a low concentration of a suitable detergent, such as Emulgen 911. Multiple forms (isozymes) must be separated from each other and purified, and the detergents must be removed before reconstitution can be carried out. Using these precautions and a combination of traditional and recent methods for protein purification, it has been possible to purify cytochrome(s) P450, as well as the NADPH-cytochrome P450 reductase from mammalian liver and lung. Various detergents have been used for solubilization, but sodium cholate is most commonly used. The two reagents most commonly used for protein precipitation are ammonium sulfate and polyethylene glycol. The materials most commonly used for column chromatography are DEAE-cellulose, CM-cellulose, hydroxylapatite and "affinity" columns based on *n*-octylamine or *n*-hexylamine, although the latter may act as hydrophobic columns rather than as true affinity columns. More recently there have been three major developments in the purification of cytochrome P450 isozymes. (1) The use of HPLC columns for the separation of proteins, including cytochrome P450. (2) The use of antibody- (polyclonal and monoclonal) based chromatography. (3) The cloning of the genes for single cytochrome P450 isozymes in an organism without other cytochrome P450s. This is the potentially most useful method. *See also* CYTOCHROME P450, ISOZYMES.

cytochrome P450, substrate specificity. An important finding from purification studies is that the lack of substrate specificity of hepatic microsomes from cytochrome P450-dependent monooxygenase activity is not due to the presence of several specific cytochromes, since many of the cytochromes isolated to date are relatively nonspecific in that all can oxidize more than one substrate. The relative activity toward different substrates and the range of substances oxidized vary greatly from one purified isozyme to another. However, the large number of isozymes and the recently discovered heterogeneity within isozyme function make this a difficult problem to resolve. Mitochondrial cytochrome P450s appear to be much more specific, usually oxidizing a narrow range of endogenous steroidal substrates and not, as with the microsomal enzymes, a wide range of lipophilic xenobiotics. Bacterial cytochrome P450, such as P450cam may be specific for a single substrate. *See also* CYTOCHROME P450, ISOZYMES.

cytochrome P450-dependent monooxygenase system. A multi-enzyme system in which cytochrome P450 forms the terminal oxidase. In the microsomal system, principally involved in the metabolism of xenobiotics, reducing equivalents are transferred from NADPH to cytochrome P450 by a flavoprotein enzyme, NADPH-cytochrome P450 reductase. The only other component essential for activity in the reconstituted system is a lipid, phosphatidylcholine, although cytochrome b_5 appears to stimulate some oxidations. In the mitochondrial system, involved primarily with the oxidation of endogenous steroids, and in the bacterial system, an additional non-heme iron protein facilitates electron transfer between a flavoprotein reductase and the cytochrome. *See also* CYTOCHROME P450; CYTOCHROME b_5.

cytolytic T cells. *See* T CELLS.

cytoplasm. The protoplasm outside the nucleus of the cell, usually containing a variety of organelles and inclusions.

cytotoxicity. Cellular injury or death caused by soluble mediators or cells of the immune system or by drugs or toxicants. Cytotoxicity is one of the effector mechanisms by which the immune system eliminates microbes and tumor cells. Soluble mediators include complement (a group of serum proteins), lymphotoxin, and tumor necrosis factor (also called cachectin). Cells capable of cytotoxicity include activated macrophages, cytotoxic T lymphocytes (Tc), and natural killer (NK) cells. The latter two cell types and the complement system kill cells by means of proteins which form trans-membrane channels. Probably the most commonly used cytotoxic drugs or toxicants are anticancer drugs which generally kill cycling cells but not G_0 cells.

cytotoxic T cells. *See* T CELLS.

cytoxan. *See* CYCLOPHOSPHAMIDE.

D

D. *See* D-AGENTS.

2,4-D ((2,4-dichlorophenoxy)acetic acid).
CAS number 94-75-7. A widely used herbicide. Acute overdose may cause weakness, stupor, hyporeflexia and muscle twitch or convulsions. 2,4-D is a peroxisome proliferator and induces CYP 4A1. A component of Agent Orange (a mixture of 2,4-D and 2,4,5-T), used as a defoliant during the Vietnam war. Reproductive and other effects seen at high doses are probably due to TCDD, until recently a common contaminant of 2,4-D and other chlorophenoxy herbicides. *See also* AGENT ORANGE; HERBICIDES; TCDD.

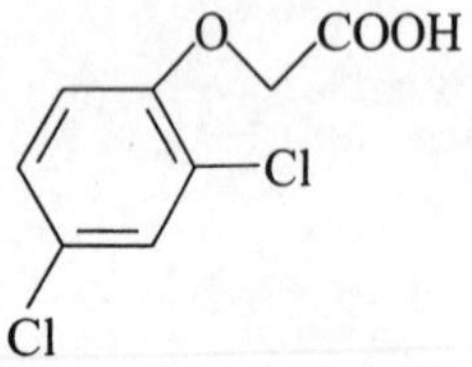

2,4-D

Dactinomycin. *See* ACTINOMYCIN D.

D-Agents (D, DC, DM). Arsenical vomiting agents, considered for use as war gases. The structure of DM (10-chloro-5,10-dihydrophenarsazine) is shown below. *See also* C-AGENTS.

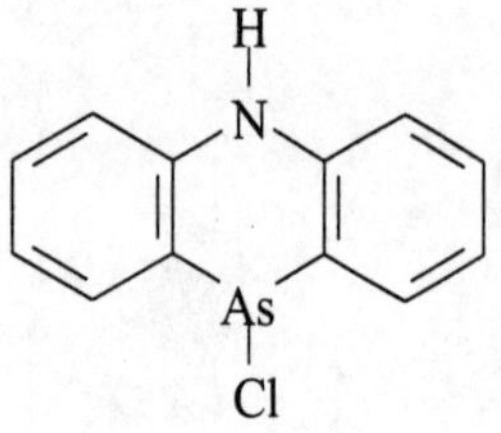

DM

daminozide. *See* ALAR.

Daphnia magna. A standard invertebrate (crustacean) used for aquatic toxicology tests; the common name is water flea. *See also* AQUATIC BIOASSAY.

Darvon. *See* PROPOXYPHENE.

databases, toxicology

Electronic

Cooper's Toxic Exposures – CD-ROM – CRC Press.

Dictionary of Alkaloids – CD-ROM – Chapman and Hall

Dictionary of Natural Products – CD-ROM – Chapman and Hall

Dictionary of Organophosphorus Compounds – CD-ROM – Chapman and Hall

Dictionary of Pharmacologic Agents – CD-ROM – Chapman and Hall

R. J. Lewis. Sax's Dangerous Properties of Industrial Materials, 8th edn, CD-ROM – Chapman and Hall

Merck Index, 12th edn, CD-ROM – Chapman and Hall

Regulated Chemicals Handbook – CD-ROM – Chapman and Hall

Printed

Complete citations may be found in the reference section.

ATSDR Summaries

Cooper's Toxic Exposures A.R. Cooper, Sr, CRC Press.

Ellenhorn Medical Toxicology

IARC Monographs

Lewis Hazardous Chemicals Desk Reference

Data Sheet Compendium. *See* ASSOCIATION OF THE BRITISH PHARMACEUTICAL INDUSTRY.

Datril. *See* ACETAMINOPHEN.

daunomycin. *See* DAUNORUBICIN.

daunorubicin ((8S-*cis*)-8-acetyl-10-[(3-amino-2,3,6-trideoxy-α-lyxo-hexapyranosyl)-oxy]-7,8,9,10-tetrahydro-6,8,11-trihydroxy-1 methoxy-5,12-naphthacenedione; **daunomycin; Rubomycin C). CAS number 20830-81-3.** An anthracycline cytotoxic antineoplastic produced by *Streptomyces peucetius*. Its LD50 in mice is 47.0 mg/kg, i.p. It is a carcinogen that inhibits DNA and RNA synthesis by intercalating in double-stranded DNA like the more potent adriamycin. Acutely, it causes nausea and vomiting, later followed by bone marrow suppression and cardiotoxicity resulting in congestive heart failure. *See also* CHEMOTHERAPY.

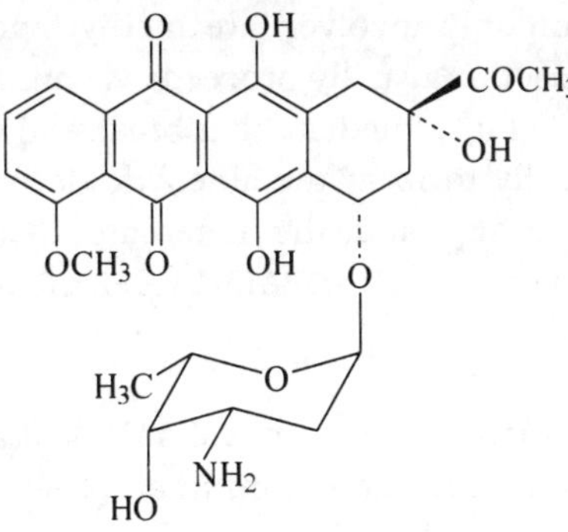

Daunorubicin

DBCP. *See* 1,2-DIBROMO-3-CHLOROPROPANE.

DBH. *See* DOPAMINE β-HYDROXYLASE.

DBP (di-*n*-butyl phthalate). *See* PHTHALIC ACID ESTERS.

DC. *See* D-AGENTS.

DDD (1,1-dichloro-2,2-bis(4-chlorophenyl)-ethane; TDE; Rhothane) CAS number 72-54-8. A DDT analog with very low mammalian toxicity; a known metabolite of DDT in mammals. Formerly used on many food crops, all registrations of DDD were cancelled in 1972, primarily because of implication in eggshell thinning in predatory birds. Its mode of action is probably the same as that of DDT. The oral LD50 in rats is 3400 mg/kg. *See also* ATSDR DOCUMENT MAY 1994; DATABASES, TOXICOLOGY; DDT; EGG-SHELL THINNING.

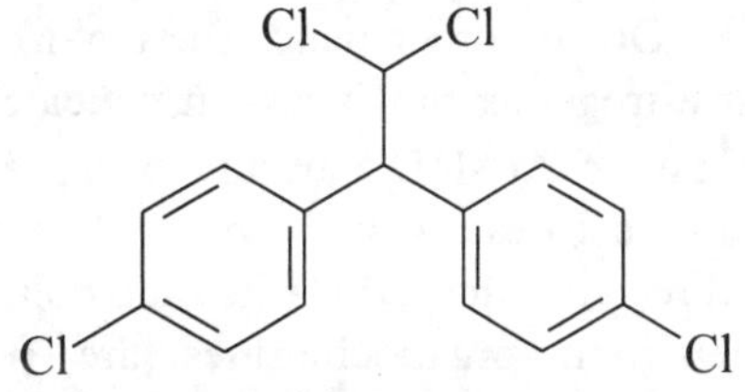

DDD

DDE (1,1-dichloro-2,2-bis(4-chlorophenyl) ethane). CAS number 72-55-9. Principal metabolite of DDT in humans and other animals. Principal long-term storage form derived from DDT in humans and other animals. Biological half-life of several years. DDE is probably related to the chronic toxic effects of DDT such as eggshell thinning. It has been suggested recently that DDT, its metabolites and other persistent organochlorines are possibly involved in cancer causation, particularly human breast cancer. *See also* ATSDR DOCUMENT, MAY 1994; DATABASES, TOXICOLOGY; DDT; DDD.

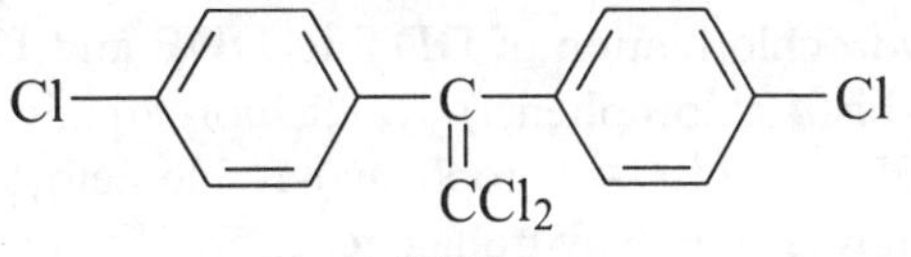

DDE

DDT (1,1,1-trichloro-2,2-bis(4-chlorophenyl) ethane; chlorophenothane). CAS number 50-29-3. The first successful organochlorine insecticide. Insecticidal properties of DDT were discovered in 1939, and the material was introduced into the USA in 1942. Because of its broad spectrum of activity and low acute mammalian toxicity, it became a very widely used insecticide on crops and domestic animals, in homes and on humans. Persistence in the environment, accumulation in fat and induction of eggshell thinning in predatory birds led to a loss in popularity of DDT, and in 1973 all registrations were cancelled by the EPA. The acute toxicity of DDT is attributed to a direct action on nerve axon membranes, increasing excitability and resulting in multiple impulses, tremors and tetanus. More specifically, DDT increases sodium conductance across nerve cell membranes, probably by a direct interaction with the sodium channel protein. The oral LD50 in rats is 113 mg/kg. The *p,p'*-isomer is the most insecticidal isomer, and it demonstrates weak estrogenic properties. On the other hand, the *o,p'*-isomer is the most estrogenic, but is less insecticidal. The estrogenicity of *o,p'*-DDT occurs because of its ability to bind to estrogen receptors. It has been suggested recently that DDT, its metabolites and other persistent organochlorines are possibly involved in cancer causation, particular human breast cancer. *See also* ATSDR DOCUMENT, MAY 1994; DATABASES, TOXICOLOGY; DDE; DDD; EGGSHELL THINNING.

p,p'-DDT

DDT dehydrochlorinase. An enzyme that has been studied most intensively in DDT-resistant houseflies, although it occurs in both mammals and insects. It occurs in the soluble fraction of homogenates, and in addition to catalyzing the dehydrochlorination of DDT to DDE and DDD (2,2-bis(4-chlorophenyl)-1,1-dichloroethane) to TDEE (2,2-bis(4-chlorophenyl)-1-chloroethylene), it catalyzes the dehydrohalogenation of a number of other DDT analogs. The reaction requires glutathione which, it was believed, serves only in a catalytic role, and does not appear to be consumed during the reaction. Recently, however, it has been suggested that DDT dehydrochlorinase is a form of glutathione *S*-transferase. The monomeric form of the enzyme has a molecular mass of about 36,000 daltons, but the enzyme normally exists as a tetramer.

DDVP. *See* DICHLORVOS.

DEA (Drug Enforcement Agency). *See* CONTROLLED SUBSTANCES ACT.

deacetylation. The removal of an acetyl group, usually from a nitrogen atom in an organic compound. Metabolic deacetylation varies widely between species, strains and individuals. Acetylation and deacetylation reactions are catalyzed by different enzymes, the relative levels of which determine the importance of acetylation as a xenobiotic-metabolizing mechanism in different species. For example, the rabbit, which has high acetyltransferase activity and low deacetylase activity, excretes significant amounts of acetylated amines, whereas the dog, in which the opposite situation exists, does not. Acetanilide, a typical substrate for the aromatic deacetylase of the liver and kidney, is deacetylated to yield aniline. *Compare* ACETYLATION.

deadly nightshade. *See* ATROPA BELLADONNA.

dealkylation. The removal or loss of alkyl groups from heteroatoms in organic compounds. Dealkylations of importance in toxicology are enzymatic, catalyzed by one or more isozymes of cytochrome P450, and involve alkyl substituents on oxygen, nitrogen or sulfur atoms. The alkyl substituents most commonly involved are methyl and ethyl, and the reaction usually proceeds via an unstable hydroxyalkyl intermediate that breaks down nonenzymatically to form the aldehyde derivative of the alkyl group and the heteroatom. *See also* *N*-DEALKYLATION; *O*-DEALKYLATION; *S*-DEALKYLATION.

***N*-dealkylation**. The removal or loss of an alkyl group from a nitrogen atom in an organic compound. *N*-Dealkylation is common in the metabolism of drugs, insecticides and other xenobiotics. Both *N*-alkyl and *N,N*-dialkyl carbamates are dealkylated, and in some cases, such as the insecticide carbaryl, the methylol intermediates are stable enough to be isolated or to be conjugated *in vivo*. *See also* CARBARYL; DEALKYLATION.

O-**dealkylation**. The removal or loss of an alkyl group from an oxygen atom in an organic compound. The best known example of metabolic *O*-dealkylation in biochemical toxicology is the demethylation of *p*-nitroanisole. Since the product, *p*-nitrophenol, can be measured spectrophotometrically, it is frequently used as a substrate for cytochrome P450. The reaction is believed to proceed via an unstable methylol intermediate that breaks down to formaldehyde and *p*-nitrophenol. The *O*-dealkylation of organophosphorus triesters involves the dealkylation of an ester rather than an ether, and is known to occur with many vinyl, phenyl, phenylvinyl and naphthyl phosphate and thionophosphate triesters. *See also* DEALKYLATION.

S-**dealkylation**. The removal or loss of an alkyl group from a sulfur atom in an organic compound. Cytochrome P450 is believed to catalyze the *S*-dealkylation of a number of thioethers, including methylmercaptan and 6-methylthiopurine. It is possible, however, that the initial attack is sulfoxidation mediated by the FAD-containing monooxygenase rather than cytochrome P450. *See also* DEALKYLATION; FLAVIN-CONTAINING MONOOXYGENASE.

deamination. The removal or loss of an amino group from an organic compound. There are several mechanisms by which amino groups can be removed from endogenous compounds, such as amino acids. The commonest are transamination reactions catalyzed by a number of different transaminases (e.g., glutamic-aspartic transaminase). Xenobiotics, on the other hand, are subjected to oxidative deamination catalyzed by cytochrome P450. *See also* OXIDATIVE DEAMINATION.

dearylation. *See* DESULFURATION AND OXIDATIVE ESTER CLEAVAGE.

debrisoquine polymorphism. *See* POLYMORPHISMS; CYTOCHROME P450, POLYMORPHISMS.

decamethrin. *See* DELTAMETHRIN.

Declaration of Helsinki. This applies to studies carried out on humans. General guidelines for such studies are that they be undertaken only when the results cannot be obtained otherwise, when the benefits to be derived are considerable, and when the risk under the conditions of the test can be estimated as close to non-existent. The Declaration of Helsinki additionally requires that these studies be carried out on properly informed volunteers and under skilled medical supervision. *See also* HUMAN TEST DATA; HUMAN TOXICITY TESTS.

DEET. *See* N,N-DIETHYL-*M*-TOLUAMIDE.

deferoxamine (*N*-[5-[3-[[(5-aminopentyl)-hydroxycarbamoyl[-propionamido]pentyl]-3-[[5-(*N*-hydroxyacetamido)-pentyl]carbamoyl]propionohydroxamic acid; Desferal). **CAS number 70-51-9**. A chelating agent used to promote iron excretion in patients suffering secondary iron overload from multiple transfusions and has also been used successfully in the treatment of dialysis encephalopathy. *See also* ALUMINUM; CHELATING AGENTS; DIALYSIS ENCEPHALOPATHY.

degradation. A deterioration or destruction. The term is largely used for the environmental destruction, either physicochemically or biologically, of toxicants, but can also be used for the destruction of xenobiotics or endobiotics by metabolism within the organism. *See also* BIODEGRADATION, METABOLISM.

dehalogenation. The removal of halogen substituents from organic chemicals. Since halogenated organic compounds are frequently toxic, dehalogenation reactions are important in biochemical toxicology. They may be enzymatic (e.g., those catalyzed by glutathione *S*-transferase or

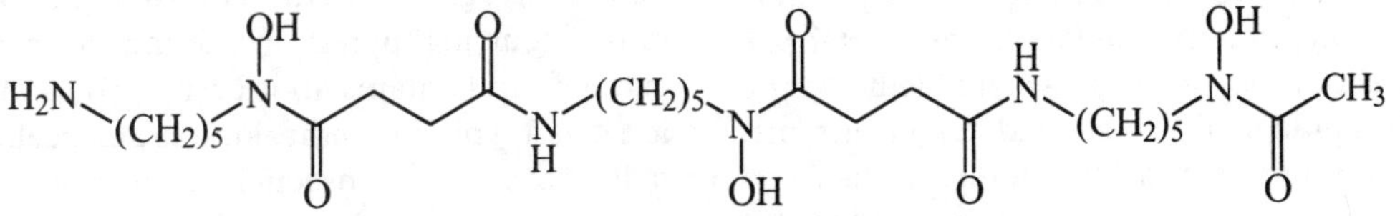

Deferoxamine

DDT dehydrochlorinase) or non-enzymatic (e.g., reaction with nucleophiles such as glutathione). *See also* DDT DEHYDROCHLORINASE; GLUTATHIONE TRANSFERASES.

DEHP. *See* DI(2-ETHYLHEXYL)PHTHALATE.

dehydration. *See* NUTRITIONAL EFFECTS ON METABOLISM, STARVATION AND DEHYDRATION.

Delaney amendment. *See* FOOD, DRUG AND COSMETICS ACT.

delayed hypersensitivity. An inflammatory response due to the presence of an activated lymphocyte population that directs a variety of associated cellular responses through the production of lymphokines. This immunological phenomenon may be recognized by the presence of a local inflammatory response. In contrast to immediate hypersensitivity, whose effects are apparent within minutes, the effects of a delayed hypersensitivity reaction are not apparent until 24–48 hours after exposure. Delayed hypersensitivity is the only type of allergic response that is mediated entirely by T cells, and the production of a delayed hypersensitivity response is used to assess the integrity of cell-mediated immunity after exposure to suspected immunosuppressive or immunomodulatory agents. *See also* ALLERGIC RESPONSE; IMMUNOTOXICITY.

delayed neuropathy. Organophosphate-induced delayed neuropathy (OPIDN) is characterized by muscular weakness, unsteady gait, ataxia and flaccid paralysis of the legs. Histological examination of nerves during progressive development of OPIDN reveals distal-to-proximal degeneration of axonal membrane followed by loss of the myelin sheath. Except in extreme cases, only the sciatic nerve and certain tracts in the nerve cord are involved. Considerable differences in sensitivity have been observed among homeothermic vertebrates, with man, chickens and cattle being among the most susceptible. No poikilothermic vertebrate or invertebrate has been shown to demonstrate OPIDN, although the suggested target enzyme, neurotoxic esterase, has been found in fish and frog brain tissue. *See also* MIPAFOX; NEUROTOXIC ESTERASE; TOCP.

delayed neuropathy tests. The delayed neurotoxic potential of organophosphates is usually tested in hens by observation of the appearance of paralysis of leg muscles or pathological examination for degeneration of the motor nerves. Recently a biochemical test involving the ratio of inhibition of cholinesterase relative to inhibition of the neurotoxic esterase has been proposed. Mature hens are used in delayed neuropathy testing because the clinical signs are similar to those in humans. Such symptoms cannot be readily elicited in the common laboratory rodents. *See also* DELAYED NEUROPATHY; NEUROTOXICITY TESTING.

delayed-type hypersensitivity T cells. *See* T CELLS.

deletions. *See* CHROMOSOME ABERRATIONS.

delirium. Toxic psychosis, acute confusional state; an altered mental state characterized by confusion, disorientation and disordered perceptions of sensory stimuli. Delusions, hallucinations, agitation and overactivity of the autonomic nervous system are often also present. Delirium characteristically has an acute onset and is of short duration. There are many causes of delirium, including exposure to certain drugs or toxic agents, alcohol withdrawal, metabolic disorders and infections. The pathophysiology of delirium is poorly understood but disruption of several neurotransmitter systems can be a contributing factor. *See also* DIAGNOSTIC FEATURES, CENTRAL NERVOUS SYSTEM; MAINTENANCE THERAPY, NERVOUS SYSTEM.

deltamethrin (Decamethrin) (δ)-d-cyano-m-phenoxybenzyl (1R,3R)-3(2,2-dibromovinyl)-2,dimethylcyclopropane-carboxylate. CAS number 52820-00-5. The most potent insecticide available, with a topical LD50 for insects of 10–30 mg/kg. It is a synthetic analog of the naturally occurring pyrethrins found in pyrethrum extract and contains an α-cyano group, designating it as a type II pyrethroid. It is an excellent contact and stomach insecticide, effective against a wide range of insects and is widely used in the control of agricultural pests. It exhibits low vertebrate toxicity; the acute oral LD50 in rats is 135–5000 mg/kg. It acts as a neurotoxicant to modify the nerve membrane sodium channel, increasing sodium permeability leading to depolarization and nerve block. There is evidence that deltamethrin also acts at the GABA receptor/ionophore complex. Symptoms in humans include gastrointestinal irritation, nausea, vomiting, diarrhea, numbness of tongue and lips, syncope, hyper-excitability, incoordination, convulsions, muscular paralysis, collapse and death due to respiratory paralysis. Treatment involves gastric lavage, emetics, cathartics, demulcents, artificial respiration, if necessary, and short-acting barbiturates for convulsions. Vijverberg, H.P.M. & van den Bercken, J. Neuropathol. Appl. Neurobiol. 8, 421–440 (1982).

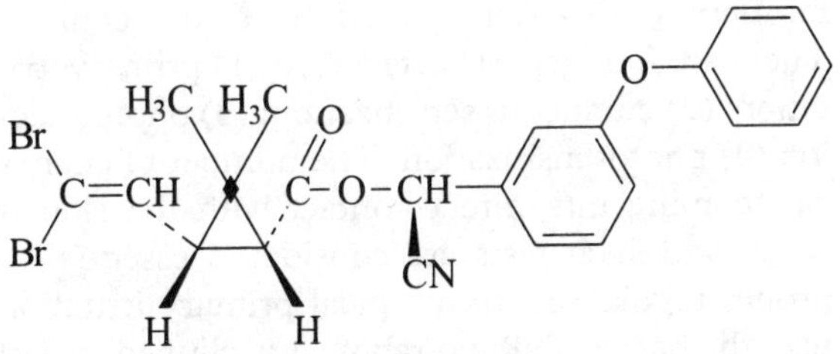

Deltamethrin

Demerol. *See* MEPERIDINE.

demethylation. A special case of dealkylation in which the alkyl group is a methyl group. Metabolic demethylation of xenobiotics is important since enzymatic demethylation by the cytochrome P450-dependent monooxygenase system usually proceeds at a faster rate than dealkylation of the higher alkyl homologs in the same series. *N*-, *O*- and *S*-demethylations are all common reactions undergone by xenobiotics. *See also* N-DEALKYLATION; O-DEALKYLATION; S-DEALKYLATION.

de minimus. A risk assessment and regulatory concept indicating that a chemical is present but that it is not of concern.

demography. The study of the characteristics of human populations including size, density distribution, etc., as well as the factors causing change in those characteristics.

demyelination. Loss of myelin. Within both the central nervous system (CNS) and peripheral nervous system (PNS), the existence of a myelin sheath allows for more rapid conduction of nerve impulses. In the CNS and the PNS, demyelination leads to loss of function. In some toxic injuries (e.g., hexachlorophene and triethyltin), a potentially reversible myelinic edema can progress to segmental demyelination (loss of myelin from an internode). Segmental demyelination can also result from injury to the myelinating cell. For example, lead may cause segmental demyelination in the PNS from a direct toxic injury to the Schwann cell. The consequences of segmental demyelination in the CNS and PNS are different. Although the myelinating cell in the PNS (i.e., the Schwann cell) can remyelinate demyelinated internodes, the CNS myelinating cell (i.e., the oligodendrocyte) cannot. Thus, segmental demyelination in the CNS is an irreversible event. *See also* MYELIN SHEATH; PERIPHERAL NEUROPATHY.

deoxycholic acid. *See* BILE ACIDS.

***d*-deoxyephedrine.** *See* METHAMPHETAMINE.

Department of Employment. A UK government department responsible for the needs of people at work and the provision of safe working conditions. Relevant divisions within the department include: Health and Safety Commission; Health and Safety Executive; Hazardous Substances Division; Technology and Air Pollution; Factory and Agricultural Inspectorates Division. *See also* HEALTH AND SAFETY COMMISSION; HEALTH AND SAFETY EXECUTIVE.

Department of the Environment. A UK government department with responsibility for the protection of the environment, including the control of water pollution, waste disposal and air pollution.

Department of Health (DH). A UK government department that is concerned with legislation covering the safety of medicines, monitoring the performance of all clinical trials for all new pharmaceuticals and cosmetics in the UK and granting product licenses. The DH also monitors good laboratory practices in UK laboratories. *See also* COMMITTEE ON SAFETY OF MEDICINES.

Department of Health and Human Services (DHHS). In the United States, a large federal cabinet-level department responsible for human health and welfare. It was previously known as the Department of Health, Education and Welfare (HEW). The agencies within DHHS of greatest interest to toxicologists are the Public Health Service, including the National Institutes of Health (NIH), the Center for Disease Control (CDC), and the Agency for Toxic Substances and Disease Registry (ATSDR).

Department of Transportation. In the United States a federal cabinet-level department responsible for regulating transportation-related issues, including the transport of hazardous substances.

Depen. *See* PENICILLAMINE.

dependence. A condition that is said to exist when equivalent or increasing doses of a drug are necessary to avoid withdrawal symptoms. Although not synonymous, dependence is often associated with drug tolerance and/or addiction. It is most often associated with the compulsive use of mood-altering drugs such as the opiates or stimulants, but dependence can develop after the repeated administration of a variety of drugs that are not used recreationally or compulsively. The symptoms comprising the withdrawal or abstinence syndrome that indicate dependence are characterized by rebound effects in the same physiological systems that were modified initially by the drug. The development of drug dependence is often associated with a behavioral preoccupation with its procurement. *See also* ALCOHOL; AMPHETAMINES; COCAINE; MORPHINE; NICOTINE; TOLERANCE.

deposition. This term has several different meanings, each particular to a different area of toxicology. In environmental toxicology it refers to the process by which a gaseous or particulate airborne pollutant becomes adsorbed onto the surface of solid or liquid media, such as plants, soil, bodies of water, etc. In pulmonary toxicology it refers to the process by which gaseous or particulate pollutants become absorbed onto the surface of the respiratory tract, that is, the amount of an aerosol or particulate that remains in the lung after expiration. The amount and site of deposition depends on inertial impaction, gravitational settling and diffusion, all of which vary with the size of the particles and their equivalent aerodynamic diameter. Retention refers to the amount deposited minus the amount cleared from the respiratory tract. *See also* ALVEOLAR CLEARANCE, AERODYNAMIC DIAMETER.

dermal administration. *See* ADMINISTRATION OF TOXICANTS, DERMAL.

dermal irritation tests. Although dermal effects may arise from systemic toxicants, there are tests for dermal irritation caused by direct contact. There are four general categories: (1) primary irritation; (2) cutaneous sensitization; (3) phototoxicity; (4) photosensitization. The number of chemicals coming into direct contact with the skin is large, and such tests are considered essential to proper regulation. In a typical primary irritation test, the backs of albino rabbits are clipped free of hair and two areas of about 5 cm^2 on each rabbit are treated with the test chemical. One of the two areas is lightly abraded before treatment. The area is covered and the body of the rabbit is wrapped to hold the material in place. After 24 and 48 hours the treated areas are evaluated for erythematous lesions and for edematous lesions, which are expressed on a numerical scale. A number of other tests exist that are variants of the above. Tests such as the mouse ear test and the guinea pig immersion test are also available, but are used much less frequently. *See also* ACUTE TOXICITY TESTING.

dermal penetration. *See* PENETRATION ROUTES, DERMAL.

dermal sensitization tests (skin sensitization tests). Tests that assess the ability of chemicals to affect the immune system, such that a second contact causes a more severe reaction than the first. The antigen involved is presumed to be formed by the binding of the chemical to body proteins. The antibodies that form to this ligand–protein complex give rise to an allergic reaction with subsequent exposure. The test animal commonly used in skin sensitization tests is the guinea pig, the animals being treated with the test compound in a suitable vehicle, with the vehicle alone or with a positive control, such as 2,4-dinitrochlorobenzene, in the same vehicle, the method of treatment being that used in dermal irritation tests. Following the initial induction treatments, the animals are rested for at least two weeks, followed by the challenge treatments. The lesions are scored on the basis of severity and the number of animals responding (incidence). Other test methods include those in which the induction phase is conducted by intradermal injection together with Freund's adjuvant and those in which the treatments are all topical, but the induction phase is accompanied by intradermal injections of Freund's adjuvant. *See also* ACUTE TOXICITY TESTING; DERMAL IRRITATION TESTS; PHOTOTOXICITY TESTS.

dermal toxicity tests. The application of a test chemical to the shaved skin of test animals, usually albino rabbits or guinea pigs, either as a single or repeated applications with or without irradiation with ultraviolet light. Such tests are not designed to evaluate systemic effects, but rather the effect of direct contact between the skin and the test chemical. Dermal tests have all been criticized. They can cause discomfort and are, to that extent, inhumane. The data generated are hard to extrapolate to humans, and some, particularly those involving intradermal injection, are regarded as unrealistic. Unfortunately none of the *in vitro* tests proposed as alternatives have yet proven applicable. Much knowledge in this area was previously obtained using human tests panels, but objections to this on ethical grounds have been almost as numerous as objections to animal studies. In view of the large number of chemicals to which human skin is exposed, it is apparent that some form of testing for dermal toxicity is necessary. *See also* ACUTE TOXICITY TESTING; DERMAL IRRITATION TEST; DERMAL SENSITIZATION TESTS; PHOTOTOXICITY TESTS.

dermatitis. Skin inflammation. May be caused by toxicants, either directly or via an immune response. It is characterized by redness, itching or lesions, and can result from reactions to toxicants or irritants, especially in cosmetics, cleaning preparations and certain plants.

dermis. *See* DIAGNOSTIC FEATURES, SKIN; PENETRATION ROUTES, DERMAL.

DES. *See* DIETHYLSTILBESTROL.

Desferal. *See* DEFEROXAMINE.

desipramine. *See* IMIPRAMINE; TRICYCLIC ANTIDEPRESSANTS.

desulfuration and oxidative ester cleavage. Phosphorothionates ($(R'O)_2P(S)OR''$) and phosphorodithioates ($(R'O)_2P(S)SR''$) are activated via an oxidative reaction in which the P=S group is converted to P=O, the resultant oxons being potent cholinesterase inhibitors. This reaction has been studied most intensively in the case of parathion and cytochrome P450. The splitting of the phosphorus ester bonds in organophosphorus insecticides is now known to be due to oxidative dearylation rather than hydrolysis. It is a typical cytochrome P450-dependent monooxygenation, and there is convincing evidence that this reaction and oxidative desulfuration involve a common intermediate of the "phosphooxithirane" type. A few organophosphorus insecticides, all phosphonates, such as fonofos, are activated by the FAD-containing monooxygenase as well as by cytochrome P450. *See also* CYTOCHROME P450-DEPENDENT MONOOXYGENASE SYSTEM; FLAVIN-CONTAINING MONOOXYGENASE; ORGANOPHOSPHORUS INSECTICIDES; PARATHION.

Phosphorothionates   Phosphorodithioates

detergents. Compounds of a large variety of different structural classes that share the ability of being amphoteric, therefore promoting a homogeneous state between otherwise incompatible materials. For this reason, detergents are used not only as cleaning aids, but also as wetting and emulsifying agents, and as solubilizers. Depending on the type of polar group on their structures, detergents are classified as anionic (sodium lauryl sulfate), cationic (tetrabutylammonium chloride) or non-ionic (sorbitan monooleate). Except for deliberate or accidental poisoning, the toxicity of these compounds is almost always limited to exposure of the eye or the skin. In the Draize test, some detergents have severe effects, whereas others can be well tolerated. In fact, many such compounds are approved as emulsifying agents for use in foods. There appears to be no correlation with the surface tension-lowering properties of these compounds and their toxicity, although cationic detergents generally present greater hazards. From an ecotoxicological perspective, detergents have been an aquatic pollutant, and the phosphates in some of these have promoted eutrophication.

detoxication. A metabolic reaction or sequence of reactions that reduces the potential for adverse effects of a xenobiotic. Such reactions or metabolic sequences normally involve an increase in water solubility which facilitates excretion and/or the reaction of a reactive compound with an endogenous substrate (conjugation) that not only increases water solubility, but also reduces the possibility of interaction with cellular macromolecules. Detoxication is not to be confused with detoxification. *Compare* DETOXIFICATION. *See also* PHASE I REACTIONS; PHASE II REACTIONS; XENOBIOTIC METABOLISM.

detoxification. Treatment by which toxicants are removed from intoxicated patients or a course of treatment during which dependence on alcohol or other drugs of abuse is reduced or eliminated. Detoxification is not to be confused with detoxication. *Compare* DETOXICATION.

developmental age. The length of different developmental stages varies with species, but in mammals they may be classified as preimplantation, organogenesis, fetal and neonatal. Each period may be further subdivided: the preimplantation stages are fertilization, cleavage, blastulation and gastrulation. Development of different organ systems proceeds at different rates during organogenesis, functional maturation and growth

in size occur during the fetal period. Since the duration of each stage as well as the duration of gestation varies with species, a knowledge of developmental age is critical to studies in teratogenesis. Each stage is sensitive to chemical insult in characteristic ways; after that stage is past, the developing organism may be quite resistant to that particular effect. Embryonic death is the most common effect during the preimplantation stage, whereas major teratogenic effects result from chemical insult during the period of organogenesis. Later effects (fetal) are more commonly growth retardation and functional deficits in various organ systems. *See also* ORGANOGENESIS.

developmental toxicity. A general term to describe any adverse effect on the developing organism. Such toxic effects may arise from toxicant exposure of the parents before conception or during prenatal development. The term is sometimes extended to include effects at any time before sexual maturity is reached. *See also* DEVELOPMENTAL AGE.

Dexedrine. *See* AMPHETAMINE.

dexflenfluramine. *See* FLENFLURAMINE.

dextromethorphan (*d*-3-methoxy-17-methyl-9α,13α,14α-morphinan). A cough suppressant. Dextromethorphan acts in the CNS to elevate the threshold for the cough reflex. Dextromethorphan is the *d*-isomer of the codeine analog levorphanol, but unlike the *l*-isomer it has no analgesic or addictive properties. Due to this insignificant potential for abuse, dextromethorphan is the most widely used non-opioid cough suppressant in over-the-counter formulations. The toxicity of dextromethorphan is low, although extremely high doses may cause depression of the CNS. *See also* CODEINE; MORPHINE.

Dextromethorphan

DFP (di*iso*propylfluorophosphate; *O,O*-di*iso*propyl phosphorofluoridate; isofluorophate). A highly toxic acetylcholinesterase inhibitor; chemically similar to the "nerve gases." In addition to its use as a pharmacological tool, it is employed in the management of glaucoma. Chronic exposure to DFP, or acute intoxication in combination with appropriate therapy, induces delayed neuropathy in hens and other sensitive species. The i.v. LD50 in monkeys is 0.3 mg/kg, and the dermal LD50 in mice is 72 mg/kg. *See also* ANTICHOLINESTERASES; DELAYED NEUROPATHY.

$$(CH_3)_2\!-\!CH \diagdown \quad \diagup O$$
$$P$$
$$(CH_3)_2\!-\!CH \diagup \quad \diagdown F$$

Diisopropylfluorophosphate

DHHS. *See* DEPARTMENT OF HEALTH AND HUMAN SERVICES.

diabetes insipidus. A disease resulting from hyposecretion of antidiuretic hormone from the neurohypophysis. As a result, inadequate amounts of water are reabsorbed from the kidney tubules, and excessive water loss in the urine occurs.

diabetes mellitus (true diabetes; sugar diabetes). A disease caused by a lack of adequate insulin secretion from the β-cells of the pancreatic islets of Langerhans or a lack of insulin sensitivity within the target tissues. As a result of diabetes mellitus, most of the cells of the body cannot absorb sufficient glucose (the brain is a notable exception), and instead they must rely on lipid metabolism for energy. Consequences include hyperglycemia, glycosuria, polyuria and acidosis. Complications include cardiovascular disturbances, cataracts, poor wound healing and weakened immune responses. Chemicals or disease that damage the pancreas can cause diabetes mellitus.

diacetylmorphine. *See* HEROIN.

diagnosis, of poisoning. Following appropriate first aid, i.e., removal of the poisoning victim from contact with the poison, prevention of further absorption of the poison, it is necessary for the physician to make a diagnosis so that the most appropriate treatment can be initiated. If the poisoning victim is a child or is comatose, it may be necessary to rely on parents, friends, eyewitnesses or an examination of the scene for useful background details. Relative to the toxicant involved, the patients fall into three classes. The first class of patients are those who have absorbed a known poison, and for whom the physican needs to initiate appropriate emergency treatment and to estimate the quantity of the poison absorbed. The second class are those known to be poisoned but the actual toxicant is unknown, usually because the poison is a complex mixture. Also identification of the toxicant is made difficult by the numerous trade names and proprietary mixtures, although some lists and reference sources are available. The nearest poison information center is a source of information, as is the manufacturer. The first person on the scene or anyone rendering first aid to a poisoning victim should send the container, properly resealed and packed, if available, with the patient when moved to the hospital or emergency center. Similarly, vomitus should be collected for analysis. If the toxicant can be identified, appropriate therapy can be initiated, otherwise the physician must rely on non-specific life support. The third class are those in which the physician needs to carry out the differential diagnosis of a disease that may or may not be the result of poisoning. This consists of a complete case history, a complete physical examination and appropriate laboratory tests. *See also* DIAGNOSTIC FEATURES; MAINTENANCE THERAPY; POISONING, EMERGENCY TREATMENT; POISONING, LIFE SUPPORT.

diagnostic features. In the absence of an authentic sample of the ingested poison and direct evidence of the amount ingested, the proper diagnosis of poisoning involves a complete analysis of the circumstances and of the physical and physiological status of the poisoning victim. General characteristics such as weight loss, lethargy and weakness are often symptoms of chronic poisoning by such toxicants as lead and mercury, whereas an elevated body temperature would be typical of poisoning with nitrophenols. Other characteristics are typical of particular organ systems. It should always be borne in mind, however, that individual variation in humans is so great that in any particular case typical signs may not be present, and individual

Table 2.   Examples of diagnostic examination of blood

	Symptom	Examples of possible causes
Appearance and cellular changes	Leukopenia, agranulocytis	Aminopyrine, phenylbutazone
	Anemia	Lead, naphthalene, chlorates, solanine and other plant poisons
	Cherry-red color	Carbon monoxide, cyanide
	Chocolate color (methemoglobin)	Nitrates, nitrites, aniline, dyes, chlorates
Blood, serum or plasma	Glucose (whole blood)	Increased after thiazide diuretics or adrenal glucocorticoids; decreased after salicylates, lead or ethanol
	Uric acid (serum)	Increased after thiazide diuretics or ethanol
	Potassium (serum or plasma)	Increased after thiazide diuretics or ethanol
Special chemical examination (analysis)	Lead and other heavy metals	Heavy metals poisoning
	Insecticides	Chlorinated hydrocarbons
	Cholinesterase	Organophosphates
	Barbiturates	Phenobarbital
	Alkaloids	Nicotine

signs may appear to be contradictory. *See also* DIAGNOSTIC FEATURES, BLOOD; DIAGNOSTIC FEATURES, CENTRAL NERVOUS SYSTEM; DIAGNOSTIC FEATURES, CIRCULATORY SYSTEM; DIAGNOSTIC FEATURES, EARS; DIAGNOSTIC FEATURES, EYES; DIAGNOSTIC FEATURES, GASTROINTESTINAL TRACT; DIAGNOSTIC FEATURES, MOUTH; DIAGNOSTIC FEATURES, NEUROMUSCULAR SYSTEM; DIAGNOSTIC FEATURES, RESPIRATORY SYSTEM; DIAGNOSTIC FEATURES, SKIN; DIAGNOSTIC FEATURES, URINARY TRACT.

diagnostic features, blood. Examination of blood cells and the chemistry of the blood are important in the diagnosis of poisoning taken in conjunction with other signs. A summary of some of the more important tests and their significance are shown in Table 2.

diagnostic features, central nervous system. Effects on the CNS may be indicated by physical, behavioral or psychological symptoms, either alone or in combination. For example, muscular twitching and convulsions may be caused by insecticides, such as nicotine, or by amphetamines, whereas headaches may arise from poisoning with such toxicants as organophosphorus insecticides or carbon monoxide. Depression, drowsiness and coma may follow barbiturate overdose or ethanol poisoning, whereas delirium or hallucinations may follow excessive alcohol, amphetamines or cocaine. Thallium, lead or mercury, as well as drugs such as antihistamines and barbiturates, may cause confusion or similar mental changes. *See also* COMA; CONVULSIONS; DELIRIUM.

diagnostic features, circulatory system. Examination of features associated with the circulatory system, such as blood pressure and pulse rate, may provide important clues to the nature of the toxicant in suspected poisoning. For example, blood pressure may be high in nicotine poisoning or low in poisoning by nitrites, arsenic or fluorides. Similarly, a fast pulse may indicate poisoning by atropine, and a slow or irregular pulse may indicate poisoning by nitrites.

diagnostic features, ears. Symptoms related to hearing or equilibrium may provide clues in poisoning cases, but are probably more variable in occurrence than many other symptoms. Tinnitus, deafness and disturbance of equilibrium may all be caused by such compounds as salicylates. *See also* TINNITUS.

diagnostic features, eyes. Blurred vision may result from poisoning with atropine, phosphate ester insecticides, cocaine or methanol, whereas double vision can result from alcohol, barbiturates, nicotine or phosphate ester insecticides. Dilated pupils can be caused by atropine and related drugs, cocaine, nicotine, solvents and depressants. Contracted pupils can be due to morphine, physostigmine or phosphate ester insecticides. *See also* MEIOSIS; MYDRIASIS.

diagnostic features, gastrointestinal tract. Vomiting, diarrhea and abdominal pain, although characteristic of poisoning in general, are so nonspecific with regard to the causative agent as to be of little diagnostic value. Others features, such as blood in the feces may be caused by coumarin anticoagulants, thallium, iron salts, salicylates and some corrosive materials.

diagnostic features, mouth. Loosening of teeth and painful teeth may be due to heavy metal poisoning, dry mouth may be associated with atropine and related drugs, and excessive salivation may be due to poisoning by phosphate ester insecticides and heavy metals.

diagnostic features, neuromuscular system. Muscular weakness or paralysis, which can be caused by lead, arsenic, thallium, etc., may be difficult to distinguish from effects on the central nervous system. Other neuromuscular effects such as tremor, muscle stiffness and muscle cramps may be useful diagnostic features.

diagnostic features, respiratory system. Respiratory difficulty, including dyspnea on exertion, chest pain and decreased initial capacity may be caused by a wide variety of toxicants, including salicylates, cyanide, carbon monoxide, atropine, strychnine and ethanol. Rapid respiration may be due to cyanide, atropine, cocaine, carbon monoxide, salicylates, alcohol or amphetamine. Slow respiration, on the other hand, may be due to such chemicals as barbiturates, morphine or antihistamines, but paradoxically may also be caused by cyanide or carbon monoxide in some patients.

diagnostic features, skin. Overt damage, such as burns or corrosion, may be caused by acids, alkalis or strong oxidizing agents (e.g., permanganate or dichromate). Other features such as cyanosis, are frequently the result of hypoxia or methemoglobinemia caused by toxicants such as nitrites or aniline. Carbon monoxide or cyanide both cause redness or flushing. A yellow color visible in the skin and the eyes may be due to jaundice from liver injury, caused by compounds such as carbon tetrachloride, or from hemolysis, caused by compounds such as aniline or arsine. *See also* CYANOSIS; JAUNDICE; METHEMOGLOBINEMIA.

diagnostic features, urinary tract. Dysfunctions of the urinary tract that may be useful in diagnosis include the following: anuria, the inability to excrete urine; proteinuria, the appearance of protein in the urine; hematuria, the appearance of blood in the urine; hemoglobinuria, the appearance of hemoglobin in the urine; myoglobinuria, the appearance of myoglobin in the urine. Anuria may result from such poisons as mercurials, oxalic acid, etc., whereas proteinuria may result from arsenic, mercurials and other toxicants. The color of the urine may also be a useful diagnostic feature. *See also* HEMOGLOBINURIA; HEMATURIA; MYOGLOBINURIA; PROTEINURIA.

dialkylhydrazines (RNHNHR′). Several dialkylhydrazines (e.g., 1,2-dimethylhydrazine, 1,2-diethylhydrazine, the antitumor agent procarbazine hydrochloride, *N*-methyl-*N*-formylhydrazine) are carcinogenic in animal test systems. Tumors that develop are commonly in the gastrointestinal tract, liver and lung.

dialysis. A technique used for the removal of toxicants from the body. It depends on the passage of the toxicant across a semipermeable membrane into a dialyzate against which the body fluids are being equilibrated. There are two types of dialysis used in the treatment of poisoning: (1) hemodialysis, in which the blood is equilibrated against a suitable solution in a dialysis machine (artificial kidney), is used to treat patients with certain types of renal failure; (2) peritoneal dialysis, in which the dialyzate is passed into and out of the peritoneal cavity, is used mostly in pediatric practice. Although dialysis is useful in some cases (e.g., phencyclidine or meprobamate poisoning), it is of little use in the case of poisoning with compounds with a large volume of distribution, a high lipophilicity or those that bind tightly to serum proteins. This principle is also used in experimental toxicology. *See also* THERAPY.

dialysis dementia. *See* DIALYSIS ENCEPHALO-PATHY.

dialysis encephalopathy (dialysis dementia). A condition with symptoms that include impaired memory, EEG changes, dementia, aphasia, ataxia and convulsions that occurs in kidney dialysis patients. It is caused by a combination of absorption of aluminum from the dialyzing solution and from decreased ability to excrete the metal. *See also* ALUMINUM.

diamine oxidases. Enzymes that oxidize amines to aldehydes with the preferred substrates being aliphatic diamines with a chain length of four (putrescine) or five (cadaverine) carbon atoms. Diamines with carbon chains longer than nine are not substrates for diamine oxidases, but are for monoamine oxidases. Secondary and tertiary amines are not substrates. Diamine oxidases are soluble pyridoxal phosphate-containing enzymes that also contain copper. They have been found in a number of tissues, including liver, intestine, kidney and placenta. *See also* AMINE OXIDASES.

2,4-diaminophenol. *See* AMINOPHENOLS.

o-**dianisidine**. *See* 3,3′–DIMETHOXYBENZIDINE.

diarrhea. Abnormally fluid discharge of feces from the large intestine. Frequently a sign of poisoning, it may be useful in eliminating the toxic material from the gastrointestinal tract. Eventually it is harmful due to the resultant fluid imbalance. Diarrhea can be treated by administering appropriate fluids or Kaopectate-Kaolin mixtures. In severe cases, drug therapy is available. *See also*

DIAGNOSTIC FEATURES, GASTROINTESTINAL TRACT; MAINTENANCE THERAPY, GASTRO-INTESTINAL TRACT; MAINTENANCE THERAPY, WATER AND ELECTROLYTE BALANCE.

diazepam (7-chloro-1,3-dihydro-1-methyl-5-phenyl-2*H***-1,4-benzodiazepin-2-one; Valium). CAS number 439-14-5.** A benzodiazepine derivative used extensively in clinical practice as an anxiolytic, muscle relaxant, sedative/hypnotic and anticonvulsant. Diazepam is also often employed in the treatment of alcohol withdrawal syndromes and as premedication in anesthesia. The prolonged use of diazepam in therapeutic doses generally results in little evidence of tolerance development or physical dependence. The abrupt cessation of the chronic administration of high doses of diazepam may precipitate marked withdrawal symptoms, including seizures. The clinical toxicity of diazepam is low, with sedation being the most often observed effects of overdosage. Although overdosage is frequent, deaths related to diazepam are very rare. The incidence of teratogenic effects of diazepam use is low, although a controversial increase in cleft deformities of the lip or palate has been suggested. Diazepam may be used to treat convulsions resulting from severe toxic insult. *See also* ANXIO-LYTICS; BENZODIAZEPINES.

Diazepam

diazinon (phosphorothioic acid, *O*,*O*-diethyl-*O*-(6-methyl-2-(1-methylethyl)-4-pyrimidinyl) ester). CAS number 333-41-5. An organophosphorus insecticide. Metabolized by cytochrome P450 to diazoxon, a potent acetylcholinesterase inhibitor. *See also* ANTICHOLINES-TERASES; DATABASES, TOXICOLOGY; OXON; ORGANOPHOSPHORUS INSECTICIDES; ORGANO-PHOSPHORUS POISONING, SYMPTOMS AND THERAPY.

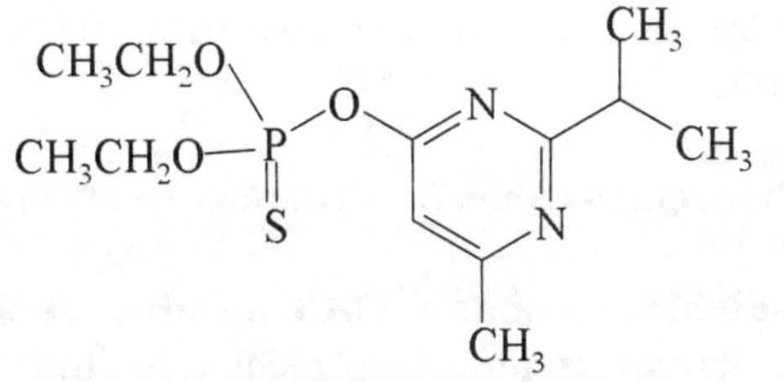

Diazinon

dibenzo[*a*,*h*]anthracene. *See* POLYCYCLIC AROMATIC HYDROCARBONS.

dibenzothiopyran. *See* THIOXANTHENE.

1,2-dibromo-3-chloropropane (DBCP). CAS number 96-12-8. A soil fumigant and nematocide. The acute oral LD50 is 170–300 mg/kg for rats and 260–400 mg/kg for mice. The acute dermal LD50 for rabbits is 1420 mg/kg. The LC50 (48 hour) is 50–125 mg/l for sunfish and 30–50 mg/l for bass. In life-time studies in which rats and mice were treated by oral gavage, it was shown to be carcinogenic. Its use has been discontinued in the USA and elsewhere because of male reproductive toxicity. Male reproductive toxicant in humans, animal carcinogen. ATSDR Document TP-91/12 (Sept. 1992). *See also* DATABASES, TOXICOLOGY.

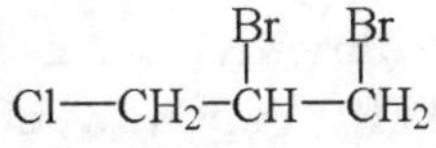

1,2-Dibromo-3-chloropropane DBCP

1,2-dibromoethane. *See* ETHYLENE DIBROMIDE.

dibromomethane. *See* METHYLENE BROMIDE.

DIBT. *See* INSTITUTE OF BIOLOGY.

dicarboxylic acid. *See* OXALIC ACID.

dichlobenil (2,6-dichlorobenzonitrile). CAS number 1194-65-6. A herbicide acting in soil used for total weed control in land that is not intended for agricultural use, cropping, and for selective weed control in orchards and forests. It is also used as an aquatic herbicide to kill floating and submerged plants in still or slow-moving water.

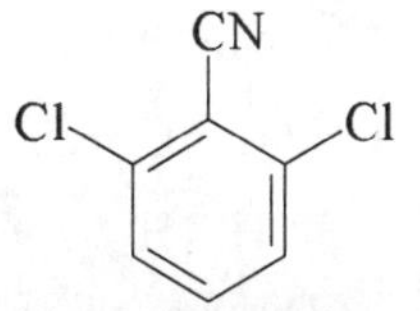

Dichlobenil

1,4-dichlorobenzene (*p*-dichlorobenzene). CAS number 106-46-7. Insect repellent used in mothballs and as a restroom deodorant. Animal carcinogen, considered a possible human carcinogen by both IARC and the US EPA. *See also* ATSDR DOCUMENT, APRIL 1993; LEWIS, HCDR, NUMBER DEP800; DATABASES, TOXICOLOGY.

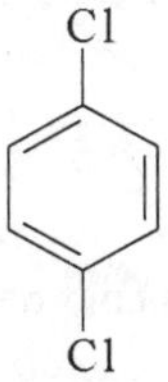

1,4-Dichlorobenzene

3,3'-*o*-dichlorobenzidine. CAS number 91-94-1. A designated animal carcinogen (IARC), hazardous waste (EPA) and priority toxic pollutant (EPA). The major uses of 3,3'-dichlorobenzidine have been in the manufacture of pigments for printing inks, textiles and plastics and as a curing agent for urethane plastics. Entry into the body is via inhalation and percutaneous absorption. This compound causes allergic skin reactions and has been shown to be a potent carcinogen in both rats and mice. Although epidemiological studies have, to the present, been largely negative, the use of dichlorobenzidine is not recommended due to its potency as an animal carcinogen.

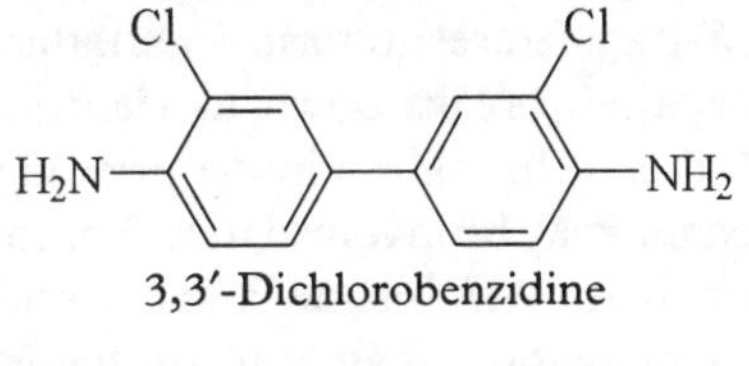

3,3'-Dichlorobenzidine

1,2-dichloroethane. CAS number 107-06-2. Chemical intermediate and degreasing agent, also known as 1,2-ethylene dichloride. No longer used for household products. Animal carcinogen. Possibly carcinogenic in humans (IARC), probable human carcinogen (EPA). *See also* ATSDR DOCUMENT, MAY 1994; DATABASES, TOXICOLOGY.

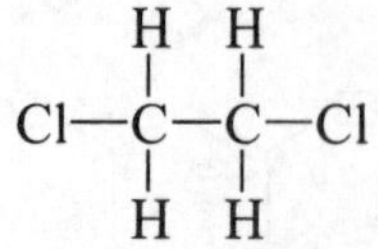

H H
| |
Cl—C—C—Cl
| |
H H

1,2-Dichloroethane

1,1-dichloroethene. **CAS number 75-35-4.** Also known as vinylidene chloride. Synthetic intermediate in the plastics and flame retardant coating industries. Although listed as a possible human carcinogen by the US EPA the evidence for either human or animal carcinogenicity is inconclusive. *See also* ATSDR DOCUMENT, MAY 1994; DATABASES, TOXICOLOGY.

Cl   H
  \   /
   C = C
  /   \
Cl   H

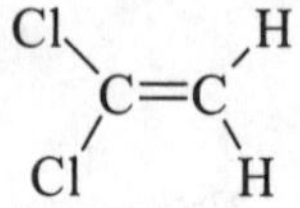

1,1 Dichloroethene

1,2-dichloroethene. Also known as acetylene dichloride. Exists as *cis* and *trans* isomers or as the isomeric mixture. Used as an industrial solvent. No evidence has been found for human or animal carcinogenicity. *See also* ATSDR DOCUMENT, AUGUST 1994; DATABASES, TOXICOLOGY.

Cl   Cl
  \   /
   C = C
  /   \
H   H

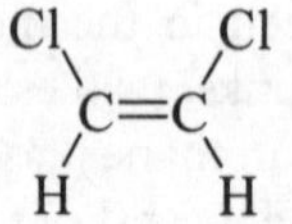

1,2-Dichloroethene

1,2-dichloroethylene. *See* 1,2-DICHLORO-ETHENE.

dichloromethane (CH$_2$Cl$_2$). CAS number 75-09-2. Dichloromethane is metabolized by glutathione S-transferases to form a glutathione conjugate that then breaks down to yield formaldehyde. Either the glutathione conjugate or formaldehyde may be involved in tumor formation in rodents. Mice which show a faster rate of glutathione conjugation than rats or hamsters are more sensitive to dichloromethane-induced tumors than the latter two species, both of which are relatively resistant. Also metabolized by CYP 2E1 in the liver, producing carbon monoxide via a formyl halide intermediate. Dichloromethane has been banned from use as a component of aerosols and is no longer used for the decaffeination of coffee.

dichloromethyl ether. *See* BIS(CHLOROMETHYL) ETHER.

dichlorophenazone. *See* CHLORAL DERIVATIVES.

1,2-dichloropropane. CAS number 78-87-5. Also known as propylene dichloride. Industrial solvent. Limited evidence for animal carcinogenicity. 1,1-Dichloropropane and 1,3-dichloropropane appear to be less toxic. *See also* LEWIS HCDR, NUMBER PNJ400.

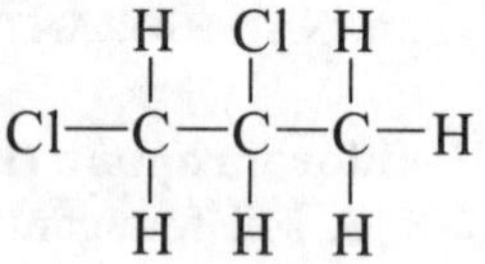

H   Cl   H
| | |
Cl—C—C—C—H
| | |
H   H   H

1,2-Dichloropropane

1,3-dichloropropene. Exists in two forms, *cis*-1,3-dichloropropene, CAS number 10061-01-5, and *trans*-1,3-dichloropropene, CAS number 10061-02-6, or as the isomeric mixture. Used as a soil fumigant (nematocide). Animal carcinogen and suspected human carcinogen. *See also* ATSDR DOCUMENT, SEPTEMBER 1992; LEWIS, HCDR, MEMBERS DDG950, DGH000 AND DGH200; DATABASES, TOXICOLOGY.

dichlorvos (*O,O*-dimethyl *O*-2,2-dichlorovinyl phosphate; DDVP; Vapona). CAS number 62-73-7. A broad-spectrum organophosphate insecticide. Dichlorvos is particularly effective for control of flies and mosquitoes. It is also of value for control of external and certain internal parasites of domestic animals. Dichlorvos can be formulated for slow release from a polymer resin to control flies and mosquitoes in buildings by fumigant action. The mode of action is inhibition of acetylcholinesterase. The oral LD50 in rats is 75 mg/kg. Possible human carcinogen. *See also* ANTICHOLINESTERASES; ORGANOPHOSPHORUS INSECTICIDES; ATSDR DOCUMENT, AUGUST 1995.

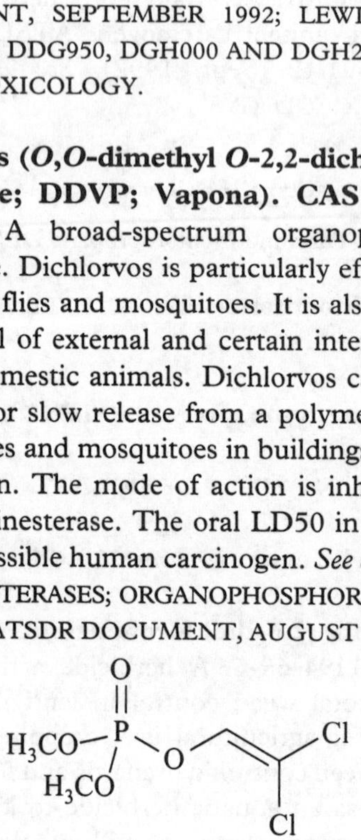

O
||
H$_3$CO—P—O   Cl
| \   /
H$_3$CO   C = C
                  \
                   Cl

Dichlorvos

dicofol (4-chloro-α-(4-chlorophenyl)-α-(trichloromethyl)benzenemethanol; FW-293; Kelthane; Mitigan; Acarin; Hifol). A nonsystemic acaricide with an oral LD50 in rats of 575 mg/kg and a dermal LD50 in rats of 1000–1230 mg/kg. It is a neurotoxicant that interferes with the function of Ca^{2+}, Na^+, K^+ and several ATPases in insects and animals. Its mode of action in mites is not known. Poisoning in humans results in nausea, vomiting, restlessness, tremor, apprehensiveness, convulsions, coma, respiratory failure or death. The therapy is gastric lavage, general supportive therapy, including anticonvulsants, and respiratory assistance, if needed. *See also* INSECTICIDES; ORGANOCHLORINE INSECTICIDES.

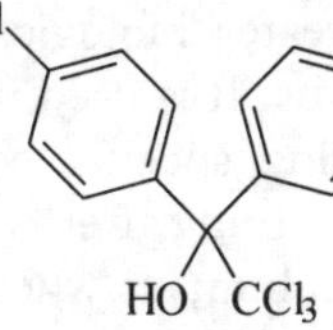

Dicofol

dicumarol (3,3'-methylenebis[4-hydroxy-2H-1-benzopyran-2-one]; 3,3'-methylenebis [4-hydroxycoumarin]). CAS number 66-76-2. A hemorrhagic agent in cattle, originally isolated from spoiled sweet clover, that is now used as an oral anticoagulant. Like the more commonly used warfarin and other anticoagulants, dicumarol antagonizes the actions of vitamin K and so reduces the activity of vitamin K-dependent clotting factors. Anticoagulant treatment can result in both pharmacodynamic and pharmacokinetic drug interactions, particularly with barbiturates and salicylates. Salicylates increase the response to oral anticoagulants, whereas barbiturates decrease the anticoagulant response by induction of hepatic microsomal enzymes. Additionally, barbiturates also interfere with the absorption of dicumarol. The side effects of dicumarol include nausea, abdominal pain and diarrhea. The oral LD50 in rats is 542 mg/kg. *See also* INDUCTION.

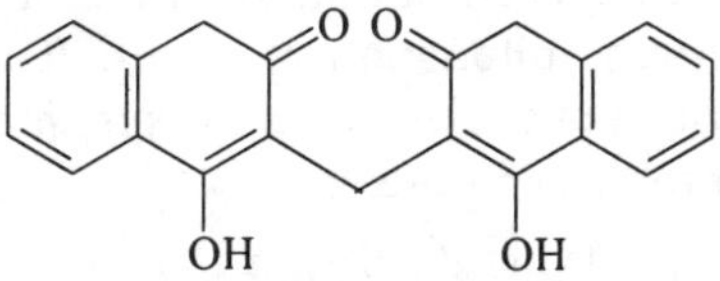

Dicumarol

dideoxy sequencing. Method for determining the primary sequence of DNA. Single-stranded DNA is copied by DNA polymerase I using the four deoxynucleoside triphosphates, including one radiolabeled with ^{32}P and another in the presence of trace amounts of its 2',3'-dideoxy equivalent. Four reactions are run in parallel with the four different precursors. Since phosphodiester bonds cannot form in the absence of the 3'-hydroxyl group, the reactions yield oligomers terminating at all the possible sites where the corresponding normal nucleosides should have been. The reaction products are then separated by gel electrophoresis, and the DNA sequence of the original template deduced from the four "step ladders" of bands thus revealed. Primary sequences several hundred nucleotides long can be determined by a single experiment. Recently, automated devices have become available for this purpose.

dieldrin. *See* CYCLODIENE INSECTICIDES.

diestrus. *See* ESTROUS CYCLE.

diet, in toxicity testing. *See* ADMINISTRATION OF TOXICANTS.

dietary effects, in toxicity testing. *See* NUTRITIONAL EFFECTS ON METABOLISM; NUTRITIONAL EFFECTS ON TOXICOLOGY.

diethyldithiocarbamate (Dithiocarb; diethylcarbamodithioic acid sodium salt). CAS number of sodium salt 148-18-5. Has been used as an immomodulator and as a chelating agent for treatment of nickel and cadmium poisoning and has also been used as a pesticide. Although diethyldithiocarbamate has been described as a "questionable" carcinogen, the evidence is either negative or equivocal. Diethyldithiocarbamate is a metabolite of disulfiram produced by disulfide reduction and is further metabolized to either a methyl ester or an *S*-glucuronide.

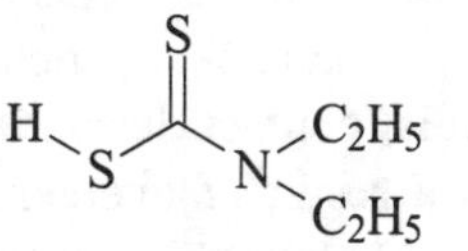

Diethyldithiocarbamate

diethyl ether. *See* ETHYL ETHER.

di(2-ethylhexyl) phthalate (DEHP). CAS number 117-81-7. A widely used plasticizer for polyvinyl chloride (PVC) products. It is especially important in medical devices, such as blood storage bags and tubing. DEHP leaches out of these plastics, since it is soluble in blood containing lipoproteins. It is a clear, colorless, odorless, oily liquid that is absorbed intact from the gastrointestinal tract. It is an eye and mucous membrane irritant. Ingestion by humans has resulted in mild gastric disturbances. It is metabolized quickly, and metabolites are excreted in the bile and urine. Animal studies have resulted in testicular atrophy, lung hemorrhage, hepatomegaly, cytotoxicity, proliferation of hepatic peroxisomes and carcinogenic and teratogenic effects. It is narcotic at high doses. DEHP and other phthalic acid esters are also environmental contaminants. The i.p. LD50 is 2.8 g/kg and 5.1 ml/kg in mice and rats, respectively; the oral LD50 in rabbits is 1 g/kg. Causes peroxisome proliferation in rodents and is a rodent carcinogen. No direct evidence for human carcinogenicity, but on the basis of animal studies, has been designated a possible (IARC) or probable (US EPA) human carcinogen. *See also* PHTHALIC ACID ESTERS; ATSDR DOCUMENT, APRIL 1993; DATABASES, TOXICOLOGY.

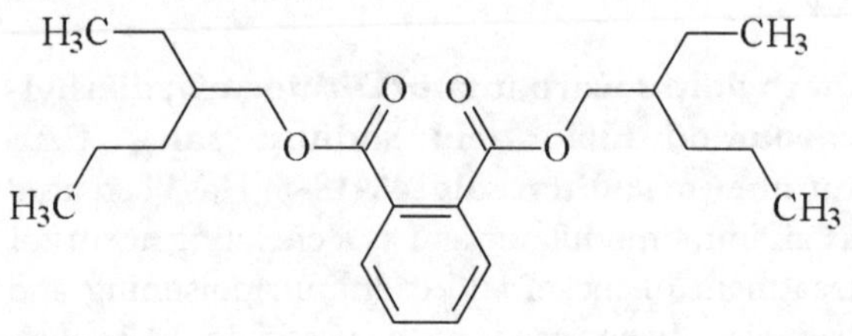

Bis(2-ethylhexyl) phthalate

1,2-diethylhydrazine. *See* DIALKYLHYDRAZINES.

***N,N*-diethyl-*m*-toluamide (DEET). CAS number 134-62-3.** Insect repellent. May have acute or chronic toxic effects, including hypotension, bradycardia, contact dermatitis, tremor, seizures, etc., as a result of overexposure. *See also* LEWIS, HCDR, NUMBER DKC800; DATABASES, TOXICOLOGY.

diethylphthalate. CAS number 84-66-2. The diethyl ester of phthalic acid, 1,2-benzenedicarboxylic acid. Used as a solvent for cellulose acetate in varnishes and denaturing alcohol. *See also* DATABASES, TOXICOLOGY.

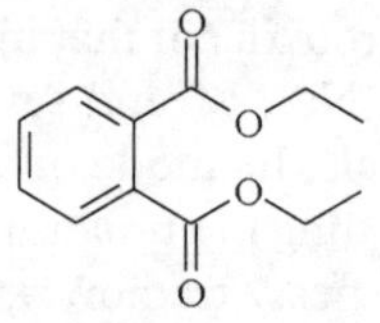

Diethylphthalate

diethylstilbestrol (DES; stilbestrol; (E)-4,4′-(1,2-diethyl-1,2-ethenediyl)bisphenol; α,α′-diethylstilbenediol; Antigestil; Stilphostrol). A synthetic, non-steroidal, orally active estrogenic compound with greater biological activity than endogenous estrogens. It is used in the treatment of carcinomas having specific estrogen-binding capacity and as a "morning after" contraceptive. It was formerly used in humans when estrogen therapy was required, but was associated with increased incidence of vaginal and cervical adenocarcinoma. It also is administered to animals, primarily feedlot cattle, to accelerate weight gain. DES is listed by the EPA as being carcinogenic, causing vaginal cancer (clear cell adenocarcinoma) in the offspring of mothers treated with DES during the first trimester of pregnancy. Reproductive effects in male offspring of DES-treated mothers have also been suggested. Acute effects include nausea and vomiting, whereas delayed effects include fluid retention, feminization and uterine bleeding. The oral LD50 in mice is 3 g/kg.

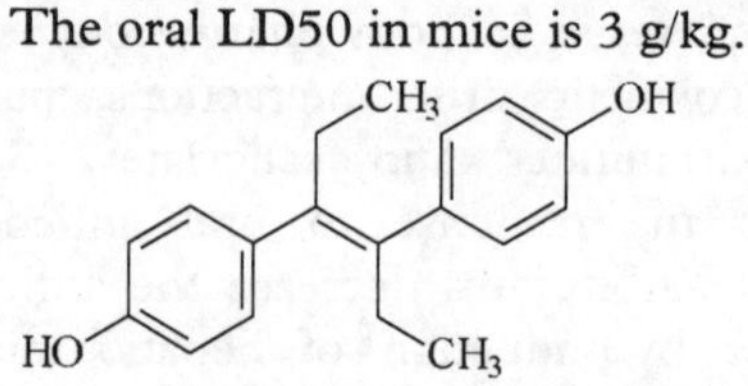

Diethylstilbestrol

diethyl sulfate (sulfuric acid diethyl ester). CAS number 64-67-5. A compound that is used as an ethylating agent, in the sulfation of ethylene and in certain sulfonation reactions. It is of low acute toxicity, but causes cancer in experimental animals on chronic exposure.

$$(CH_3CH_2)_2SO_4$$

Diethyl sulfate

difference spectra, optical. *See* OPTICAL DIFFERENCE SPECTRA.

differentiation. Process by which previously unspecialized cells become specialized for particular functions. Embryonic cells of animals and meristematic cells of plants are relatively unspecialized in both form and function, but during growth and development they give rise to cells with discrete specialization, such as muscle cells, neurons or stomatal guard cells. Cells with characteristic specialization are said to belong to distinct types, each type consisting of a population of cells with identical patterns of specialization. The state of differentiation is usually very stable, once acquired, and is faithfully passed on at cell division to daughter cells. Experimental evidence from tissue-grafting experiments reveals that frequently a stage of commitment or determination precedes the onset of overt differentiation. The biochemical mechanisms underlying the process of differentiation are poorly understood. Although cells of different differentiated types can be shown to express unique sets of genes, each set being a highly restricted portion of the total genome, the mechanism that engineers this choice of selective gene expression is unclear, although it is often presumed to be itself an aspect of gene regulation.

diffusion. The movement of molecules from a region of high concentration to one of lower concentration due to random molecular motion. Diffusion of gases in other gases is most rapid, but diffusion of solutes in solvents occurs, and solids are capable of diffusing into each other, although at extremely slow rates. Diffusion is important in respiratory toxicology since oxygen and carbon dioxide pass across the alveolar wall between the alveolar lumen and the capillary blood by passive diffusion. The length of the diffusion path may be changed by lung fibrosis. Pulmonary diffusing capacity may be changed by an increased diffusion path or a decreased area for exchange or both.

diffusion capacity. *See* DIFFUSION.

diffusion trapping. *See* EXCRETION, RENAL.

diflubenzuron (*N*-[[(4-chlorophenol)-amino] carbonyl]-2,6-difluorobenzamide; Dimilin). CAS number 35367-38-5. A non-systemic stomach and contact insecticide, larvicide and ovicide. The acute oral LD50 in mice is greater than 4640 mg/kg; the intraperitoneal LD50 in mice is greater than 2150 mg/kg; the percutaneous LD50 in rabbits is greater than 2000 mg/kg. In two-year feeding trials, the "no effect" level for rats was 40 mg/kg diet. No effect was observed in teratogenic, mutagenic and oncogenic studies. No toxic signs were observed in mallard ducks and bobwhite quail at 4640 mg/kg diet. The LC50 (96 hours) is 135 mg/kg for bluegill and 140 mg/l for rainbow trout. Insecticidal activity is as a growth regulator, affecting cuticle development. It interferes with chitin synthesis and deposition, and blocks DNA synthesis.

Diflubenzuron

digitalis (foxglove; purple foxglove; digifortis; digitora). The dried leaves of *Digitalis purpurea*. Its active principles are a mixture of alkaloids including digitoxin, digitonin, digitalin, digitalosmin and digitoflavone. The extract works as a cardiotonic glycoside, with the therapeutic dose being close to the toxic dose. The compounds act principally by inhibiting Na^+/K^+-ATPase associated with the membrane-bound sodium pump, resulting in alteration of cardiac electrical function with resulting premature atrial beats, atrial fibrillation, atrioventricular block, ventricular tachycardia and ventricular fibrillation. Symptoms in humans include arrhythmia, anorexia, nausea, vomiting, diarrhea, disorientation and hallucinations. The therapy may include administration of parenteral potassium and antiarrhythmia drugs such as lidocaine, phenytoin or propranolol. Suicidal overdoses may necessitate treatment with digitalis antibodies or Fab fragments of such antibodies. *See also* DIGITOXIN.

digitoxigenin. *See* DIGITOXIN.

digitoxin (3-[(*O*-2,6-dideoxy-β-D-ribo-hexo-pyranosyl-(1,4)-*O*-2,6-dideoxy-β-D-ribo-hexopyranosyl-(1,4)-2,6-dideoxy-β-D-ribo-hexoyranosyl)oxy]-14-hydroxycard-20(22)-enolide; **Cardidigin; Digisidin; Digitaline Nativelle; Digitophyllin**). A secondary glycoside extracted from *Digitalis purpurea*. The aglycone is digitoxigenin (see structure). It is cardiotonic and is used to increase cardiac contractility in the treatment of heart failure. The steroid nucleus and lactone ring are necessary for activity; other constituents influence pharmacokinetic variables. Its oral LD50 is 60 mg/kg in guinea pigs and 0.18 mg/kg in cats. It acts by inhibiting Na^+/K^+-ATPase associated with the membrane-bound "Na pump." It causes an alteration of cardiac electrical function, resulting in premature atrial beats, atrial fibrillation, atrioventricular block, ventricular tachycardia and ventricular fibrillation. Symptoms include arrhythmia, anorexia, nausea, vomiting, diarrhea and disorientation. The therapy for acute poisoning may include administration of parenteral potassium and antiarrhythmia drugs such as lidocaine, phenytoin or propranolol. Suicidal overdoses may necessitate treatment with glycoside antibodies or Fab fragments of such antibodies. *See also* DIGITALIS.

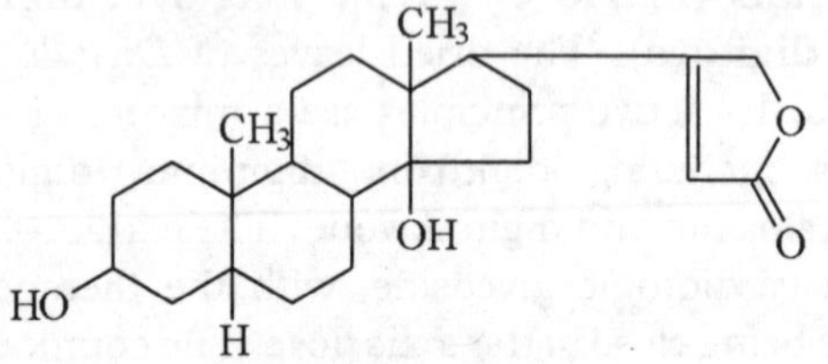

Digitoxigenin

digoxin. CAS number 20830-75-5. A secondary glycoside extracted from *Digitalis purpurea* similar to digitoxin. *See also* DIGITOXIN.

dihydrodiols. Dihydroxy compounds in which the hydroxy groups are on adjacent ring carbon atoms with the carbon-carbon bond between the two hydroxyl substituted carbons being saturated. Dihydrodiols are not to be confused with diphenols (catechols) in which the carbon-carbon bond retains its aromatic character. Dihydrodiols are produced by the action of epoxide hydrolase on arene oxides. *See also* EPOXIDE HYDRATION; EPOXIDES.

dihydrophenytoin. *See* PHENYTOIN.

dihydroxybenzene. *See* CATECHOL.

L-3,4-dihydroxyphenylalanine. *See* L-DOPA.

diisopropylfluorophosphate. *See* DFP.

diisopropylphosphofluoridate. *See* DFP.

γ-diketone neuropathy (hexacarbon neuropathy). The γ-diketone 2,5-hexanedione is the ultimate neurotoxic metabolite of *n*-hexane and methyl *n*-butyl ketone. Other γ-diketones are similarly neurotoxic (e.g., 2,5-heptanedione and 3,6-octanedione), whereas α-, β- and γ-diketones are not. The γ-diketone metabolite appears to exert its toxicity through reaction with lysyl amino groups of proteins to yield 2,5-dimethylpyrrolyl derivatives. It has been hypothesized that the pyrrole rings undergo autoxidation, leading to covalent cross-linking of proteins. Furthermore, the stability of the neurofilament appears to predispose this protein to extensive derivatization and cross-linking during chronic intoxication with γ-diketones or hydrocarbons that can be metabolized to γ-diketones.

Dilantin. *See* PHENYTOIN.

dill. *See* ESSENTIAL OILS.

dimercaprol. *See* 2,3-DIMERCAPTO-1-PROPANOL.

2,3-dimercapto-1-propanol (British Anti-Lewisite; BAL; dimercaprol). CAS number 59-52-9. Used alone, or with other drugs, as a metal chelator. It is effective in the treatment of arsenic, gold, mercury and lead poisoning. Therapy is most effective when applied as soon as possible after intoxication. Because BAL-metal complexes break down in acid environments, urine should be kept alkaline during therapy. BAL

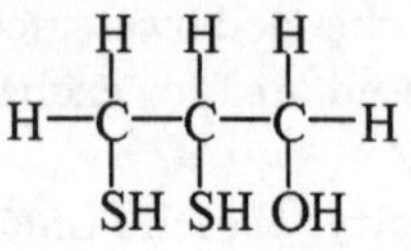

Dimercaprol

causes a transient tachycardia and increase in blood pressure after injection. *See also* ARSENIC; CHELATION AGENTS.

dimethoate (phosphorodithioic acid *O*,*O*-dimethyl *S*-[2-(methylamino)-2-oxoethyl] ester; Cygon; Rebelate; Perfekthion). CAS number 60-51-5. A systemic and contact insecticide and acaricide with an LD50 to rats of 250 mg/kg. It is a neurotoxicant by virtue of its ability to inhibit cholinesterase. *See also* INSECTICIDES; ORGANOPHOSPHATE POISONING, SYMPTOMS AND THERAPY; ORGANOPHOSPHORUS INSECTICIDES.

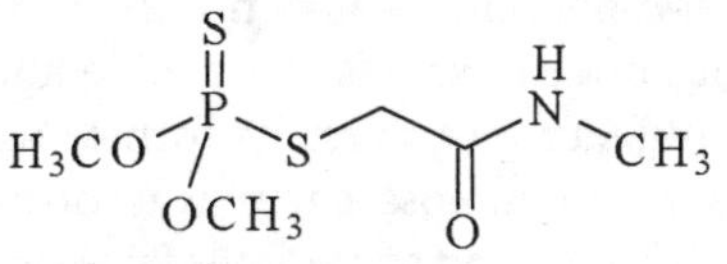

Dimethoate

3,3′-dimethoxybenzidine (*o*-dianisidine). CAS number 119-90-4. A probable carcinogen used in the manufacture of azo dyes. *See also* BENZIDINE.

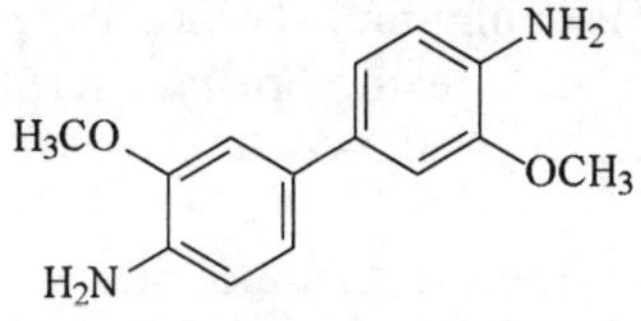

Dianisidine

dimethoxymethylamphetamine. *See* DOM.

4-dimethylaminoazobenzene. *See* AZO COMPOUNDS; BUTTER YELLOW.

dimethylaniline (dimethylaminobenzene). CAS number 121-69-7. Toxic action similar to aniline, a central nervous system depressant, although it is less toxic than aniline. The original substrate used for the characterization of the flavin-containing monooxygenase (FMO) which forms the *N*-oxide. *See also* DATABASES, TOXICOLOGY; FLAVIN-CONTAINING MONOOXYGENASE.

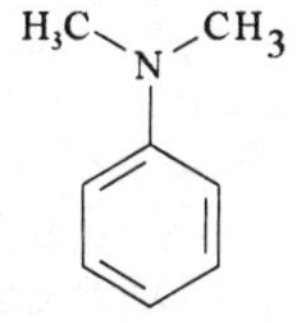

Dimethylaniline

dimethylbenzanthracene. *See* POLYCYCLIC AROMATIC HYDROCARBONS.

dimethyl carbamoyl chloride. CAS number 79-44-7. A designated animal carcinogen (IARC) and hazardous waste (EPA); a suspected carcinogen in humans. It is a liquid boiling at 165 °C that is used primarily in the manufacture of drugs and pesticides. Dimethyl carbamoyl chloride is extremely toxic.

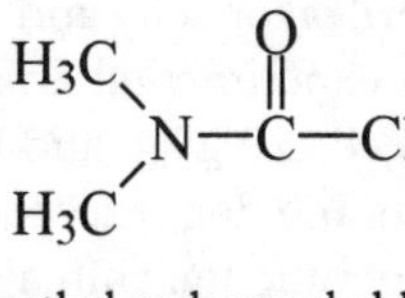

Dimethyl carbamoyl chloride

N-dimethylnitrosamine. The prototypical nitrosamine; a known potent mutagen and carcinogen in many animal systems. The primary target organ is the liver or kidney, depending on the exposure regimen, and in primates, may lead to liver cancer very rapidly. Toxicity requires that the parent compound undergoes a hydroxylation–demethylation reaction, and the resultant unstable nitroso structure yields an unstable intermediate which decomposes to an alkylating carbonium ion. Diets or drugs that decrease the initial phase I reaction reduce the toxicity of *N*-dimethylnitrosamine. *See also* NITROSAMINES.

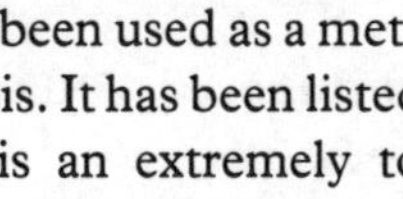

N-Dimethylnitrosamine

dimethyl sulfate (DMS; sulfuric acid dimethyl ester). CAS number 77-78-1. A compound that has been used as a methylating agent in organic synthesis. It has been listed as a carcinogen (EPA). DMS is an extremely toxic compound. Acute poisoning can occur via percutaneous uptake, which is rapid, or by inhalation of vapors. Topically the liquid causes blistering of the skin, whereas the vapors can cause inflammation and necrosis of the mucous membranes of the mouth, eyes and respiratory tract; pulmonary damage may be fatal. Acute systemic effects are extensive, involving damage to the liver and kidneys. The symptoms include convulsions, delirium and coma.

$$H_3C-O-\overset{\displaystyle O}{\underset{\displaystyle O}{\overset{\|}{\underset{\|}{S}}}}-O-CH_3$$

Dimethyl sulfate

dimethyl sulfoxide (DMSO). CAS number 67-68-5. An effective solvent that allows toxicants, drugs and allergens to penetrate the skin easily. It can produce redness, swellings and blisters by affecting membrane permeability and, therefore, ionic balance. Corneal opacity and lens alterations have occurred in experimental animals. The oral LD50 in rats exceeds 20 g/kg, and the i.p. and i.v. LD50 in mice, rats and dogs exceed 15 g/kg. Acute lethal doses in experimental animals leads to rapid breathing, restlessness, coma, hyperthermia, and rapid death, or death after several days because of renal failure. Repeated exposures lead to renal and hepatic lesions. Dermal exposures can result in disturbances of color vision, photophobia, headache and diarrhea. Inhalation by experimental animals has resulted in chemical pneumonia, hepatic swelling and renal toxicity. Teratogenicity has been suggested, but results are not conclusive. DMSO is used as an antifreeze, hydraulic fluid and a paint and varnish remover. It has been proposed for clinical use as an anti-inflammatory agent, an analgesic and a pharmaceutical solvent. Additional effects include nerve blockade, bacteriostasis, diuresis, mild cholinesterase inhibition, some reduction in fibrotic masses and vasodilatation.

$$\begin{array}{c} H_3C \\ H_3C \end{array}\!\!\!\! S\!=\!O$$

Dimethyl sulfoxid (DMSO)

dimethyltryptamine. *See* DMT.

1,3-dimethylxanthine. *See* THEOPHYLLINE.

3,7-dimethylxanthine. *See* THEOBROMINE.

Dimilin. *See* DIFLUBENZURON.

dinitrobenzenes. Exists as three isomers; *m*-**dinitrobenzene, CAS number 99-65-0,** *o*-**dinitrobenzene, CAS number 528-29-0,** and *p*-**dinitrobenzene, CAS number 100-25-4.** The mixture is assigned **CAS number**

25154-54-5, and is described as a suspected carcinogen, as are each of the individual isomers. *See also* DATABASES, TOXICOLOGY.

Dinitrobenzenes

dinitro-*o*-cresol (DNOC; 4,6-dinitro-*o*-cresol). A designated hazardous waste (EPA) and priority pollutant (EPA). It exists in nine isomeric forms of which the most important in commerce is 4,6-dinitro-*o*-phenol, CAS number 534-52-1. DNOC has boeen used as a pesticide and is used in the manufacture of dyes. Its former use, in the 1930s, as a weight loss agent was discontinued because of serious and sometimes fatal side effects. It is an uncoupling agent that blocks the formation of ATP in mitochondria with the energy being released as heat. Initial signs of poisoning are elevation of basal metabolic rate and high body temperature followed by fatigue, sweating and dehydration. Poisoning may eventually progress to tachycardia and death. *See also* ATSDR DOCUMENT, AUGUST 1995; DATABASES, TOXICOLOGY.

dinitro pesticides. Compounds whose molecules contain a dinitro group and that are used as contact herbicides, fungicides and insecticides (e.g., dinoseb, dinocap, dnoc). They are highly toxic to plants and animals, and may be harmful to humans in very small doses so their use is under review. They degrade rapidly after application and so cause no delayed environmental contamination. *See also* DINOCAP.

2,4-dinitrophenol (2,4-DNP). CAS number 51-28-5. A designated hazardous substance (EPA), hazardous waste (EPA) and priority toxic pollutant (EPA). There are six isomers of dinitrophenol of which the 2,4-isomer is the most important. 2,4-DNP is used in the manufacture of dyes, wood preservatives, photographic developers and as an intermediate in many chemical syntheses. It has also been used as an insecticide and herbicide. Entry into the body is by ingestion or by percutaneous absorption. 2,4-DNP uncouples oxidative phosphorylation, as does dinitro-*o*-cresol, causing increased heat production and oxygen uptake. Less severe poisoning results in nausea, anorexia, weakness and sweating, whereas severe poisoning leads to a dramatic rise in body temperature, tachycardia and possibly death. The use of 2,4-DNP to induce weight loss is extremely hazardous. See also oxidative phosphorylation inhibitors.

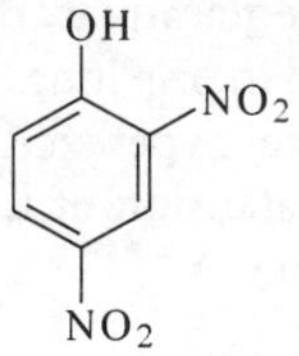

2,4-Dinitrophenol

2,4-dinitrotoluene (1-methyl-2,4-dinitrobenzene). CAS number 121-14-2. Suspected carcinogen based on assays with experimental animals. On acute exposure can cause anemia, methemoglobinemia, cyanosis and liver damage. *See also* DATABASES, TOXICOLOGY.

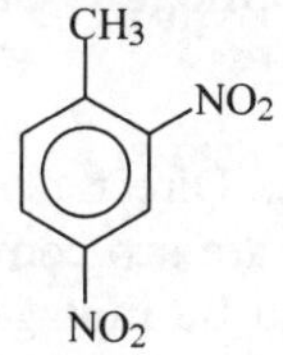

Dinitrotoluene

di-*n*-octyl phthalate. CAS number 117-84-0. A designated hazardous waste (EPA) and priority toxic pollutant (EPA). It is used as a plasticizer in the manufacture of plastics. Di-*n*-octyl phthalate has been shown to be teratogenic in experiments with rats. There is no direct evidence of its carcinogenicity or mutagenicity, but it is known to cause peroxisome proliferation. *See also* PEROXISOME PROLIFERATION; PHTHALIC ACID ESTERS; ATSDR DOCUMENT, JUNE 1994.

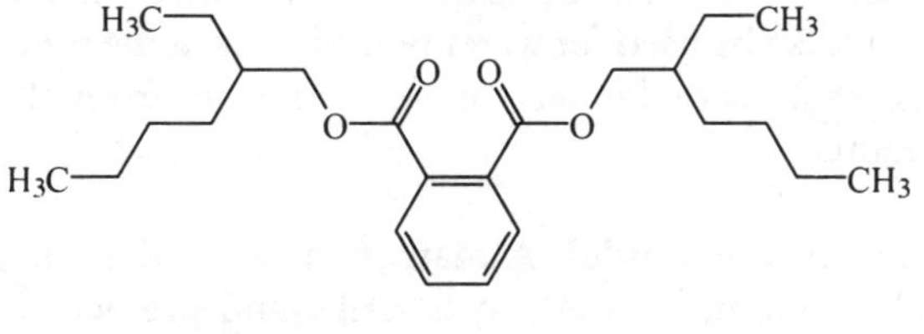

Di-*n*-octyl phthalate

di-*n*-octyltin. *See* ORGANOTINS.

dinocap (DNOCP). A dinitro fungicide and acaricide dinitro group used to control powdery mildew in horticulture and to suppress red spider mites. It can be irritating to the eyes and skin, and is harmful to fish.

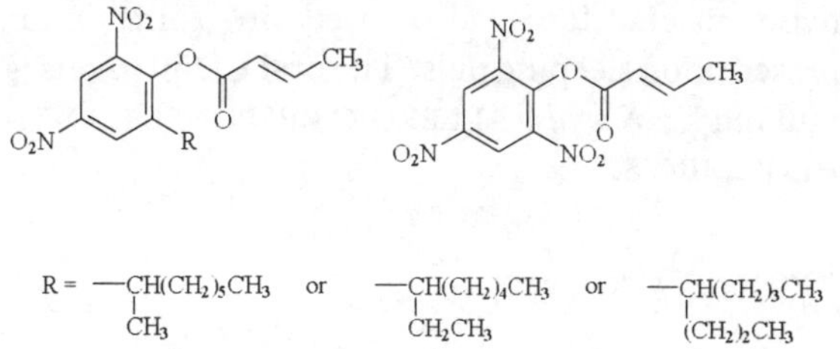

$$R = -CH(CH_2)_5CH_3 \quad or \quad -CH(CH_2)_4CH_3 \quad or \quad -CH(CH_2)_3CH_3$$
$$CH_3 CH_2CH_3 (CH_2)_2CH_3$$

Dinocap DNOCP

1,4-dioxane (*p*-dioxane). CAS number 123-91-1. A designated animal carcinogen (IARC) and hazardous waste. It is a volatile colorless liquid that is used primarily as a solvent for cellulose acetate and for dyes, fats and waxes. In the home and elsewhere, it is used for stripping paint and varnish and as a wetting agent in a variety of industrial applications. Entry into the body may be via inhalation of the vapor and either ingestion or percutaneous absorption of the liquid. Acute exposure may cause drowsiness, nausea and liver and kidney damage. Chronic exposure probably results in carcinogenesis.

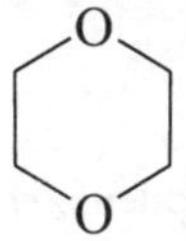

Dioxane

dioxin. Commonly, and inaccurately, used as a synonym for TCDD (2,3,7,8-tetrachlorodibenzo-*p*-dioxin). More accurately dioxins are a class of compounds based on substituted dioxane. *See also* 1,4-DIOXANE; TCDD.

Dip. Tox. *See* ROYAL COLLEGE OF PATHOLOGISTS.

diphenhydramine (2-(diphenylmethoxy)-*N,N*-dimethylethylamine; Benadryl). CAS number 58-73-1. An antihistamine used to treat perennial and seasonal rhinitis and mild allergic reactions, and as an adjunctive therapy for more severe allergic or anaphylactic responses. It is often used to treat the allergic responses to chemical exposures or insect bites. Because of its anticholinergic properties, overdosing often causes atropine-like symptoms. Therapy for overdosage includes emesis or gastric lavage, and vasopressors to treat hypotension. It is also used in some non-prescription sleeping pills. The oral LD50 in rats is 500 mg/kg. *See also* ALLERGIC RESPONSES; ANTI-HISTAMINES.

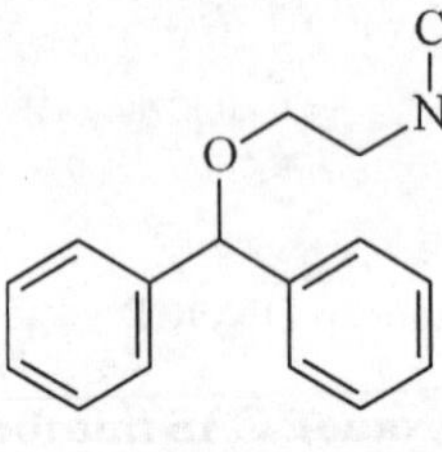

Diphenhydramine

diphenoxylate (1-(3-cyano-3,3-diphenylpropyl)-4-phenyl-4-piperidinecarboxylic acid ethyl ester). CAS number 915-30-0. An antiperistaltic, antidiarrheal drug that is also listed as a controlled substance (opiate). *See also* OPIATES.

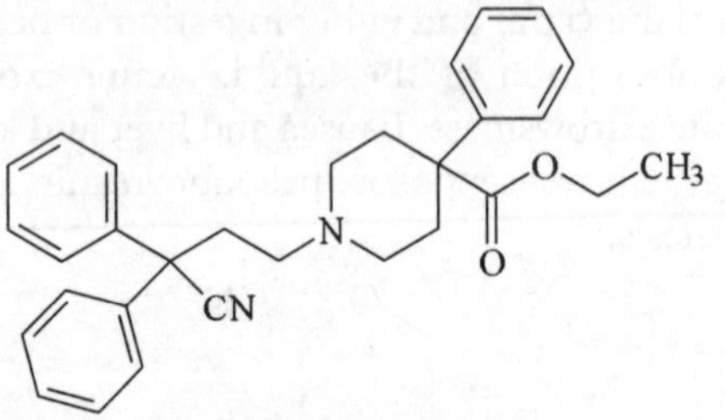

Diphenoxylate

diphenylmethane diisocyanate. *See* TOLUENE DIISOCYANATE.

diphtheria toxin. *See* PERTUSSIS TOXIN.

diploid. Having a dual set of chromosomes, one paternally and one materally derived. This is the normal chromosomal composition of the somatic cells, in contrast to the haploid content of the germ cells. *Compare* HAPLOID.

Diplomate in Toxicology. *See* ROYAL COLLEGE OF PATHOLOGISTS.

diquat (6,7-dihydrodipyrido[1,2-*a*:2′,1′-*c*]-pyrazinediium dibromide; Aquacide; Reglone). CAS number 85-00-7. A contact herbicide used as a defoliant. Its oral LD50 in rats is 231 mg/kg and in mice is 125 mg/kg. It is a convulsant, and its herbicidal and toxic actions may be mediated by free radical reactions similar to those of paraquat. Unlike paraquat, diquat is not toxic to, and not retained in, the lung. Acute diquat poisoning causes acute hyperexcitability leading to convulsions and distension of the gastrointestinal tract. *See also* PARAQUAT.

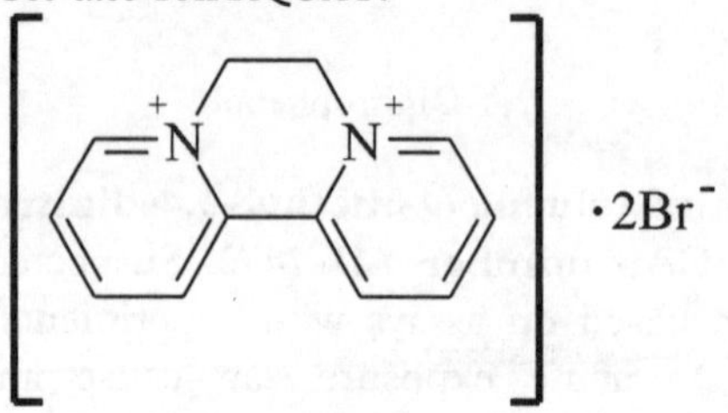

Diquat

direct-acting carcinogen. *See* CARCINOGEN, PRIMARY.

direct black dyes. Direct dyes such as direct black 6, 38 and 95 are azo compounds, many of which are known to be mutagenic and carcinogenic. *See also* AZO COMPOUNDS.

discontinuous variable. A variable when the theoretical range of values is limited. For example, if animals were ranked on the basis of a behavioral effect of a toxicant, this variable would be considered discontinuous. Discontinuous variables are often dichotomous (e.g., gender). *See also* STATISTICS, FUNCTION IN TOXICOLOGY.

disinfectants. *See* ANTIMICROBIALS.

dispersion. Movement and subsequent distribution. Used most often in airborne pollution but may also be used for water pollution or in the more general sense for any movement away from the source.

dispersion model. A mathematical model, usually computer based, to describe and predict the movement and distribution of airborne pollutants from the source or point of emission into the atmosphere

disposition. The fate of a chemical within the body, and includes absorption, transport, storage, and excretion.

dispositional tolerance. *See* METABOLIC TOLERANCE.

dissociation. In toxicology, of particular importance in the transport of toxicants and/or their metabolic products by blood proteins. Once a molecule binds to a plasma protein, it circulates until it dissociates from the protein either for attachment to another molecule or at a site of low concentration of unbound ligand. Dissociation occurs when the affinity of another molecule or medium is greater than that of the protein to which the toxicant was originally bound. Concentration differential, innate affinity, pH change, ionic strength and temperature change may all be involved. If dissociation is to occur, the forces of association must be strong enough to establish the initial interaction, but weak enough to permit dissociation at another site. If binding is reversible, in order to maintain equilibrium, redistribution will occur whenever the concentration of any one pool (blood or tissue) is diminished. *See also* AFFINITY CONSTANT; BINDING; BINDING SITES AND TRANSPORT; COMPETITIVE BINDING AND TRANSPORT; DISTRIBUTION OF TOXICANTS; K_D.

dissociation constant (K_D). A quantitative measure of the strength of the interaction in ligand binding. The dissociation constant is the reciprocal of the association constant K_A. Traditionally, values of K_D were determined using the Scatchard plot (more properly, the Rosenthal– Scatchard plot). Toxicants with modes of action that involve high affinity interaction with specific macromolecules usually have K_D's in the range of 0.001–10 nM. *See also* ASSOCIATION CONSTANT; BINDING; BINDING AFFINITY; K_D; SCATCHARD PLOT.

distress. Defined as "The animal puts substantial effort (resources) into the adaptive response. It is probably aware of the effort and may be considered to be suffering. The diversion of effort is to the detriment of other biological processes, e.g., growth and the response may have detrimental side-effects," in Sanford, et al. Vet. Rec. 118, (334). *See also* STRESS EFFECTS.

distribution of toxicants. Distribution refers both to the movement of a toxicant from the portal of entry to the tissue and also to the description of different concentrations reached in different locations. The first involves the study of transport mechanisms, primarily in the blood, and both are subject to mathematical analysis in toxicokinetic studies.

disulfide bond (S-S bond). A covalent bond between two sulfur heteroatoms. Disulfide bonds are important in establishing crosslinks between polypeptide chains or between loops of a single polypeptide chain and serve to stabilize the three-dimensional structure of proteins. They are formed by the oxidation of the sulfhydryl groups of two cysteine moieties, thus forming a cystine residue.

disulfide reduction. Some disulfides, such as the drug disulfiram (Antabuse), are reduced to their sulfhydryl constituents. These reactions are often three-step sequences, the last step catalyzed by glutathione reductase. *See also* REDUCTION.

$$XSSX + GSH \longrightarrow XSSG + XSH$$

$$XSSG + GSH \longrightarrow GSSG + XSH$$

$$GSSG + NADPH + H^+ \longrightarrow 2GSH + NADP^+ + 2GSH$$

Disulfide reduction

disulfiram (bis(diethyldithiocarbamoyl)disulfide; Antabuse). CAS number 97-77-8. Used in the treatment of chronic alcoholism, markedly altering the intermediary metabolism of ethanol. It is converted to diethydithiocarbamate, which is a strong chelator of copper and thus an inhibitor of copper-dependent enzymes. Normally, ethanol is metabolized by alcohol dehydrogenase in the liver to form acetaldehyde which in turn is rapidly oxidized by aldehyde dehydrogenase. Disulfiram inhibits the activity of aldehyde dehydrogenase, resulting in the accumulation of acetaldehyde to blood concentrations five to ten times higher than normal. Disulfiram, by itself, is a relatively non-toxic substance, but when given in combination with ethanol it produces marked signs and symptoms of toxicity attributed to the increased circulating concentration of acetaldehyde. Vasodilation, headache, respiratory distress, nausea and vomiting, hypotension, sweating and confusion are commonly observed sequelae of this drug combination. More extreme forms of this acetaldehyde-related toxicity include respiratory failure, cardiac arrhythmias, congestive heart failure, convulsions and death. When treated with disulfiram, the alcoholic must avoid the inadvertent administration of alcohol in the form of sauces, cough syrups and aftershave lotions. *See also* DIETHYLDITHIOCARBAMATE; ETHANOL.

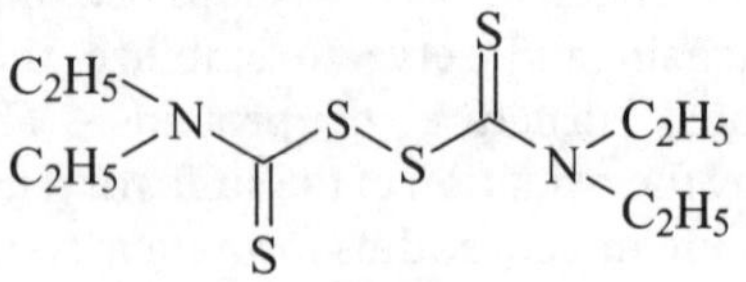

Disulfiram

disulfoton (**O,O-diethyl S-[2-(ethylthio) ethyl]phosphordithioate**). **CAS number 298-04-4**. Organophosphorus insecticide used primarily in agriculture, although use is decreasing. Cholinesterase inhibitor. *See also* ORGANOPHOSPHORUS INSECTICIDES; ORGANOPHOSPHORUS POISONING, SYMPTOMS AND THERAPY; ATSDR DOCUMENT, OCTOBER 1993; DATABASES, TOXICOLOGY.

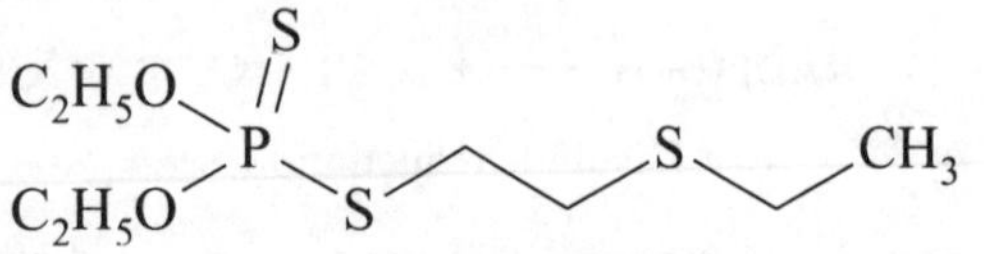

Disulfoton

diuresis. Increased urine production by the kidneys or urine passage by the bladder. Diuresis may be a consequence of chemical toxicity.

diuretics. Compounds that increase the rate of urine formation. These include a number of different classes of compounds each with different potentials for unwanted toxicity. A common toxicity problem of diuresis is the disturbance of ionic balance, including potassium depletion, magnesium depletion, etc., with resultant effects on the cardiovascular and muscular systems.

diuron. *See* UREA HERBICIDES.

DM. *See* D-AGENTS.

DMBA (dimethylbenzanthracene). *See* POLYCYCLIC AROMATIC HYDROCARBON.

DMN. *See* N-DIMETHYLNITROSAMINE.

DMS. *See* DIMETHYL SULFATE.

DMSO. *See* DIMETHYL SULFOXIDE.

DMT (**N,N-dimethyltryptamine**). **CAS number 61-50-7**. A hallucinogenic (psychedelic) agent that may catalyze the onset of emotional problems or psychosis in predisposed individuals. The mechanism of action for hallucinogens is not understood at the present time, and DMT is perhaps one of the least studied of the hallucinogens. It causes perceptual alterations and illusions, including changes in touch, taste and odor. The thinking process is substantially altered; there are hallucinations and loss of contact with reality. There have been no overdose deaths attributed to the direct effects of DMT. The drug is very short-acting, with a duration of effect of about half an hour or less. *See also* HALLUCINOGENS.

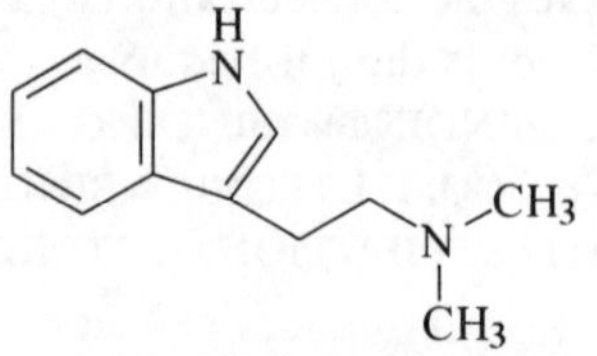

N,N-Dimethyltryptamine

DNA (deoxyribonucleic acid). The molecule that carries the genetic code through which genotypic characters are inherited. In somatic cells, it carries the code for the synthesis of all of the protein constituents of the cell. DNAs are long, linear macromolecules consisting of an invariable structural backbone of deoxyribose molecules linked by phosphodiester bridges (3′-5′ bridges). The variable portions are purines and pyrimidines in the 1′-position, the particular sequence of bases comprising the genetic code. The three-dimensional structure of DNA is a double helix of two such chains, in which the chains wind around each other in opposite directions with the bases on the inside. Hydrogen bonding between purine and pyrimidine bases holds the chain together. Adenine is paired with thymine, and guanine with cytosine. The two chains are thus complementary, a fact that permits them to act as templates for each other during DNA replication. This structure was discovered by James Watson and Francis Crick, who thus laid the basis for the recent rapid development of molecular biology and biotechnology. In toxicology, knowledge of DNA structure and metabolism is essential for the study of carcinogenesis and mutagenesis. *See also* CARCINOGENESIS; CHROMOSOME ABERRATIONS; DNA ADDUCTS; DNA DAMAGE AND REPAIR TESTS; DNA OXIDATIVE DAMAGE; DNA REPAIR; MUTAGENESIS; MUTATION.

DNA adducts. Compounds formed by the reaction of electrophiles with nucleophilic sites on DNA molecules. Most carcinogens are either electrophiles or are metabolized to electrophiles, and DNA adduct formation has been associated with both carcinogenesis and mutagenesis. Many different DNA adducts can be formed with different sites having varying susceptibilities, depending not only on their intrinsic reactivity, but also on the nature of the reactive electrophile. For example, such alkylating agents as methyl- or ethylmethane sulfonate react most avidly with the N-7 position of guanine residues. They also react with the N-1, N-3 and N-7 of adenine, the N-3 and O-6 of guanine, the N-3 of cytosine and the O-4 of thymine. Other carcinogens, such as the epoxide of aflatoxin B_1 or the dihydrodiol epoxide of benzo[*a*]pyrene, also react at several sites. It is becoming clear that all of these sites are not equally important in carcinogenesis, and currently attention is being directed to the determination of which particular adduct is associated with the carcinogenesis caused by specific chemicals. In light of current knowledge of oncogenes, it is possible that adduct formation is involved in the activation of proto-oncogenes.

DNA cloning. Technique whereby DNA from one source is inserted into a cloning vector and then introduced into a host organism (usually a bacterium). The DNA for cloning may be prepared by partial or total digestion with the restriction endonucleases and inserted into a cloning vector that has been cleaved by the same restriction endonuclease, or an enzyme that yields complementary single-stranded termini. Alternatively DNA may be prepared for insertion by mechanical shearing, deoxyribonuclease digestion or tailing. Loose ends are religated using DNA ligase to produce a coherent recombinant DNA molecule. Recombinant DNA molecules are introduced into a host bacterium (usually *E. coli*) by transformation if a plasmid vector is used, or if the cloning vector is bacteriophage-based by transfection or infection (following *in vitro* packaging).

DNA crosslinks. A DNA lesion brought about when a chemical covalently binds to two nucleotide residues, one in each strand of a DNA molecule. DNA crosslinking generally prevents duplication and thus is lethal to dividing cells.

DNA damage and repair tests. The most widespread test for DNA damage by monitoring repair is the unscheduled DNA synthesis test using cultured primary rat hepatocytes. Other ways of studying DNA damage are by assessing covalent binding of the test chemical to DNA or by measuring DNA breakage following *in vivo* or *in vitro* exposure of DNA to the test chemical. Strains of the bacterium *Escherichia coli* that are deficient in DNA polymerase cannot repair DNA damaged by mutagens as effectively as strains displaying normal polymerase levels. *In vitro* test systems use this principle to detect mutagens by monitoring retarded growth of the bacterium in the presence of mutagens. *See also* BACTERIAL MUTAGENESIS; COVALENT BINDING TESTS; EUKARYOTE MUTAGENICITY TESTS.

DNA fingerprinting. Technique in which the banding pattern of DNA fragments is compared and can be used in many species, including the human, to indicate relatedness. DNA is digested with restriction enzymes, run on an electrophoretic gel, and blots made from the gel (*see* SOUTHERN BLOTTING). Such blots are then hybridized with radiolabeled probe DNA consisting of cloned sequences of the short interspersed repeat sequences (such as the ALU sequences in the human) which are common in vertebrate genomes. Autoradiography then provides a distinct banding pattern of DNA fragments containing such DNA sequences.

DNA, genomic. DNA of the genome, which, in bacteria, is a single, circular loop, and in eukaryotic cells is the entire haploid nuclear complement of DNA. Non-genomic DNA includes, in bacteria, the DNA of plasmids, and in eukaryotes the DNA of viruses or other contaminants. Note that in eukaryotes the mitochondrial genome and chloroplast genome are often considered separately from the nuclear genome.

DNA hybridization. Production of double-stranded DNA or DNA-RNA hybrid molecules from single-stranded molecules from different sources by the formation of hydrogen bonds at complementary nucleotide sequences. Some hybridization reactions are performed as a mixed phase with one of the nucleic acid strands immobilized to a solid support. This technology has been used extensively to study gene structure, genome organization and the control of gene expression. Normally a fragment of DNA is radiolabelled and then used as a hybridization "probe" to detect homologous or nearly homologous sequences that have been immobilized onto a solid supporting matrix (i.e., by Southern blotting). Hybrid formation is a complex reaction depending on the type of probe used. Using a single-stranded probe the rate of hybridization follows first-order kinetics and is affected by probe strand length, complexity, ionic strength, temperature, pH and viscosity. Annealing of nucleic acid strands to form hybrids is a reversible process. The stability of perfectly or imperfectly matched duplexes depends on clearly defined criteria. Hence, sequence relatedness of hybrid duplexes can be determined by changing these criteria in a procedure known as stringent washing.

DNA library (DNA bank). Collection of cloned DNA fragments that represents part or all of the genome of an organism. Most libraries are partial simply as a result of the method of formation and the comparative rarity of some gene sequences. Genomic and cDNA libraries differ in that the former comprises pieces of genomic DNA and therefore include introns and non-coding sequences, whereas the latter, being complementary to mRNA, contain only coding sequences.

DNA ligases. One of the enzymes involved in DNA replication in prokaryotes. The enzymes from *E. coli* and bacteriophage T4 have been characterized. The enzyme catalyses the formation of phosphodiester bonds between adjacent 5'-phosphate and the free 3'-hydroxy groups in DNA duplexes. It is used in sealing restriction fragments together at Eco RI sticky ends generated, for example, by the restriction enzyme Eco RI.

DNA ligation. Joining of adjacent nucleotides in a strand of DNA by formation of a phosphodiester bond. The process is catalyzed by DNA ligases and occurs during DNA replication and DNA repair, and in recombinant DNA technology.

DNA melting. Denaturation of double-stranded DNA to yield single-stranded DNA. Melting, which can be induced by increased temperatures when DNA is dissolved in a suitable salt solution, results in a reduction of viscosity and an increase in ultraviolet absorption. This increase in light absorption is the hyperchromic effect. Melting can be followed by annealing or renaturation, which involves specific hybridization between sister strands and is used in the derivation of cot plots.

DNA methylation. Attachment of a methyl group to cytosine residues of eukaryotic DNA to form 5-methylcytosine. Usually the cytosine residues that become methylated are in a C-G pair in the DNA. In prokaryotes and lower eukaryotes, some adenine residues are also methylated. DNA methylation is a post-replicational modification to the DNA, and in bacterial cells the methylation of the genomic DNA serves to preserve it from the attack by native restriction endonucleases which rapidly degrade invading viral DNA. Thus the restriction/modification system of bacteria uses DNA methylation as a protective measure to ensure preservation of the genome and destruction of foreign DNA. In cells of some eukaryotes (e.g., *Drosophila*) no methylation has been detected, but in higher eukaryotes much of the DNA contains a proportion of methylcytosine residues. There is a strong, but not absolute, correlation between high levels of methylation and transcriptional inactivity. The pattern of methylation in a sequence is normally passed on faithfully at DNA replication (through preference of DNA methylase for half-methylated sites), but can be inhibited by the addition of the base analogue 5'-azacytidine. There is also evidence that methylation of cytosine residues in DNA may fundamentally change the conformation of the double helix, leading to a preferential transition from B form to Z form (left-handed DNA).

DNA, native. Double-stranded, nondenatured DNA in a preparation that has been extracted from a particular known biological source (viral, bacterial or eukaryotic tissue) as distinct from any additional material added as a probe or marker.

DNA oxidative damage. A postulated important mechanism of radiation-induced carcinogenesis. The effect of ionizing radiation on cells is initiated by the absorption of energy sufficient to expel electrons from molecules, resulting in the formation of positively charged ions. The expelled electrons react with nearby molecules to form negatively charged ions. Since water is the principal component of the cell, it absorbs most of the ionizing radiation forming free radicals that react with each other, with other water molecules, and/or with cellular macromolecules. These "active" oxygen species (e.g., superoxide ($O_2^{\bullet}$), hydroperoxy radical ($HO_2^{\bullet}$), hydroxyl radical ($OH^{\bullet}$), hydrogen peroxide (H_2O_2)) cause oxidative damage to cellular macromolecules, including DNA. *See also* FREE RADICALS; OXYGEN, REACTIVE SPECIES; SUPEROXIDE.

DNA polymerases (DNA-dependent DNA polymerases). Enzymes responsible for the synthesis of DNA from nucleotide precursors using single-stranded DNA as a template. A number of different DNA polymerases can be recovered from eukaryotic cells, some of which are repair enzymes which polymerize short pieces of DNA where sections have been deleted from a sequence or help to substitute correct bases for incorrect bases. But at least one enzyme species (and probably more than one) is responsible for the polymerization of new DNA in the replication process. *See also* DNA REPAIR; DNA REPLICATION; REVERSE TRANSCRIPTASE.

DNA repair. Enzymes exist within cells that can repair many of the mutations that may occur to the original DNA molecule. Consequently, fewer mutations are retained in the replicated DNA molecules than originally occurred. If the mutation is not so repaired, the incorrect information may be transcribed into RNA, and the mutation expressed as an altered protein, such changes being critical or insignificant, depending on the position of the amino acid in the protein or the amount and function of the protein affected. The protein that repairs O^6-methylguanine is a methyltransferase which removes the methyl group and restores the DNA structure in a single step. Other enzymes that repair DNA are glycosylases which split the bond between the N-9 position of the purine and the deoxyribose forming an apurinic site in the DNA. These sites and those generated by spontaneous hydrolysis of methylated bases are then restored by the action of an endonuclease which breaks the DNA chain, excising three or four nucleotides, including the damaged site. Subsequently, the gap is filled by nucleotide polymerization using DNA polymerase followed by closing of the strand using DNA ligase. *See also* DNA DAMAGE AND REPAIR TESTS.

DNA replication. Process of DNA synthesis whereby a parent DNA molecule is faithfully copied, giving rise to two identical daughter molecules. DNA replication is semiconservative. Polymerization of the nucleotide forming the new strand is catalyzed by DNA polymerase, and a number of steps are involved. First, the double helix is destabilized and opened up to permit each strand to serve as a template for the polymerase enzyme. Second, a short primer sequence of RNA is synthesized, followed by the DNA sequence. The RNA primer later is cleaved out and replaced with DNA. Finally, the DNA is replicated only in one direction since the DNA strands are polarized, synthesis proceeding from a 5'- to a 3'-direction, that is, the parent strand is read in the 3'- to 5'-direction. The last observation introduces a complication, since only one of the two parent strands can be continuously read in the required direction. In order to overcome this the new DNA on the so-called lagging strand is synthesized discontinuously in short Okazaki fragments, later to be joined up by DNA ligases. Synthesis on the leading strand appears to be continuous. This pattern of DNA replication is followed in both prokaryotes and eukaryotes but, in prokaryotes, where the bacterial genome is circular, synthesis proceeds from a single initiation point in both directions around the circle. DNA synthesis is also continuous throughout the prokaryotic cell cycle. In contrast, eukaryotic DNA synthesis is discontinuous, and proceeds only during the S phase of the cell cycle. The DNA is replicated from many separate initiation points along the length of a chromosome, again in both directions, and eventually the separate replicons join up to yield the two complete daughter strands.

DNA restriction endonuclease. Most important class of restriction endonucleases, class II, which cut double-stranded DNA molecules only at sites characterized by a specific nucleotide sequence. Restriction enzymes are isolated from bacterial cells, and are tools for molecular biologists. Several hundred restriction enzymes are now known, each with a specific sequence requirement dictating where it will cut DNA. Most recognize sequences between four and six base pairs long, which, in turn, are likely to occur by chance once every few hundred to once every few thousand nucleotides along a DNA molecule. Some, such as Hin dIII, make staggered cuts leaving "sticky ends" three nucleotides long protruding on one strand from each severed terminus; others make clean cuts in both strands at the same place and thus generate "blunt ends." Digesting DNA with a restriction enzyme therefore creates a characteristic set of fragments, which can be isolated by electrophoresis and subsequently analyzed.

DNA-RNA hybridization. Pairing of DNA with RNA molecules by specific hydrogen bonding between complementary bases. DNA-RNA association by annealing can be favored relative to DNA-DNA association by appropriate manipulation of the conditions.

DNase (deoxyribonuclease). Family of enzymes that degrade DNA, either by cutting the molecule one nucleotide at a time from the ends (an exonuclease) or by cutting it internally, sometimes at specific sequences (an endonuclease). Enzymes that degrade both DNA and RNA are termed simply nucleases. Some DNases cut only single strands of DNA, even if the DNA is in duplex form; others cut both strands. An enzyme that is widely used to introduce nicks into DNA is DNase I, a bivalent metal ion-requiring enzyme derived from bovine pancreas. Enzymes referred to as DNase II, which may be derived from mammalian spleen or thymus, or from bacteria (now termed staphylococcal nuclease, previously referred to as micrococcal nuclease) have no metal requirement, but operate at a rather acid pH. They have been widely used for the digestion of chromatin to yield nucleosomes. S1 nuclease is an endonuclease from *Aspergillus* that cuts single-stranded DNA selectively.

DNA sequencing. Technique used to determine the precise sequence of bases in length of DNA. The first complete nucleotide sequence, which was not for DNA but for the comparatively small alanine tRNA was published in 1965, but since that time the technical difficulties in sequencing DNA have been overcome. The problems of cutting DNA at specific points, not only to dissect out the required section and to cut the DNA into manageable lengths, but also to perform the sequencing analysis, were solved by the discovery and isolation of the restriction endonucleases. These enzymes are also essential in the preparation of sufficient quantities of particular fragments by DNA cloning. For particular methods, *see* DIDEOXY SEQUENCING.

DNA vector. System, such as a plasmid or a virus, that is used as a vehicle to transfer DNA from one cell to another.

DNOC. *See* DINITRO-*O*-CRESOL.

2,4-DNP. *See* 2,4-DINITROPHENOL.

DOB (bromo-DMA; 2,5-dimethoxy-4-bromo-amphetamine; 1-(2,5-dimethoxy-4-bromo-phenyl)-2-aminopropane). A hallucinogenic (psychedelic) agent that is obtained by chemical synthesis. It may catalyze severe emotional problems or psychosis in predisposed individuals, and in large doses, produces peripheral arterial spasm which, if not treated, can lead to gangrene. DOB is a potent serotonin 5-HT$_2$ agonist, and although the underlying mechanism of action for hallucinogens is not well understood, this may be related to its actions in the CNS. Symptoms include hyperreflexia, restlessness, perceptual alterations and illusions, including changes in touch, taste and odor, and the thinking process is substantially altered. At high doses, it causes hallucinations, loss of contact with reality and pain and coldness in the extremities at toxic levels. Therapeutically, peripheral arterial spasm has been treated with intraarterial tolazoline hydrochloride. Its LD50 is in mice 80 mg/kg, i.v., in rats 8 mg/kg, i.p., in dogs 4 mg/kg. i.v., and in monkeys 2 mg/kg, i.v. *See also* AMPHETAMINES; HALLUCINOGENS.

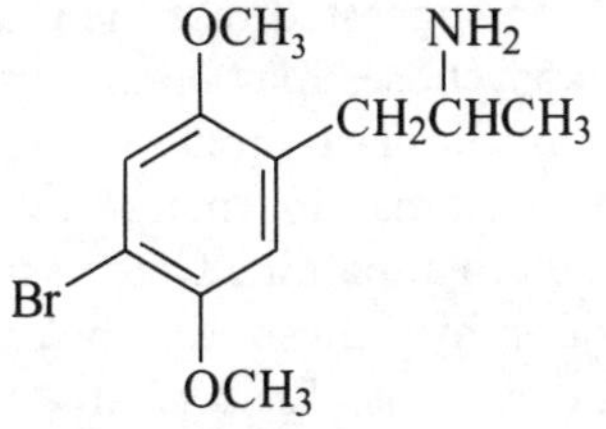

DOB

DOM   (1-(2,5-dimethoxy-4-methylphenyl)-2-aminopropane; 2,5-dimethoxy-4-methylamphetamine; STP). A hallucinogenic (psychedelic) agent. It may catalyze the onset of emotional problems or psychosis in predisposed individuals. Although the mechanism of action for hallucinogens is not understood, DOM is believed to act by being an agonist at serotonin 5-HT$_2$ receptors. It causes hyperreflexia, restlessness and perceptual alterations in illusions, including changes in touch, taste and odor, and the thinking process is substantially altered. At high doses, hallucinations and loss of contact with reality result. The duration of action may be 16–24 hours. Its LD50 is in mice 36 mg/kg, i.v., in rats 32.5 mg/kg, i.p., in dogs 7.2 mg/kg, i.v., and in monkeys 8 mg/kg, i.v. *See also* AMPHETAMINES; HALLUCINOGENS.

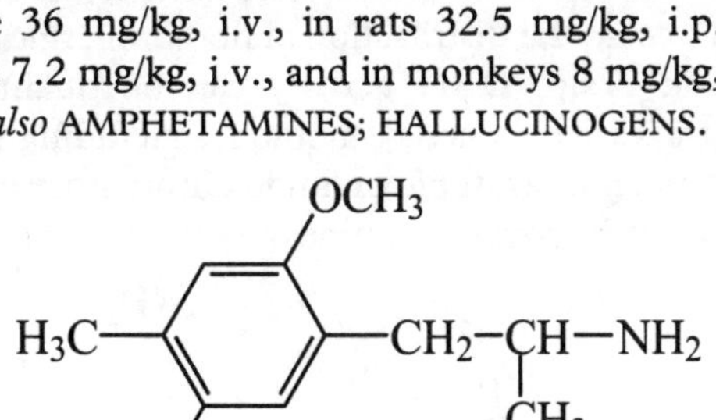

DOM

domestic animals. *See* POLLUTION, EFFECTS ON DOMESTIC ANIMALS.

domestic sewage. The used water of a community exclusive of industrial wastewater and storm water run-off that requires treatment before discharge into the environment. The average biochemical oxygen demand (five days, 20 °C) is 250 mg O$_2$/l. The composition varies from minute to minute. Components in domestic sewage include large objects, heavy materials (e.g., rocks, glass), oil and grease, suspended solids, dissolved organic and inorganic matter, and a large number of microorganisms including some pathogenic species.

domestic wastes. *See* POLLUTION, DOMESTIC AND MUNICIPAL WASTES.

dominant lethal (rodent) test. An *in vivo* test that assesses the ability of a suspected mutagen, which has proved positive in an *in vitro* screen, to cause dominant lethal mutations in rats, mice or hamsters. Male rodents are treated with the test agent and are then mated to groups of naive females over several weeks to test for effects occurring at all stages of spermatogenesis. Following sacrifice, the females are evaluated for the following: fertility index; numbers of implantations; numbers of corpora lutea; preimplantation losses; dead implantations. Negative and positive controls are run concurrently. *See also* CHROMOSOME ABERRATION TESTS.

dominant visible mutation. A dominant mutation that produces a visible phenotype in the heterozygote. *See* MUTATION, DOMINANT VISIBLE.

domoic acid (2S-(2α,3β,4β(1Z,3E,5S*))-2-carboxy-4-(5-carboxy-1-methyl-1,3-hexadienyl)-3-pyrrolidineacetic acid). **CAS number 14277-97-5.** An excitory amino acid isolated from the red alga *Chondria armata*. A structural analog

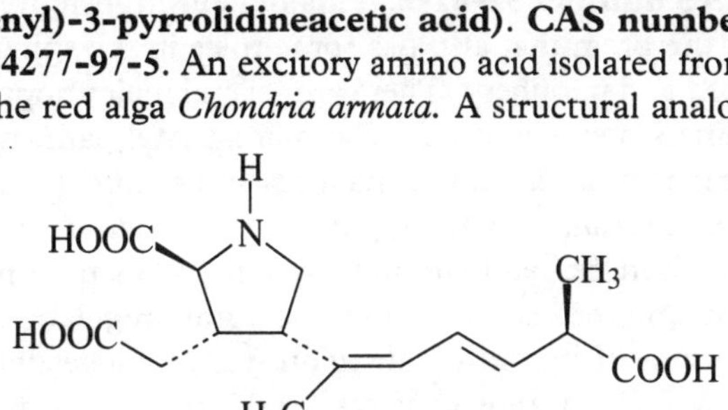

Domoic acid

of kainic acid, domoic acid has been shown to be responsible for the shellfish poisoning associated with eating certain cultured blue mussels. *See also* NEUROTOXICITY.

donated drugs. The donation of past "expiry date" or otherwise surplus medicines for use in disasters or in other aspects of aid work has resulted in frank toxicities in recipients. In one reported case closantel was supplied without package leaflets, and misidentified.

Donora. *See* ENVIRONMENTAL DISASTERS.

L-dopa   (L-3,4-dihydroxyphenylalanine). **CAS number 59-92-7**. The amino acid intermediate for the catecholamine neurotransmitters dopamine, norepinephrine and epinephrine. It is formed by decarboxylation of tyrosine by the enzyme tyrosine hydroxylase, and its formation is the rate-limiting step in catecholamine biosynthesis. It is used therapeutically to treat idiopathic or chemical parkinsonism, often in combination with a peripheral aromatic amino acid decarboxylase inhibitor and/or a direct-acting dopamine agonist. *See also* CATECHOLAMINES; DOPAMINE; EPINEPHRINE; NOREPINEPHRINE; PARKINSONISM; TYROSINE HYDROXYLASE.

L-Dopa

dopamine   (L-3,4-dihydroxyphenethylamine; 2-(L-3,4-dihydroxyphenyl)aminoethane). **CAS number 51-61-6**. A major neurotransmitter of the brain that also has some roles in the spinal cord and periphery. There are several major dopamine systems in brain. The nigrostriatal pathway originates in the substantia nigra and terminates in the striatum (caudate-putamen). Because this field is in the extrapyramidal system, it functions in fine motor control and postural regulation. Lesions of this terminal region (e.g., by ingestion of MPTP) or disease states (Parkinsonism) result in motor dysfunction. Another major dopamine system is the mesolimbic–mesocortical system.

These neurons also originate in the midbrain region and project to parts of the limbic system and defined areas of the cortex. The functions regulated include activity and emotionality. Some toxicants (e.g, triethyllead) that cause profound effects on behavior, including psychotic reactions, may affect the function of these systems. Finally, the tuberoinfundibular dopamine system is intrinsic within the hypothalamus, and plays a role in neuroendocrine regulation. Toxicants affecting these neurons (e.g., large doses of monosodium glutamate during development) alter neuroendocrine function by affecting, in part, these neurons. Because the clinical effectiveness of antipsychotic drugs correlates with blockade of dopamine receptors, it has been suggested that the primary lesion in idiopathic psychoses may be in dopamine neurotransmission. Similarly, toxic insult that causes psychotic symptoms in man, or behavioral changes related to dopamine systems in laboratory animals, is often hypothesized to be due to effects on dopamine systems. *See also* ANTIPSYCHOTIC DRUGS; DOPAMINE RECEPTORS; MANGANESE; 1-METHYL-4-PHENYL-1,2,3,6-TETRAHYDROPYRIDINE; PARKINSONISM.

dopamine β-hydroxylase (DBH; EC 1.14. 17.1). An enzyme in the catecholamine biosynthetic pathway that converts dopamine to norepinephrine. It is a copper-containing monooxygenase that requires ascorbic acid as a cofactor and molecular oxygen to add a hydroxyl group to the β-carbon on the side chain of dopamine. DBH is localized in storage vesicles in noradrenergic and adrenergic neurons and adrenal medulla cells. Because copper is involved in the reaction, copper chelators are potent inhibitors of DBH, as are disulfiram and fusaric acid. DBH activity has been used to map the distribution of noradrenergic neurons in brain. DBH activity can be quantified using a variety of assay methods, including photometric, radioisotopic or liquid chromatographic. Typically, phenylethylamine or tyramine is used as

Dopamine

the substrate and phenylethanolamine or octopamine as the product. *See also* CATECHOLAMINES; NOREPINEPHRINE.

dopamine receptors. Receptors for the neurotransmitter dopamine are located on pre- and postsynaptic sites of the CNS, as well as in other locales, including the pituitary, area postrema (chemoreceptor trigger zone) and in the peripheral vasculature. Direct- or indirect-acting dopamine agonists elicit behaviors or physiological sequelae controlled by these different areas of the CNS (called D_1, D_2, D_3, D_4 and D_5). There are few genes that encode multiple dopamine receptors (including some splice variants), although all are in the G-protein-coupled receptor superfamily. Many drugs and toxicants (antipsychotic drugs, amphetamines, ergot alkaloids, etc.) work directly or indirectly via actions at dopamine receptor. *See also* ANTIPSYCHOTIC DRUGS; DOPAMINE.

Doriden. *See* GLUTHEMIDE.

dosage. The amount of a toxicant, drug, or other chemical administered or taken, expressed as some function of the organism and of time (e.g., mg/kg body weight/day). Finding the most appropriate dosage is of critical importance in all types of toxicity testing. For examples of appropriate dosage under various conditions *see also* CARCINOGENICITY TESTING; CHRONIC TOXICITY TESTING; MAXIMUM TOLERATED DOSE; REPRODUCTIVE TOXICITY TESTING; TERATOLOGY TESTING; SUBCHRONIC TOXICITY TESTING. *Compare* DOSE.

dose. The total amount of a toxicant, drug or other chemical administered to, or taken by, the organism. *Compare* DOSAGE.

dose response. In toxicology, the quantitative relationship between the amount of a toxicant administered, or taken, and the incidence or extent of the adverse effect.

dose-response assessment. A major step in the risk assessment process that characterizes the relationship between the dose of a chemical administered to a population of test animals and the incidence of a given adverse effect. Typically it involves mathematical modeling techniques to extrapolate from the high-dose effects observed experimentally in test animals to estimate the effects expected to result from exposure to the usually low doses encountered by humans. *See also* RISK ASSESSMENT.

dose-response curve. The graphical relationship between the dose of a toxicant and the toxic response. It assumes a causal relationship between the toxicant in question and the effect being measured. It implies that not only is there an active site for the toxicant, and that the production of a response is related to the concentration of the toxicant at that site, but also that the concentration at the active site is related to the dose administered or to the time and concentration of exposure. These implications are not fundamental, however, to the dose-response curve, that requires only that there be available an accurate method to administer the dose and an accurate method to measure the response. The meaning of "curve," as expressed in the above implications, may in part be inferred from the shape of the curve itself or may require additional studies. Nonlinear plots of dose-response are not easily extrapolated, and various mathematical transformations are used to provide straight (i.e., extrapolatable) lines. Dose is almost always expressed on a logarithmic scale, whereas response may be expressed directly or in probability units (probits). Comparison of dose-response curves can provide additional information beyond median effective doses (ED50, LD50, LC50, etc.), including separate comparisons of efficacy and potency, as well as permitting calculation of such values as the therapeutic index and the margin of safety. *See also* LOW-DOSE EXTRAPOLATION; MARGIN OF SAFETY; THERAPEUTIC INDEX.

dose-response curve, in risk analysis. *See* DOSE-RESPONSE CURVE; LOW-DOSE EXTRAPOLATION.

dose surrogate. *See* DOSIMETER.

dosimeter (dose surrogate). A measure of exposure (e.g., mg/kg, AUC, plasma concentration peak height, metabolite level, etc.).

dosimetry. Measurement or modeling of the amount, rate and distribution of a toxicant in the body, particularly as it relates to mode of toxic action.

dosing. The procedure by which the appropriate dose is administered to the test organism. *See also* ADMINISTRATION OF TOXICANTS.

DOT. *See* DEPARTMENT OF TRANSPORTATION.

doxepin. *See* TRICYCLIC ANTIDEPRESSANTS

doxorubicin (10-[(3-amino-2,3,6-trideoxy-α-L-lyxohexopyranosyl)oxy]-7,8,9,10-tetra-hydro-6,8,11-trihydroxy-8-(hydroxyacetyl)-1-methoxy-5,12-naphthacenedione; adriamycin). CAS number 23214-92-8. An anthracycline cytotoxic antineoplastic that is produced by *Streptomyces peucetius*. The LD50 in mice is 9.4 mg/kg, i.v. It is a carcinogen that inhibits DNA and RNA synthesis by intercalating in double-stranded DNA with the amino sugar in the minor groove and the 9'-OH group of the anthracycline ring hydrogen-bonded to the adjacent guanine. It also alters membrane fluidity and ion transport, and generates free radicals through a cytochrome P450-mediated reductive process. In humans, it causes alopecia, stomatitis, nausea, vomiting, diarrhea, cardiotoxicity (manifested by tachycardia) and potentially fatal congestive heart failure.

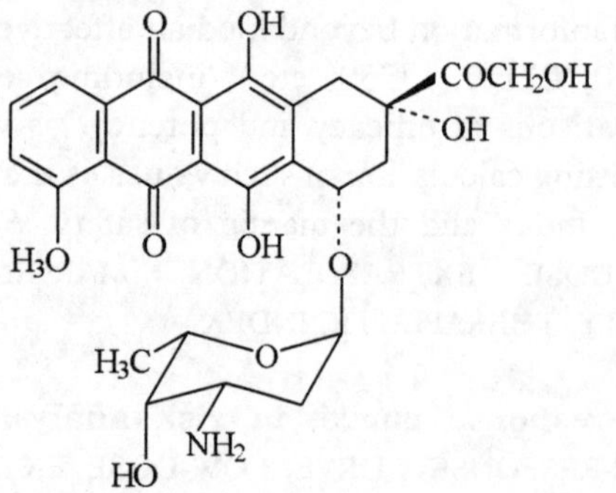

Doxorubicin

doxylamine (*N*,*N*-dimethyl-2-[1-phenyl-1-(2-pyridinyl)ethoxy]ethanamine; Benedictin). An antihistamine that formerly was used in pregnant women for antihistaminic and sedative properties. Although it has excellent sedative proper-ties, it has been implicated in teratogenesis and in causing neurobehavioral toxicity, and is therefore no longer used.

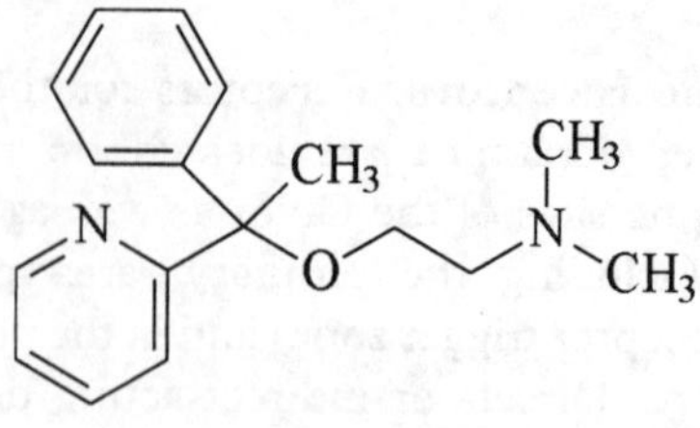

Doxylamine

Draize test. *See* EYE IRRITATION TEST.

drift, environmental. The movement of chemicals in the environment as a result of atmospheric transport. The distance a chemical will be carried depends on meteorological conditions such as winds and precipitation, topography and vegetation, as well as the chemical state (gaseous, vapor or particulate) of the compound.

drinking water. *See* ADMINISTRATION OF TOXICANTS, ORAL.

Drosophila melanogaster. The fruit fly, a dipterous insect used in mutagenicity testing. *See also* SEX-LINKED RECESSIVE MUTATION TEST.

drug abuse. The repeated use of a legal or illicit drug for its reinforcing properties that occurs at the expense of the physiological and/or psychological well-being of the person. *See also* ALCOHOL; AMPHETAMINES; COCAINE; DEPENDENCE; MORPHINE; NICOTINE; TOLERANCE.

Drug Enforcement Administration. *See* CONTROLLED SUBSTANCES ACT.

drug metabolizing activity. *See* XENOBIOTIC METABOLISM.

drugs, therapeutic. Essentially, all therapeutic drugs can be toxic at some dose. The danger to the individual patient is dependent upon the nature of the toxic response, the dose necessary to produce the toxic response and the relationship between the therapeutic and the toxic dose. Drug toxicity is affected by all of those factors that affect the toxicity of any xenobiotics, including individual (genetic) variation, diet, age and the presence of other exogenous chemicals. The risk of toxic side effects from a particular drug must be weighed against the expected benefits. The use of a quite dangerous drug with only a narrow tolerance between the therapeutic and toxic doses might well be justified if it is the sole treatment for an otherwise fatal disease. The three principal classes of cytotoxic agents used in the treatment of cancer all contain known carcinogens (e.g., melphalen, a nitrogen mustard; adriamycin, an antitumor antibiotic; methotrexate, an antimetabolite). Toxic effects of drugs have been associated with almost every organ system. The stiffness of the joints accompanied by optic nerve damage (SMON, subacute myelooptic neuropathy), common in Japan in the 1960s, was apparently a toxic side effect of chloroquinol, an antidiarrhea drug. Skin effects (dermatitis) are common side effects of drugs, as in the case of topically applied corticosteroids. Toxic effects on the blood have also been documented, including agranulocytosis caused by chlorpromazine, hemolytic anemia caused by methyldopa and megaloblastic anemia caused by methotrexate. *See also* THERAPEUTIC INDEX.

drugs of abuse. Although all drugs are toxic at some dose and may have deleterious effects on humans, drugs of abuse either have no medicinal function or are taken at higher than therapeutic doses. Some drugs of abuse may affect only higher nervous functions (mood, reaction time and coordination), but many produce physical dependence and have serious physical effects, with fatal overdose being a not uncommon occurrence. The drugs of abuse include CNS depressants (e.g., ethanol, methaqualone, secobarbital), CNS stimulants (e.g., cocaine, methamphetamine, caffeine, nicotine), opioids (e.g., heroin, morphine, meperidine), and hallucinogens (e.g., lysergic acid diethylamide, phencyclidine, tetrahydrocannabinol, the most important active principle of marijuana). *See also* HALLUCINOGENS; OPIOIDS; AMPHETAMINES.

dry-cleaning solvents. Compounds such as tetrachloroethylene; 1,1,1-trichloroethane; trichloroethylene are used as solvents for dry cleaning and in other industrial processes. Although less toxic than chloroform, they may produce many of the

same toxic effects, including hepatic tumors and angiosarcomas. *See also* CHLOROFORM; METHYLCHLOROFORM; TETRACHLOROETHYLENE; TRICHLOROETHYLENE.

Duncan's multiple range test. An *a posteriori* test that employs a procedure by which *post hoc* comparisons can be made for all possible pairs of treatment means with the alpha level applied to the collection of tests rather than individual tests. For example, suppose six treatment conditions were being compared within a single experiment. If a significant main effect was found for treatments using ANOVA, the multiple range test allows all possible pairs of means (A vs B, A vs C, B vs C, etc.) to be tested to determine which pairs of means differ significantly one from the other. The computational procedures in the Duncan test are the same as those used to compute Newman-Keuls, with the exception that the critical value is found in special tables. *See also* STATISTICS, FUNCTION IN TOXICOLOGY.

duodenum. *See* INTESTINE.

duplications. *See* CHROMOSOME ABERRATIONS.

dust. The largest particulate matter contributing to air pollution, with particle diameter of about 100 μm. The particles come directly from a substance under use, such as coal, cement, grain, ash or sawdust. *See also* DUST, RESPIRABLE.

dust, non-proliferative. Dusts other than those listed as proliferative (asbestos, coal, cotton and silica) are classified as non-proliferative. They do not induce fibrotic modifications of the lung, and their effects are generally reversible due to phagocytic action. *Compare* DUST, PROLIFERATIVE. *See also* DUST.

dust, proliferative. Dusts that are not readily removed by phagocytosis or other pulmonary defense mechanisms. They accumulate in the lung and cause lung involvement in the form of fibrotic hardening. The general term for this type of irreversible lung damage is pneumoconiosis. Free silica gives rise to a proliferative condition know as silicosis, asbestos to one called asbestosis. Asbestosis is not to be confused with the lung cancer that is also associated with inhalation of asbestos. Similar conditions are caused by inhalation of cotton dust (byssinosis) and coal dust, which gives rise to a diffuse fibrosis and accompanying bronchitis and emphysema. *Compare* DUST, NON-PROLIFERATIVE. *See also* ASBESTOSIS; DUST; PNEUMOCONIOSIS.

dust, respirable. Particulate matter which is of small enough size to be taken into the respiratory tract by inhalation.

Dyfonate. *See* FONOFOS.

dynamic chambers. *See* DYNAMIC EXPOSURE.

dynamic exposure. In inhalation toxicity testing, exposure to the toxicant in chambers through which the toxicant, in a stream of air, flows continuously. The air stream consists of clean air at constant temperature and humidity to which the toxicant is added by a metering device. Dynamic chambers are the most common type used.

dysosmia. An abnormal sense of smell, usually manifested as a reduced ability to detect odorants, and caused by some olfactory toxicants.

dysplasia. A disordered growth or development. The term is used most commonly with reference to the growth patterns of cells. It does not necessarily imply precancerous changes (e.g., some forms of dwarfism are due to bone dysplasias). Dysplasia is often used interchangeably with atypia when referring to cells with morphological characteristics that fall short of outright anaplasia.

dyspnea. Labored breathing, shortness of breath, respiratory distress. Although dyspnea is frequently due to cardiac insufficiency or other pathological conditions, it may also be due to the toxic effects of chemicals such as those inducing acidosis, irritant aerosols or histamine.

E

E102. *See* TARTRAZINE.

E123. *See* AMARANTH.

E127. *See* ERYTHROSINE.

E132. *See* INDIGO CARMINE.

Eadie–Hofstee plot. One of several ways to linearize enzyme- or receptor-binding data based on derivations of the law of mass action (with appropriate assumptions). Based on rearrangement of the Michaelis–Menten equation, the equation for the Eadie–Hofstee plot is:

$$\frac{1}{v} = K_{m} * \left(\frac{v}{[S]} \right) + V_{max}$$

Experimentally, if $\frac{1}{v}$ is plotted versus $\left(\frac{v}{[S]} \right)$ (where v is the initial velocity of the enzyme reaction in the presence of a given concentration of substrate [S]), the intercept on the ordinate is V_{max} and the slope of the line is K_{m}. This permits one to estimate experimentally the apparent K_{m} and the apparent maximum velocity (V_{max}). The equation is essentially identical for radioreceptor assays, except that B (amount bound) is equivalent to v (the initial velocity), [F] (concentration of free ligand) to [S] (concentration of substrate); K_{D} (dissociation constant) to K_{m} (Michaelis constant) and B_{max} (theoretical number of sites) to V_{max} (maximal theoretical velocity). *See also* ENZYME KINETICS; K_{D}; K_{m}; LINEWEAVER–BURK PLOT; METABOLITE INHIBITORY COMPLEXES; MICHAELIS–MENTEN EQUATION; RADIORECEPTOR ASSAYS; WOOLF PLOT; XENOBIOTIC METABOLISM, INHIBITION.

ears. The organs of hearing and balance. Both hearing and balance depend upon minute hairs, the movement of which stimulates sensory cells that communicate with the CNS via the auditory nerve. In mammals, the ear consists of an outer ear, a tympanic membrane, a middle ear through which sound is conducted by three very small bones (malleus, incus and stipes) to the inner ear. The inner ear contains the semicircular canals and the cochlea, the latter containing the sensory receptors. The ears are important in toxicology primarily as an aid in diagnosis, since acute toxicants may affect equilibrium and/or hearing. *See also* DIAGNOSTIC FEATURES, EARS.

EC. *See* EFFECTIVE CONCENTRATION.

ECETOX. *See* EUROPEAN CHEMICAL INDUSTRY ECOLOGY TESTING CENTER.

E. coli. *See* ESCHERICHIA COLI.

ecological effects. Environmental pollutants can affect ecosystems by reduction of the productivity of producers, creation of eutrophication or reduction in certain species through toxicity or effects on reproductive success. The last effect causes changes in the species composition of an ecosystem, with frequently a shift toward more opportunistic species. The communities affected can be plant, animal or microbial. *See also* ECOLOGICAL EFFECTS, FIELD TESTS; ECOLOGICAL EFFECTS, LABORATORY TESTS; ECOLOGICAL EFFECTS, MODEL ECOSYSTEMS; ECOLOGICAL EFFECTS, SIMULATED ECOSYSTEM; ECOLOGICAL EFFECTS, SIMULATED FIELD TESTS; POLLUTION.

ecological effects, field tests. Ecological tests in which test chemicals are applied to a section of unaltered environment for determination primarily of effects on natural populations and, secondarily, the fate of the toxicant. Although a similar untreated section of environment or the test environment prior to treatment can serve as controls, there is no assurance that either of these controls is comparable to a laboratory control. Long-term ecological effects can be characterized, although bias can result from emigration or immigration. *Compare* ECOLOGICAL EFFECTS, LABORATORY TESTS; ECOLOGICAL EFFECTS, MODEL ECOSYSTEMS; ECOLOGICAL EFFECTS, SIMULATED ECOSYSTEM; ECOLOGICAL EFFECTS, SIMULATED FIELD TESTS.

ecological effects, laboratory tests. Laboratory tests can be used to estimate potential ecological effects, such as toxicity at various life stages, physiological and reproductive effects, and bioaccumulation. A closer approximation of the environmental situation can be made using model ecosystems. Laboratory tests control extraneous factors to the greatest extent and typically can allow replication, but are the farthest removed from real environmental conditions. *Compare* ECOLOGICAL EFFECTS, FIELD TESTS; ECOLOGICAL EFFECTS, SIMULATED ECOSYSTEM; ECOLOGICAL EFFECTS, SIMULATED FIELD TESTS.

ecological effects, model ecosystems. Artificial test systems set up in the laboratory for monitoring the environmental fate and effects of toxicants in a controlled situation that has many of the constituents of the environment. The most widely used system has an aquatic phase with vertebrates, invertebrates and plankton, and a terrestrial phase with substrate, plants and herbivores. The bioconcentration and degradation of a radiolabeled test compound can be determined. More elaborate models involving such aspects as drainage, rainfall or tides, as well as strictly terrestrial model ecosystems have also been devised. *See also* AQUATIC ECOSYSTEM; ECOLOGICAL EFFECTS; SIMULATED ECOSYSTEM; TERRESTRIAL–AQUATIC ECOSYSTEMS.

ecological effects, simulated ecosystem. An artificial ecosystem set up in the environment, such as a small test pond, that is stocked with appropriate plant and animal species, but is open to migration, weather effects and other natural conditions. Such systems can be used to study the fate (e.g., bioaccumulation, metabolism, microbial degradation, deposition in sediments) or

effects (acute or chronic toxicity, including mortality, reproductive, physiological or pathological effects, shifts in population density) of a test material. This is a more natural setting than isolated laboratory tests or model ecosystems, but is still limited in scope and more closely controlled than a field test. *See also* ECOLOGICAL EFFECTS, SIMULATED FIELD TESTS.

ecological effects, simulated field tests. Ecological tests that expose the test chemical to both biological and environmental influences. The test chemical is applied in a greenhouse, test plot, small natural section of environment or simulated ecosystem for monitoring primarily the fate of the chemical and secondarily for effects on populations that cannot migrate into or out of the test area. *See also* ECOLOGICAL EFFECTS, SIMULATED ECOSYSTEM.

ecological risk assessment. *See* RISK ASSESSMENT, ENVIRONMENTAL.

ecology. The study of the relationship of populations and communities of living organisms with their physical and biological environments.

ecorisk. A term formed by contraction of the term ecological risk, it refers to the issues involved in ecosystems risk assessment.

ecosystems. Ecological units consisting of a specified environment with interactive communities of producers, consumers and saprophytes. *See also* AGROECOSYSTEM; AQUATIC ECOSYSTEM; ESTUARINE ECOSYSTEM; TERRESTRIAL–AQUATIC ECOSYSTEM; TERRESTRIAL ECOSYSTEM.

ecotoxicology. The study of the effects of environmental toxicants on populations and communities of living organisms. *See also* ENVIRONMENTAL TOXICOLOGY.

ecstasy. *See* MDMA.

ECVT. *See* EUROPEAN COLLEGE OF VETERINARY TOXICOLOGY.

ED. *See* EFFECTIVE DOSE.

edema. The accumulation of an excessive amount of interstitial fluid in subcutaneous or other body tissue. The extracellular fluid volume may increase depending on a variety of factors, including increased venous pressure, decreased osmotic pressure gradient across the capillary (e.g., due to increases in osmotically active substances), increased capillary permeability, inadequate lymphatic drainage, or decreased plasma protein concentration. Capillary damage due to toxicants may cause an increase in interstitial fluid.

EDTA (ethylenediaminetetraacetic acid). CAS number 60-00-4. A widely used chelating agent. Experimentally, it is used in *in vitro* experiments for regulation of metal ion concentrations and availability. Clinically it is used in the treatment of heavy metal poisoning, principally lead. It is usually administered as the calcium disodium form ($CaNa_2EDTA$), since the exchange of lead for calcium minimizes physiological calcium depletion. *See also* CHELATING AGENTS; HEAVY METAL POISONING, THERAPY.

$$HOOCCH_2 \diagdown \qquad \diagup CH_2COOH$$
$$\qquad\quad N-CH_2-CH_2-N$$
$$HOOCCH_2 \diagup \qquad \diagdown CH_2COOH$$

EDTA (ethylenediaminetetraacetic acid)

EDTA, Ca. *See* EDTA.

EEC. *See* EUROPEAN ECONOMIC COMMUNITY.

effective concentration (EC). The concentration of a compound that causes a specific magnitude of response in an *in vitro* system. It almost always is used with a numerical modifer relating to the percentage of response (e.g., EC50 is the concentration that causes 50% of maximal response). EC provides a way for comparing the potencies of various toxicants in eliciting a specific effect. *See also* ENZYME KINETICS; RADIORECEPTOR ASSAYS.

effective dose (ED). The amount of a toxicant (or drug) required to cause a given functional change in the intact organism, in isolated tissue or at a biochemical site. It almost always is used with a numerical modifer relating to the percentage of response (e.g., ED50 is the dose that causes 50% of maximal response). The relationship between the effective dose and the administered dose is affected by toxicokinetic phenomena, such as metabolism (both activation and inactivation), distribution and elimination, and by toxicodynamic events (e.g., tolerance).

effector cells. The muscle cells (skeletal, cardiac or smooth) or glandular cells that function to bring about actions resulting from nervous activity, such as from a reflex.

eggshell thinning. A controversial potential effect of organochlorine pollutants on avian physiology, resulting in reduced avian reproduction. DDT is the compound primarily implicated, although other organochlorine compounds have also been suggested. Absolute correlations between residues and degree of thinning, however, cannot be made, nor can the implicated compounds consistently produce this effect in the laboratory. Although the significance of organochlorine residues in the reproduction of natural bird populations has not been accurately assessed, eggshell thinning was one of the important factors leading to the banning of DDT in the USA. *See also* DDT.

EHCs. *See* ENVIRONMENTAL HEALTH CRITERIA DOCUMENTS (113).

EIA. *See* ENVIRONMENTAL IMPACT ASSESSMENT.

EIS. *See* ENVIRONMENTAL IMPACT STATEMENT.

Ekofisk Bravo 14. *See* ENVIRONMENTAL DISASTERS.

Elapidae. A family of venomous snakes containing such snakes as coral snakes (*Micrurus*), cobras (*Naja*), kraits (*Bungarus*) and mambas, whose venoms are primarily neurotoxic. *See also* α-BUNGAROTOXIN; β-BUNGAROTOXIN.

electromagnetic spectrum. Range of energies of electromagnetic radiation. All of the spectroscopic methods listed are of use in analytical toxicology, particularly for the quantitation and identification of toxicants, their metabolites and their environmental degradation products.

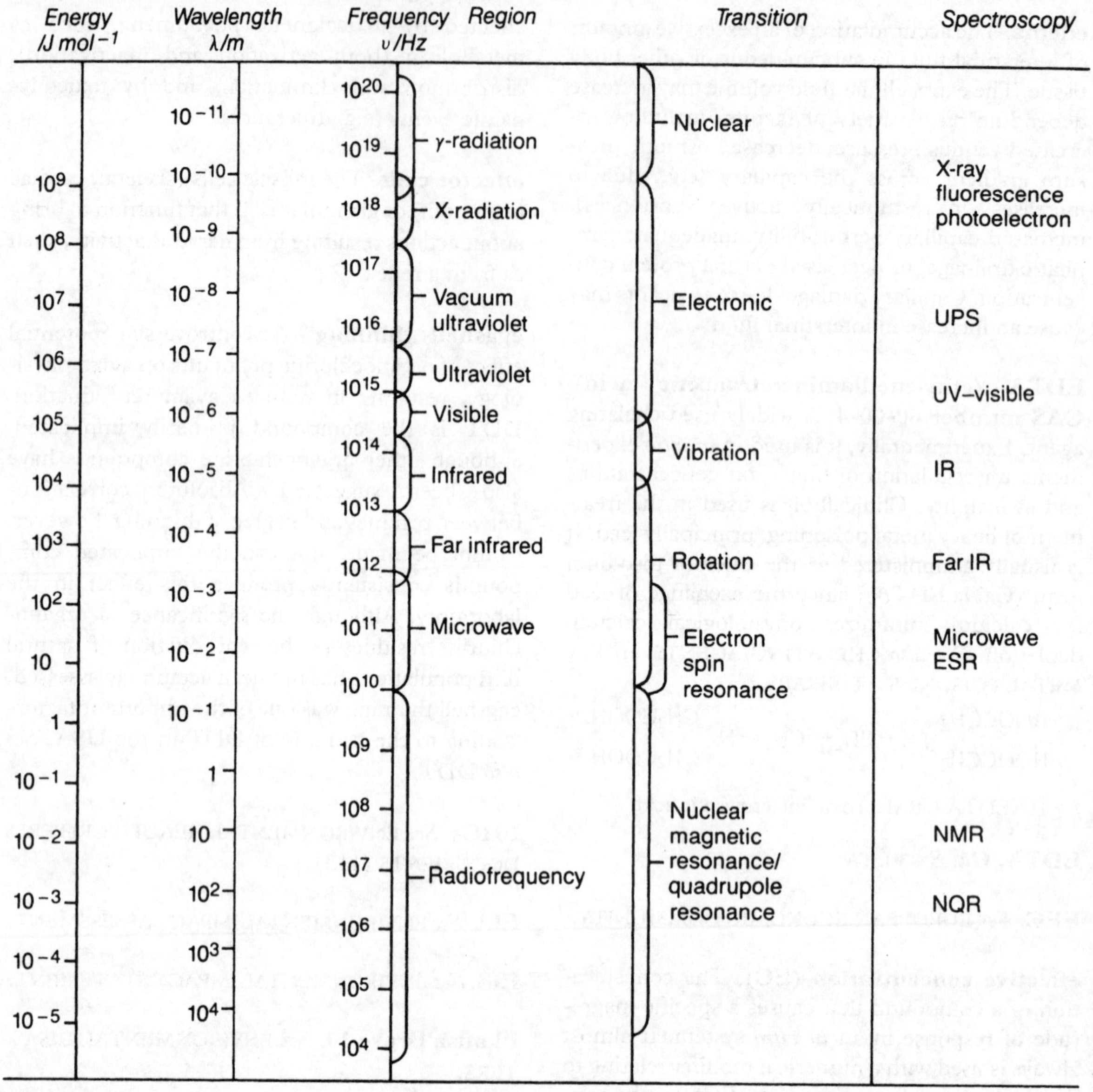

Energy $/J\ mol^{-1}$	Wavelength λ/m	Frequency υ/Hz	Region	Transition	Spectroscopy
	10^{-11}	10^{20}		Nuclear	
10^9	10^{-10}	10^{19}	γ-radiation		X-ray fluorescence photoelectron
10^8	10^{-9}	10^{18}	X-radiation		
10^7	10^{-8}	10^{17}	Vacuum ultraviolet	Electronic	UPS
10^6	10^{-7}	10^{16}	Ultraviolet		UV–visible
10^5	10^{-6}	10^{15}	Visible		
10^4	10^{-5}	10^{14}	Infrared	Vibration	IR
10^3	10^{-4}	10^{13}	Far infrared		Far IR
10^2	10^{-3}	10^{12}		Rotation	
10	10^{-2}	10^{11}	Microwave	Electron spin resonance	Microwave ESR
1	10^{-1}	10^{10}			
10^{-1}	1	10^9			
10^{-2}	10	10^8		Nuclear magnetic resonance/ quadrupole resonance	NMR
10^{-3}	10^2	10^7	Radiofrequency		NQR
10^{-4}	10^3	10^6			
10^{-5}	10^4	10^5			
		10^4			

Electromagnetic spectrum

electron spin resonance spectrometry. *See* SPECTROMETRY, ELECTRON SPIN RESONANCE.

electron transport. In biology, the enzymatic transfer of electrons from electron donors, such as NADPH, via one or an integrated series of reactions, to the final electron acceptor of the series, usually resulting in the reduction of oxygen to water. The energy lost during such oxidation/reduction sequences may be conserved in the form of high-energy intermediates, such as ATP, to be utilized for other metabolic functions. The electron transport systems of importance include the mitochondrial electron transport system, the cytochrome P450-dependent monooxygenase system and photosynthesis. Inhibition of mitochondrial electron transport or photosynthesis is an important mechanism of toxicity in animals and plants. The cytochrome P450-dependent monooxygenase system catalyzes many of the most important phase I reactions in xenobiotic metabolism. *See also* CYTOCHROME P450; CYTOCHROME P450-DEPENDENT MONOOXYGENASE SYSTEM; ELECTRON TRANSPORT SYSTEM, MITOCHONDRIAL.

electron transport system, mitochondrial (ETS; respiratory chain; cytochrome chain). A series of cytochromes and other electron carriers arranged in the inner mitochondrial membrane. These components transfer the electrons obtained from the NADH or $FADH_2$, generated in fuel oxidations, to oxygen, the final electron acceptor, through a series of alternate oxidations and reductions. The energy that these electrons lose during these transfers is used to pump H^+ from the matrix into the intermembrane space, creating an electrochemical proton gradient that drives oxidative phosphorylation. The electron carriers in the ETS include ubiquinone (coenzyme Q), five different cytochromes and proteins bound to copper, flavin or iron-sulfur complexes. The carriers are organized into three major respiratory enzyme complexes: (1) the NADH dehydrogenase complex which transfers electrons from NADH to ubiquinone; (2) the b-c complex which transfers electrons from ubiquinone to cytochrome c; (3) the cytochrome oxidase complex (cytochrome a-a₃) which transfers electrons from cytochrome c to oxygen. A relatively large drop in free energy occurs as the electrons pass through each of these complexes and is responsible for the pumping of protons across the membrane. *See also* ELECTRON TRANSPORT SYSTEM INHIBITORS; OXIDATIVE PHOSPHORYLATION; OXIDATIVE PHOSPHORYLATION INHIBITORS.

electron transport system inhibitors. Each of the three major respiratory enzyme complexes of the mitochondrial electron transport system can be blocked by specific inhibitors. For example, rotenone inhibits the NADH dehydrogenase complex, antimycin A inhibits the b-c complex, and cyanide and carbon monoxide inhibit the cytochrome oxidase complex. In contrast to the oxidative phosphorylation inhibitors, which prevent phosphorylation while allowing electron transfers to proceed, the electron transport system inhibitors prevent both electron transport and ATP production. *See also* ELECTRON TRANSPORT SYSTEM, MITOCHONDRIAL; OXIDATIVE PHOSPHORYLATION; OXIDATIVE PHOSPHORYLATION INHIBITORS.

electrophilic. Describing chemicals that are attracted to, and react with, electron-rich centers in other molecules. Many activation reactions produce electrophilic intermediates such as epoxides, that exert their toxic action by forming covalent bonds with nucleophilic substituents in cellular macromolecules such as DNA or proteins.

electrophoresis. Separation of macromolecules or cells according to their overall charge by placing them in an electric field. For macromolecules, the separation is performed in a supporting gel, usually polyacrylamide gel and thus the technique is known as polyacrylamide gel electrophoresis (PAGE). In some cases gradient gels may be used in which the concentration of the gel increases and the pore size decreases along the length of the gel. This allows the separation of substances according to molecular size. The detergent sodium laurel (dodecyl) sulfate (SDS) may be incorporated into the gel. Electrophoresis is used for the separation of molecules from mixtures (preparative electrophoresis) or for the identification of molecules. The latter makes use of the fact that molecules migrate at constant rates in defined conditions and so can be ascribed R_f values (i.e., the ratio of the distance migrated compared with that of a dye) to enable their identification. Proteins or other substances of known molecular weights may be added to the sample before separation to act as reference markers. Electrophoresis can be combined with other techniques. In immunoelectrophoresis, molecules are first separated by electrophoresis and are then identified by precipitation with antisera. Electrophoresis can also be combined with radiolabeling methods. Following separation the gel may be sliced, and the radioactivity in each slice determined by scintillation counting. Alternatively, the gel slab may be exposed to a photographic emulsion and the position of radiolabeled substances visualized by autoradiography.

elimination. *See* KINETIC EQUATIONS.

elimination of toxicants. Simple forms of life eliminate toxicants into the surrounding medium, which is usually water. As organisms evolved, elimination became a complex regulatory function, and elimination of toxicants became a part of a specialized system of elimination functioning also in the maintenance of salt and water balance. Xenobiotics are not readily eliminated until they are in a form similar to that utilized for the elimination of endogenous substances. Thus, they are first metabolized by one or more reactions to progressively more polar forms, a process that permits their eventual excretion, primarily by renal and hepatic routes. Other minor routes of excretion may also serve to eliminate the parent compounds without metabolism. *See also* EXCRETION; XENOBIOTIC METABOLISM.

ELISA (enzyme-linked assay; enzyme-linked immunosorbent assay; adsorption assay; enzyme-linked immunoassay). A binding assay, usually performed in the solid phase, making use of a ligand and a binding protein that can be an antibody (most commonly), lectin, receptor, etc. Either the ligand or the binding protein is conjugated to an enzyme. Following separation of the antibody ligand complex from free ligand and free binding protein, a substrate of the enzyme is added. These substrates may generate colored, insoluble or fluorogenic products, the presence of which is proportional to the amount of bound ligand. Three common types of ELISA exist. (1) Simple competitive, where the antibody is adsorbed to a surface, and the test ligand competes with a known quantity of labeled ligand. (2) Sandwich, where cold antibody is adsorbed to a surface and then test ligand and cold ligand are added, followed by labeled antibody to form a "sandwich." The enzyme product is proportional to ligand concentration. (3) Immunoenzymometric, where unlabeled ligand is adsorbed to a surface, labeled antibody and test ligand are free in solution, and the labeled antibody bound to the surface is inversely proportional to the amount of free test ligand. *See also* IMMUNOASSAY.

embryo. The young of any species in an early stage of development. In mammals it is the stage between formation of the embryonic disc and the beginning of the fetal stage during which the principal organ systems are differentiated. In humans it lasts from the second to the eighth week of pregnancy. The embryo is particularly sensitive to the effects of teratogenic chemicals. *See also* DEVELOPMENTAL AGE.

embryo–fetal toxicity. In teratology testing, it is important to measure embryo–fetal toxicity as a separate parameter. Embryo–fetal toxicity is determined from the number of dead fetuses and resorption sites relative to the number of implantation sites. In addition to the possibility of lethal malformations, such toxicity may be due to maternal toxicity, stress or direct toxicity to the embryo or fetus that is not related to developmental malformations. A high level of embryo–fetal toxicity may also obscure teratological effects that might have occurred at a lower dose. Thus, in tests that result in a high level of embryo–fetal toxicity at a particular dose, the next lower dose level should be evaluated with care and, if necessary, the study repeated with additional dose levels. Fetal weight and fetal size may also be a measure of toxicity, but should not be confused with the variations seen as a result of differences in the number of pups per litter. *See also* MATERNAL TOXICITY; REPRODUCTIVE TOXICITY TESTING; TERATOLOGY TESTING.

embryogenesis. The phase of development that results in the formation of the fully formed embryo. In humans, embryogenesis lasts from the end of the second week of gestation to the end of the eighth week, after which the fully formed embryo becomes a fetus. *See also* DEVELOPMENT AGE; EMBRYO.

embryotoxicity. The deleterious effects exhibited by an embryo (i.e., an animal from the blastula through the completion of organogenesis; the time equivalent to the first trimester in human development) as a result of exposure to a toxic agent. In the broadest sense embryotoxic manifestations include: (1) lethality; (2) growth impairment; (3) structural anomalies; (4) metabolic or physiological dysfunctions. In a more restrictive sense, it refers to growth retardation (sublethal effect) or death of an embryo (embryo lethality), thereby segregating embryotoxicity from teratogenicity and/or neural toxicity.

EMEA. *See* EUROPEAN MEDICINES EVALUATION AGENCY.

Emergency Planning and Community Right-to-Know Act (EPCRA). Title III of the US Superfund Amendments and Reauthorization Act of 1986 requires state and local governments to develop appropriate mechanisms to handle information on hazardous chemicals and to prepare for emergencies involving such chemicals. Facilities that manufacture, process or use designated chemicals must provide chemical information to state and local government agencies and make this information available to the general public.

emesis. The act of vomiting. The induction of emesis is a frequently used treatment following toxicant ingestion. The drugs of choice for inducing emesis (i.e., emetics) are syrup of ipecac (30 ml for adults, 10–15 ml for children) or the direct-acting dopamine agonist apomorphine. Although apomorphine has a more rapid onset of action, toxicant recovery is approximately the same with each method. Apomorphine produces CNS depression in children at doses that induce emesis; this effect is presumably mediated by dopamine autoreceptors. Apomorphine may also result in protracted vomiting. It is estimated that 30% of the toxicant can be recovered 60 minutes after ingestion of the emetic. Emesis is contraindicated if toxicant ingestion has resulted in coma or seizures, or if the victim has lost the gag reflex. If the toxicant ingested is a strong acid or base, emesis is also contraindicated to prevent further damage to esophageal tissue. Generally, ingestion of petroleum distillate hydrocarbons would also be a contraindication to emesis. Emesis can also occur following stimulation of the chemoreceptor trigger zone in the area postrema of the medulla by such drugs as morphine or its derivatives. *See also* ANTIEMETICS; AREA POSTREMA; IPECAC, SYRUP OF.

emetics. Agents that cause emesis. *See also* EMESIS.

EMIT. *See* ELISA.

emphysema. Chronic respiratory disease involving distended or ruptured alveoli in the lung, along with a loss of lung elasticity and of surface area and a diminution of lung function. Total surface area for gas exchange is reduced. It is one of the adverse effects associated with tobacco smoking and with air pollution.

EMTD. *See* ESTIMATED MAXIMUM TOLERATED DOSE.

endangerment assessment. A site-specific risk assessment of the actual or potential danger to human health and the environment caused by the release of hazardous chemicals. Such assessments are required for enforcement actions under CERCLA or RCRA. *See also* CERCLA; RCRA.

end-labeling. Attachment of a radiolabel, usually ^{32}P, to either the 5′- or the 3′-end of a DNA molecule.

endocrine. Any aspect of physiology or toxicology related to hormones, their function or the glands that produce them.

endocrine disruptors. Chemicals which have the potential to cause effects within the endocrine system and thereby alter physiology, including development and reproduction. Such compounds as xenoestrogens, anti-androgens and thyroid hormone mimics have been identified, and include some insecticides, fungal and plant chemicals, and some industrial chemicals, among others. *See also* ESTROGENS, ENVIRONMENTAL.

endocrine system. The anatomical/physiological system consisting of the endocrine glands, secretory organs which release their secretions into the blood stream. These secretions (hormones) then exert their effects in distant tissues. Important endocrine glands include the pituitary (hypophysis), thyroid, parathyroid, pancreas and sex organs.

endocrine toxicity. *See* ADRENAL GLAND TOXICITY; PANCREATIC TOXICITY; PITUITARY GLAND TOXICITY; REPRODUCTIVE TOXICITY; THYROID GLAND TOXICITY.

endocytosis. *See* ENTRY MECHANISMS, ENDO-CYTOSIS.

endogenous. Produced or arising from within a cell or organism. *Compare* EXOGENOUS.

endometrium. The inner glandular layer of the uterus that responds to the ovarian hormones, estrogen and progesterone, to become a vascular, secretory tissue suitable for implantation of the embryo. The endometrium undergoes cyclic changes of proliferation and secretory activity with the cycle of the ovarian hormones. If there is no fertilization or implantation, the developed endometrium is shed (menstruation) or resorbed (estrus cycle) with the decline of the hormones of the regressing corpus luteum. If there is implantation, the endometrium fuses with the embryonic chorion to form the placenta.

endoplasmic reticulum (ER). An extensive branching and anastomosing double membrane distributed in the cytoplasm of eukaryotic cells. The ER is of two types: (1) rough ER (RER) which contains attached ribosomes on the cytosolic surface; and (2) smooth ER (SER) which is devoid of ribosomes. The ribosomes of the RER are involved in protein biosynthesis, and the RER is especially abundant in cells specialized for protein synthesis. Membrane-bound enzymes that metabolize hormones, drugs and many lipophilic xenobiotics are integral components of both SER and RER, such as the cytochrome P450-dependent monooxygenase system and the FAD-containing monooxygenase, although the specific content is usually higher in SER. The SER and associated enzymes of the cytochrome P450 monooxygenase system can be induced by a number of foreign compounds, such as phenobarbital, 3-methylcholanthrene and TCDD. After removal of the inducing agent, the SER returns to normal, usually within five days. When tissue or cells are disrupted by homogenization, the ER is fragmented into many smaller (100 nm diameter) closed vesicles called microsomes, which can be isolated by differential centrifugation.

endorphins. Derived from "endogenous morphines" α, β and γ-endorphin are some of the endogenous opioid peptides that function as neuromodulators in the nervous system. It is the receptors for these peptides on which narcotic drugs, in part, act. *See also* NARCOTIC ANTAGONISTS; NARCOTICS; OPIOIDS.

endosulfan   (6,7,8,9,10,10-hexachloro-1,5,5a,6,9,9a-hexahydro-6,9-methano-2,4,3-benzodioxathiepin-3 oxide). **CAS number 115-29-7**. A cyclodiene insecticide, not persistent in humans or the environment. No significant evidence of human or other carcinogenicity. *See also* CYCLODIENE INSECTICIDE; DATABASES, TOXICOLOGY; LEWIS, HCDR, NUMBER EAQ750.

endothelium. An epithelium lining an organ or vessel. Important examples include the epithelium lining the heart and blood vessels.

endotoxins. *See* MICROBIAL TOXINS.

Endoxan. *See* CYCLOPHOSPHAMIDE.

endpoints. *See* TOXIC ENDPOINTS.

endrin. *See* CYCLODIENE INSECTICIDES.

energy sources. *See* POLLUTION, ENERGY SOURCES.

energy supply. In biological systems, energy is usually supplied via the high-energy phosphate bonds of adenosine triphosphate (ATP), although for some reactions other nucleotides may be important (e.g., guanosine triphosphate, GTP) or energy may be stored in other high-energy phosphate compounds (e.g., creatine phosphate). ATP for muscle contraction, chemical synthesis and other energy-requiring processes is produced primarily from oxidative phosphorylation in the mitochondria from intermediates generated during glycolysis, the pentose cycle and the tricarboxylic acid cycle. Any toxicant that inhibits any of these processes is, potentially, a potent acute toxicant or in lower doses may have chronic or subacute effects. Examples include cyanide which inhibits cytochrome oxidase, fluoroacetate which blocks the tricarboxylic cycle and dinitrophenol which uncouples oxidation and phosphorylation. Effects on energy supply have been postulated as causes of teratogenic defects. *See also* ATP; OXIDATIVE PHOSPHORYLATION; TERATOGENIC MECHANISMS, ENERGY SUPPLY.

enflurane (2-chloro-1-(difluoromethoxy)-1, 1,2-trifluoromethane; Ethrane). CAS number 13838-16-9. A gaseous anesthetic introduced in 1973 that has been widely used because of lower toxicity than agents such as halothane. Because less of an administered dose of enflurane is metabolized (about 3%) than with halothane, hepatitis is less of a risk. The resulting fluoride produced from enflurane may be of concern, however, when it is used with patients having compromised renal status, although fluoride concentrations will usually be less than half the threshold for renal toxicity. Because enflurane may cause increased seizure activity, especially when there is hypocarbia, its use should be avoided in patients having epilepsy or pre-existing EEG abnormalities. *Compare* HALOTHANE. *See also* ANESTHETICS.

$$ \begin{array}{ccccc} & F & & F & Cl \\ & | & & | & | \\ H-&C&-O-&C&-C-H \\ & | & & | & | \\ & F & & F & F \end{array} $$

Enflurane

enkephalins. Peptides occurring naturally in the brain that have similar properties to opiates such as morphine and codeine. Met-enkephalin is the pentapeptide H-Tyr-Gly-Gly-Phe-Met-OH while Leu-enkephalin is H-Tyr-Gly-Gly-Phe-Leu-OH. *See also* OPIOIDS.

enterohepatic circulation. The excretion of a compound into the bile and its subsequent reabsorption from the small intestine and transport back to the liver, where it is available again for biliary excretion. The most important mechanism is conjugation in the liver, followed by excretion into the bile. In the small intestine, the conjugation product is hydrolyzed, either non-enzymatically or by the microflora, and the compound is reabsorbed to become a substrate for conjugation and re-excretion into the bile.

enterotoxin. *See* MICROBIAL TOXINS.

Enterovioform. *See* CHLOROQUINOL.

entry mechanisms, endocytosis. The general process by which a cell membrane invaginates or flows around a toxicant, thereby internalizing a vacuole into the interior of the cell. This permits more ready transfer across membranes for both liquids (pinocytosis) and solids (phagocytosis). Only in such isolated instances as absorption of carrageenens ($Mr = 40,000$) in the gut have these mechanisms been found to be important in initial entry. However, once inside the body, endocytosis is a rather common mechanism, and engulfment of compounds in the lung is common (lung phagocytosis).

entry mechanisms, filtration. There are often pores in membranes that permit compounds with molecular weights of 100 daltons, or less, to traverse more quickly. Larger molecules are excluded except in more highly porous tissues, such as kidney and liver. As many toxicants are relatively large molecules, this pathway is of limited importance.

entry mechanisms, passive transport. A mechanism of entry into the body that predominates for most toxicants. With compounds of appropriate water:lipid partition coefficients, simple diffusion largely determines the rate of movement. The rate may vary considerably among compounds and is not always predictable. Compounds in the ionized form do not move readily by passive diffusion due to ionic interactions among xenobiotics, lipids and proteins. In addition, the ionized form tends to have reduced lipid solubility; high lipid solubility is a necessary attribute for efficient membrane diffusion.

entry mechanisms, special transport. Special transport systems, particularly in the gastrointestinal tract, aid in the transport of endogenous compounds or nutrients across membranes. Such processes may require energy and permit passage against a concentration gradient (i.e., active transport) or may not require energy and be unable to move compounds against a gradient (i.e., facilitated transport). In both cases, a carrier protein is postulated that associates with the toxicant, moves from one side of the membrane to the other and, on the other side, dissociates from the toxicant. Such penetration is more rapid than simple diffusion and, in the case of active transport, may proceed beyond the point where concentrations are equal on either side of the membrane. The special transport of toxicants is not common, but is most likely to occur in the gastrointestinal tract. These mechanisms become of much greater importance in the elimination of toxicants, in which special transport is important in the removal of xenobiotics and their metabolites. Special transport systems, when operative, often permit movement of compounds with lesser lipid solubility that would ordinarily be expected to move slowly through lipid membranes.

ENU. *See N-ETHYL-N-NITROSOUREA*.

E numbers. A number prefixed by the letter E is assigned to any food additive assessed as safe for use in the EC. This assessment is made by the scientific committee for food, under five EC Directives covering antioxidants, colors, emulsifiers and stabilizers, extraction solvents, and preservatives. *See also* COLORING MATTER IN FOOD REGULATIONS.

environment, for chronic toxicity tests. *See* CHRONIC TOXICITY TESTING; TESTING VARIABLES, NON-BIOLOGICAL.

Environmental Defense Fund. A US non-governmental organization, formed primarily by environmentalists and lawyers. It monitors environmental issues and initiates legal action for environmental protection.

environmental disasters. The most common environmental disasters of toxicological concern are oil spills. According to the Oil Spill Intelligence Report (http://www.cutter.com/osir/biglist.htm) there were more than 60 oil spills involving 10 million or more gallons between 1960 and 1996. Table 3 lists the major pollution and other environmental incidents that have occurred in recent years. They are arranged alphabetically with dates and brief details.

environmental drift. *See* DRIFT, ENVIRONMENTAL.

environmental effects on xenobiotic metabolism, altitude. Altitude can increase or decrease toxicity. For example, at altitudes of 5000 feet or higher the lethality of digitalis or strychnine to mice is decreased, whereas that of *d*-amphetamine is increased. It has been suggested that these effects are related to the metabolism of the toxicant, but this has not been established.

environmental effects on xenobiotic metabolism, ionizing radiation. Ionizing radiation causes a reduction in the rate of metabolism of xenobiotics as measured *in vivo* or in enzyme preparations isolated from animals that have been irradiated. This has been seen in the hydroxylation of steroids, in the development of oxidative desulfuration activity in young rats and in glucuronide formation in mice.

environmental effects on xenobiotic metabolism, light. Many enzymes, including some of those involved in xenobiotic metabolism, show a diurnal pattern that can be keyed to the light cycle. There is a diurnal rhythm in the activity of hydroxyindole *O*-methyltransferase in the pineal gland, which is the highest at night. Cytochrome P450 and monooxygenase activity show a diurnal rhythm in both rat and mouse, with the greatest activity occurring at the beginning of the dark phase.

environmental effects on xenobiotic metabolism, moisture. Although such effects are unknown in vertebrates, they have been seen in invertebrates such as insects. Housefly larvae maintained on diets containing reduced moisture levels have up to four times more heptachlor epoxidase activity than larvae reared in saturated media.

environmental effects on xenobiotic metabolism, noise. A stress factor that has been shown to affect the rate of metabolism of a xenobiotic, 2-naphthylamine, causing a slight increase in the rat.

environmental effects on xenobiotic metabolism, temperature. Temperature variations in homeothermic animals are a form of stress and as a result can produce changes mediated by hormonal interactions, such effects being mediated through

Table 3. Some examples of extensive environmental disasters. Adapted from the Directory of the Environment. M.A. Allaby

Incident	Year	Place	Details
Amoco Cadiz	1978	French coast	Oil spill, severe pollution
Bhopal	1984	Bhopal, India	Industrial accident, 2500 people killed, 200,000 injured
Castillo de Bellver	1983	Cape of Good Hope, South Africa	Oil tanker fire, soot contamination on-shore
Cavtat	1974–78	Adriatic Sea	Ship sank with a cargo of tetraethyllead that later leaked
Chernobyl	1986	Ukraine	Explosion at a nuclear reactor, 31 people killed, widespread contamination
Donora	1948	Pennsylvania, USA	Air pollution, 18 deaths, 5900 people ill
Ekofisk Bravo 14	1977	North Sea	Blow-out on an oil platform releasing oil, little coastal pollution
Esso Bernicia	1979	Shetland	Tanker collided with jetty, severe contamination, bird deaths and harm to sheep
Exxon Valdez	1989	Alaska, USA	Oil tanker ran aground, severe coastal pollution
Iraq Mercury	1971–72	Iraq	Consumption of alkylmercury-treated seed grain. c. 6500 victims and 450 deaths
Irene Serenade	1980	Greece	Oil tanker sank, severe coastal pollution
Ixtoc 1	1979	Mexico	Oil well blew out, released 3 million barrels of oil
James River	1975	Virginia, USA	Chlordecone contamination of soil and river estuary – 76 cases diagnosed, 0 deaths
London	1952, 1962	London	Smog lasting 4 days in 1952, 5 days in 1962, 4000 people died in 1952, 700 in 1962
Love Canal	1978	Niagara, New York, USA	Leak from industrial waste dump, more than 200 familes evacuated
Meuse Valley	1930	France	Air pollution, 60 people died, hundreds ill, many cattle slaughtered
Minamata	1953–60	Japan	Mercury poisoning due to industrial pollution, 43 deaths, many injuries, teratogenic consequences
Poza Rica	1950	Mexico	Air pollution by hydrogen sulfide, 22 deaths, 320 people made ill
Sangara	1980	Nigeria	Oil well blew out into Niger River, contaminating water supplies and fish
Seveso	1976	Italy	Factory explosion releasing dioxin, 700 people evacuated, livestock destroyed, crops burnt
Tanio	1980	English Channel	Oil tanker sank, broke in half and leaked a large amount of oil, causing severe pollution to beaches in Britanny
Three Mile Island	1979	Pennsylvania, USA	Nuclear reactor failed, small radioactive release, no injuries to the public
Times Beach	1982	Missouri, USA	Dioxin contamination from wastes, town evacuated and declared unfit for human habitation
Torrey Canyon	1967	Scillies, UK	Oil tanker sank, world's first major oil spill, contaminated beaches

the pituitary–adrenal axis. There are two types of temperature effect on toxicity: (1) an increase in toxicity at both high and low temperatures; (2) an increase in toxicity with increasing temperature. For example, both high and low temperatures increase the toxicity of caffeine to mice, but *d*-amphetamine toxicity is low at reduced temperatures and increases as the temperature increases.

environmental estrogens. *See* ESTROGENS, ENVIRONMENTAL.

environmental factors, in toxicity testing. *See* TESTING VARIABLES, NON-BIOLOGICAL.

environmental fate. The final disposition of a pollutant after release into the environment. Usually used in such a way as to include all of the physical, chemical and biological processes leading to the final disposition.

environmental health criteria documents (EHCs). A series of documents published under the sponsorship of the UN Environment Programme and the World Health Organization. Each is concerned with a chemical or group of chemicals that adversely affects human health. The series includes mycotoxins, metals, agricultural chemicals, radiation, etc.

environmental impact assessment (EIA). The identification and evaluation of the environmental consequences of a proposed development and of the measures intended to minimize adverse effects. The EIA was introduced first in the USA, where it is a legal requirement of development. Impacts are identified and listed according to their significance. The technique is largely subjective, since not all impacts can be predicted, not all cause-and-effect relationships are understood, and decisions on the relative importance of each impact are a matter of opinion. Thus the system invites manipulation, and claims for its scientific objectivity are dubious. *See also* ENVIRONMENTAL IMPACT STATEMENT.

environmental impact statement (EIS). A detailed study of the adverse and beneficial effects that construction, maintenance and operation of a proposed development or land use change will have on the environment, including people. It must include all probable and beneficial impacts, considerations of alternative or mitigating courses of action, and comparisons of the long- and short-term impacts. An EIS is a requirement imposed by the US National Environmental Policy Act since 1970 for all projects receiving federal funding, as well as by some states for private projects. In many other countries organizations planning new projects are also required by law to conduct such studies and produce an EIS, which can then be examined critically, sometimes in public.

Environmental Mutagen Society. *See* UNITED KINGDOM ENVIRONMENTAL MUTAGEN SOCIETY.

environmental pollution. The contamination of the environment (air, water or soil) by pollutants, resulting primarily from industrial, agricultural or energy-generating processes. These pollutants can affect organisms directly and also can become incorporated into the food chain and, therefore, can affect a variety of higher trophic levels following bioaccumulation. *See also* AIR POLLUTION; BIOACCUMULATION; ECOLOGICAL EFFECTS; POLLUTION; WATER POLLUTION.

Environmental Protection Agency (EPA). The most important US federal agency for the regulation of toxic chemicals. Formed in 1970, it is involved in both research and regulation, as well as being responsible for the formulation of regulations authorized by several major legislative acts and the enforcement of those acts. These include the Federal Insecticide, Fungicide and Rodenticide Act (FIFRA), the Toxic Substances Control Act (TSCA), the Resource Conservation and Recovery Act (RCRA), the Clean Air Act and the Clean Water Act.

environmental risk. *See* RISK, ENVIRONMENTAL.

environmental risk assessment. *See* RISK ASSESSMENT, ENVIRONMENTAL.

environmental run-off. *See* RUN-OFF, ENVIRONMENTAL.

environmental toxicology. A branch of toxicology that is concerned with the source of toxicants or potential toxicants in the environment, their transformations under environmental conditions, their movement within the environment and through food chains, and their effect on population dynamics of affected species. *See also* BIOACCUMULATION; ECOLOGICAL EFFECTS; ECOSYSTEMS; ENVIRONMENTAL IMPACT STATEMENT.

environmental xenobiotic cycles. The recycling of xenobiotics in the environment, or biosphere, as a result of atmospheric, geochemical and biological processes. The constant movement of water above (precipitation), on (overland flow) and below (infiltration) the Earth's surface maintains a cycling of xenobiotics in the environment.

enzyme inhibition. Inhibition of enzyme activity by specific small molecules is important in cell function because it can serve as a control mechanism for the system that includes the enzyme in question. In toxicology, enzyme inhibition can be important in mode of toxic action or in metabolism of xenobiotics. As a consequence of the lack of specificity of xenobiotic-metabolizing enzymes, it can be critical in interactions between toxicants. *See also* ENZYMES; INHIBITION; XENOBIOTIC METABOLISM, IRREVERSIBLE INHIBITION; XENOBIOTIC METABOLISM, REVERSIBLE INHIBITION.

enzyme kinetics. A branch of biochemistry that deals with all of the factors that affect the rate of enzymatic reactions. This includes the formation and breakdown of enzyme–substrate or inhibitory complexes, characteristics of the active site and the effect of pH, ionic strength, temperature, activators, etc. The study of enzyme kinetics is concerned with both qualitative evaluation of biological mechanisms and quantitative description and derivation of constants that describe these reactions. Enzyme kinetics can be a powerful tool for elucidation of mechanisms and sequelae of toxicity. *See also* EADIE–HOFSTEE PLOT; K_D; K_M; LINEWEAVER–BURK PLOT; METABOLITE INHIBITORY COMPLEXES; MICHAELIS–MENTEN EQUATION; RADIORECEPTOR ASSAYS; WOOLF PLOT; XENOBIOTIC METABOLISM, INHIBITION.

enzyme-linked immunosorbent assay. *See* ELISA; ENZYME KINETICS; IMMUNOASSAY.

enzymes. Proteins, present in all living organisms, responsible for catalyzing most cellular reactions with extraordinary specificity and power. The presence of a non-protein component is often required for enzymic activity; if combined with the protein it is known as a prosthetic group (e.g., the heme group of catalase) and if loosely attached it is a coenzyme (e.g., NAD+). Certain metals may also be required as activators (cofactors) in a combined form (e.g., copper, magnesium).

Enzymes are susceptible to a wide variety of inhibitors. (1) Noncompetitive inhibitors react with functional groups on the enzyme causing chemical transformation of the enzyme (e.g., heavy metal ions, alkylating agents). (2) Competitive inhibitors, molecules similar in shape and size to the substrate, block the active site and prevent access by the substrate (e.g., sulfonamides block *p*-aminobenzoic acid sites in the synthesis of folic acid). This type of inhibition is reversible on the addition of more substrate. (3) Uncompetitive inhibitors bind reversibly to the enzyme–substrate complex to yield an inactive enzyme–substrate-inhibitor complex. This type of inhibition is uncommon with one-substrate systems.

Classification of enzymes is according to the reactions which they catalyze; they were formerly named by the addition of the suffix "-ase" to the substrate or process of the reaction. The confusing nomenclature has been clarified in a recommendation of IUB and IUPAC in which each enzyme has a specific code number. The old nomenclature is still retained, however, and trivial names are usually given in discussion of a particular enzyme. Six main types of enzyme are recognized.

1. Oxidoreductases. Enzymes catalyzing redox reactions in which the reduced form of the substrate (MH_2) is oxidized by an electronic transfer process, often involving the presence of a coenzyme (e.g., NAD^+)

$$MH_2 + NAD^+ \rightarrow M^+ + NADH_2$$

(e.g., dehydrogenases, oxidases, peroxidases, hydrogenases, and hydrolyases).

2. Transferases. Enzymes catalyzing the transfer of a group from one compound to another (e.g., transaminases, transpeptidases, kinases).

3. Hydrolases. Enzymes catalyzing the hydrolytic cleavage of C-O, C-N and C-C bonds, (e.g., esterases, glucosidases, proteinases, lipases) and also some other bonds (e.g., sulfatases, phosphatases).

4. Lyases. Enzymes that cleave C-C, C-O, C-N and some other bonds by elimination leaving double bonds or conversely which add groups across a double bond (e.g., decarboxylases, lyases, anhydrases, synthases).

5. Isomerases. Enzymes catalyzing structural or geometrical changes within a molecule (e.g., epimerases, rotases, isomerases, mutases, racemases).

6. Ligases. Enzymes catalyzing the reaction of two molecules with the elimination of a pyrophosphate bond (e.g., synthetases).

EPA. *See* ENVIRONMENTAL PROTECTION AGENCY.

EPCRA. *See* EMERGENCY PLANNING AND COMMUNITY RIGHT TO KNOW ACT.

ephedrine (α-[1-(methylamino)ethyl]-benzene-methanol; 2-methylamino-1-phenyl-1-propanol). CAS number 299-42-3. An indirect-acting sympathomimetic that is used as a bronchodilator and vasoconstrictor, CNS stimulant and mydriatic agent. A host of similar compounds have either been isolated from plant sources or synthesized, including *d*- and *l*-ephedrine and *d*- and *l*-pseudoephedrine. The i.p. LD50 in mice is about 150 mg/kg. Therapy for overdoses includes the administration of β-adrenergic antagonists. The parent alkaloid (now made synthetically) first came from *Ephedra vulgaris*, a tall shrub-type plant whose branches and stems first were used by ancient Chinese "doctors" to make "ma huang" tea for use as a decongestant. The Utah Mormons were introduced to a related American plant by native Americans in the nineteenth century, leading to a drink called "Mormon Tea." *See also* AMPHETAMINES.

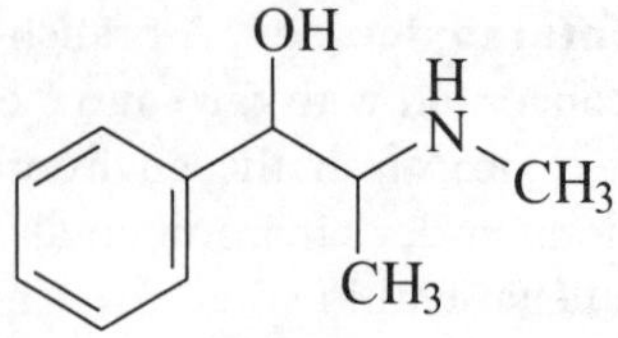

Ephedrine

epichlorohydrin (1-chloro-2,3-epoxypropane). CAS number 106-89-8. A designated animal carcinogen (IARC), hazardous substance (EPA) and hazardous waste (EPA). It is used in the manufacture of epoxy resins, as well as cellulose esters and ethers, paints, varnishes and lacquers. Entry into the body may be via ingestion, inhalation or through the skin. It is acutely irritating to skin and eyes, causing blistering and sometimes dermatitis. Systemic poisoning symptoms are initially gastrointestinal, with subsequent cyanosis and pneumonitis. In animals, lung, kidney and liver damage have all occurred on chronic exposure.

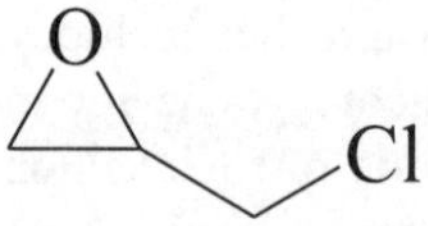

Epichlorohydrin

epidemiological studies, case control. In case control studies subjects are selected on the basis of disease status and compared with matched disease-free control subjects. Case control studies are all retrospective. Controls are matched for as many variables as possible: age, gender, occupation, etc. However, given the large number of possible variables, the selection of study populations of large enough size to permit meaningful interpretation of the results is a significant problem in all case control studies.

epidemiological studies, cohort. Studies of a group or groups of people who have had a common insult (e.g., exposure to an agent suspected of causing disease such as viral hepatitis or a chemical or a common disease such as diabetes). If groups of people are compared where one group serves as a control, the groups may be matched for a number of variables such as sex, age and socioeconomic status or the group may be compared with the general population.

epidemiological studies, cross-sectional. Studies of a group or groups with a particular characteristic, such as exposure to a chemical or to chemicals at one point in time. An example might be the study of a population that had ingested fish highly contaminated with chlorinated compounds.

epidemiological studies, prospective. Cohort studies in which the pertinent observations are made on events occurring after the start of the study. A group is followed over time. An example is the Framingham study, in which a random sample of persons was identified and followed to determine the frequency of coronary heart disease and factors related to it.

epidemiological studies, retrospective. Cohort studies are based on a group of persons known to have been exposed at some time in the past. Data are collected from routinely recorded events, up to the time the study is undertaken. For instance, a cohort of patients given X-ray therapy for ankylosing spondylitis between 1934 and 1954 was assembled. Death from leukemia or aplastic anemia between 1935 and 1954 was determined. Retrospective cohort studies are generally more economical and produce results more quickly than prospective studies, but they are limited to causal factors that can be ascertained from existing records and/or examining survivors of the cohort.

epidemiology. (1) The determination of the relationships of various factors modifying the frequency and distribution of diseases in a human community. (2) The field of medicine concerned with the determination of the etiology of localized outbreaks of infection, such as viral hepatitis, of toxic disorders, such as lead poisoning, or any other disease of recognized etiology.

epidermis. *See* PENETRATION ROUTES, DERMAL.

epigenetic carcinogen. *See* CARCINOGEN, EPIGENETIC.

epilepsy. *See* SEIZURES.

epinephrine (4-[1-hydroxy-2-(methylamino)-ethyl]-1,2-benzenediol; 1-(3,4-dihydroxy-phenyl)-2-(methylamino)ethanol; adrenaline). CAS number 51-43-4. A catecholamine formed by the action of the enzyme phenethylamine *N*-methyltransferase on its immediate precursor norepinephrine. It has a predominantly hormonal function, like the other catecholamines norepinephrine and dopamine, although it does have a role as a minor neurotransmitter. It is released from chromaffin granules in the adrenal medulla in response to splanchic stimulation and may be released from chromaffin in response to hypoglycemia. Its secretion is stimulated by the nervous system under conditions of stress, pain, fear and a fall in blood sugar. Although it is a minor neurotransmitter of the CNS, it plays an important role in peripheral events. The most important effects are on dilation and constriction of blood vessels and carbohydrate metabolism, resulting in stimulated blood flow and high glucose levels. Epinephrine is synthesized from catechol, m.p. 212 °C. It is included in local anesthetics to constrict blood flow locally. It is also a powerful brochodilator used in treatment of bronchial asthma. The naturally occurring (–)-form is about 20 times more active than the (+)-form. The oral LD50 in mice is 50 mg/kg. *See also* CATECHOLAMINES; RECEPTOR.

Epinephrine

epithelial cell, ciliated. A cell with contractile cilia, the beating of which serves to move fluids across the surface of the cell. Those in the tracheobronchial region of the lung, for example, are important in lung clearance since they move mucus, containing trapped particles and dissolved toxicants upwards and out of the lung. *See also* EPITHELIUM.

epithelium. The layer of cells forming the surface membranes of the skin. The cells rest on a basement membrane and may form a simple, single layer or a stratified layer several cells thick. The cells may be flat (squamous), cuboidal or columnar in form and may be ciliated or glandular, depending upon the function of the membrane and the cell. Epithelia in general are important in toxicology as they occur in all portals of entry and must be crossed by toxicants entering the body. They may also be targets for toxic action. *See also* PENETRATION ROUTES, DERMAL.

EPN (phenylphosphonothioic acid *O*-ethyl *O*-*p*-nitrophenyl ester; Santox). **CAS number 2104-64-5**. An insecticide and acaricide, sometimes used in combination with methyl parathion. It has oral LD50s in male and female rats of 36 and 7.7 mg/kg, respectively. It is a neurotoxicant by virtue of its ability to inhibit acetylcholinesterase. *See also* INSECTICIDES; ORGANOPHOSPHATE POISONING, SYMPTOMS AND THERAPY; ORGANOPHOSPHORUS INSECTICIDES.

EPN

epoxidation and aromatic hydroxylation. Epoxidation is an important reaction in toxicology and is catalyzed by cytochrome P450 isozymes. Stable and environmentally persistent epoxides can be formed, as well as arene oxides, the highly reactive intermediates of aromatic hydroxylations. Many of these highly reactive intermediates are involved in chemical carcinogenesis. Naphthalene oxidation was one of the earlist examples known of an epoxide intermediate in aromatic hydroxylations. The ultimate carcinogens produced by the metabolic activation of benzo[*a*]pyrene are stereoisomers of benzo[*a*]pyrene-7,8-diol-9,10-epoxide. In addition to reactions with cellular macromolecules that may result in toxicity such epoxides can rearrange non-enzymatically, can interact with epoxide hydrolase to yield the corresponding dihydrodiol or can interact with glutathione *S*-transferase to yield the glutathione conjugate that is ultimately metabolized to a mercapturic acid. *See also* ALIPHATIC EPOXIDATION; BENZO[*A*]PYRENE-7,8-DIOL-9,10-EPOXIDES; CYTOCHROME P450-DEPENDENT MONOOXYGENASE SYSTEM.

epoxide hydratase. *See* EPOXIDE HYDRATION.

epoxide hydration. Epoxides are frequently unstable and are hydrated by water to form dihydrodiols. Metabolically, epoxide derivatives of alkene and arene compounds are hydrated by enzymes known as epoxide hydrolases, the enzyme from animals forming the corresponding *trans*-diols, although microbial hydrolases may form *cis*-diols. In some cases, such as benzo[*a*]pyrene, the hydration of an epoxide is a step in an activation sequence which ultimately yields highly toxic *trans*-dihydrodiol epoxides. Reactive epoxides may also be detoxified by either glutathione *S*-transferase or epoxide hydrolase. The reaction probably involves a nucleophilic attack by -OH on the oxirane carbon. The most studied epoxide hydrolase is microsomal, and this enzyme has been purified from hepatic microsomes of several species. Soluble epoxide hydrolases with different substrate specificities have also been described. Well-known examples of epoxide hydrolase reactions are the formation of styrene 7,8-glycol from styrene oxide and the above-mentioned activation sequence for benzo[*a*]pyrene. *See also* EPOXIDATION AND AROMATIC HYDROXYLATION; EPOXIDES.

epoxide hydrolase. *See* EPOXIDE HYDRATION.

epoxides. Organic compounds in which there is an oxygen bridge between two carbon atoms that are also connected by a carbon–carbon bond, thus forming a C-O-C ring substituent. If the carbon–carbon bond is aromatic, the epoxides are known as arene oxides. Many epoxides, arene oxides in particular, are strong electrophiles and thus reactive metabolites important in toxic action (e.g., epoxides of polycyclic aromatic hydrocarbons). Others, however, such as the epoxides of cyclodiene insecticides such as aldrin (dieldrin) or heptachlor (heptachlor epoxide) are stable, relatively unreactive, metabolic products. *See also* DIHYDRODIOLS; EPOXIDE HYDRATION.

EPP (erythrocyte protoporphyrin). *See* FREE ERYTHROCYTE PROTOPORPHYRIN.

EPS. *See* EXTRAPYRAMIDAL SIDE EFFECTS.

Equanil. *See* MEPROBAMATE.

equilibrium. That condition in which processes operating in opposite directions are exactly balanced. This term is widely used in toxicology to describe many different phenomena. For example, the homeostasis of many body processes is dependent upon equilibrium processes that can be disturbed by toxicants. Similarly, body burden of a toxicant may be in equilibrium when the rate of uptake is equal to the sum of the rates of the processes that lead to elimination.

equilibrium dialysis. The method usually used to measure binding of toxicants to macromolecules, particularly plasma proteins. The unbound ligand equilibrates across the dialysis membrane, whereas the bound ligand does not. Thus the excess ligand on the side of the membrane with the protein in solution represents the bound ligand. Radiolabeled ligands are generally used. The analytical method consists simply of counting radioactivity inside and outside the membrane after equilibrium has been reached. The nature of the binding, affinity constants, etc. can be evaluated by the use of the Scatchard equation. *See also* AFFINITY CONSTANT; BINDING; PROTEIN BINDING; SCATCHARD PLOT.

ergolines. *See* ERGOT ALKALOIDS.

ergosterol (24-methyl-5,7,22-cholestatrien-3β-ol). CAS number 57-87-4. Plant sterol (m.p. 168 °C) isolated from the ergots of rye and many fungi and yeasts. UV radiation yields vitamin D_2.

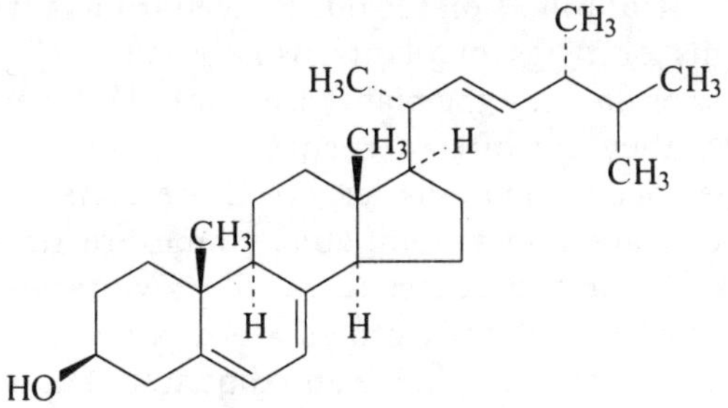

Ergosterol

ergot alkaloids. Compounds derived from the parasitic fungus *Claviceps purpurea*, which grows on rye as well as other grains. Ergot alkaloids are often divided into (1) amine alkaloids (e.g.,

lysergic acid, ergonovine and methylergonovine, methylsergide, lergotrile) and (2) amino acid alkaloids (e.g., ergotamine, bromocriptine) and have a wide range of physiological effects. These effects are largely due to their agonist, partial agonist and/or antagonistic effects at biogenic amine receptor sites. Ergot alkaloids increase uterine motility, have complex effects on cardiovascular function, suppress prolactin secretion and are used in the treatment of migraine, postpartum hemorrhage and Parkinson's disease. The ergot alkaloids are highly toxic and can result in nausea, vomiting, decreased circulation, rapid and weak pulse and coma. Historically, ingestion of contaminated grain, particularly rye, was responsible for epidemic poisoning. *See also* BROMOCRIPTINE; D-LYSERGIC ACID; METHYLERGONOVINE; DOPAMINE RECEPTORS.

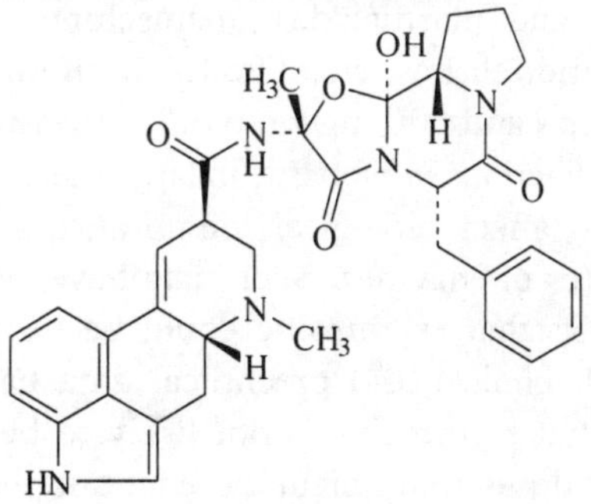

Ergotamine

EROD. *See* ETHOXYRESORUFIN *O*-DEETHYLASE.

erythema. A redness of the skin caused by dilation of superficial capillaries as a result of a nervous mechanism, inflammation or an external mechanism such as sunburn.

erythrocytes (red blood cells). Enucleate, biconcave disc-like cells containing hemoglobin but with no internal membranes. The number of erythrocytes in the average adult is 5,000,000 per mm^3. The primary function of erythrocytes is oxygen transport. They also transport significant amounts of carbon dioxide, and they contribute to acid/base balance through the carbonic anhydrase reaction and the buffering ability of hemoglobin. They are formed by the process of erythropoiesis in the red bone marrow and circulate for an average of 120 days. At this point they become fragile and burst; the membrane fragments are phagocytosed primarily by the spleen. The released hemoglobin is processed by the liver for excretion in the bile. An increase in erythrocyte numbers is called polycythemia and results primarily from hypoxia. A decrease in erythrocyte numbers is called anemia and can result from damage to the red bone marrow, such as by radiation, or from interference with the ability of DNA to replicate itself, such as by alkylating agents or antimetabolites.

erythromycins. *See* ANTIBIOTICS.

erythrosine (FD&C Red No. 3; E127; disodium or dipotassium salt of 2,4,5,7-tetra-iodofluoroscein). A food color formerly approved for use in the USA and Europe. It is used primarily in jams and marmalades, maraschino cherries, pickles and relishes, etc. The LD50 in rats is 150 mg/kg, i.p., and 600 mg/kg, p.o. Erythrosine has a variety of actions *in vitro* due in large measure to its ability to affect biological membranes and lipophilic sites of enzymes. Such data have led to the hypothesis that erythrosine could be neurotoxic, but both clinical and preclinical data have suggested that erythrosine is not likely to be neurotoxic at doses that might be encountered. Two other toxicological issues have been raised with this food color. It has been suggested to be a potential, if weak, carcinogen, and it may also contribute to potential thyroid toxicity resulting from release of iodine. *See also* FOOD COLORS.

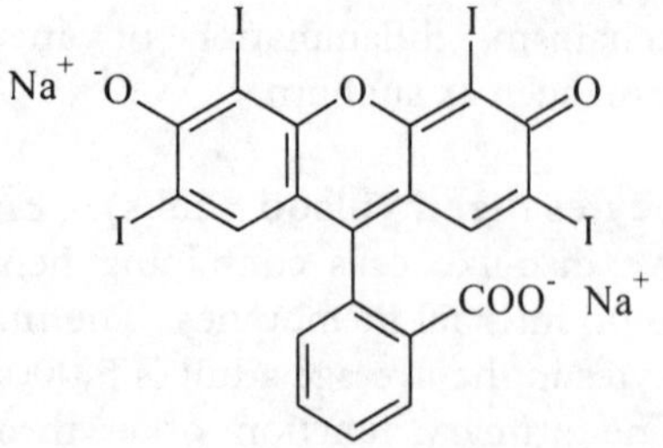

Erythrosine

Escherichia coli. Selected strains of this microorganism with aberrations in tryptophan, nicotinic acid, arginine or galactose metabolism or deficiencies in DNA polymerase are used in prokaryote mutagenicity tests to detect chemicals with the ability to cause forward or reverse mutations. *See*

also BACTERIAL MUTAGENESIS; DNA REPAIR; MUTATION; PROKARYOTE MUTAGENICITY TESTS.

eserine (3a,S-*cis*-1,2,3,3a,8,8a-hexahydro-1, 3a,8-trimethylpyrrolo[2,3-*b*]inol-5-olmethyl-carbamate; physostigmine). CAS number 57-47-6. The toxic principle of Calabar bean (*Physostigma venenosum*); the first known acetylcholinesterase inhibitor. Elucidation of its structure led first to the synthesis of clinically useful carbamates and later to more lipophilic insecticidal carbamates. Its potency as a cholinesterase inhibitor with little or no activity towards other serine esterases makes eserine an invaluable pharmacological tool. It also has limited use in treatment of glaucoma. The oral LD50 in mice is 4.5 mg/kg. *See also* ANTICHOLINESTERASES.

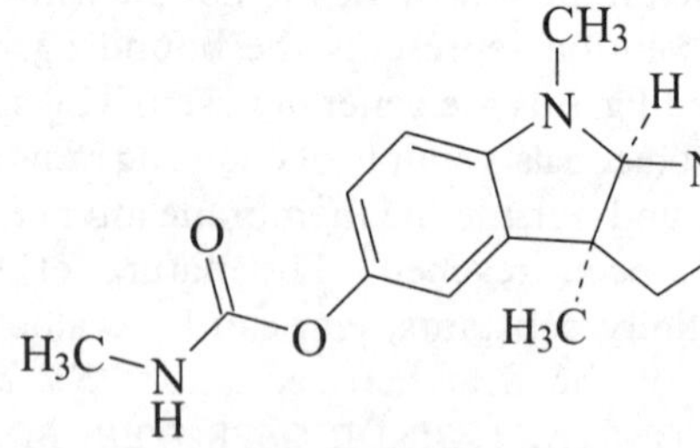

Eserine (physostigmine)

ESR. *See* SPECTROMETRY, ELECTRON SPIN RESONANCE.

ESRA. *See* EUROPEAN SOCIETY OF REGULATORY AFFAIRS.

essential oils. Volatile oils derived from leaves, stems or twigs of plants usually carrying the odor or flavor of the plant (see Table 4). Chemically they are often terpenes, but many other types occur. The oils, except those containing esters, are non-saponifiable. Some are nearly pure single substances (e.g., oil of wintergreen (methyl salicylate)); others are mixtures (e.g., oil of turpentine (pinene and dipentene) and oil of bitter almonds (benzaldehyde and hydrocyanic acid)). They have a pungent taste and odor; are usually colorless when fresh, but become darker and thicker on an exposure to air; are insoluble in water, but are soluble in organic solvents. Typical essential oils are those

Table 4.   Essential oils

Oil of	Natural source	Main compenent(s)	Uses
Anise	*Illicium verum*	Anethole	Carminative, ingredient of cough lozenges, flavoring
Bay	*Laurus nobilis*	Myrcene	Astringent, perfume
Bergamot	*Citrus bergamia*	Linalool, limonene	Perfume flavoring
Camphor	*Carum carvi*	Carvone	Relief of flatulence
Cinnamon	*Cinnamonum zeylanicum*	Cinnamic aldehyde	Carminative, antiseptic, flavoring, perfume
Cloves	*Eugenia caryophillus*	Eugenol	Antiseptic, local anesthetic in dentistry
Coriander	*Coriandrum sativum*	Coriandrol	Stimulative
Dill	*Anethum graveolens*	Carvone	Relief of flatulence in infants
Eucalyptus	*Eucalyptus* sp.	Cineole, α-pinene	Medicinal, perfume
Jasmine	*Jasminum officinale*	Jasmone, benzyl ethanoate	Perfume
Peppermint	*Mentha piperita*	Menthol, menthyl esters	Aromatic carminative, relief of flatulence
Thyme	*Thymus vulgaris*	Thymol	Perfume, antiseptic
Turpentine	Variety of pines	α-Pinene	Paint thinner

obtained from cloves, roses, lavender, citronella, eucalyptus, peppermint, camphor, sandalwood, cedar and turpentine. They are widely used as food flavorings, solvents, and in perfumery and medicines.

Esso Bernicia. *See* ENVIRONMENTAL DISASTERS.

esterases. *See* HYDROLYSIS.

ester cleavage. *See* HYDROLYSIS; DESULFURATION AND OXIDATIVE ESTER CLEAVAGE.

esters. Organic compounds formed by the combination of an acid, usually the carboxyl group of an organic acid (-COOH) and the hydroxyl group of an alcohol or a phenol (-OH) with the elimination of the elements of water.

$$RCOOH + ROH \longleftrightarrow R-\overset{\overset{\displaystyle O}{\|}}{C}-O-R \ + H_2O$$

Ester-type bonds can also be present in such compounds as organophosphorus esters and amides. Many esters are important in toxicology, including phthalic acid esters (plasticizers), phenoxy acid esters (herbicides), pyrethroids (insecticides) and organophosphate ester insecticides. As a consequence esterases have been widely studied and are known to be important in xenobiotic metabolism. *See also* HYDROLYSIS.

estimated maximum tolerated dose (EMTD). The maximum tolerated dose for chronic toxicity studies estimated from the results of shorter-term studies. Frequently a series of such studies (acute, 14–30-day, 90-day) is used for estimating purposes. *See also* MAXIMUM TOLERATED DOSE.

estradiol-17β-(1,3,5(10)-estratriene-3,17β-diol. CAS number 50-28-2. The most potent naturally occurring estrogen in mammals. It is synthesized primarily in the ovary, but also in the testis, adrenal gland and placenta, and to a limited extent by peripheral tissues (e.g., liver, fat, skeletal muscle) from androstenedione and testosterone. It is responsible for the development of secondary sex characteristics in the female at puberty (i.e., growth and development of the vagina, uterus and fallopian tubes, enlargement of the breasts and growth and maturation of long bones). *See also* ESTROGENIC; ESTROGENS.

Estradiol

estrogenic. Describing any compound having an action similar to that of an estrogen. Such compounds may occur naturally in mammals (e.g., estradiol), in plants (e.g., phytoestrogens such as coumestrol and genistein) and as mycotoxins (e.g., zearalinone from *Fusarium graminearum*). Synthetic non-steroidal estrogens include diethylstilbestrol and certain synthetic chlorinated insecticides such as chlordecone and *o,p'*-DDT. *See also* ESTROGENS.

estrogens. Substances, either naturally occurring or synthetic, that exert biological effects characteristic of estradiol-17β, the most potent naturally occurring estrogen in mammals. Estrogens were originally named because of their ability to induce estrus in lower mammals, but they are now recognized to produce a variety of effects involving cellular proliferation and growth in estrogen-sensitive tissues, leading to the stimulation of secondary sex characteristics in the female. Estrogens act by binding to a specific receptor, forming a complex that binds tightly to nuclear chromatin and influencing gene transcription. They can induce tumors of the breast, uterus, testis, kidney, bone and other tissues in various animals, including humans, when administered chronically. Estrogens may also be teratogenic and can induce reproductive disorders resulting in infertility. Estrogen therapy is associated with cholestasis, gallbladder disease, hypertension and cardiovascular and thromboembolic disease. *See also* ESTROGENIC.

estrogens, conjugated. (1) A mixture of conjugated estrogens obtained from urine of pregnant mares and consisting of 50–65% estrone sulfate and 20–35% equilin sulfate. Therapy utilizing conjugated estrogens can increase the incidence of cardiovascular and thromboembolic disorders, as well as toxicities described under estrogens. (2) Any glucuronide or sulfate conjugate of the major estrogens (estrone, estradiol, estriol); D-ring glucuronide conjugates of estradiol and estriol are cholestatic. *See also* ESTROGENIC; ESTROGENS.

estrogens, environmental. A variety of chemicals in several chemical and use classes which exert estrogenic action, either directly or indirectly, and thereby can impact the sexual development and/or function of animals. This is the group most prominent among the endocrine disruptors. Some of these chemicals, or their metabolites, have been shown to interact with the vertebrate estrogen receptor and activate it. They typically have much lower affinities for the estrogen receptor than endogenous estrogen does. Certain organochlorine insecticides (such as chlordecone, *o,p'*-DDT and methoxychlor) and industrial chemicals (such as nonylphenol and PCBs) among numerous others have been characterized or implicated as environmental estrogens. Environmental estrogens have been suggested to be responsible for some human health concerns, such as breast cancer, and reproductive problems noted in wildlife populations. However, phytoestrogens are also implicated in some of these disorders. This topic is a currently controversial one, and is based on relatively sparse data sets. *See also* ENDOCRINE DISRUPTORS.

estrone (3-hydroxyestra-1,3,5(10)-trien-17-one). CAS number 53-16-7. An oxidized metabolite of the most abundant and most potent estrogen, estradiol-17β. It is used in the preparation of 19-norsteroids and as the estrogen in a variety of therapeutic preparations. *See also* ESTROGENS.

Estrone

estrone sulfotransferase. *See* SULFATE CONJUGATION.

estrous cycle. In sub-primate female mammals, the time interval between physiological events that begin at estrus and culminate at the following estrus. The estrous cycle is divided into four phases. (1) Estrus is the period of sexual receptivity, during which ovulation and the beginning of corpus luteum formation occur in most species. (2) Metestrus is the postovulatory phase in which the corpus luteum develops and begins secreting progesterone. (3) Diestrus is the period when the corpus luteum is fully functional. (4) Proestrus encompasses the period when the corpus luteum fails, progesterone decreases and follicular growth and estrogen production increase.

estrus. *See* ESTROUS CYCLE.

estuarine ecosystem. An ecosystem in an estuary containing brackish water and organisms tolerating the wide range of salinities occurring in estuaries. Estuarine ecosystems are subject to pollution from domestic sewage, agriculture and industry.

ethanol (ethyl alcohol). **CAS number 64-17-5**. A liquid used in alcoholic beverages in appropriate dilutions, as a solvent and dehydrating agent in laboratory and industrial applications, in the manufacture of perfumes and pharmaceuticals, and as an antiseptic agent. The TLV has been set at 1000 ppm, and the widely accepted blood level for intoxication is approximately 0.1%. Ethanol is a CNS depressant having anesthetic properties. It causes disinhibition, as well as motor and cognitive impairment at relatively low doses. At increased blood levels, ethanol results in anesthetic effects, loss of sensory acuity, impaired coordination, nausea and vomiting, hypothermia and loss of consciousness. Chronic use results in pharmacokinetic and pharmacodynamic tolerance, and dependence. Ethanol can also have teratogenic effects causing a fetal alcohol syndrome, that includes mental retardation, craniofacial anomalies, irritability and microcephaly. The mechanism of action of ethanol in the CNS is not clear, although alterations in membrane fluidity appear to be of importance. In addition to its CNS effects, ethanol affects most other systems of the body, including the liver. Although toxic effects on liver may be secondary to nutritional deficiencies, ethanol also appears to have direct toxic effects on liver. Ethanol–drug interactions also occur with ethanol potentiating many centrally acting agents (sedative–hypnotics, anticonvulsants, antidepressants, anxiolytics, etc.).

Ethanol

ethchlorvynol (1-chloro-3-ethyl-1-penten-4-yl-3-ol; Placidyl). **CAS number 113-18-8**. A tertiary alcohol that has been used as a sedative–hypnotic. Ethchlorvynol has a rapid onset and short duration of action and, like other sedative–hypnotics, may cause respiratory depression. Long-term use or abuse of ethchlorvynol may cause the expected tolerance and dependence, and abrupt withdrawal may lead to symptoms similar to those seen with ethanol or the barbiturates, and may include convulsions. Withdrawal can be treated by substituting decreasing doses of a barbiturate such as phenobarbital, and psychotic symptoms can be treated with a phenothiazine. The oral and s.c. LD50 in rats are 290 and 240 mg/kg, respectively. *See also* SEDATIVE–HYPNOTICS.

Ethchlorvynol

ethene. *See* ETHYLENE.

ethenylbenzene. *See* STYRENE.

ether (1,1'-oxybisethane; ethyl ether). *See* ETHYL ETHER.

ethers. Compounds in which an oxygen atom forms a stable covalent bridge between carbon atoms in two other functional groups. *See also* ETHYL ETHER.

ethidium bromide (3,8-diamino-5-ethyl-6-phenylphenanthridinium bromide; homidium bromide). CAS number 1239-45-8. Intercalating dye widely used to stain DNA in gels and gradients. The DNA can be visualized readily by irradiation with ultraviolet light, as little as 0.5 µg of DNA being detectable by such methods. Ethidium bromide is also added to cesium chloride density gradients, since as an intercalating molecule it binds more readily to linear DNA than to closed colinear circles of DNA (such as plasmids). Binding of ethidium bromide reduces the density of DNA, thus covalent circles of DNA have higher densities at saturating concentrations of ethidium bromide, permitting the separation of plasmid DNA. Ethidium bromide is a putative carcinogen.

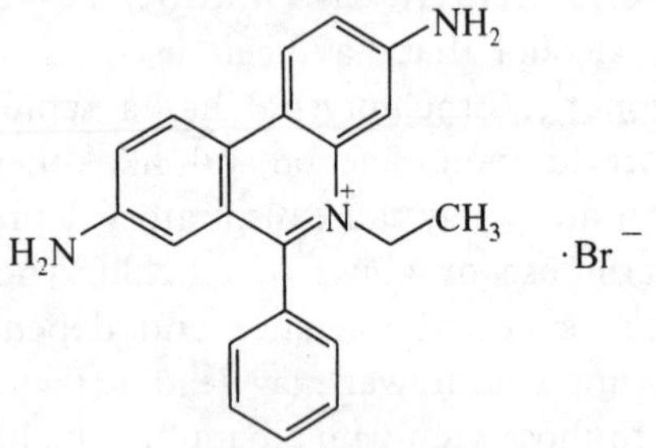

Ethidium bromide

ethionine (2-amino-4-(ethylthio)butyric acid). CAS number 13073-35-3. The *S*-ethyl analog of methionine. It is a carcinogen and hepatotoxic agent once proposed as an antineoplastic agent. It inhibits the incorporation of methionine and glycine into proteins and substitutes for methionine in transmethylation reactions, the ethyl group appearing in the products in place of the methyl groups of methionine (e.g., ethylcholine is formed instead of choline). Ethionine is currently used only as an experimental compound in studies of hepatotoxicity and methionine metabolism and nutrition.

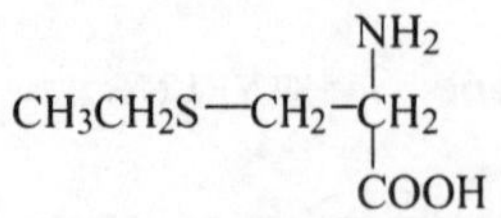

$$CH_3CH_2S-CH_2-\underset{\underset{COOH}{|}}{\overset{\overset{NH_2}{|}}{CH_2}}$$

Ethionine

ethoxyresorufin. Various alkyl resorufins are used as model substrates for cytochrome P450 and in some cases they show specificity for particular CYP isoforms. Of these ethoxyresorufin is probably the most significant.

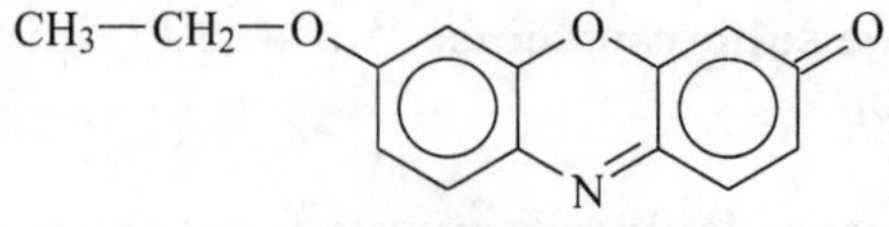

Ethoxyresorufin

ethoxyresorufin *O*-deethylase (EROD). A cytochrome P450-mediated activity associated primarily with CYP1A, which is highly inducible by polycyclic aromatic hydrocarbons, such as 3-methylcholanthrene, and by TCDD. The induction of this enzyme activity results from xenobiotic interaction with the Ah receptor. This is used as a marker of CYP1A activity and induction and has been used as a biomarker of environmental pollution in a number of species.

Ethrane. *See* ENFLURANE.

ethyl alcohol. *See* ETHANOL.

ethyl chloride (chloroethane). CAS number 75-00-3. A gas with anesthetic and narcotic properties; it was once used as an anesthetic. It is no longer used because it is flammable. In addition it causes some non-specific sympathoadrenal release. *See also* ANESTHETICS.

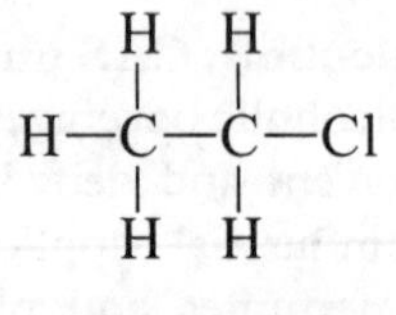

Ethyl chloride

ethylene (ethene). CAS number 74-85-1. The monomer used in the synthesis of polyethylene. It is a gas with low blood solubility that is rapidly excreted and does not seem to be significantly metabolized. Potential toxicity is from its asphyxiant properties, rather than local toxicity.

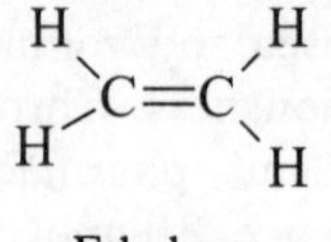

Ethylene

ethylene dibromide (EDB; 1,2-dibromoethane). CAS number 106-93-4. A compound used principally as a soil fumigant, as a fumigant for milling machinery and grain storage facilities, and as a gasoline additive. The fumigant uses, however, have been discontinued in the USA. It has been designated an animal carcinogen (IARC), a hazardous substance (EPA), and a hazardous waste (EPA). It is positive in essentially all *in vitro* mutagenicity tests and animal carcinogenicity tests, although human epidemiological studies have not been conclusive. Uptake into the body is primarily by inhalation, but dermal absorption also occurs. Although prolonged skin contact with the liquid may produce blistering, ulcers and skin sensitization and inhalation of the vapor may cause respiratory injury and CNS depression, it is the potential carcinogenesis that has lead to increasing regulation of this chemical.

$$Br-\overset{\overset{\displaystyle H}{|}}{\underset{\underset{\displaystyle H}{|}}{C}}-\overset{\overset{\displaystyle H}{|}}{\underset{\underset{\displaystyle H}{|}}{C}}-Br$$

Ethylene dibromide

1,2-ethylene dichloride. *See* 1,2-DICHLORO-ETHANE.

ethylene glycol (HOCH₂CH₂OH). CAS number 107-21-1. An antifreeze; also used in hydraulic fluids, condensers and heat exchangers, as well as a solvent and chemical intermediate. The principal route of entry into the body is by inhalation of aerosols or vapor or by accidental ingestion. Since the boiling point is high and the vapor pressure at room temperature is low, the accidental ingestion is the more likely route in poisoning. Inhalation causes CNS depression, whereas ingestion causes depression followed by respiratory, cardiac and renal failure. Ethylene glycol is a substrate for alcohol dehydrogenase, and its toxicity may be due to the aldehyde produced by this reaction. *See also* ALCOHOL DEHYDROGENASE; ATSDR DOCUMENT, MAY 1993; LEWIS, HCDR, NUMBER EJC500; DATABASES, TOXICOLOGY.

$$HO-\overset{\overset{\displaystyle H}{|}}{\underset{\underset{\displaystyle H}{|}}{C}}-\overset{\overset{\displaystyle H}{|}}{\underset{\underset{\displaystyle H}{|}}{C}}-OH$$

Ethylene glycol

ethylene oxide. CAS number 75-21-8. A designated hazardous waste (EPA). It exists as a flammable liquid or a colorless gas and is used as an intermediate in the synthesis of such compounds as ethylene glycol, glycol ethers, acrylonitrile, plastics, drugs and pesticides. It is also used as a sterilant, a fungicide and a fumigant. Uptake is primarily by inhalation, although aqueous solutions are irritating to the skin, producing blisters and, occasionally, dermatitis. Inhalation of ethylene oxide can cause nausea and irritation of the mucous membranes of the nose, throat and lungs, leading to pulmonary edema. Ethylene oxide is an experimental mutagen and has been shown to cause cancer in female mice.

Ethylene oxide

ethylene-2-thiourea (ETU; 2-imidazoline-thione). CAS number 96-45-7. A breakdown product of ethylene bis-dithiocarbamate fungicides such as Zineb and Maneb. It has also been used as an organic rodenticide. The oral LD50 in rats is 545 mg/kg and in mice is 3000 mg/kg. Ethylene-2-thiourea is a carcinogen in both rats and mice and a possible teratogen in rats.

Ethylene thiourea

ethyl ether (diethyl ether; 1,1-oxybisethane; ether). CAS number 60-29-7. A highly volatile liquid that is the prototype of the modern anesthetic agents, although it is no longer used because it presents an explosion hazard in the operating room. Its use was characterized by prolonged induction and emergence, and by a high incidence of postoperative vomiting and nausea. Other agents in this group include the chemically related

Ethyl ether

compound vinyl ether and several structurally dissimilar ones including ethyl chloride, fluroxene and cyclopropane. *See also* ANESTHETICS.

ethylenimine (aziridine). CAS number 151-56-4. A monomer for the polymerization of polyethylenimine, used as a flocculant in wastewater treatment and as a wet strength additive in the textile and paper industries. It has an oral LD50 in rats of 15 mg/kg and a dermal LD50 in guinea pigs of 14 mg/kg. It is a carcinogen and potent cytotoxin that alkylates DNA. In humans, it is cytotoxic to liver, kidney and myocardium, respiratory tract and skin irritation.

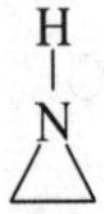

Ethylenimine

ethyl isocyanide (ethyl isonitrile). Principal use in toxicology is in the characterization of cytochrome P450 isozymes. Ethyl isocyanide and the reduced cytochrome form a characteristic optical difference spectrum with two peaks in the Soret Region (type III). The pH equilibrium point (the pH at which the two peaks are of equal height) varies between different isozymes. *See also* CYTOCHROME P450, OPTICAL DIFFERENCE SPECTRA.

$$CH_3CH_2NC$$

Ethyl isocyanide

ethyl isonitrile. *See* ETHYL ISOCYANIDE.

***N*-ethyl-*N*-nitrosourea (ENU).** A carcinogen that is effective in producing brain tumors, a rare type of chemically induced cancer, as well as other types of tumors. Like other nitrosoureas, it does not have to be metabolically activated to be an alkylating agent, so it is a transplacental carcinogen (although it is less potent transplacentally than *N*-methyl-*N*-nitrosourea). *See also* NITROSOUREAS.

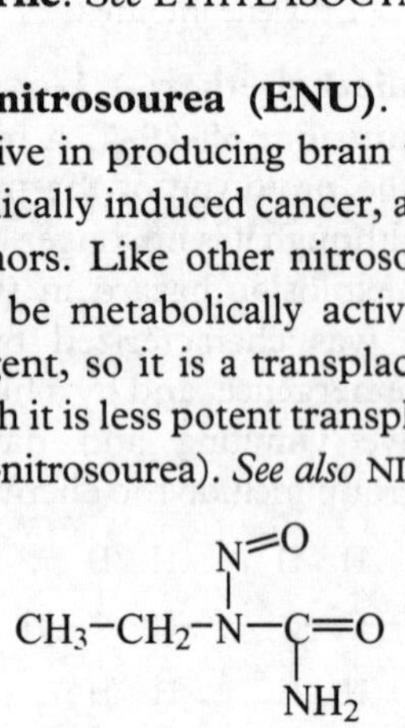

N-ethyl-*N*-nitrosourea (ENU)

ethynylestradiol (19-nor-17α-pregra-1,3,5(10)-trien-20-yne-3,17-diol). CAS number 57-63-6. Synthetic estrogen with potent activity (inhibition of ovulation), widely used in oral contraceptives. Manufactured from natural estrogen, estrone, by reaction with potassium acetylide (HC≡CK) in liquid ammonia. The synthetic 17α-ethynyl derivative of estradiol-17β. The 17α-ethynyl group increases the *in vivo* potency of estradiol-17β by blocking the action of 17β-dehydrogenase, a major pathway of estradiol-17β metabolic inactivation. It is thus active orally and is among the most potent of the known estrogenic compounds.

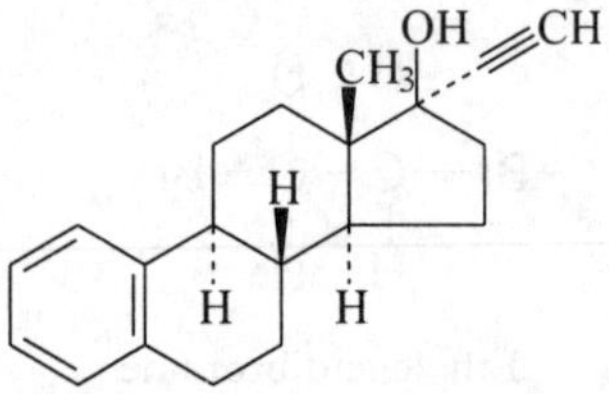

Ethynylestradiol

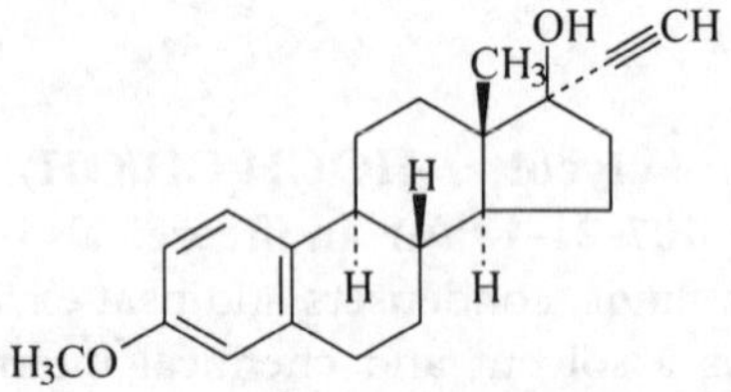

Ethynylestradiol 3-methyl ether

etorphine (4,5α-epoxy-3-hydroxy-6-methoxy-α,17-dimethyl-α-propyl-6,14-ethenomorphinan-7α(R)-methanol). CAS number 14521-96-1. A potent neuroleptanalgesic used as a veterinary anesthetic and remote tranquilizing ("darting") agent. Causes profound (potentially fatal) opioid depression in humans.

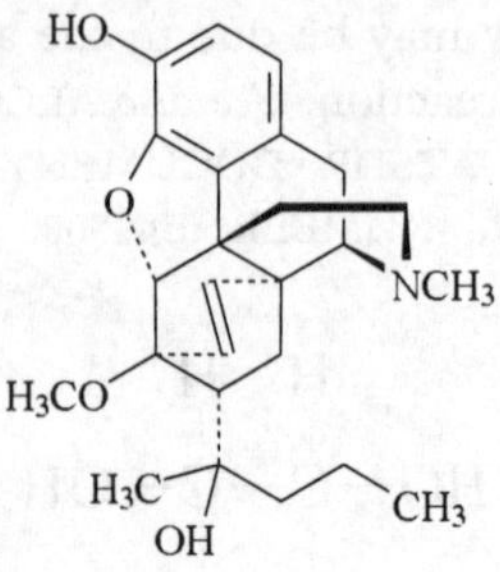

Etorphine

ETS. *See* ELECTRON TRANSPORT SYSTEM.

ETU. *See* ETHYLENE-2-THIOUREA.

eucalyptus. *See* ESSENTIAL OILS.

eucaryote. *See* EUKARYOTE.

eukaryote. A type of cell having a nucleus. In addition to the presence of a nuclear envelope, the DNA is linear and is associated with histones. A variety of organelles may be present, such as the endoplasmic reticulum, Golgi apparatus, lysosomes, secretory vesicles, mitochondria and cytoskeletal elements. Eukaryote cells include protozoa, yeasts and cells of animals and plants. *Compare* PROKARYOTE.

eukaryote mutagenicity tests. Short-term tests that use eukaryotic cell cultures or lower eukaryotic organisms to test for the mutagenic potential of chemicals. These tests include mutations to the HGPRT, TK or ouabain loci in cultured mammalian cells, the sex-linked recessive lethal test in *Drosophila*, yeast mutation tests and the specific locus test in mice. *See also* MAMMALIAN CELL MUTATION TESTS; HGPRT LOCUS; SEX-LINKED RECESSIVE MUTATION TEST; TK LOCUS; YEAST MUTATION TESTS.

Eureceptor. *See* CIMETIDINE.

European Chemical Industry Ecology and Toxicology Centre (ECETOC). An office established by the chemical industries of Europe. The secretariat is in Brussels.

European College of Veterinary Toxicology (ECVT). The professional body for Veterinary Toxicology in the EC and adjacent countries, established under the auspices of the EC's Board of Veterinary Specialization to act as the authenticating and examining body as well as encouraging scholarship, research and other contributions to the discipline.

European Economic Community (EEC). A group of initially six, but now of 12 countries (Belgium, Denmark, France, Greece, Ireland, Italy, Luxembourg, Netherlands, Portugal, Spain, UK and Germany) formed to promote free trade among members. Wider social and political objectives include the construction and implementation of coordinated policies for environmental improvement and the conservation of species, habitats and natural resources.

European Federation of Animal Health. Trade association of the European veterinary pharmaceutical industry, composed of individual members, and national associations: Belgium— AGIM; Denmark—MEFA; Germany—Bft; France—SIMV; Ireland—FICI; Italy—AISA; The Netherlands—FIDIN; Portugal— APIFARMA; Spain—VETERINDUSTRIA; Switzerland— SGCI; United Kingdom—Noah.

European Medicines Evaluation Agency (EMEA). Proposed body to take over central functions for the authorization of (human and veterinary) medicines within the EC. Much authorization (particularly for "conventional" products) would remain at the national level. Establishment awaits agreement of the agency's location.

European Society of Regulatory Affairs (ESRA). European body with same purposes and currently same offices as British Institute of Regulatory Affairs.

eutrophication. The natural or artificial enrichment of nutrients, particularly nitrogen, phosphorus and carbon, and the effects of this enrichment on lakes, streams and estuaries. A eutrophic body of water is characterized by large populations of both flora and fauna, often leading to depletion of the oxygen supply. Natural eutrophication occurs slowly as a consequence of the accumulation of silt; eutrophication is accelerated in those bodies of water that accumulate waste due to human activity.

eutrophy. *See* EUTROPHICATION.

excess risk. Term used in risk assessment to describe an increased risk of a deleterious effect above that estimated to occur in the absence of the toxicant in question.

excision repair enzymes. *See* DNA REPAIR.

excitatory amino acids. Amino acids that increase the firing rate of neurons having appropriate receptors for the compound in question. Some of these compounds can cause neuronal death, presumably by causing sustained neuronal firing. Such compounds have sometimes been called "excitotoxins" and include natural amino acid neurotransmitters like glutamate, as well as various analogs such as kainic acid. *See also* GLUTAMATE.

excitotoxins. *See* EXCITATORY AMINO ACIDS.

excretion. The process by which the end products of metabolism are eliminated from the body. The primary organs involved are the kidney, for urinary excretion, and the liver, for excretion via the bile duct. The kidney, in addition to its role in eliminating nitrogenous wastes such as urea or uric acid, plays a vital role in maintaining salt and water balance. Both kidney and liver play an important role in the elimination of the end products of xenobiotic metabolism, and there are also several minor routes of excretion. *See also* ELIMINATION OF TOXICANTS; EXCRETION, ALIMENTARY; EXCRETION, HEPATIC; EXCRETION, MINOR ROUTES; EXCRETION, PULMONARY; EXCRETION, RENAL.

excretion, alimentary. Toxicants in body fluids that have the lipophilicity necessary to traverse membranes may move through the alimentary canal into the lumen. There is also some evidence for active transport of penicillin in the salivary glands and ammonia compounds in the intestine, but alimentary excretion is more often passive. Although passive elimination in the alimentary canal is usually unimportant it may, in some cases, be an important route of elimination. The contaminant chlordecone, for example, appears to be primarily eliminated in the intestine, although the rate is slow. The therapy for chlordecone poisoning is the administration of cholestyramine, which binds chlordecone and prevents its reabsorption, thus permitting appreciable amounts of chlordecone to be eliminated.

excretion, hepatic (biliary excretion). The most significant route of elimination after the renal route. Bile was first recognized as a route of excretion for xenobiotics over 100 years ago, but only in recent years has it been recognized as a major mechanism and now over 200 foreign compounds have been detected in bile. The liver is an important locus for the metabolism of both endogenous and exogenous compounds, and the products of metabolism may be released either into the circulating blood or excreted into the bile. The walls of the liver sinusoids are permeable to relatively large molecules, and solutes may be transferred from the hepatic cells to the bile or blood by either active or passive processes. There is little transfer of lipophilic compounds, however, prior to metabolism to more water-soluble forms. The compounds actively secreted by bile are usually amphipathic, having both polar and non-polar moieties. Bile salts are examples of endogenous amphipathic molecules, whereas conjugates of lipophilic xenobiotics are examples of amphipathic molecules of exogenous origin. As the pK of most conjugates is 3–4, they are almost completely ionized at physiological pH, thus facilitating active transport. Compounds representing nearly every class of toxicant appear in bile to some extent, generally as metabolites. Biliary excretion has been known to occur in most common laboratory animals, fish, several domesticated and wild animals, and in humans, although there is considerable variation from one species to another. A major factor that determines the ratio between renal and hepatic elimination is the molecular weight of the excretory product. A threshold exists below which compounds are excreted primarily in the urine and above which they are excreted primarily in the bile. The approximate molecular weight threshold is 325 in rats, 400 in guinea pigs, 475 in rabbits and 500–700 in humans. In each case an intermediate range of molecular weights exists that may be excreted in both urine and bile to appreciable extents. *See also* ENTEROHEPATIC CIRCULATION; LIVER.

excretion, minor routes. Minor routes of excretion may be important in specific instances. Excretion of some compounds is linked to reproductive functions of the female. When the mother has accumulated, in fatty depots, considerable quantities of highly lipid-soluble toxicants that are refractory to metabolism, such as DDT or PCBs, they may be eliminated in milk. This is due to an exchange between fatty deposits and blood of those toxicants that readily cross the mammary cell membrane. The growing list of potentially adverse compounds that have been shown to occur in milk includes caffeine, alcohol, drugs, vitamins, hormones and a number of pesticidal and industrial chemicals. For compounds with long half-lives, this may be an important mechanism of elimination. In studies with chlorinated insecticides in cows, over 25% of the administered dose was eliminated in the milk. In some South American countries, the DDT content of human milk is close to the acceptable daily intake for DDT recommended by the World Health Organization. Adverse effects on infants have been reported when nursing mothers were accidentally exposed to high concentrations of either hexachlorobenzene or polychlorinated biphenyls. Another sex-linked route of excretion is the eggs of birds. With polar toxicants and metabolites, adverse effects are transient or not noted while lipophilic compounds may be eliminated into the egg yolk and, in some cases, have adverse effects on hatching and viability of the chicks. The placental barrier is no longer considered an important barrier to lipophilic compounds, and they may pass from the mother to the fetus. Although the fetus contains relatively small amounts of toxicants in most cases, the teratological effects of thalidomide, the toxic effects of mercury, and carcinogenic effects of diethylstilbestrol are all well documented. Finally, elimination of toxicants may also involve some very obscure and little-understood routes. Since any part of the body can provide the opportunity for diffusion of toxicants across cell membranes, hair, feathers, oil glands, sweat glands, etc. may all be expected to eliminate small quantities of lipophilic compounds. Such elimination might also be possible when components of the body are continuously removed, for example, in the sloughing of skin. Compounds such as mercury, selenium, arsenic and, more recently PCBs, are toxicants associated with hair.

excretion, pulmonary. Although the renal and biliary systems are the most important routes of elimination, many volatile compounds are eliminated via the respiratory system. The alveoli, with their great surface area and thin membranes, are a highly specialized part of the lung with the primary function of exchanging oxygen and carbon dioxide, but any toxicant in the blood with adequate volatility may also pass from blood to air for

elimination. A well-known example is ethanol. The rate of elimination of volatile toxicants depends upon the solubility in blood, the rate of respiration and the blood flow to the lungs. The best known examples of respiratory elimination are among the anesthetic gases, but pesticide fumigants, many volatile organic solvents and volatile metabolites of non-volatile toxicants are also eliminated to a significant extent by the lungs.

excretion, renal. Elimination via the kidneys accounts not only for most by-products of normal metabolism, but also for excretion of polar xenobiotics and the hydrophilic metabolites of lipophilic xenobiotics. The initial step in urine formation is glomerular filtration. The plasma, under pressure from the heart, is passively filtered as it passes through numerous glomerular pores 70–100 Å in diameter. No specificity is shown except for molecular size; any solute in the plasma small enough to pass the pores appears in the ultrafiltrate. Molecules too large to pass, or those bound to proteins, do not appear in the filtrate and must either be further altered or be eliminated by other routes. The second major process occurring in the kidney is tubular reabsorption. A large number of solutes necessary for normal body function (water, amino acids, glucose, salts, etc.) are recovered from the glomerular filtrate by this process. The proximal segment of the tubule accounts for about 75% of reabsorption from the glomerular filtrate. Both active and passive mechanisms operate and permit varying degrees of selective action. Reabsorption of xenobiotics is usually passive and regulated by the same principles that permit passage of similar endogenous molecules. Lipophilic compounds are able to traverse cell membranes more readily than polar compounds, and therefore passive reabsorption of lipophilic toxicants is greater than reabsorption of more polar ones, resulting in a relatively lower renal excretion of lipophilic xenobiotics. Another major mechanism whereby solutes may be excreted by the kidney is tubular secretion. This mechanism permits transport of solutes from the peritubular fluid to the lumen of the tubule, and the process may be active or passive. One active mechanism permits secretion of a number of organic acids, including glucuronide and sulfate conjugates, whereas a second active process secretes strong organic bases. Passive secretion of some weak basic and acidic organic compounds may occur as a result of pH differences. The un-ionized, and therefore more lipophilic, form is readily diffusible through the tubule walls. If the pH in the tubular lumen is such that the compounds become ionized, they are unable to diffuse back across the cell wall. This mechanism, called diffusion trapping, is very sensitive to fluctuations in the pH of urine, and modification of the urine pH can, in some cases, be used to help eliminate unwanted compounds. Thus toxicants are excreted by the same mechanisms that eliminate endogenous substances. Polar xenobiotics of a size permitting glomerular passage are removed from the plasma and concentrated in the tubules. Minimal tubular reabsorption of such polar compounds occurs, and they are readily excreted.

exhaust emissions. *See* POLLUTION, EXHAUST EMISSIONS.

exogenous. Originating outside the organism (e.g., xenobiotics or foreign compounds). *Compare* ENDOGENOUS.

exon. *See* GENE.

exotoxin. *See* MICROBIAL TOXINS.

exposure. Toxicants cannot exert their deleterious effects unless they first come in contact with the organism, are absorbed and reach the site of action. Exposure to toxicants is thus a primary consideration in overall toxicity and the study of exposure or the means by which an organism comes in contact with the toxicant is of critical importance in risk assessment and in industrial toxicology. The events subsequent to exposure are considered under many headings, including penetration, portals of entry, distribution, metabolism and several modes of toxic action. Factors that affect the availability of the toxicant to the organism include its concentration, its physical form and other chemicals with which it might be formulated or mixed. Duration and frequency are also key characteristics of exposure in any consideration of risk or potential toxicity. *See also* EXPOSURE, ACUTE; EXPOSURE, CHRONIC; EXPOSURE, INTEGRATED; EXPOSURE, SUBACUTE; EXPOSURE, SUBCHRONIC; EXPOSURE ASSESSMENT.

exposure, acute. Exposure to a chemical for less than 24 hours. Experimentally such exposures may be a single injection (i.p., i.v., s.c. or i.m.), a single dose by gavage or a single dermal application. Although acute is often taken to mean a single exposure, in fact repeated doses within a short time period (24 hours) are also regarded as acute. In the industrial setting, an increase in ambient air levels for a period up to 24 hours is regarded as an acute exposure. *Compare* EXPOSURE, CHRONIC; EXPOSURE, SUBACUTE.

exposure, chronic. As with subchronic exposure, the doses may be repeated discrete doses (e.g., by injection or gavage) or continuous dosing in food, drinking water or air. However, the time frame is even longer, being longer than three months. In experimental animals, chronic exposure is often extended for periods close to the expected lifetime for the species. In industrial situations and epidemiological studies, any exposure of humans longer than three months is considered chronic. *Compare* EXPOSURE, ACUTE; EXPOSURE, SUBCHRONIC.

exposure, cumulative. A computation or assessment of all of the exposure to a toxicant which has been experienced by the organism or population up until a specific point in time.

exposure, integrated. For estimations of exposure or permitted exposures in the workplace, the concentration of the chemical in the ambient air is not considered alone, rather it is integrated with some expression of time of exposure. For example, the threshold limit value-time-weighted average (TLV-TWA) is not a maximum concentration, but a concentration that should not be exceeded on average during an eight-hour working day. If not inappropriate for other reasons, excursions above this limit are permitted if compensated for by excursions below the limit. Again the excursions are not estimated by concentration alone, but by an integrated expression of time and concentration. *See also* THRESHOLD LIMIT VALUE, TIME-WEIGHTED AVERAGE.

exposure, subacute. This resembles acute exposure except that the number of doses is greater and the time of exposure longer. One definition is that of 13–40 doses extended over a period of several days. Another refers to repeated exposure for a month or less. *Compare* EXPOSURE, ACUTE; EXPOSURE, CHRONIC; EXPOSURE, SUBCHRONIC.

exposure, subchronic. Repeated doses spread over an intermediate time range (i.e., one to three months). Doses may be repeated single doses or continous low-level doses in food, drinking water or air. *Compare* EXPOSURE, ACUTE; EXPOSURE, CHRONIC; EXPOSURE, SUBACUTE.

exposure assessment. A major component of risk assessment that establishes the number of individuals likely to be exposed to a chemical in the environment or in the work place and estimates the intensity, frequency and duration of human exposure. Exposure assessment techniques may also be employed to evaluate various technologies directed toward reducing and/or controlling human exposure to chemicals. National Academy of Sciences Risk Assessment in the Federal Government: Managing the Process (National Academy Press, Washington, DC, 1983). *See also* RISK ASSESSMENT.

exposure chambers. The unique difficulties inherent in inhalation toxicity testing require specially designed exposure chambers. Although exposure chambers of many shapes and sizes have been designed, all are intended to provide: (1) space for a number of animals adequate for the particular test; (2) a uniform concentration of the airborne toxicant; (3) access for sampling or for the probes necessary for continuous monitoring; (4) viewing facilities; (5) safe ventilation of test atmospheres. *See also* ADMINISTRATION OF TOXICANTS, INHALATION; ATMOSPHERE GENERATION; ATMOSPHERIC ANALYSIS.

exposure coefficient. Quantitative estimate of the amount of contaminated medium contacted by a living organism per day.

extraction. The transference of a substance from a more complex to a more simple matrix by chemical or physical action prior to its qualitative identification or quantification. Extraction techniques generally utilize the physicochemical properties (e.g., polarity, acid/base) of the compound of interest to impart an affinity for an adsorbent resin or to effect a partitioning into an added solvent. In quantitative analytical techniques, it is important that the recovery of the compound of interest from the assayed matrix be defined for a given extraction method. Ideally, loss of compound during extraction should be monitored by the incorporation of internal standards. *See also* ANALYTICAL TOXICOLOGY; CHROMATOGRAPHY; SOLVENT PARTITIONING; SPECTROSCOPY.

extrapolation. The use of data obtained under one set of conditions to predict the result that would have been obtained under a different set. In toxicology, extrapolation between species and from high to low doses is a necessary part of the risk assessment process. *See also* ABCW EXTRAPOLATION; CARCINOGENESIS, EXTRAPOLATION TO HUMANS; LOW-DOSE EXTRAPOLATION; SPECIES EXTRAPOLATION.

extrapolation, to humans. Extrapolation from the results of toxicity tests conducted on other species in order to predict the effect of the same test chemical on humans. Extrapolation to humans is of particular concern in considerations of carcinogenesis, but is necessary for all forms of toxicity evaluated for regulatory purposes. *See also* ABCW EXTRAPOLATION; CARCINOGENESIS, EXTRAPOLATION TO HUMANS; LOW-DOSE EXTRAPOLATION; SPECIES EXTRAPOLATION.

extrapyramidal side effects (EPS). Acute neurological sequelae, include dystonias, akathesia and pseudoparkinsonism, that can occur from perturbation of the basal ganglia in the brain. They are a common toxic side effect of antipsychotic drug treatment. Dystonias involve abrupt muscle contractions, typically of the head and neck. These muscle contractions may result in torticollis (head turned to the side) or retrocollis (head turned to the back). Dystonic reactions can also include facial grimacing, tongue protrusion, throat spasms, oculogyric crisis and scoliosis. Anticholinergic agents such as diphenhydramine or benztropine given i.v. or i.m. will rapidly suppress these drug-induced reactions. Akathesia refers to a state of agitation and motor restlessness or hyperactivity. Akathesia can be attenuated with β-adrenergic antagonists. Drug-induced parkinsonism involves tremor of the extremities, flat facial expression, muscular or "cogwheel" rigidity, decreases in voluntary movement, stooped posture and shortened, shuffling gait. Excessive salivation and "pill rolling" may also occur. Decreasing the dose of the antipsychotic drug or coadministration of an anticholinergic agent will eliminate such side effects. *See also* ANTIPSYCHOTIC DRUGS; DOPAMINE; PARKINSONISM.

Exxon Valdez. *See* ENVIRONMENTAL DISASTERS.

eye irritation tests. All regions of the eye may be subject to systemic toxicity, however, this is usually chronic and is revealed in chronic or subchronic toxicity tests. Eye irritation tests, on the other hand, test for irritancy of compounds applied topically to the eye. These tests are variations of the Draize test, and the experimental animal is the albino rabbit. The test consists of adding the material to be tested directly into the conjunctival sac of one eye of each of several albino rabbits, the other eye serving as the control. Grading of effects after one, two and three days is subjective and based on the appearance of the cornea, particularly as regards opacity; the iris, as regards both appearance and reaction to light; the conjunctiva, as regards redness and effects on blood vessels; and the eyelids, as regards swelling. Fluorescein may be used to assist visual examination. This test is probably the most controversial of all routine toxicity tests, being criticized primarily on the grounds that it is inhumane. Since both concentrations and volumes used are high, and the results show high variability, it has also been suggested that these tests cannot be extrapolated to humans. Since visual impairment is a critical toxic endpoint, however, tests for ocular toxicity are essential. Attempts to solve the dilemma have taken two forms: (1) to find substitute *in vitro* tests; (2) to modify the Draize test so that it becomes not only more humane, but also more predictive for humans. Attempts to use cultured cells or eyes from slaughtered food animals have not yet produced an acceptable routine test. Using smaller volumes and lower concentrations of test materials does, however, appear to reduce variability. *See also* ACUTE TOXICITY TESTING.

eyes. Organs of light perception. In mammals the lens of the eye focuses light on the retina. Light-sensitive cells in the retina generate nerve impulses in sensory cells that result in impulse transmission to the CNS via the optic nerve. The eyes are important in toxicology for several reasons: (1) the importance of eye function and the possibility of eye damage by chemicals has given rise to regulatory requirements for eye irritation tests, including the controversial Draize test; (2) effects on vision (blurred vision, light sensitivity, etc.) may be important indicators of systemic poisoning. *See also* DIAGNOSTIC FEATURES, EYES; EYE IRRITATION TESTS.

F

F_1. First filial generation obtained when two organisms are mated. The parental generation that produced the F_1 generation is termed P_1, and breeding between members of the F_1 generation produces F_2, the second filial generation. Recessive genes are not expressed in the F_1 generation if one parent is homozygous recessive and the other homozygous dominant for a particular locus (a classic test cross), but homozygous recessive individuals can be expected in the F_2.

F_2. Second filial generation, obtained when two organisms from an F_1 generation are mated. These progeny of the F_1 can be expected to provide phenotypic expression of recessive genes in a classic test cross (P_1 generation homozygous recessive and homozygous dominant for a given trait), since some will be homozygous for such genes. The ratios of phenotypic expression in the F_2 can be used to determine the true genotype of the parental generation.

FAC. *See* FOOD ADVISORY COMMITTEE.

FACC. *See* FOOD ADDITIVES AND CONTAMINANTS COMMITTEE.

facilitated diffusion. *See* FACILITATED TRANSPORT.

facilitated transport (facilitated diffusion). A process similar to active transport in that it is carrier-mediated and proceeds at a more rapid rate than passive diffusion. Unlike active transport, however, it does not move chemicals against a concentration gradient, nor is it metabolic energy-dependent. *See also* ACTIVE TRANSPORT; ENTRY MECHANISMS, SPECIAL TRANSPORT.

facilities, for chronic toxicity testing. *See* ANIMAL ENVIRONMENT; TESTING VARIABLES, NON-BIOLOGICAL.

Faculty of Occupational Medicine (FOM). A faculty of the Royal College of Physicians (London), acting as a professional body for medical practitioners in occupational medicine.

FAD (flavin adenine dinucleotide). CAS number 146-14-5. Biochemical intermediate that is derived from the vitamin riboflavin. A key part of the structure of FAD is its isoalloxazin ring which is able to gain two hydrogen atoms, thus producing the reduced form $FADH_2$. FAD is the prosthetic group of some membrane-bound flavoprotein dehydrogenases such as succinate dehydrogenase as well as flavin-containing monooxygenase. It is also the prosthetic group of some oxidases that react directly with oxygen, the two hydrogen atoms of $FADH_2$ reacting to give hydrogen peroxide. Examples of these are D-amino acid oxidase and yeast alcohol oxidase. *See also* FLAVIN CONTAINING MONOOXYGENASE.

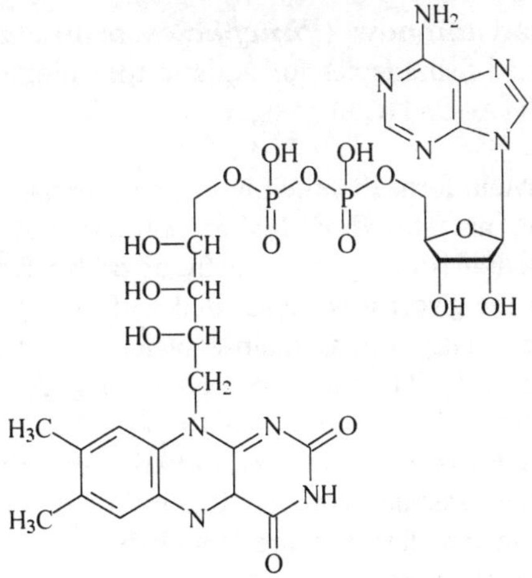

FAD

FAE. *See* FETAL ALCOHOL EFFECTS.

FAO. *See* FOOD AND AGRICULTURE ORGANIZATION.

Farm and Garden Chemicals Regulations. UK regulations, published in 1971, which require that preparations retailed for use in gardens and on farms must be labeled stating the pesticides and other substances contained within the preparation.

FAS. *See* FETAL ALCOHOL SYNDROME.

FASEB. *See* FEDERATION OF AMERICAN SOCIETIES FOR EXPERIMENTAL BIOLOGY.

fast and slow acetylators. Individuals that display a genetic polymorphism in the metabolism of drugs such as isoniazid, the differences being related to the rate of acetylation of isoniazid. Slow acetylators are homozygous for a recessive gene, and this is believed to lead to the lack of the hepatic acetyltransferase, which in normal homozygotes or heterozygotes (rapid acetylators) acetylates isoniazid. Human populations show marked differences in the frequency distribution of the recessive gene. It is low in Eskimos and Japanese, with 80–90% of these populations being rapid acetylators, whereas only 40–60% of Blacks and some European populations are rapid acetylators. Rapid acetylators often develop hepatotoxicity and polyneuritis during treatment with isoniazid. *See also* ACETYLATION; ISONIAZID.

fathead minnow (*Pimephales promelas*). A standard fish species for aquatic toxicology tests. *See also* AQUATIC BIOASSAY.

fats. Main form in which lipids, a potential energy source, are stored in higher animals and some plants. Fat is composed chiefly of triglycerides, in which the glycerol is substituted with one or more different fatty acids, mainly oleic, palmitic and stearic acids. They are hydrolyzed to glycerol and the fatty acids by acids, alkalis and by the action of lipases. Fats can be extracted from tissues with ether or other organic solvents. Lipophilic xenobiotics partition into fats and are stored there. The term fat(s) is often used is a more general sense to apply to all lipids. *See also* LIPID.

fatty acids. Alkyl carboxylic acids, so-called because of their occurrence in natural fats. They may be saturated or have one, two, three or more double bonds. These are esterified to glycerol to form triglycerides or phospholipids.

fatty acyl CoA synthetase. *See* AMINO ACID CONJUGATION.

fatty liver. A liver containing more than 5% by weight of lipid with visible lipid accretions in the cells visible under light microscopy. It may be caused by chemical toxicity (e.g., ethionine, cyclohexamide) or nutritional deficiency (e.g., low choline). *See also* HEPATOTOXICITY, BIOTRANSFORMATION AND REACTIVE METABOLITES.

favism. Type of hemolytic anemia (i.e., anemia involving breakage of erythrocytes) that results from the consumption of broad beans by individuals who suffer a genetically based deficiency of glucose-6-phosphate dehydrogenase.

FCF. *See* FOOD COLORS.

FDA (Food and Drug Administration). A federal agency in the USA that approves the use of food additives and drugs and establishes criteria for toxicity testing.

FD&C (Food, Drug and Cosmetic). An abbreviation that is used as a prefix for food or cosmetic colors. *See also* FOOD COLORS; FOOD, DRUG AND COSMETIC ACT.

FD&C red No. 2. *See* AMARANTH.

FD&C red No. 3. *See* ERYTHROSINE.

FD&C yellow No. 5. *See* TARTRAZINE.

Federal Environmental Pesticide Control Act. *See* FEDERAL INSECTICIDE, FUNGICIDE AND RODENTICIDE ACT.

Federal Food, Drug & Cosmetic Act (FFDCA). *See* FOOD, DRUG AND COSMETIC ACT.

Federal Hazardous Substances Act. An act in the USA that authorizes the Consumer Products Safety Commission to regulate products that are toxic, corrosive, combustible or radioactive. *See also* CONSUMER PRODUCTS SAFETY COMMISSION.

Federal Insecticide, Fungicide and Rodenticide Act (FIFRA). The basic US law under which pesticides and other agricultural chemicals distributed in interstate commerce are registered and regulated. First enacted in 1947, FIFRA placed the regulation of agrochemicals under control of the US Department of Agriculture. In 1970, this responsibility was transferred to the newly created Environmental Protection Agency (EPA). Subsequently, FIFRA has been extensively revised by the Federal Environmental Pesticide Control Act (FEPCA) of 1972 and by the FIFRA amendments of 1975, 1978 and 1980. FIFRA is a complex statute that seeks to balance the social and economic benefits derived from the use of pesticides against the potential costs/risks to humans and the environment. Under FIFRA all new pesticide products used in the USA must be registered with EPA. This requires the registrant to submit information on the composition, intended use and efficacy of the product along with a comprehensive database establishing that the material can be used without causing unreasonable adverse effects on humans or the environment. If it is an unacceptable risk to human health or the environment, the EPA may initiate cancellation or suspension proceedings to remove the material from commerce. Arbuckle, J.G. et al. Environmental Law Handbook, 8th edn (Government Institutes, Rockville, 1985). *See also* AGRICULTURAL CHEMICALS; CANCELLATION, UNDER FIFRA; SUSPENSION, UNDER FIFRA; TOXIC SUBSTANCES CONTROL ACT.

Federal Water Pollution Control Act. A US statute enacted into law in 1972 for the prevention of water pollution. Subsequently amended by the Clean Water Act. *See also* CLEAN WATER ACT.

Federation of American Societies for Experimental Biology (FASEB). An association of ten US societies in the area of biomedicine, with a joint office in Bethesda, Maryland, USA. The Life Science Research Office (LSRO) was established within FASEB to analyze specific problems in biomedicine confronting federal agencies. LSRO reviews the GRAS (Generally Recognized as Safe) list for the Food and Drug Administration. Other LSRO reports include the Scientific Report on Evaluation of the Evidence of Carcinogenicity and Genotoxicity of Drugs and Cosmetic Ingredients. The ten constituent societies are the American Physiological Society, American Society for Biochemistry and Molecular Biology, American Society for Investigative Pathology, American Society for Nutritional Sciences, American Association of Immunologists, American Society for Cell Biology, Biophysical Society, American Association of Anatomists, and Protein Society.

Federation of European Laboratory Animal Science Association (FELASA). A grouping of national associations, holds a European meeting each fourth year.

FEDESA. *See* EUROPEAN FEDERATION OF ANIMAL HEALTH.

feed. The convention that feed is fed to animals, while food is eaten by man, is a useful if not universally employed distinction. *See also* FOOD.

Feingold hypothesis. A hypothesis proposed by Benjamin Feingold, a pediatrician, in a book published in 1973 entitled "Why Your Child Is Hyperactive". He hypothesized that the combination of natural and artificial salicylates in the diet, coupled with artificial food colors, caused neurotoxicity expressed as profound behavioral changes. Feingold stated that more than half of all children with attention deficit disorder ("hyperactivity") were helped by his diet. Although receiving extensive support from open trials, most controlled studies have found only rare, idiosyncratic effects. *See also* ERYTHROSINE; FOOD COLORS; HYPERACTIVITY; TARTRAZINE.

FEL. *See* FRANK EFFECT LEVEL.

FELASA. *See* FEDERATION OF EUROPEAN LABORATORY ANIMAL SCIENCE ASSOCIATION.

fence line concentration. A term used in regulatory toxicology to describe the concentration of a pollutant at the boundary of the property on which it is being released.

fenfluramine (*N*-ethyl-α-methyl-3(trifluoromethyl)benzeneethanamine; Redux). CAS number 458-24-2. Fenfluramine is an amphetamine analog that acts to release serotonin, and to a lesser extent dopamine, from nerve terminals in the brain. It has been available both as a racemate (fenfluramine) and as the active enantioner *d*-fenfluramine (dexfenfluramine). There have been several toxicological controversies surrounding this drug. Chronic administration of fenfluramine to various animal species has been reported to cause toxicity to serotonin neurons, evidenced by a loss of serotonin in brain and disappearance of protein markers for the serotonin neurons. Patients have reported memory loss and depression, but PET scans on humans have not detected damage. An issue of special toxicological concern has been the combination known as "fen-phen", the concomitant use of fenfluramine ("fen") and "phenteramine" as appetite suppressants. In animal studies, the fen-phen combination has been found to increase the amount of neurotoxicity caused by fenfluramine alone. Fen-phen also has been implicated in causing primary pulmonary hypertension (PPH), an otherwise rare condition in healthy individuals. In PPH, the vessels in the lungs constrict and pressure in the pulmonary artery rises for no apparent reason, and the right ventricle to the heart is damaged as it pumps harder to get the blood through the constricted vessels in the lungs. In the most severe stage of the disease, both the heart and lungs fail. Recently, heart valve disease was reported in patients taking fen-phen; the diseased valves were found to have distinctive features similar to those seen in carcinoid syndrome. The cluster of unusual cases of valve disease in fen-phen users suggested that there might be an association between fen-phen use and valve disease. *See also* AMPHETAMINE NEUROTOXICITY; PHENTERMINE; SEROTONIN.

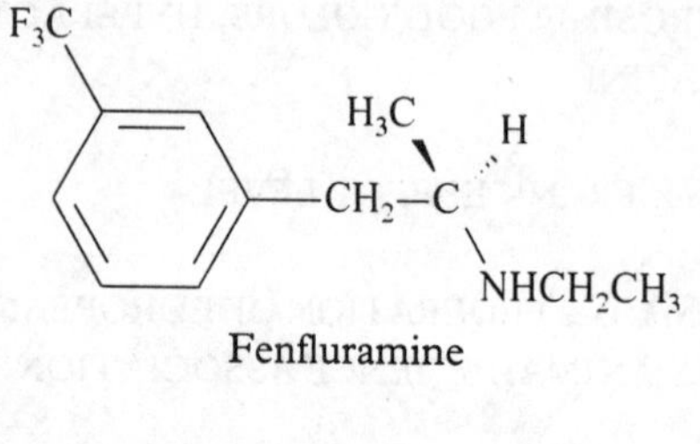

fenitrothion (o,o-dimethyl o-(3 methyl-4-nitrophenyl)phosphorothioate. CAS number 122-14-5. An organophosphorus insecticide used to control aphids and caterpillars in fruit crops, moths and weevils in peas, and leather jackets in cereals. It is also used to control beetle pests in grain stores. Cholinesterase inhibitor. *See also* DATABASES, TOXICOLOGY; ORGANOPHOSPHORUS INSECTICIDES; ORGANOPHOSPHORUS POISONING, SYMPTOMS AND THERAPY.

fen-phen. Fen-phen refers to the use of a combination of two prescription medications (phenteramine and fenfluramine) as appetite suppressants for the short-term management of obesity. The safety of this combination has been questioned due to both neurotoxicity and cardiovascular toxicity. *See also* FENFLURAMINE; PHENTERAMINE.

fenvalerate (cyano(3-phenoxyphenyl)-methyl-4-chloro-α-(1-methylethyl)benzene acetate; pydrin; sumicidin; Belmark). CAS number 66230-04-4. A broad-spectrum contact insecticide with an oral LD50 in rats of 451 mg/kg and an i.v. LD50 in rats of 75 mg/kg. It is a neurotoxicant affecting both the peripheral and central nervous systems, producing axonic disturbances by its effect on sodium channels. Poisoning in humans results in incoordination, tremors, excessive salivation, vomiting, diarrhea, hypersensitivity to sound and touch, convulsions and death. Treatment is symptomatic since no specific therapy is known. In cases of oral ingestion, gastric lavage is used with care to avoid aspiration. *See also* INSECTICIDES; PYRETHROID INSECTICIDES.

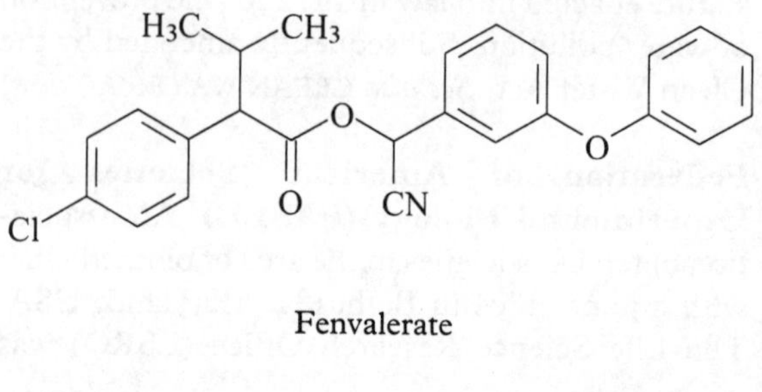

Fenfluramine

Fenvalerate

FEP. *See* FREE ERYTHROCYTE PROTOPOR-PHYRINS.

FEPCA (Federal Environmental Pesticide Control Act). *See* FEDERAL INSECTICIDE, FUNGICIDE AND RODENTICIDE ACT.

ferric oxide (Fe$_2$O$_3$). An iron oxide that is used as a pigment in rubber, paper, glass, ceramics and linoleum, in paint for iron, as a polishing agent, in electrical resistors and semiconductors, as a catalyst and in magnets and magnetic tapes. Inhalation of the ferric oxide dust can cause benign pneumoconiosis. *See also* PNEUMOCONIOSIS.

fertility. The ability to conceive and produce viable offspring. In toxicity testing is usually expressed numerically, e.g. number of offspring per litter. Fertility can be adversely affected by reproductive toxicants acting on either males or females.

fertility index. A numerical expression of mating success used in reproductive toxicity testing. It is the number of pregnancies expressed as a percentage of the number of matings. *See also* GROWTH INDEX; REPRODUCTIVE TOXICITY TESTING; SEX RATIO; VIABILITY INDEX; WEANING INDEX.

fertility test. In general, any test of the ability of an organism to initiate a reproductive sequence leading to fertilization of the ovum. Colloquially and in medicine, the term is used more loosely to mean any test of the ability of an organism to initiate a successful reproductive sequence (i.e., leading to live birth of normal offspring). In reproductive toxicity testing, in which examination of offspring is the desired endpoint, the term refers to dose range-finding studies designed to ensure that the dose of the test compound is low enough for sufficient numbers of offspring to be available for examination. *See also* REPRODUCTIVE TOXICITY TESTING.

fertilization. The fusion of the male and female pronuclei to form the zygote to trigger development.

fetal abnormalities. The results of teratogenic effects on the fetus. These differ from those that occur on exposure of the embryo. Characteristically they are growth retardation and functional deficits rather than anatomical birth defects. *See also* DEVELOPMENTAL AGE.

fetal alcohol effect (FAE; alcohol-related birth defects; ARBD). The full range of alcohol-related teratology from its mildest, least severe presentation to the fully characterized fetal alcohol syndrome (FAS). Current knowledge regarding the teratogenic effects of alcohol suggests that alterations within the fetus resulting from alcohol exposure are varied and wide ranging. At the far end of the spectrum of ethanol-related teratology is the pattern of developmental effects designated fetal alcohol syndrome (FAS). In the absence of full diagnostic criteria which qualify for the designation of FAS, the symptomatology resulting from alcohol exposure during development is classified as fetal alcohol effects (FAE). The characteristic features occurring in FAE fall into the same three major categories as FAS and include: (1) prenatal and/or postnatal growth retardation; (2) CNS involvement; (3) characteristic facial dysmorphology. *See also* FETAL ALCOHOL SYNDROME.

fetal alcohol syndrome (FAS). The pattern of symptomatology that lies at the far end of the spectrum of ethanol-related teratology in humans. Minimal criteria for diagnosis of FAS have been recommended by members of the Fetal Alcohol Study Group of the Research Society of Alcoholism. This group recommended that FAS be diagnosed "only when the patient has signs in each of three categories:" (1) prenatal and/or postnatal growth retardation (weight, length, and/or head circumference below the tenth percentile when corrected for gestational age); (2) central nervous system involvement (signs of neurologic abnormality, developmental delay, or intellectual impairment); or (3) characteristic facial dysmorphology with at least two of these three signs: microcephaly (head circumference below third percentile), microophthalmia and/or short palpebral fissures, or poorly developed philtrum, thin upper lip, and flattening of the maxillary area. *See also* FETAL ALCOHOL EFFECT.

FETAX (frog embryo teratogenesis assay, Xenopus). A developmentally relevant, time- and resource-effective, short-term test system that uses early embryos of the African-clawed frog *Xenopus laevis*. This *in vitro* screening assay for embryotoxic and teratogenic effects exposes early- to mid-blastula embryos at 23 °C for 96 hours (i.e., through organogenesis) to toxic agents in aqueous solution. Following exposure, a number of endpoints are quantitated including survivors, both normal and abnormal, relative teratogenic index (i.e., the ratio of lethality to abnormality), embryo length (i.e., growth) and developmental stage attained. In addition, gross, histological and ultrastructural pathology can be examined and biochemical markers monitored.

fetotoxicity. The deleterious effects exhibited by a fetus (i.e., an animal from the completion of organogenesis to birth, the time equivalent to the second and third trimester of human development) as a result of exposure to a toxic agent. Fetotoxicity manifestations include: (1) lethality; (2) growth impairment (e.g., reduced birth weight); (3) physiological dysfunctions.

fetus. A mammal *in utero* from the completion of organogenesis to birth, the time equivalent to the second and third trimesters of human development.

FEV. *See* FORCED EXPIRATORY VOLUME.

FFDCA. *See* FOOD, DRUG AND COSMETIC ACT.

FHSA. *See* FEDERAL HAZARDOUS SUBSTANCES ACT.

fibrillary gliosis. *See* GLIOSIS.

fibroblast. A cell in connective tissue that is responsible for the formation of fibers.

fibrosarcoma. A sarcoma containing much connective tissue. *See also* SARCOMA.

fibrosis (scarring). The deposition of collagen within an organ or tissue. The collagen deposition is generally preceded by proliferation of fibroblasts. Fibrosis is a common tissue response to acute or chronic injury and is the hallmark of the repair phase of the inflammatory response.

Ficks law of diffusion. *See* PENETRATION, RATE.

field tests. *See* ECOLOGICAL EFFECTS, FIELD TESTS.

FIFRA. *See* FEDERAL INSECTICIDE, FUNGICIDE AND RODENTICIDE ACT.

filtration. *See* ENTRY MECHANISMS, FILTRATION.

first aid. *See* POISONING, EMERGENCY TREATMENT.

first-order kinetics. A process in which the rate of a reaction is proportional to the amount present. It is represented by a proportionality constant relating the rate of elimination to the amount. This elimination rate constant has units of reciprocal time (e.g., min^{-1}, hr^{-1}). Many pharmacokinetic processes of absorption, distribution and elimination occur by passive transfer and can be described by first-order kinetics. The term can also be applied to enzyme reactions where the velocity of the reaction (i.e., product formed per unit time) is proportional to substrate concentration. *See also* KINETIC EQUATIONS; PHARMACOKINETICS; TOXICOKINETICS.

first-pass effect. A phenomenon in which a substance is removed from the blood by the liver before reaching the systemic circulation. It occurs because, anatomically, blood from the upper portion of the gastrointestinal tract passes through the liver before reaching the venous system. As a result, the measured systemic bioavailability may be less than the fraction of the dose absorbed from the gastrointestinal tract. This effect can be considered a form of presystemic metabolism along with metabolism in the lumen or wall of the gastrointestinal tract. *See also* CLEARANCE; KINETIC EQUATIONS; KINETIC EQUATIONS, HEPATIC CLEARANCE; PHARMACOKINETICS; TOXICOKINETICS.

Fischer's exact probability test. A statistic that is designed to test the independence of frequency data classified on two dichotomous variables (2×2 contingency table). This test is generally used with small samples where the chi-square test is inappropriate. *See also* CHI-SQUARE TEST; STATISTICS, FUNCTION IN TOXICOLOGY.

flame photometry. A spectrophotometric method similar to atomic absorption spectroscopy. A sample is atomized in a flame, and a photometer detects the characteristic narrow bands of electromagnetic radiation emitted by the element in question. The amount of light detected should be proportional to the number of atoms emitting light in the flame. Although flame photometry is not as sensitive as atomic absorption spectroscopy, this technique is rapid, inexpensive and is routinely used for measuring alkali metals such as sodium, potassium and lithium. A major problem is interference from other elements or compounds. *See also* SPECTROMETRY, ATOMIC ABSORPTION.

flash point. The lowest temperature at which a flammable chemical or mixture will ignite.

flavin-containing monooxygenase (FMO). Tertiary amines such as trimethylamine and dimethylaniline have long been known to be metabolized to *N*-oxides by an amine oxidase that is microsomal but is not dependent on cytochrome P450. This enzyme is now known to have a much wider substrate specificity than formerly supposed and is known as the microsomal flavin-containing monooxygenase (FMO). It is dependent upon NADPH and oxygen, has a monomeric molecular mass of about 65,000 per mole of FAD and has been purified to homogeneity from pig and mouse liver microsomes. It oxidizes tertiary and secondary amines and sulfur compounds, such as sulfides, thioethers, thiols and thiocarbamates. This enzyme has been shown recently to attack organophosphorous compounds, catalyzing the oxidation of phosphines to phosphine oxides and phosphonates to their oxons. Many substrates for the flavin-containing monoxygenase are also known to be substrates for cytochrome P450. The enzyme is now known to have multiple isoforms that are expressed differently in different tissues. *See also* CYTOCHROME P450-DEPENDENT MONOOXYGENASE SYSTEM; FLAVOPROTEINS; NADPH-CYTOCHROME P450 REDUCTASE.

flavoproteins. Proteins that contain the cofactor flavin adenine dinucleotide (FAD) and/or flavin mononucleotide (FMN). The flavin prosthetic group may be used for the transfer of electrons. Examples of flavoproteins important in toxicology include the flavin-containing monooxygenase, which catalyzes the oxidation of many tertiary and some secondary amines as well as sulfur and phosphorus compounds. This enzyme is similar to cytochrome P450 in that it is also located in the microsomes and is dependent upon NADPH and oxygen. Another flavoprotein of toxicological importance is the NADPH-cytochrome P450 reductase, which contains one mole each of FAD and FMN and is responsible for the transfer of electrons from NADPH to cytochrome P450. *See also* CYTOCHROME P450-DEPENDENT MONOOXYGENASE SYSTEM; FLAVIN-CONTAINING MONOOXYGENASE; NADPH-CYTOCHROME P450 REDUCTASE.

floxuridine. *See* ABNORMAL BASE ANALOGS.

fluid balance. In poisoning, fluid loss may be excessive due to vomiting or diarrhea, or fluid retention may be excessive due to impaired kidney function. It is important that maintenance therapy be carried out in such a way as to minimize or correct such effects on fluid balance and not be carried out in a manner likely to cause such effects. Fluid balance may, and usually does, also involve effects on salt balance. *See also* MAINTENANCE THERAPY, GASTROINTESTINAL TRACT; MAINTENANCE THERAPY, URINARY TRACT; MAINTENANCE THERAPY, WATER AND ELECTROLYTE BALANCE.

fluid retention. A common concomitant of acute poisoning in which urine discharge from the urinary tract is drastically reduced. The most common cause is impaired kidney function. Fluid retention can have important consequences on both water and electrolyte balance and is treated symptomatically during maintenance therapy. *See also* MAINTENANCE THERAPY, GASTRO-

INTESTINAL TRACT; MAINTENANCE THERAPY, URINARY TRACT; MAINTENANCE THERAPY, WATER AND ELECTROLYTE BALANCE; NEPHRO-TOXICITY.

flumeturon. *See* UREA HERBICIDES.

fluorides. Inorganic fluorides, such as sodium, zinc or barium fluoride, can be highly irritating and toxic. The rat oral LD50 for sodium fluoride is 80 mg/kg and for sodium monofluorophosphate (MFP) is 75 mg/kg; calcium fluoride is considerably less toxic. Large doses of fluoride can cause nausea, vomiting, diarrhea, cramps and irritation of the skin, eyes and mucous membranes. The primary cause for concern, however, is the development of fluorosis (sclerosis of bone and mottled teeth) following chronic exposure as, for example, in cryolite mining or in cattle following the use of high-fluoride fertilizers. Fluorine gas (F_2) is also highly irritating and at high concentrations can be lethal due to lung damage. Hydrogen fluoride, hydrofluoric acid is also dangerous because of the severe acid burns induced. *See also* ATSDR DOCUMENT, APRIL 1993.

fluorine (F). *See* FLUORIDES.

fluorimetry. A technique in which a fluorescent chemical can be quantified. The compound may be a substrate, product or cofactor in a reaction or a label placed on a macromolecule, such as an antibody. The fluorescent moiety is excited at its excitation wavelength and observed at its emission wavelength. *See also* ANALYTICAL TOXICOLOGY.

fluoroacetamide (compound 1081). CAS number 640-19-7. A moderately fast-acting rodenticide. Fluoroacetamide is formulated primarily as a food bait. Probably not toxic as such, fluoroacetamide is hydrolyzed to fluoroacetate and further metabolized to fluorocitrate. The oral LD50 in rats is 15 mg/kg. *See also* FLUOROACETATE; FLUOROCITRATE.

$$F-CH_2-\overset{\overset{\textstyle O}{\|}}{C}-NH_2$$

Fluoroacetamide

fluoroacetate (compound 1080). CAS number 144-49-0. One of the most toxic of all pesticides in use in the USA. Formulated as a food bait or in water, it is a fast-acting rodenticide and is licensed for use by governmental agencies and registered pest control operators only. Apparently, fluoroacetate is rapidly metabolized to fluorocitrate, a potent inhibitor of the mitochondrial citric acid (Krebs) cycle. Unlike the anticoagulant rodenticides, carcasses of fluoroacetate-killed rodents may be highly toxic to dogs, cats, etc. The oral LD50 in rats is 0.2 mg/kg. *See also* ACONITASE; FLUOROCITRATE; LETHAL SYNTHESIS.

$$F-CH_2-\overset{\overset{\textstyle O}{\|}}{C}-OH$$

Fluoroacetate

fluorocarbons. Hydrocarbons in which some or all of the hydrogen atoms are replaced by fluorine. Fluorocarbons have different properties from the other halogenated hydrocarbons, largely due to the strength of the carbon-fluorine bond. The lower alkyl fluorides are stable, but fluoropentane and above spontaneously decompose into an alkene and hydrogen fluoride. 1,2-Difluoroalkanes are also unstable. Because of the increasing strength of the carbon-fluorine bond with the numbers of fluorine atoms, however, perfluorocompounds are chemically inert. Polytetrafluoroethene (PTFE) is widely used where resistance to chemical attack is required. Inert fluorocarbon oils, greases and dielectrics are also of importance. Other uses are as refrigerants, fire extinguishers and propellants for aerosols. These agents, along with other trace gases, are believed to be depleting the ozone layer of the Earth's atmosphere. Without the protection from ultraviolet radiation that ozone provides, additional cases of skin cancer and cataracts, damage to polymeric materials and losses of crops and marine life could be expected. *See also* FREONS; OZONE LAYER.

fluorocitrate. A highly toxic material that kills by disrupting energy metabolism. Specifically, fluorocitrate inhibits aconitase, the enzyme responsible for conversion of citrate to isocitrate in the citric acid (Krebs) cycle. It is likely that the toxicities of fluoroacetamide and fluoroacetate can be attributed to their conversion *in vivo* to fluorocitrate.

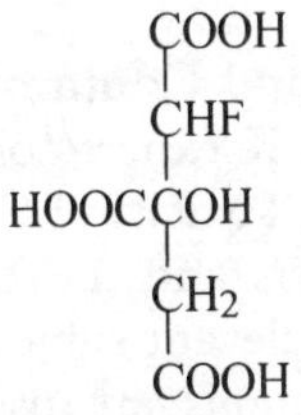

$$\begin{array}{c} COOH \\ | \\ CHF \\ | \\ HOOCCOH \\ | \\ CH_2 \\ | \\ COOH \end{array}$$

Fluorocitrate

5-fluorodeoxyuridine. *See* ABNORMAL BASE ANALOGS.

fluorosis. Two adverse effects of high levels of fluoride in the drinking water are dental fluorosis (mottling of the teeth) and skeletal fluorosis (increased bone density). The latter effect can be beneficial, although at extremely high levels of fluoride crippling can occur.

5-fluorouracil (FU; 5-FU; 5-fluoro-2,4(1H,3H) pyrimidinedione). CAS number 51-21-8. A cytotoxic antineoplastic agent with an i.p. LD50 in mice of 260 mg/kg. It is clastogenic, embryotoxic and teratogenic, and inhibits DNA synthesis. It inhibits the conversion of dUMP to thymidine by thymidylate synthetase, resulting in a lack of substrate for DNA synthesis. In humans, it causes bone marrow depression, toxicity to the epithelium of the gastrointestinal tract and oral mucosa, cardiotoxicity and neurotoxicity. Danenberg, P.V. Biochim. Biophys. Acta 473, 73–92 (1977).

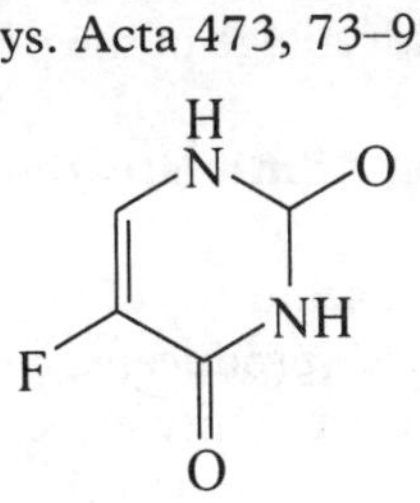

Fluorouracil

fluoxetine. *See* SELECTIVE SEROTONIN RE-UPTAKE INHIBITORS.

fly ash. Non-burnable by-products of combustion, primarily resulting from energy-generating and industrial processes. *See also* POLLUTION, ENERGY SOURCES.

FMO. *See* FLAVIN-CONTAINING MONOOXYGENASE.

fog. Aerosols with liquid dispersed phases that are formed by condensation; either a normal meteorological phenomenon if uncontaminated or, in addition, a form of air pollution if chemically contaminated. *See also* MIST; SMOG.

Folex. *See* METHOTREXATE.

folic acid (N-(4-(((2-amino-1,4-dihydro-4-oxo-6-pteridinyl)methyl)amino)benzoyl)-L-glutamic acid). CAS number 59-30-3. A water-soluble vitamin required in the diet of mammals. Sulfonamide drugs are selectively toxic to bacteria because they inhibit the incorporation of *p*-aminobenzoic acid into folic acid, a biosynthetic process in bacteria. Folic acid deficiency adversely affects prenatal development in humans. Dietary supplementation with folic acid dramatically reduces the incidence of neural tube defects in humans. Folic acid deficiency may also contribute to the causes of megaloblastic macrocytic anemia and a consequence of this is that this disease can be induced, as a side effect, when methotrexate, a folic acid antagonist, is used in cancer chemotherapy.

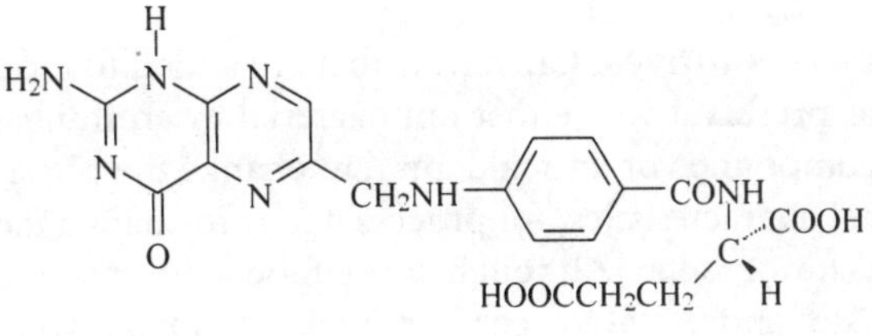

Folic acid

follicle-stimulating hormone (FSH). A glycoprotein gonadotropic hormone from the adenohypophysis (anterior pituitary) that stimulates development of the primary ovarian follicle in the vertebrate female and stimulates spermatogenesis in the male. Its secretion is stimulated by gonadotropin-releasing hormone (GnRH) from the hypothalamus. FSH and LH are usually released and act synergistically. Major component in treatment of infertility.

FOM. *See* FACULTY OF OCCUPATIONAL MEDI-CINE.

fonofos (*O*-ethyl *S*-phenyl ethylphosphono-dithioate; Dyfonate). CAS number 944-22-9. An insecticide used primarily in agriculture. The name is derived from the presence of a phosphon-ate (P–C) bond in the molecule. Due to this struc-tural feature fonofos, unlike organophosphorus insecticides lacking this structure, is activated to the oxon by the flavin-containing monooxygenase (FMO) as well as cytochrome P450. Organophos-phorus compounds lacking the P–C bond are acti-vated only by cytochrome P450. *See also* DATA-BASES, TOXICOLOGY; ORGANOPHOSPHORUS INSECTICIDES; ORGANOPHOSPHATE POISON-ING, SYMPTOMS AND THERAPY.

Fonofos

food. By convention humans eat food, other ani-mals, particularly domestic and experiment ani-mals are said to eat feed. *See also* FEED.

food additives. Chemicals that are added to food as preservatives (either antibacterial or antifungal compounds or antioxidants), to change the physi-cal characteristics, for processing, or to change the taste or odor. Although most food additives are safe and without chronic toxicity, many were introduced when toxicity testing was relatively unsophisticated, and some have been shown sub-sequently to be toxic. The most important inor-ganic additives are nitrate and nitrite. It should be noted that there are certainly hundreds, and possi-bly thousands, of food additives in use worldwide. Well-known examples include the antioxidant butylated hydroxyanisole (BHA), fungistatic agents such as methyl-*p*-benzoic acid, the emulsi-fier propylene glycol, sweeteners such as saccharin and aspartame, and dyes such as tartrazine and erythrosine. Not all toxicants in food are synthetic food additives; many examples of naturally occurring toxicants in the human diet are known, including both carcinogens and mutagens. *See also* FOOD COLORS; FOOD CONTAMINANTS.

Food Additives and Contaminants Commit-tee (FACC). A UK expert committee that with the Committee on Toxicity of Chemicals in Food, Consumer Products and the Environment pub-lishes reports on relevant subjects. The Commit-tee's recommendations are used as a basis for regulation on food safety issued by the Ministry of Agriculture, Fisheries and Food.

Food Advisory Committee (FAC). A UK non-statutory body, consisting of representatives in equal proportions from industry and retailing; consumer and enforcement bodies; and the medi-cal and academic community. It is concerned with advising on the need for novel agents in food. If it establishes a need the matter is referred to an expert committee (e.g., committee on toxicity) for advice.

Food and Agriculture Organization of the United Nations (FAO). One of the first of the UN specialist agencies to be formed, its headquar-ters are in Rome. Its aim is to increase food pro-duction and availability among those sections of the world population where hunger is prevalent. In addition to agriculture and trade, its operations extend into fisheries, forestry and nutrition. It con-ducts many field projects, initiates and cooperates in research and seeks to reform world food-trading policies to the advantage of the poor.

Food and Drug Administration. *See* FDA.

food chain. The sequence of organisms of differ-ent trophic levels (producers, herbivores, carni-vores) within a community or ecosystem through which energy is transferred by the process of eating and being eaten. A food web is an interconnected series of food chains. The energy transferred from one trophic level to another is usually a small per-centage of the potential energy available; the bal-ance is lost to metabolic maintenance and heat production. Consequently, organisms at each tro-phic level pass on less energy than they receive, thereby setting a limit on the number of trophic levels supported in a single food chain.

Compounds that are not easily metabolized or eliminated are concentrated in succeeding trophic levels because the transfer efficiency may be near 100%. *See also* BIOACCUMULATION.

Food Chemicals Codex. A document, prepared by the National Research Council of the US National Academy of Sciences; a compilation of specifications and descriptions of agents that are used as food additives. It provides standardization of the food additives manufactured and utilized by the food industry and thereby provides a way to help ensure the safety of food in which these chemicals are used. *See also* FDA; FOOD ADDITIVES.

food colors. Compounds added to foods and other products (e.g., pharmaceuticals) to increase consumer acceptance or to differentiate between products. Food colors are usually characterized by high water solubility, the ability to produce many different shades of color and relative stability in foods. Most of the compounds presently used are based on coal tar dyes and contain sulfonate and/or azo groups. Prior to the establishment of the FDA, about 80 of the nearly 700 dyes derived from coal tar were used in foods. The FDA narrowed this list to seven, and an additional 10 were added by 1929. In the intervening time, the majority of these have been removed from the approved list principally because of animal data which suggested that they were potential carcinogens. In addition to these synthetic colors, there are also other preparations that are used for coloring, including fruit and vegetable juices and extracts. The number of approved colors varies from country to country, ranging from several dozen in Denmark to none in Greece. Generally, approved compounds have very low levels of acute or subacute toxicity, with p.o. LD50s in the g/kg range and i.p. LD50s ranging from 500 mg/kg and

Sunset yellow (FCF)

higher. The most common toxicological concern with these food colors has been their potential carcinogenicity, but allergic responses (e.g., tartrazine) and even possible neurotoxicity (e.g., erythrosine) have been suggested. It should be noted that the specification for these colors usually calls for purities in the range of 85–90%. Thus, the large percentage of structurally related compounds present in the commercial product greatly complicates toxicological considerations with food colors. *See also* AMARANTH; AZO DYES; CITRUS RED; COAL TAR DYES; ERYTHROSINE; FOOD ADDITIVES; TARTRAZINE.

food consumption, in chronic toxicity testing. *See* TOXIC ENDPOINTS.

food consumption, in subchronic toxicity testing. *See* TOXIC ENDPOINTS.

food contaminants. Those compounds that are included inadvertently in foods, either raw, cooked or processed. They include bacterial toxins, such as the exotoxin of *Clostridium botulinum*, mycotoxins, such as aflatoxins from *Aspergillus flavus*, plant alkaloids, animal toxins, pesticide residues, residues of animal food additives, such as diethylstilbestrol and antibiotics, and a variety of industrial chemicals, such as polychlorinated biphenyls and polybrominated biphenyls. *Compare* FOOD ADDITIVES.

Food, Drug and Cosmetic Act. An act passed by the US Congress in 1938 and modified several times thereafter. This legislation establishes policy for the use of food additives, cosmetic components and drugs. It was a successor to the original Food and Drug Act of 1906. The Food, Drug and Cosmetic Act sets criteria for drug safety for both human and animal use, and requires manufacturers to prove efficacy as well as safety. Administered by the Food and Drug Administration (FDA), it authorizes that agency to define the required toxicity testing for each product. One important component of the early acts was the Delaney clause, which states that food additives that cause cancer in humans or animals at any level shall not be considered safe and are, therefore, prohibited from such use. This law also empowers the FDA to establish and modify a list of food additives that are "generally recognized as safe" (GRAS) and to establish good laboratory practice (GLP) rules. *See also* GOOD LABORATORY PRACTICES.

Food Safety Council. A group of experts supported by the food industry of the USA. The Scientific Committee of the Food Safety Council has published recommendations for chronic toxicity testing of food additives and for a "decision tree" approach for toxicity testing that includes exposure assessment and *in vivo* tests, as well as acute and chronic toxicity tests. Food Safety Council, Scientific Committee. Fd. Cosmet. Toxicol. (suppl.) 16(2), 1–136 (1978).

Food Standards Committee Report on Colouring Matter. Provides a review of the classification of dyes used in food in the UK according to their toxicities. *See also* REPORT ON THE REVIEW OF FLAVOURINGS IN FOOD.

food web. *See* FOOD CHAIN.

Forane. *See* ISOFLURANE.

forced expiratory volume (FEV). A measure of lung function, the FEV is the amount of air that can be forcefully exhaled in a given time, usually one second.

forced vital capacity (FVC). A measure of lung function, the FVC is the total amount of air that can be forcefully exhaled following maximum inhalation.

forensic studies, tissue sampling. In forensic studies, a primary concern is the identification of the cause and circumstances of poisoning and/or death and the legal issues arising therefrom. The toxicologist is often presented with many problems, such as lack of familiarity of medical personnel with requirements for sampling, storage and identification, as well as decay or other alteration of the victim's tissues subsequent to death. Samples should be clearly tagged, and an unbroken chain of possession maintained. If a death is involved, tissue sampling usually occurs during or at the conclusion of the autopsy or necropsy. Sufficient numbers and quantities of tissue should be

taken and preserved at this time, since later sampling may be impossible (cremation) or difficult (exhumation). *See also* SAMPLING, TISSUES.

forensic toxicology. The study of the medicolegal aspects of the adverse effects of chemicals on humans and animals. Although primarily devoted to the identification of the cause and circumstances of death and the legal issues arising therefrom, forensic toxicologists also deal with sublethal poisoning cases. The analytical methods utilized may also be applicable in clinical toxicology, to assist in diagnosis of the cause of poisoning.

formaldehyde. CAS number 50-00-0. A designated carcinogen, hazardous substance (EPA) and hazardous waste (EPA). It is a colorless, pungent gas, commonly sold and used as an aqueous solution containing 30–50% formaldehyde and 0–15% methanol (formalin), the latter being added to prevent polymerization. Formaldehyde has found extensive industrial use as a fungicide and bacteriocide and was also used in embalming fluids. It is used as an intermediate in drug and pesticide manufacture, in the manufacture of melamine resins, dyes, cellulose esters and compounds such as phenol, urea and thiourea. It may enter the body by inhalation, ingestion and percutaneous absorption. Locally the gas may irritate the mucous membranes of the respiratory tract, eyes, etc., high concentrations causing difficulty in breathing and pulmonary edema. Formaldehyde has been found to be a mutagen and an animal carcinogen, and its use is coming under increasing regulation. May be formed as a metabolite, by both alcohol dehydrogenase and cytochrome P450.

$$\begin{matrix} H \\ \\ H \end{matrix} \!\! > \!\! C = O$$

Formaldehyde

formalin. *See* FORMALDEHYDE.

formamidines. This class of compounds is best represented, in toxicology, by an acaricide, chlordimeform. Chlordimeform, N'-(4-chloro-*o*-tolyl)-N,N-dimethylformadine, CAS number 6164-98-3, is used in the control of mites and ticks and in some cases, insects. Moderately toxic to humans.

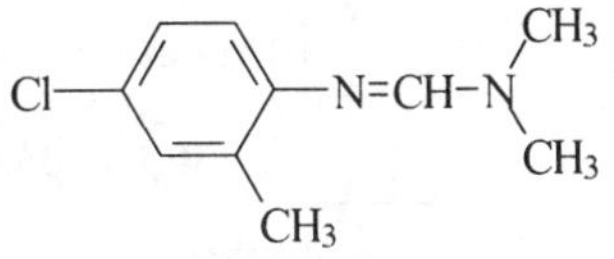

Chlordimeform

formic acid. CAS number 64-18-6. A designated hazardous substance (EPA) and hazardous waste (EPA). It is a colorless, flammable liquid with a pungent odor. It is used in the synthesis of acetic acid, allyl alcohol, phenolic resins, insecticides and drugs. Formic acid is a strong oxidizing agent that can enter the body by inhalation of the vapor, by percutaneous absorption or by ingestion of the liquid. Locally it causes severe irritation of the skin and mucous membranes. Ingestion of formic acid can be fatal. Formic acid generated *in vivo* from methanol by the action of alcohol dehydrogenase and aldehyde dehydrogenase is believed to be the cause of the acute acidosis that occurs following methanol ingestion. Formic acid is also a major component of the venom of some ants, and is largely responsible for the pain ant stings elicit.

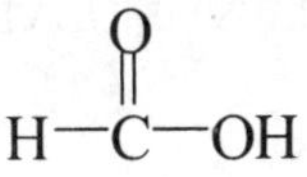

Formic acid

formulation. A UK term, synonymous with composition of medicine.

forskolin. Alkaloid derived from *Coleus forskolin* that directly activates the enzyme adenylate cyclase via actions at the catalytic subunit and by effects on the interaction of the enzyme with G-proteins. *See also* ADENYLATE CYCLASE; G-PROTEINS.

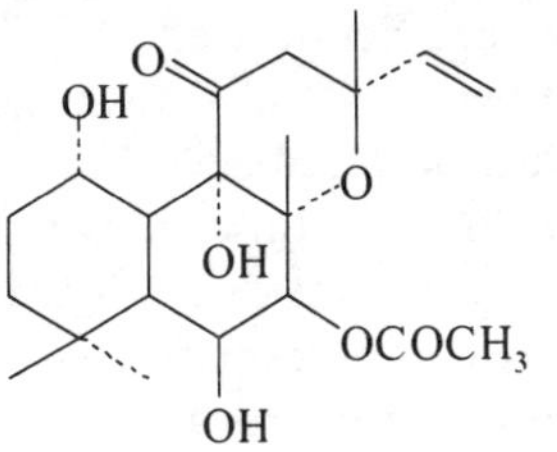

Forskolin

forward mutation. A mutation that causes a wild-type organism to display a new characteristic or a mutant form. *See also* AMES TEST; MUTATION.

fossil fuels. Energy sources from geological formations, such as crude oil, natural gas and coal, formed by the reduction of chemical remains of prehistoric life. *See also* OIL SPILLS; POLLUTION.

foxglove. A plant, *Digitalis purpura* in the family Scrophulariaceae. It contains the cardioactive agent digitalis. *See also* DIGITALIS; DIGITOXIN.

frameshift mutations. Addition or deletion of a base in the DNA molecule puts the triplet code out of sequence and results in a frameshift mutation. If the addition of another base follows in close proximity to a deletion, the production of functional or partially functional proteins may occur. Some chemicals (e.g., acridine) are known to induce frameshift mutations. Errors occurring during chromatid cross-over may also lead to frameshift mutations. *Compare* POINT MUTATION. *See also* CHROMOSOME ABERRATIONS; MUTATION.

frank effect level (FEL). A level of exposure to a chemical or mixture that provides an acute, unequivocal deleterious effect. *See also* NO OBSERVED EFFECT LEVEL (NOEL); NO OBSERVED ADVERSE EFFECT LEVEL (NOAEL).

F ratio. The ratio of two mean squares (estimates of the sample variance). The hypothesis being tested is that the samples are derived from population variances that are equal. In a single-factor experiment the F ratio is compared with an F critical value to determine whether a difference among treatment means (main effect) is significant. In a two-factor ANOVA, three F ratios are generated: one to test whether there is a significant difference on factor A, one to test for significant main effects for factor B, and a third F ratio to test the interaction between factors A and B. *See also* ANALYSIS OF VARIANCE; STATISTICS, FUNCTION IN TOXICOLOGY.

free erythrocyte protoporphyrin (FEP; erythrocyte protoporphyrin; EPP). An indirect measure of lead levels in blood. Protoporphyrin is formed in the mitochondrion during the differentiation of the erythrocyte in the bone marrow. The conversion to heme requires the insertion of iron into the protoporphyrin ring. As blood lead increases, there is an exponential increase in inhibition of porphobilinogen synthase (aminole-vulinic acid dehydratase; ALAD) which results in decreased production of porphobilinogen (proto-porphyrin precursor). Lead also inhibits ferroche-latase, which causes accumulation of inactive hemoglobin molecules which contain zinc proto-porphyrin (ZPP) instead of heme. This analysis, based on the fluorescence of ZPP, is technically much simpler than the measurement of lead in blood and is not affected by possible lead contami-nation during sampling. The use of this method is recommended for screening purposes at blood lead concentrations greater than 20 mg/100 ml blood. *See also* LEAD.

free radicals. Molecules that have unpaired electrons. Free radicals may be produced metabolically from xenobiotics and, since they are extremely reactive, may be involved in inter-actions with cellular macromolecules, giving rise to adverse effects. Examples include the tri-chloromethyl radical ($CCl_3^{\bullet}$) produced from carbon tetrachloride or the carbene radical ($RC^{\bullet\bullet}$) produced by oxidation of the acetal carbon of methylenedioxyphenyl synergists.

Freons (Arctons). Polyhalogenated derivatives of methane and ethane containing fluorine and, in most examples, chlorine and bromine. They com-bine chemical and thermal stability, low boiling points, low viscosity, low surface tension and low toxicity. They are used as refrigerants, propellants for aerosols, fire extinguishers, solvents and as intermediates in polymerization. Examples include the following:

Freon	Structure
11	Cl_3CF
12	Cl_2CF_2
12	$ClCF_3$
13B1	$BrCF_3$
22	$HClCF_2$
113	$ClCF_2CClF_2$
113B2	$BrCF_2CBrF_2$

Freon	Structure
114	$ClCF_2CCl_2F$
142	CH_3CClF_2

See also FLUOROCARBONS.

Freund's adjuvant. Freund's complete adjuvant is a water-in-oil emulsion containing detergent and killed mycobacteria (usually *M. tuberculosis*). Incomplete Freund's adjuvant does not contain any killed bacteria or bacterial products. Freund's adjuvant is thought to enhance antibody response by retarding antigen clearance from the site of innoculation. It tends to also induce an influx of leukocytes, leading to non-specific lymphoid system activation. *See also* ADJUVANT.

frog embryo teratogenesis assay, *Xenopus*. *See* FETAX.

FSC. *See* FOOD SAFETY COUNCIL.

FSH. *See* FOLLICLE-STIMULATING HORMONE.

F test. *See* F RATIO.

FU. *See* 5-FLUOROURACIL.

fuel oils. Petroleum products used as fuels for engines, in lamps, in stoves and in furnaces. Fuel oils may also be used as solvents. Since fuel oils are refined from crude oil to different specifications for many different purposes, there are numerous fuel oils, although they have many characteristics in common. Some important fuel oils are: fuel oil number 1 or kerosene, including jet fuels (JP-5) and a widely used deodorized fuel oil (Deobase); fuel oil number 2 (also known as diesel fuel number 1); fuel oil number 3 (home heating oil); and fuel oil number 4 (also known as diesel fuel number 2), a heavy residual oil used in marine engines. All are complex mixtures of aliphatic, ali-cyclic and aromatic hydrocarbons with traces of sulfur compounds and frequently various addi-tives. Inhalation of fuel oil vapor has many acute effects, primarily on the nervous system, including headache, drowsiness, etc. Chronic inhalation can have nephrotoxic effects. Ingestion of fuel oils can have effects on the gastrointestinal system, including nausea and vomiting, large amounts may cause coma, convulsions and death. Marine diesel oil can cause skin and liver cancer in mice. Little is known of the potential to cause cancer in humans. IARC has designated exposure during refining as probably carcinogenic to humans, but this is not specific for fuel oils. *See also* ATSDR DOCUMENT, MAY 1993.

fugu. *See* PUFFERFISH.

fumes. Small particulate matter contributing to air pollution, with particle diameter less than 1 μm. Fumes of zinc or lead oxides, for example, result from metallurgical or chemical processes. *See also* AIR POLLUTION.

fumigants. Pesticides that volatilize and enter via the respiratory system. Common fumigants are ethylene dibromide and methyl bromide.

functional residual capacity. The difference between the minimum of the tidal volume and the lung without any gas content; one of several measures of lung capacity.

fungi. A number of fungi produce pharmacologically and/or toxicologically active agents, mycotoxins. Some of these fungi grow on edible plants and can exert their effects on the animals and humans that ingest these crops by the mycotoxins they produce. A number of mushrooms contain highly toxic agents, and others contain psychoactive compounds which have been used for recreational purposes. Some of the most notable of toxicologically important fungi follow. *Claviceps purpurea* (ergot) which is parasitic on grains of rye, and causes vasoconstriction of blood vessels, leading to gangrene, then to a darkening of tissue called "St. Anthony's fire"; ergot alkaloids are derivatives of lysergic acid. *Acremonium coenophialum* also contains lysergic acid derivatives and is symbiotic with grass and causes "fescue toxicosis" in cattle and horses. *Fusarium* species produce fumonisins. *F. moniliforme* grows on corn and can produce in horses "moldy corn poisoning" or equine leukoencephalomalacia, or hepatotoxicity and toxicity to other organs in several species such

as horses, pigs and chickens. *Fusarium* and *Tricoderma* species produce tricothecenes, the most famous of which is T-2 toxin. *Aspergillus flavus* and related fungi produce aflatoxins, which are common on corn and peanuts, and are potent hepatotoxicants and carcinogens. *Amanita muscaria* and *A. pantherina* contain ibotenic acid, an excitatory amino acid, muscimol and small amounts of muscarine. Ingestion of these mushrooms leads to CNS depression, ataxia, hysteria and hallucinations. *A. phalloides* (the death cap) and *A. ocreata* (the death angel) produce phylloidin, a cyclic heptapeptide, and amatoxins, bicyclic peptides, and α-amanitin, which binds to RNA polymerase II and leads to hepatotoxicity and nephrotoxicity. *Inocybe* and *Clitocybe* contain large amounts of muscarine, which leads to numerous parasympathetic signs such as diarrhea, sweating, salivation and lacrimation. *Lepiota* (the parasol mushroom) also produces amatoxins. *See also* AFLATOXINS; ERGOT ALKALOIDS; MYCOTOXINS; TRICOTHECENES.

fungi, hallucinogenic. *See* ERGOT ALKALOIDS.

fungicides. Chemicals produced for the control of pathogenic fungi, primarily those affecting food and ornamental plants, although a few drugs are available to treat fungal diseases of humans and animals. With the exception of the mercury-containing fungicides, they are of low acute toxicity to animals. Fungicides are a diverse group drawn from several different chemical classes. They include dicarboximides such as captan and folpet, substituted aromatics such as pentachlorophenol, dithiocarbamates such as ziram or maneb, nitrogen heterocycles such as benomyl and mercury compounds such as methylmercury. *See also* CAPTAN; METHYLMERCURY; PENTACHLOROPHENOL.

FVC. *See* FORCED VITAL CAPACITY.

FW-293. *See* DICOFOL.

FWPCA. *See* FEDERAL WATER POLLUTION CONTROL ACT.

G

GA. *See* TABUN.

GABA (γ-aminobutyric acid). CAS number 56-12-2. A ubiquitous inhibitory transmitter in the CNS, its inhibitory effects being due to increased Cl⁻ flux. GABA appears to mediate the inhibitory actions of local interneurons, and there is a major GABAergic pathway descending from the caudate nucleus to the substantia nigra. GABA is also released by spinal cord interneurons and depolarizes axon terminals of primary afferent fibers, resulting in presynaptic inhibition of motor neurons. The anatomical localization of GABAergic neurons has been accomplished by the use of immunocytochemical methods for identifying glutamic acid decarboxylase (GAD), the enzyme that converts glutamate to GABA. Benzodiazepines potentiate GABA actions, as most GABA receptors are part of a macromolecular complex that includes a benzodiazepine-binding site. The GABA receptors are also presumably the target for many of the chlorinated cyclodiene insecticides which compete for the picrotoxinin binding site and antagonize GABA action. The GABA receptor site is also presumably the target for many of the chlorinated cyclodiene insecticides which compete for the picrotoxinin binding site and antagonize GABA action. The biosynthetic pathway for GABA involves what is referred to as the GABA shunt. This is a closed loop whereby α-ketoglutarate, an intermediate in the Krebs cycle, is transaminated to glutamic acid by GABA-α-ketogluturate transaminase (GABA-T). Glutamic acid is decarboxylated by glutamic acid decarboxylase (GAD) to form GABA. GABA, in turn, is converted by GABA-T to succinic semialdehyde and, then, via succinic semialdehyde dehydrogenase, to succinate which re-enters the Krebs cycle. In this way GABA remains available in high concentrations. Inhibition of GABA synthesis (e.g., by 3-mercaptoproprionic acid) or blockade of GABA transmission (e.g., by bicuculline or picrotoxin) can result in convulsions. *See also* γ-AMINOBUTYRIC ACID TRANSAMINASE; BENZODIAZEPINES; GLUTAMIC ACID DECARBOXYLASE.

$$\underset{H}{\overset{H}{{>}}}N-CH_2-CH_2-CH_2-\overset{\overset{O}{\|}}{C}-OH$$

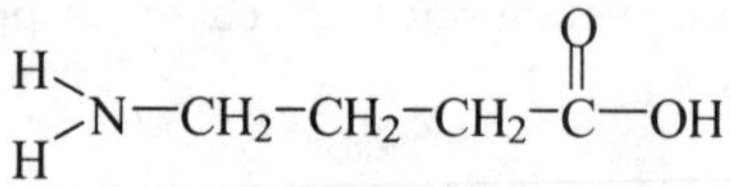

Gamma-aminobutyric acid (GABA)

GABA-T. *See* γ-AMINOBUTYRIC ACID TRANSAMINASE.

GAD. *See* GLUTAMIC ACID DECARBOXYLASE.

G agents. A group of potent organophosphorus cholinesterase inhibitors synthesized and investigated by the German discoverers (notably G. Schrader) prior to and during World War II as chemical warfare nerve gas (G gas). The three most active compounds among them are tabun, sarin and soman, designated as GA, GB and GD, respectively. These G agents are highly volatile liquids, thus permitting them to be disseminated in vapor form. They are generally colorless to light brown, odorless (faint fruity odor for GA) and readily absorbable through the lungs, eyes, skin and gastrointestinal tract. A brief exposure may be fatal, and death usually occurs in minutes following exposure to high concentrations. The aging of the GD-AChE complex occurs within minutes and thus is refractory to reactivation of AChE by oximes. The aging is slower after exposure to GA or GB (in hours) and thus is treatable with oximes such as 2-PAM and with atropine. *See also* ACETYLCHOLINESTERASE, AGING; ANTICHOLINESTERASES; ORGANOPHOSPHORUS INSECTICIDES; SARIN; SOMAN; TABUN.

gall bladder. A sac-like organ of smooth muscle that accumulates and concentrates the bile produced by the liver. It contracts and delivers the bile, via the common bile duct, into the duodenum in response to the duodenal hormone cholecystokinin, which is secreted in response to the presence of fat in the duodenum.

Gallium (Ga). A metal of atomic weight 69.72 and atomic number 31. Three valence states. Non-radioactive gallium is used in cancer chemotherapy for the treatment of Hodgkins disease and non-Hodgkins lymphoma and also for the treatment of hypercalcemia. There do not appear to be any recorded adverse effects from occupational exposure and the side effects from therapeutic use are relatively mild. In animal studies neuromuscular effects and renal damage have been noted.

gamete. The mature germ cell, either an ovum or a spermatozoan, which contains the haploid number of chromosomes. It is produced by the process of gametogenesis during which meiosis occurs, bringing about a halving of the chromosome number.

gametogenesis. The process of spermatogenesis or oogenesis, which produces spermatozoa or ova, respectively. In vertebrates, gametogenesis is dependent upon follicle-stimulating hormone (FSH) and luteinizing hormone (LH), both hormones from the adenohypophysis. Agents affecting the normal feedback systems controlling hormone production, such as oral contraceptives, can suppress gametogenesis.

gamma-aminobutyric acid. *See* GABA.

gamma counting. *See* SPECTROMETRY, GAMMA.

gamma-diketone neuropathy. *See* γ-DIKE-TONE NEUROPATHY.

gamma multi-hit model. *See* LOW-DOSE EXTRAPOLATION.

ganglia. Plural of ganglion; an accumulation of nervous tissue outside the CNS, comprising mainly nerve cell bodies, dendrites and synapses, such as the dorsal root ganglia of spinal nerves or the autonomic ganglia of autonomic nerves.

gap junction. Junctions between adjacent cells comprised of protein bound channels through which small chemicals can migrate for the purpose of intercellular communication. Interference with normal gap junction function is considered a possible mechanism of carcinogenesis for some carcinogens.

gaps. *See* CHROMOSOME ABERRATIONS.

gas chromatography. *See* CHROMATOGRAPHY, GAS.

gas–liquid chromatography. *See* CHROMA-TOGRAPHY, GAS–LIQUID.

gasoline (petrol). A flammable liquid petroleum distillate that contains mainly C_4–C_{12} aliphatic hydrocarbons. Some formulations contain an appreciable amount of aromatic hydrocarbons, and the toxicity of the gasoline is related to the benzene content. The boiling point range is from 40 to 255 °C. It is used as a fuel for motor vehicles with internal combustion engines, as well as a diluent and industrial solvent. Gasoline is an irritant of skin, conjunctiva and mucous membranes, and prolonged exposure can result in dermatitis from defatting of the skin, and blistering. The vapors act as CNS depressants. Possible symptoms include flushing of the face, stagger, confusion, slurred speech, unconsciousness, coma and even death. Acute exposures can also lead to vomiting, pancreatic hemorrhage, hepatic and renal degeneration, splenic congestion, hematopoietic changes, chemical pneumonitis, cyanosis and pulmonary edema. Its volatility and flammability make it a serious fire hazard. To increase the octane rating, tetraethyllead is sometimes added to gasoline, and this introduces the possibility of lead poisoning from repeated exposures. Gasoline is normally not a toxic hazard even to those occupationally exposed. Gasoline has been sniffed to produce euphoria. There is no evidence to date that gasoline causes cancer in humans. Long-term animal inhalation studies caused kidney tumors in male rats and liver tumors in female mice. The former have been attributed to a male rat specific mechanism involving the alpha 2u-globulin and are probably not relevant to human risk while the latter may be mediated via an estrogen-dependent mechanism. *See also* ATSDR DOCUMENT, JUNE 1995.

gastric. Pertaining to the stomach.

gastric gavage. *See* ADMINISTRATION OF TOXICANTS, ORAL.

gastric intubation. A technique for introducing toxicant or vehicle into an animal by injecting the material directly into the stomach using a rounded-tip intubation needle.

gastric lavage. The washing of the stomach usually with saline solutions via a lavage tube. It is used as a rapid method to remove stomach contents in poisoning cases, particularly in cases in which emesis is not recommended. Special precautions are taken in the case of corrosives, since the lavage tube may damage the esophagus, or, in the case of petroleum derivatives, when the trachea should be intubated with a tube having an inflatable cuff. In convulsing patients, the convulsions should first be controlled. Materials used for gastric lavage include milk (for corrosives or to retard uptake), lemon juice (for alkali poisoning), activated charcoal suspension, saline, sodium bicarbonate or milk of magnesia. Sodium bicarbonate is never given in the case of poisoning by acids since the carbon dioxide generated may damage the stomach. *See also* POISONING, EMERGENCY TREATMENT.

gastrointestinal. Pertaining to the digestive tract. In humans, this consists of the buccal cavity, esophagus, stomach, small intestine (duodenum, jejunum and ileum), large intestine (colon and rectum), with various associated glands and accessory structures. The gastrointestinal tract is important in toxicology as a major site of absorption of toxicants, as a site of xenobiotic metabolism and as a site of toxic action.

gastrointestinal penetration. *See* PENETRATION ROUTES, GASTROINTESTINAL.

gastrointestinal tract. *See* DIAGNOSTIC FEATURES, GASTROINTESTINAL TRACT.

Gastromet. *See* CIMETIDINE.

gastrotomy. An incision into the stomach. Its only use in clinical toxicology is for the removal of large amounts of solid toxic materials that, having formed a solid mass in the stomach, cannot be removed by gastric lavage or vomiting.

gavage. *See* ADMINISTRATION OF TOXICANTS, ORAL.

GB. *See* SARIN.

GC/MS. *See* SPECTROMETRY, MASS.

GD. *See* SOMAN.

gel filtration chromatography. *See* CHROMATOGRAPHY, GEL FILTRATION.

GEMS. *See* GRAPHICAL EXPOSURE MODELING SYSTEMS.

gene. A functional hereditary unit consisting of a sequence of DNA and occupying a specific locus within the genome. Most eukaryotic genes consist of coding regions (exons) interrupted by noncoding regions (introns). Genes contain not only the coding sequences for the production of specific proteins (via RNA intermediates) but sequences responsible for the control of gene expression. Chemical toxicity is often mediated through the modification of DNA, and hence genes, by reactive intermediates. *See also* GENOTOXICITY.

gene library (gene bank). Collection of cloned genes, frequently comprising most or all of the genes from a particular species. Such libraries may consist of genomic sequences or cDNA sequences, the latter having been made from messenger RNA and lacking intron sequences. Libraries are made by cutting purified DNA with selected restriction endonucleases, followed by the cloning of the fragments into viral or bacterial plasmid vectors. Gene libraries can be searched using a homologous sequence from a related organism in order to identify the clone within the library which represents the desired gene. *See also* NUCLEIC ACID HYBRIDIZATION. *Compare* GENOMIC LIBRARY.

gene mutation tests. *See IN VITRO* TOXICITY TESTS.

gene pool. The available genes within a population that could be acquired by individuals that are the reproductive offspring of the population. A larger gene pool yields greater diversity of traits within the population and therefore gives the population a better probability of withstanding toxic or other stress.

generally recognized as safe. *See* FOOD, DRUG AND COSMETIC ACT.

gene splicing. *See* RECOMBINANT DNA.

genes, transformation. *See* CELL TRANSFORMATION.

genetic code. Information for the synthesis of proteins coded in the structure of the DNA. The addition of a particular amino acid to a polypeptide chain is determined (coded) by a specific sequence(s) of three nucleotides (codons) in the DNA molecule. As 64 (i.e., $4 \times 4 \times 4$) codons are possible using the two purine and two pyrimidine bases and only 20 amino acids are used, each amino acid may be specified by more than one triplet. The initiation of protein synthesis is signaled by the codon AUG; in the middle of a message this codon also codes the introduction of a methionyl residue in the normal way. Termination is signaled by UAA, UAG or UGA. The genetic code is universal and is the basis of the hereditary information contained in nucleic acids.

genetic differences in xenobiotic metabolism. In the same way that differences in xenobiotic-metabolizing ability in different animal species are usually due to different enzymes and, therefore, different genetic constitutions, different strains within a species may also differ in their ability to metabolize xenobiotics. In this case, however, genetic crosses can be utilized to investigate the inheritance of the enzymes. *See also* CYTOCHROME P450, POLYMORPHISMS; GENETIC DIFFERENCES IN XENOBIOTIC METABOLISM, ENZYME DIFFERENCES; GENETIC DIFFERENCES IN XENOBIOTIC METABOLISM, *IN VIVO* TOXICITY; GENETIC DIFFERENCES IN XENOBIOTIC METABOLISM, METABOLITE PRODUCTION; POLYMORPHISMS.

genetic differences in xenobiotic metabolism, enzyme differences. Although differences are known to exist, the nature and amount of xenobiotic-metabolizing enzymes have only recently been extensively studied in different strains of the same vertebrate. Since resistance is often due to high oxidase activity, the differences in microsomal cytochrome P450 between insecticide-resistant and insecticide-susceptible strains of the housefly have been studied intensively, and there is strong evidence for both qualitative and quantitative differences between strains. At least four genes, three on chromosome II and one on chromosome V, are required to explain the spectral variations (presumably isozymes).

genetic differences in xenobiotic metabolism, *in vivo* toxicity. The toxicity of organic compounds has been found to vary between different strains of laboratory and other animals. For example, Harvard and wild Norway rats are 11 and 335 times, respectively, more resistant to thiourea than rats of the Hopkins strain. Another example is the development of strains of insects resistant to insecticides that is known to have occurred in over 200 species, the level of resistance being as high as several hundred-fold.

genetic differences in xenobiotic metabolism, metabolite production. Genetic differences may also be apparent in metabolite production. For example, strain variation in response to hexobarbital may depend upon its degradation rate. Male mice of the AL/N strain are long sleepers, a trait correlated with slow inactivation of the drug. CFW/N mice, on the other hand, have a short sleeping time correlated with rapid hexobarbital oxidation. Induction of the cytochrome P450 isozymes responsible for aryl hydrocarbon hydroxylase activity is controlled by a single gene locus: Ah^b represents the allele for responsiveness, Ah^d the allele for non-responsiveness. Phase II reactions may also show interstrain differences. The Gunn rat, a mutant strain of the Wistar rat, is characterized by a severe, genetically determined defect of bilirubin glucuronidation.

genetic predisposition. *See* PREDISPOSITION.

genetic toxicology. The study of adverse effects on the process of heredity. Studies of genetic toxicology have given rise to a number of testing procedures designed to assess the effects of chemicals on genetic mechanisms and the consequent risk to organisms, including humans. Of equal importance are studies of the mechanisms by which adverse genetic effects are mediated and epidemiological studies of the frequency of genetic effects relative to chemical exposure. *See also IN VITRO TOXICITY TESTS.*

Geneva Convention on Long-Range Transboundary Air Pollution. An international convention, drawn up under the auspices of the United Nations, in force since 1983. It calls for collaboration in research into air pollution and exchange of information among signatories regarding pollutants, especially new ones.

genitourinary system. *See* EXCRETION, RENAL.

genome. The complement of genes contained in the haploid set of chromosomes.

genomic library. DNA sequences of genomic origin, held in cloning vectors. It differs from a cDNA library since the latter contains only sequences complementary to mRNA, and therefore contains only DNA coding sequences without introns or regulatory sequences. *See also* GENE LIBRARY.

genotoxic. Having a specific adverse effect on the genome of living cells. *See also* GENOTOXICITY.

genotoxic carcinogen. *See* CARCINOGEN, GENOTOXIC.

genotoxicity. A specific adverse effect on the genome of living cells that, upon the duplication of the affected cells, can be expressed as a mutagenic or a carcinogenic event because of specific alteration of the molecular structure of the genome through translocation of proto-oncogenes. It results from a reaction with DNA that can be measured either biochemically or, in short-term tests, with endpoints that reflect on DNA damage.

genotoxicity tests. Screening tests for toxic effects on the genome. The ones most commonly used are tests for mutagenicity, the best known of which is the Ames test which utilizes reverse mutations in *Salmonella* as an endpoint. Other mutagenicity tests include the measurement of either forward or reverse mutations in the fungus *Neurospora* and forward mutations in a variety of human and other mammalian cell lines. Several tests for mutations are also carried out using intact animals, primarily either *Drosophila* or the mouse. In addition to mutagenicity tests there are several tests for effects at the chromosome level. They include tests for chromosome breaks, aneuploidy, sister chromatid exchange and for effects on DNA repair mechanisms.

genotype. The genetic composition of an individual.

gentamicin (gentamycin). **CAS number 1403-66-3**. An antibiotic complex that is formed from the fermentation of *Micromonospora purpurea* or *Micromonospora echinospora*. This complex is made up of gentamicins C1, C2, C1a (*O*-3-deoxy-4-C-methyl-3-(methylamino)-β-L-arabinopyranosyl-(1,6)-*O*-[2,6-diamino-2,3,4,6-tetradeoxy-α-D-erythro-hexopyranosyl-(1,4)]-2-deoxy-*d*-streptamine) and gentamicin A (*O*-2-amino-2-deoxy-α-D-glucopyranosyl-(1,4)-*O*-[3-deoxy-3-(methylamino)-α-D-xylopyranosyl-(1,6)] 2-deoxy-D-streptamine). Gentamicin is used in the treatment of serious gram-negative bacterial infections. Like other aminoglycosides, gentamicin can cause irreversible ototoxicity and even greater nephrotoxicity than other drugs in this class. *See also* AMINOGLYCOSIDES; ANTIMICROBIALS; ANTIBIOTICS.

Geomet. *See* PHORATE.

geosmin (*trans*-1,10-dimethyl-*trans*-9-decalol). Geosmin and other volatile compounds are produced by a variety of bacteria, cyanobacteria, algae and fungi. They are responsible for some of the odors of water supplies and food sources. Odor production is greatest when nutrient production and dissolved oxygen are high. *See also* ODOROUS COMPOUNDS, IN WATER.

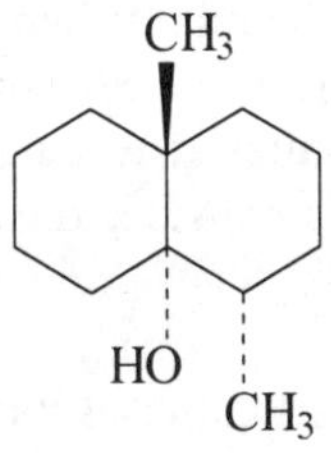

Geosmin

germanium (Ge). An element that has use in construction of infrared sensing and identification systems, the microelectronics industry and a few pharmaceuticals and cosmetics. The inorganic compounds of germanium are of relatively low toxicity, but some organic forms (e.g., trialkylgermanium compounds) are notably neurotoxic. Germanium forms compounds in the +2 and +4 oxidation states. Germanium(II) compounds are strongly reducing and convert readily to germanium(IV). The thermal decomposition of GeH_4 to germanium and hydrogen at 280 °C is used in the semi-conductor industry to lay down a thin film of germanium. Some alkyl and aryl germanium compounds are known.

germ cell. *See* GAMETE.

germ cell toxicity. The toxic effects on cells in the germ line (i.e., spermatozoa or their precursors, spermatids, spermatocytes or spermatogonia and ova or their precursors, secondary and primary oocytes and oogonia).

germ risk assessment assays. Tests that are specific for toxic effects on cells in the germ line, producing heritable defects. Such tests include the rodent-specific locus test, the heritable translocation test and the *Drosophila* sex-linked recessive lethal test.

Gesellschaft fur Versuchtierkunde, Society of Laboratory Animal Science (GV-SOLAS). A bilingual (German, English) society for the study of laboratory animal science, with a predominantly German-speaking membership in central Europe.

gestation. In mammals, the length of time from conception to birth.

gestation index. The number of live fetuses per litter relative to the total number of fetuses. *See also* REPRODUCTIVE TOXICITY TESTING.

GFR. *See* GLOMERULAR FILTRATION RATE.

G gas. *See* G AGENTS.

Gila monster. *Heloderma suspectum*, a venomous lizard of the southwestern United States and Mexico. Its venom is high in hyaluronidase and low in proteolytic enzymes.

gills. Respiratory structures in aquatic animals (both vertebrates and invertebrates). Gills possess a large surface area for extensive gas exchange. Some toxicants can alter gill structure, reducing available surface area. Other toxicants, such as petroleum, can physically occlude the gills, preventing gas exchange.

ginger jake. A form of illegal alcoholic drink, flavored with ginger extract, sold during prohibition in the USA. In the early 1930s, cases of delayed paralysis (ginger jake paralysis) were first reported due to the use of ginger extract contaminated with cresyl phosphates used in the extraction process. *See also* DELAYED NEUROPATHY; TOCP.

gingival hyperplasia. A proliferation of the epithelium and connective tissue of the gums associated with administration of the antiepileptic drug phenytoin. This toxic effect occurs in approximately 20% of patients receiving chronic administration of the drug and is the most frequently observed toxic sign in children and adolescents. The overgrowth of tissue is thought to be due to perturbations in collagen metabolism. Drug discontinuation is not required as this condition can be controlled with good oral hygiene. *See also* PHENYTOIN.

ginseng. A native American plant, *Panax quinquefolium*, of the family Araliaceae. The dried root of the plant is primarily exported to the orient where it is preferred, for medicinal purposes, to the oriental ginseng, *P. pseudoginseng*, although US consumption has recently increased. Has been used in traditional Chinese medicine for several millenia for cardiovascular problems, fatigue, anemia, cancer, etc. Ginseng contains several saponin glycosides, some of which appear to have an estrogenic-like effect. Chronic excessive consumption has caused hypertension, insomnia, skin eruptions and diarrhea.

GLC. *See* CHROMATOGRAPHY, GAS–LIQUID.

gliosis (astrogliosis, fibrillary gliosis). An increase in the number of non-neoplastic, glial filament-filled astrocytes within an area of the CNS or retina. The accumulation of glial filaments within astrocytes is usually preceded by proliferation (astrocytosis) and enlargement (hypertrophy) of the astrocytes. Gliosis is a common response of neural tissue to acute or chronic injury.

Global 2000 Report to the President. A report drawn up in 1980 by the Council on Environmental Quality and the Department of State at the request of US President Carter. It maintained that severe problems would arise from pollution, resource depletion and the extinction of species unless steps were taken urgently to prevent them.

Global Environment Monitoring System (GEMS). The organization established by the United Nations Environment Program as part of Earthwatch to acquire monitoring data needed for the rational program environmental management. GEMS monitors changes in climate, renewable resources, human health, the long-range transport of pollutants and the oceans.

globefish. *See* PUFFERFISH.

glomerular filtration. *See* EXCRETION, RENAL.

glomerular filtration rate (GFR). The rate (volume per unit time) at which glomerular ultrafiltrate is formed in the kidney tubules (Bowman's capsules) from the glomerular capillaries. The normal rate in adult humans is 115–125 ml/min. The GFR is regulated by the sympathetic nervous system and by renal autoregulation. Measurement of the GFR to test for kidney function can be accomplished by measuring the excretion of inulin, a fructose polymer, which is filtered by the glomeruli, but which is not subject to tubular reabsorption.

glomerulus. The capillary bed in the nephron. The functional unit of the vertebrate kidney, from which the blood is filtered as the glomerular filtrate into the Bowman's capsule, the initial portion of the kidney tubule.

GLP. *See* GOOD LABORATORY PRACTICES.

glucagon. CAS number 9007-92-5. A straight-chain polypeptide (29 amino acid residues) hormone secreted by the α-cells of the pancreatic islets of Langerhans that causes the catabolism of glycogen with a subsequent increase in blood glucose. It acts via cyclic AMP by a cascade mechanism to ultimately activate phosphorylase. Glucagon secretion is elicited by hypoglycemia or exercise, thus, it antagonizes effects of insulin.

glucose tolerance test. A clinical test for diabetes or hypoglycemia in which the subject ingests or receives an i.v. injection of a glucose solution and the concentration of glucose in the blood is subsequently monitored.

glucoside formation. Glucosides of xenobiotics are uncommon in vertebrates, but are common in both insects and plants. Formed from uridine diphosphate glucose, similar to the glucuronides, they occur as *N*-, *O*- and *S*-derivatives. *See also* GLYCOSIDE CONJUGATION; PHASE II REACTIONS.

β-glucuronidase. An enzyme that hydrolyzes glucuronides in the β-configuration, the configuration characteristic of the glucuronides of xenobiotics. It occurs in the intestinal microflora and is involved in enterohepatic recirculation of xenobiotics excreted as glucuronides in the bile. β-Glucuronidase also occurs in lysosomes and is used as a marker enzyme for this fraction by means of an assay utilizing *p*-nitrophenyl β-glucuronide as a substrate. *See also* ENTEROHEPATIC CIRCULATION.

N-glucuronide. A glucuronic acid conjugate (glycone) formed from the UDP-glucuronosyltransferase catalyzed reaction of UDPGA with xenobiotics containing a nitrogen-containing functional group such as aromatic amino groups, sulfoamide groups, carbamyl groups, heterocyclic nitrogen atoms or aliphatic tertiary amines. The mechanism involves transfer of the glucuronyl moiety from uridine diphosphate glucuronic acid to the acceptor, forming a *N*-glucuronide. *See also* URIDINE DIPHOSPHATE GLUCURONIC ACID.

O-glucuronide. A glucuronic acid conjugate formed from the UDP-glucuronosyltransferase catalyzed reaction of UDPGA with xenobiotics containing an alcohol or acid functional group. They include the following: (1) ether type, formed from phenolic compounds, primary, secondary or tertiary alcohols; (2) ester type, formed from carboxylic acids; (3) enol type, formed from pseudo acids (i.e., 4-hydroxycoumarin, pK_a = 5.8); (4) hydroxylamino types. *See also* URIDINE DIPHOSPHATE GLUCURONIC ACID.

S-glucuronide. A glucuronic acid conjugate formed from the UDP-glucuronosyltransferase catalyzed reaction of uridine diphosphate glucuronic acid with xenobiotics containing a thiol functional group including thiols and dithioic acids such as thiophenol, 2-mercaptobenzothiazole and disulfiram (Antabuse). *See also* URIDINE DIPHOSPHATE GLUCURONIC ACID.

glucuronide formation. The reaction of uridine diphosphate glucuronic acid (UDPGA) with an aglycone, in many cases, a xenobiotic. The reaction is a nucleophilic displacement (SN2 reaction) of the functional group of the substrate. Although UDPGA is in the α-configuration, the glucuronide formed is in the β-configuration due to the accompanying Walden inversion. The enzyme involved, glucuronosyltransferase, occurs in the microsomal fraction of liver, kidney and other tissues, and appears to exist as a family of closely related isozymes. Homogeneous glucuronosyltransferase exists as a single polypeptide chain of about 59,000 daltons, apparently containing carbohydrate, that requires microsomal lipid for maximum activity. There appears to be an absolute requirement for UDPGA, related UDP-sugars will not suffice. A wide variety of reactions are mediated by glucuronosyltransferases. *O*-Glucuronides, *N*-glucuronides and *S*-glucuronides have all been identified. *See also* GLYCOSIDE CONJUGATION; *N*-GLUCURONIDE; *O*-GLUCURONIDE; *S*-GLUCURONIDE; PHASE II REACTIONS; URIDINE DIPHOSPHATE GLUCURONIC ACID.

glucuronosyltransferase. *See* GLUCURONIDE FORMATION.

glue sniffing. The practice of inhaling the vapors of glue, presumably for their CNS effects. Although there may be multiple solvents in glue, the alkylbenzene toluene is usually a major constituent. Even at low concentrations, toluene produces fatigue, weakness and confusion. Inhaled alkylbenzenes cause acute toxicity in animals, the LC50 in mice, for example, being 5320 ppm/8 hr. Acidosis, potentially due to acidic metabolites of toluene, has been reported in humans abusing glue solvents. Inhalation of the vapors of glue containing benzene or hexane may result in hematological effects or peripheral neuropathies. *See also* TOLUENE.

glutamate (monosodium glutamate, MSG). CAS number 142-47-2. An excitatory amino acid neurotransmitter. It has been demonstrated that neonatal animals are sensitive to large doses of glutamate, which cause permanent lesions of the hypothalamus, resulting in profound neuroendocrine deficits. Toxicity presumably involves increased availability of glutamate due to an immaturity of the blood–brain barrier or removal mechanisms, followed by death of neurons due to prolonged excitatory stimulation. Infantile mice are also reported to have retinopathies after large doses of glutamate. Some humans are sensitive to ingestion of large amounts of glutamate added as a food flavor enhancer and experience headaches or "Chinese restaurant syndrome." *See also* CHINESE RESTAURANT SYNDROME; EXCITATORY AMINO ACIDS.

Glutamate (Monosodium glutamate)

glutamic acid. *See* GLUTAMATE.

glutamic acid decarboxylase (GAD; E.C. 3.1.1.15). An enzyme that is responsible for converting glutamic acid to the inhibitory neurotransmitter, γ-aminobutyric acid (GABA). GAD has a molecular weight of 85,000 and requires pyridoxal phosphate (vitamin B_6) as a cofactor. The K_m for glutamic acid is 0.7 mM and 0.05 mM for the cofactor. Inhibitors of the enzyme have been shown to have convulsant properties. Immunocytochemical methods for localization of GAD have been used to identify GABA-ergic neurons. In addition to mapping GABA-ergic neurons, a significant reduction in GAD activity in substantia nigra and globus pallidus has been reported in Huntington's disease. *See also* γ-AMINOBUTYRIC ACID TRANSAMINASE; GABA.

glutamic-oxaloacetic transaminase. *See* LIVER ENZYMES, IN BLOOD.

glutamic-pyruvic transaminase. *See* LIVER ENZYMES, IN BLOOD.

glutamine conjugation. An uncommon form of amino acid conjugation seen in humans and certain other primates. *See also* AMINO ACID CONJUGATION; PHASE II REACTIONS

γ-glutamyl transpeptidase. A membrane-bound glycoprotein necessary for the formation of mercapturic acids from glutathione conjugates. It has been purified from human and rat liver and from the kidney of several species. The kidney enzyme has a molecular weight of 68,000–90,000 daltons, and the enzyme consists of two unequal subunits; the different forms appear to differ in the degree of sialylation. This enzyme has a number of acceptor amino acids and catalyzes three reactions. *See also* ACETYLATION; CYSTEINYL GLYCINASE; GLUTATHIONE TRANSFERASES; MERCAPTURIC ACIDS.

Hydrolysis

γ–Glu —X + H_2O ⟶ γ–Glu + HX

Transpeptidation

γ–Glu —X + acceptor ⟶ gluc-acceptor + HX

γ–Glu–X + γ–Glu— X ⟶ γ–Glu–γ–Glu — X + HX

γ-glutamyl transpeptidase

glutathione. CAS number 70-18-8. A tripeptide of glycine, cysteine and glutamic acid with the γ-carboxyl group of glutamine being involved in the peptide bond with glycine. It is involved in many reactions in which the nucleophilic sulfhydryl group reacts with electrophilic groups, generally in reactions mediated by glutathione-*S*-transferase. Since the monooxygenation of xenobiotics often leads to reactive electrophilic intermediates, this is an important reaction in the detoxication of these potentially toxic products. It is the first in a series of reactions leading to mercapturic acids. *See also* GLUTATHIONE TRANSFERASES; MERCAPTURIC ACIDS.

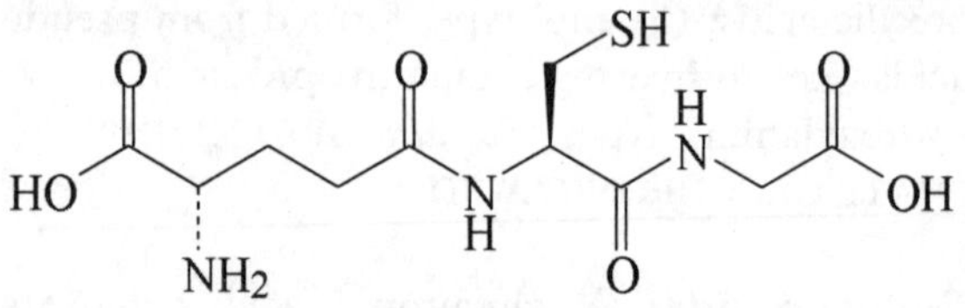

Glutathione

glutathione, and oxidative damage. Glutathione is involved in protection from oxidative damage in several ways. For example, superoxide anion may be metabolized to hydrogen peroxide by superoxide dismutase. The hydrogen peroxide may then be further metabolized to water by glutathione peroxidase, a reaction involving the oxidation of glutathione. Glutathione is also involved in the detoxication of peroxidase-generated free radicals of organic compounds. *See also* OXIDATIVE STRESS.

glutathione, and reactive metabolites. *See* GLUTATHIONE; GLUTATHIONE TRANSFERASES.

glutathione transferases. Enzymes that catalyze the conjugation of xenobiotics having electrophilic substituents with glutathione. If a mercapturic acid is to be formed, this is followed by transfer of the glutamate to an acceptor amino acid by γ-glutamyl transpeptidase, then by the loss of glycine via cysteinyl glycinase and finally by acetylation of the cysteine amino group. The glutathione *S*-transferase reaction is extremely important in toxicology since it protects vital nucleophilic groups in macromolecules such as proteins and nucleic acids by removing reactive electrophiles. The mercapturic acids formed are excreted either in the bile or urine. The glutathione transferases are a family of isozymes found in essentially all groups of living organisms. Found primarily in the soluble fraction of mammalian liver, they also occur in microsomes. All forms appear to be highly specific for glutathione, but non-specific with respect to the xenobiotic substrate, although the relative rates for different substrates can vary between isozymes. The types of reactions catalyzed are: alkyl transferase; aryl transferase; aralkyl transferase; alkene transferase; epoxide transferase. The presence of multiple forms of glutathione transferase has been demonstrated in the liver of rat, mouse and human; they also occur in insects. The various isozymes have molecular weights in the range 45,000–50,000 daltons, and each consists of two subunits. They are usually identified and named from their chromatographic behavior. One of them, form B, appears to be identical to the binding protein ligandin. *See also* ACETYLATION; CYSTEINYL GLUCINASE; γ-GLUTAMYL TRANS-PEPTIDASE; MERCAPTURIC ACIDS.

gluten, wheat. A condition called celiac sprue or gluten-induced enteropathy is seen in susceptible individuals consuming gluten. Ingestion of gluten causes flattening of the mucosal surface and infiltration of the epithelial layer and lamina propria with inflammatory cells. This leads to malabsorption and a syndrome characterized by diarrhea, steatorrhea, bloating and weight loss. The gluten is believed to cause these effects both by direct toxic effects on the mucosa of susceptible individuals and by activation of immunological responses. A gluten-free diet causes significant improvement.

gluten-induced enteropathy. *See* GLUTEN, WHEAT.

glutethimide (3-ethyl-3-phenyl-2,6-piperidine-dione; 2-ethyl-2-phenylglutarimide; Doriden). **CAS number 77-21-4**. Glutethimide, and a structurally similar compound methyprylon, has been used occasionally as a sedative-hypnotic, although glutethimide's use for longer than three days is not recommended. Glutethimide causes a skin rash in nearly 10% of those using it, and although it was once thought to produce less respiratory depression than the barbiturates its overdose fatality record is not good. Much of the drug's action can

be attributed to 4-hydroxyglutethimide, which is more than twice as potent and has a long half-life. Like many other sedative-hypnotics, abrupt withdrawal after chronic use or abuse resembles that of ethanol or the barbiturates and must be managed accordingly. *See also* METHYPRYLON; SEDATIVE-HYPNOTICS.

Glutethimide

glycine conjugation. *See* AMINO ACID CONJUGATION; PHASE II REACTIONS.

glycol ethers. A class of aliphatic compounds containing both a hydroxyl group (-OH) and an ether (-C-O-C-) linkage (e.g., ethylene glycol monomethyl ether, $HOCH_2CH_2OCH_3$). Widely used as solvents, they are miscible with water and organic solvents. Glycol ethers are not toxic acutely, but toxicity of some members of the series has been noted in both humans and animals.

glycols. *See* ALCOHOLS, POLYHYDROXY.

glycoprotein. *See* P-GLYCOPROTEIN.

glycoside conjugation. A phase II reaction; the formation of a water-soluble conjugate of a sugar with a xenobiotic having an appropriate substituent group. Such compounds are often the product of phase I reactions. The two reactions of importance in toxicology are glucuronide formation and glucoside formation. An activated intermediate, either uridine diphosphate glucose (UDPG) or uridine diphosphate glucuronic acid (UDPGA), is required for these reactions. The enzymes involved in these syntheses occur in the soluble fraction of the liver and other organs, as illustrated. *See also* GLUCOSIDE FORMATION; GLUCURONIDE FORMATION; URIDINE DIPHOSPHATE GLUCOSE; URIDINE DIPHOSPHATE GLUCURONIC ACID.

Uridine triphosphate (UTP) + glucose-1-phosphate $\xrightarrow[\textit{Pyrophosphorylase}]{\textit{UDPG}}$

Uridine diphosphate glucose (UDPG) + pyrophosphate

$$UDPG + 2NAD^+ + H_2O \xrightarrow[\textit{Dehydrogenase}]{\textit{UDPG}}$$

Uridine diphosphate glucuronic acid (UDPGA) + 2NADH$_2$

UDPGA formation

glycosuria. An excess of glucose in the urine indicating that the blood levels of glucose have exceeded the renal threshold and that more glucose is entering the glomerular filtrate than can be reabsorbed by the renal tubule. Because of the osmotic effect of glucose, excess water loss in the urine occurs. This is a common symptom in uncontrolled diabetes mellitus and is an effect of diabetagenic chemicals.

glycosylase. An enzyme which recognizes and removes physically or chemically modified bases (e.g., alkyl purines) from the sugar phosphate DNA chain leaving behind a hole (an abasic site).

GMP. *See* CYCLIC GMP.

gonad. The ovary or the testis; the sex organ that produces both gametes and sex hormones. It is the target of many toxicants that adversely affect reproduction.

gonadal. Pertaining to the gonads. *See also* GONAD.

gonadal toxicology. *See* REPRODUCTIVE TOXICITY.

good laboratory practices (GLP). Laws and regulations governing good laboratory practices are in effect in both the USA and OECD. They cover all phases of toxicity testing, including facilities, personnel training, data gathering, laboratory inspections, animal health and welfare, chemical analysis and sample preparation. Experiments conducted to generate data for regulatory purposes must be carried out in conformation with good laboratory practices as laid down by the appropriate regulatory agency.

gossypol (1,1′,6,6′,7,7′-hexalydroxy-3,3′-dimethyl-5,5′-bis(1-methylethyl) [2,2′-binaphthalene]-8,8′-dicarboxaldehyde). **CAS number 303-45-7**. A secondary plant product produced by some varieties of cotton and found in cottonseed meal and cottonseed oil from those varieties. Affects the male reproductive system and has potential use as a male contraceptive agent. May be irritating to the GI tract. In animal studies large doses caused lung edema and paralysis.

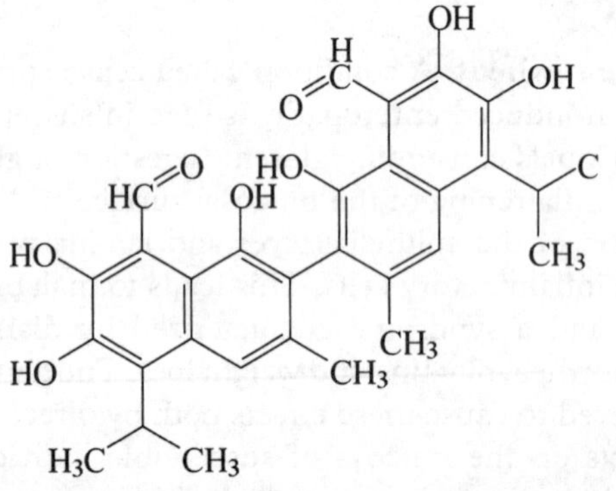

Gossypol

G-protein-coupled receptors (GPCRs). A large superfamily of extracellular receptors that often are 400–600 amino acids in length, contain seven transmembrane spanning regions, and often have a ligand-binding dopamine in a hydrophilic pocket formed by a circle of the transmembrane regions. These receptors couple to specific G-proteins, and activate them after binding a ligand. There are more than 200 known GPCRs for neurotransmitters and hormones, as well as more than 1000 different odorant receptors of this class. This class of proteins is an important target for toxicants including morphine, atropine, LSD, muscarine, etc. *See also* DOPAMINE RECEPTORS; G-PROTEINS; MUSCARINIC RECEPTORS; OPIOIDS.

G-proteins (guanine nucleotide-binding proteins). A series of heterotrimeric proteins consisting of three subunits: α, β and γ. The α subunit has a binding site for the guanine nucleotides GTP and GDP, as well as GTPase enzymatic activity. G-proteins bind to members of a receptor superfamily called the G-protein coupled receptors. When these receptors are activated, the G-protein dimerizes into its α, β and γ subunits, each of which can modulate numerous intracellular events. There are dozens of individual G-protein subunits expressed in cells that can have both stimulatory and inhibitory effects on target enzymes. They serve important regulatory roles in cells and were first characterized as the regulatory proteins involved in the coupling of hormone or neurotransmitter receptors to adenylate cyclase. It is now known that many variants of these proteins exist, that they serve wider roles as intracellular messengers and that they may be tissue-specific. Several of the G-proteins are known to be the site of action of certain toxicants such as pertussis or cholera toxin. In addition to these intercellular messengers, there is a large and important superfamily of structurally different intracellular G-proteins, related to tyrosine kinases, that are important regulators of gene expression and cell cycle regulation. *See also* ADENYLATE CYCLASE; CHOLERA TOXIN; PERTUSSIS TOXIN.

gramicidins. *See* ANTIBIOTICS; OXIDATIVE PHOSPHORYLATION INHIBITORS.

granulocytopenia. *See* AGRANULOCYTOSIS.

Granutox. *See* PHORATE.

Graphical Exposure Modeling System (GEMS). A composure model of exposure that integrates several discrete tools, such as environmental fate and transport models, chemical property estimation models and statistical methods, into a single interactive model. Developed by the US Environmental Protection Agency for use in regulatory toxicology.

GRAS (Generally Recognized as Safe). *See* FOOD, DRUG AND COSMETIC ACT.

Graves' disease. *See* THYROID GLAND TOXICITY.

grayanotoxins (andromedotoxin; rhodotoxin; dodecahydro-1,1,4a,8a-tetramethyl-7,9aa H-cyclopenta[b]heptalene-2,4,8,11,11-aa,12(1H)-hexol-12-acetate (GTX-I); GTX-II; GTX-III). Grayanotoxins are found in the leaves and flowers of plants of the Ericaceae family, such as rhododendron (*Rhododendron maximum*) and mountain laurel (*Kalmia latifolia*). Three toxic components exist: GTX-I, GTX-II and GTX-III. GTX-I and GTX-III are most potent with the LD50s in male mice of 1.28 and 0.91 mg/kg, i.p., respectively. The complex actions arise from a reversible increase in membrane permeability to Na^+, resulting in depolarization, which can be blocked by tetrodotoxin. This mechanism is the basis of the membrane depolarization in squid axon, the positive inotropic effect in mammalian myocardium and may involve the Na^+/Ca^{2+} exchange system. Grayanotoxins affect both cardiovascular and respiratory systems. Symptoms include a burning sensation in the mouth and pharynx, anoxia, salivation, emesis, muscular weakness, dimness of vision and bradycardia followed by severe hypotension, respiratory paralysis, coma and death. Therapy in acute poisoning consists of supportive care with oxygen, external application of heat and nikethamide. Cardiovascular effects respond to sympathomimetic amines, whereas the bradycardia is refractory to atropine. Gastric lavage is suggested if spontaneous emesis does not occur.

	R_1	R_2	R_3
Grayanotoxin I	OH	CH_3	$COCH_3$
Grayanotoxin III	OH	CH_3	H
Grayanotoxin II	CH_2	CH_2	H

greenhouse effect. A possible warming of the Earth's surface from an accumulation of carbon dioxide and other so-called greenhouse gases in the atmosphere as a result of the increased burning of fossil fuels. Atmospheric carbon dioxide is presumed to better insulate the Earth and to prevent heat loss from the surface. A possible ramification could be partial melting of the polar ice caps, with a resulting rise in ocean levels.

green technology. A colloquialism referring to processes which are less likely than traditional technology to pollute or otherwise harm the environment.

griseofulvin ((2S-trans)-7-chloro-2′,4,6-trimethoxy-6′-methylspiro[benzofuran-2(3H),1′[2] cyclohexene]-3,4-dione). CAS number 126-07-8. An antifungal agent produced by *Penicillium* strains that has a low acute toxicity (the oral LD50 in rodents is greater than 10 g/kg). It is used as a fungistatic drug in humans and is also used to control fungal diseases agriculturally. Typical minor side effects in humans include headache and gastrointestinal distress. Experimental studies in rats have resulted in liver cell necrosis and other hepatic aberrations, as well as teratogenicity (since it acts as a spindle poison) and carcinogenicity.

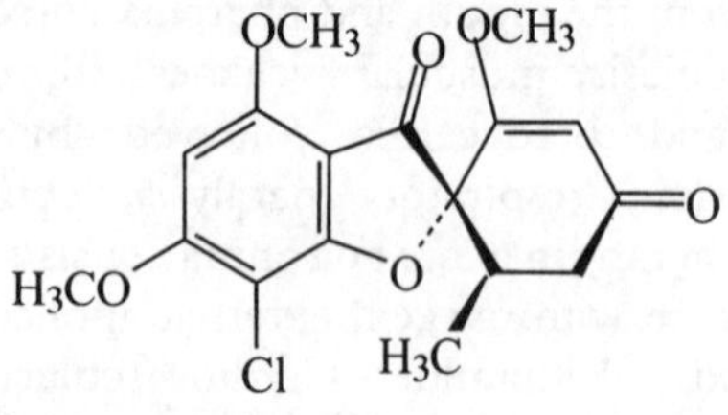

Griseofulvin

ground water (spring water; well water). Water below the surface of the ground, which is under pressure greater than atmospheric pressure. It is water below the water table, in the zone of saturation where it fills all intergranular pores in soil or rock or in the fractures within rock. Contamination of ground water with such toxicants as insecticides or nitrate is currently a cause for concern. Ground water below sandy soils, which do not readily absorb toxicants, is more likely to become contaminated than water below soils with a high clay or organic matter content.

growth. Growth of an organism includes both increase in size, usually expressed as body weight, and development or progress towards the mature form (differentiation). In the immature organism, from birth to puberty, these two processes

normally occur together, although either one can occur in the absence of the other. In the mature animal, increases in size can occur in the absence of development. In reproductive toxicity testing, growth is often used to refer to increase in size only.

growth hormone (somatotropin). A protein hormone produced by the adenohypophysis (anterior pituitary) in response to the hypothalamic hormone growth hormone-releasing hormone. It promotes a number of metabolic pathways that favor growth, and it causes prepubertal elongation of long bones and also bone elongation. Deficiencies in growth hormone result in dwarfism, in which individuals fail to achieve their genetically dictated height. Therapy with growth hormone prior to epiphyseal closure at puberty will allow the person to achieve normal or near normal height. Excess growth hormone before puberty causes gigantism and after puberty, acromegaly.

growth index. An expression of growth used in reproductive toxicity testing; the body weight of the offspring at preselected intervals (e.g., in rodents at birth and at 4, 7, 14 and 21 days postpartum). It is an expression of weight gain only, not including development. *See also* FERTILITY INDEX; REPRODUCTIVE TOXICITY TESTING; SEX RATIO; VIABILITY INDEX; WEANING INDEX.

growth rate, in chronic toxicity testing. *See* TOXIC ENDPOINTS.

growth rate, in subchronic toxicity testing. *See* TOXIC ENDPOINTS.

GTX. *See* GRAYANOTOXINS.

guanine nucleotide-binding proteins. *See* G-PROTEINS.

guanosine-3′,5′-cyclic monophosphate. *See* CYCLIC GMP.

guanylate cyclase (guanyl cyclase). The enzyme that synthesizes cyclic GMP from GTP. Because cyclic GMP can act as a second messenger, this enzyme has a potentially important regulatory role. In a few well-characterized systems, the enzyme has been shown to be linked to a polymeric complex with a hormone or neurotransmitter receptor. However, despite the very high concentrations of cyclic GMP in most cells, the regulation and physiological significance of this enzyme is not as well characterized as that of adenylate cyclase. Some toxicants (e.g., nitroprusside) can directly cause large increases in the activity of the enzyme. *See also* ADENYLATE CYCLASE; SECOND MESSENGERS.

guanyl cyclase. *See* GUANYLATE CYCLASE.

Guide for Laboratory Animal Facilities and Care. The original name (1963, 1965 and 1968 editions) of the US Public Health Service publication, called since 1972 the "Guide for the Care and Use of Laboratory Animals". *See also* GUIDE FOR THE CARE AND USE OF LABORATORY ANIMALS.

Guide for the Care and Use of Laboratory Animals (The Guide). A booklet issued by the Division of Research Resources, National Institutes of Health, US Public Health Service (PHS). The booklet is prepared by the Committee on the Care and Use of Laboratory Animals of the Institute of Laboratory Animal Resources, National Research Council. Publication is authorized by the Health Research Extension Act of 1985 (PL 99–158). The Guide was published in 1963, 1965 and 1968 as the "Guide for Laboratory Animal Facilities and Care". Editions under the present title followed in 1972, 1978 and 1985. The Guide assists institutions in caring for and using laboratory animals (including large, domestic species) in ways that are professionally and humanely appropriate. The PHS requires institutions to use The Guide as a basis for developing and implementing programs and activities involving animals. Topics covered include institutional policies, husbandry, veterinary care, physical plant and hazardous agent usage.

Guidelines for Reproductive Studies for Safety Evaluation of Drugs for Human Use. A publication of the Food and Drug Administration published in 1966. *See also* REPRODUCTIVE TOXICITY TESTING; TERATOLOGY TESTING.

guinea pig (cavy; *Cavia procellus*). A hystricomorph rodent of South American origin. Caviidae have reduced tails, capacious ceca, one pair of mammary glands and three or four digits. Hair coat varieties include one, two or three colors, the English or short-haired Duncan-Hartley and Hartley outbred and inbred (2 and 13) strains, the Abyssinian pattern of hair whorls and the long-haired Peruvian. Guinea pigs are gregarious, herbivorous, coprophagus and crepuscular, and are fastidious eaters. They lack the hepatic enzyme *l*-gulonolactone oxidase and are therefore dependent on dietary vitamin C. They have open-rooted teeth, a subcutaneous thymus, a vaginal closure membrane, precocious young and a relative resistance to the effects of steroids. They are used for studies of antigen-induced respiratory anaphylaxis, delayed hypersensitivity, immunology (and as a complement source), the ear, infectious diseases, nutrition, optic neuropathies, ulcerative colitis and antibiotic effects on intestinal flora. Respiratory and intestinal diseases are common. Neoplasia is rare.

guinea pig, in skin testing. *See* DERMAL SENSITIZATION TESTS; DERMAL TOXICITY TESTS; GUINEA PIG.

guinea pig ileum test. A technique to measure the effect of chemicals on contractility of smooth muscle of the gastrointestinal tract. A segment of isolated ileum is mounted in an organ bath and bathed in Tyrode's solution in such a way as to permit measurement of contraction. Test compounds are added to the bath and can be removed by washing. Typically the concentration is varied so as to permit the determination of the ED50 of the added chemical. *See also* GUINEA PIG.

Gulf War Syndrome. A complex set of neuromuscular, psychological, reproductive and other symptoms reported by US veterans of the Gulf War. To date there has been no consistent explanation of the potential cause although most theories involve synergistic effects between various chemicals to which US troops were exposed, either deliberately for prophylactic or therapeutic reasons or accidentally in the course of destroying Iraqi facilities containing nerve gases. Chemicals in the first category include pyridostigmine bromide, the insecticide chlorpyrifos and the insect repellent DEET, while sarin is believed to be a component of the second category, perhaps the only one. A further complication is the known exposure of troops to additional adverse environmental effects including burning oil wells and

petroleum products. Despite some preliminary evidence there is little to confirm or deny any of the hypotheses based on chemical exposure.

gut. *See* GASTROINTESTINAL; DIAGNOSTIC FEATURES, GASTROINTESTINAL TRACT.

H

Haber's rule. Where C is the concentration and T is the time, then the product K (toxic effect) is constant.

$$C \cdot T = K$$

Haber's rule is applied to gaseous toxicants and is approximated in many, but not all, cases.

haem. *See* HEME.

HAL. *See* HEALTH ADVISORY LEVEL—DRINKING WATER.

half-life. The period of time necessary for one-half of a substance to disappear. In toxicology this may refer to such phenomena as the disappearance of a toxicant from the blood stream or from the body or the time necessary for one-half of the total amount of a toxicant to be metabolized or to penetrate the skin. It is a particularly important value since the rate of such events is seldom linear with time. The time for completion is almost impossible to determine with accuracy, and often the mathematical relationship is so complex that accurate extrapolation is impossible. In these circumstances the half-life $(T_{0.5})$ is frequently the best standard for comparison between chemicals or between different experimental conditions.

hallucinations. *See* DIAGNOSTIC FEATURES, CENTRAL NERVOUS SYSTEM; HALLUCINOGENS.

hallucinogens (psychedelic agents; psychotomimetic agents). Compounds that produce changes in thought, perception and mood, without causing major disturbances in the autonomic nervous system. Stupor, narcosis or excessive stimulation is not an integral part of the action. Drugs such as LSD, mescaline and psilocybin are considered to be classical representatives of the action of this class of drugs. *See also* AMPHETAMINE; BOD; DMT; LSD; MESCALINE; PSILOCYBIN.

halogenated hydrocarbons. A very general term including any aliphatic or aromatic hydrocarbon in which one or more of the hydrogen atoms is substituted by any of the halogens. Within this group of compounds are substituted alkanes and alkenes, many of which are used as industrial solvents, pesticides, chemical intermediates and anesthetics. The group also includes a number of carcinogens (e.g., vinyl chloride, dichloroethane), hepatotoxicants (e.g., carbon tetrachloride), nephrotoxicants (e.g., chloroform) and immunotoxicants (e.g., polychlorinated biphenyls, TCDD).

haloperidol. *See* BUTYROPHENONES.

halothane (2-bromo-2-chloro-1,1,1-trifluoroethane). CAS number 151-67-7. A fairly high-potency, non-flammable, extremely lipid-soluble inhalational anesthetic. It is frequently used with i.v. thiopental for induction followed by halothane for maintenance of anesthesia. It is popular because it permits easy change of the depth of anesthesia, a rapid awakening when administration is ceased and a relatively low incidence of toxic side effects. Relaxation of skeletal muscles is frequently needed in surgical procedures. Halothane causes some muscle relaxation through central mechanisms and also increases the duration and magnitude of relaxation provided by agents such as *d*-tubocurarine. The margin of safety with halothane is not large, however, because of profound reductions in blood pressure that halothane may cause. This hypotension is a result of direct effects on the myocardium (resulting in decreased cardiac output) and a reduction in baroreceptor-mediated tachycardia. Another effect sometimes seen with halothane is tachyar-rhythmias, some of these being of the re-entrant type. Adequate ventilation and the absence of car-diac disease, hypoxia or acidosis or electrolyte imbalance will effectively prevent this side effect. A rare side effect of halothane and related anesthet-ics is malignant hyperpyrexia. It is characterized by a rapid rise in body temperature and increase in oxygen consumption, frequently leading to death. Malignant hyperpyrexia is believed to be mediated in muscles. It appears that the occurrence of malignant hyperpyrexia is related to a pre-existing muscle defect. Halothane hepatitis may also be caused by other potent inhalation agents. It occurs very infrequently, but when it does, begins with fever, anorexia and vomiting starting two to five days after surgery. This is subsequently followed by other signs characteristic of hepatitis, and fre-quently results in liver failure and death. Normally about 80% of absorbed halothane is eliminated unchanged in exhaled air. About 15% is biotrans-formed, and these products have been implicated in halothane hepatitis. Although halothane pro-vides sleep, agents to cause additional muscle relaxation and suppression of visceral responses are often also needed during halothane anesthesia. Halothane does not cause much analgesia, and other drugs (such as opiates or nitrous oxide) are used for this purpose.

$$F-\underset{\underset{F}{|}}{\overset{\overset{F}{|}}{C}}-\underset{\underset{H}{|}}{\overset{\overset{Cl}{|}}{C}}-Br$$

Halothane

halothane hepatitis. *See* HALOTHANE.

haploid. The condition of having half the normal diploid number of chromosomes. In vertebrates and many other animals the haploid condition is characteristic of germ cells, whereas the diploid condition is characteristic of all other cells, includ-ing both mature somatic cells as well as undifferen-tiated embryonic cells. In certain insects the males are haploid, whereas the females are diploid. *Com-pare* DIPLOID.

hapten. *See* ANTIGEN.

hashish. *See* CANNABIS SATIVA.

hazard. The qualitative description of the adverse effect resulting from a particular toxic chemical, physical effect or inappropriate action without regard to dose or exposure. For example, carcino-genesis is a hazard, as is asphyxiation. *See also* HAZARD CONTROL; HAZARD IDENTIFICATION; RISK.

hazard control. The elimination of the exposure of humans or animals to the causes of hazard. This is of particular concern in the industrial setting or in animal facilities. Such control may involve new handling protocols, substitution of less hazardous material for material whose hazard has been iden-tified or physical modification of facilities. A more appropriate concept is that of risk management, risk being the probability of harm under defined exposure conditions. *See also* HAZARD; HAZARD IDENTIFICATION; RISK MANAGEMENT.

hazard identification. The qualitative determi-nation of whether exposure to a chemical causes an increased incidence of an adverse effect (e.g., cancer, birth defects) in a population of test ani-mals and an evaluation of the relevance of this information to the potential of the chemical for causing similar effects in humans. It involves char-acterizing the nature and strength of all available evidence relating to the causation of the adverse effect. This is considered to be the first step in the process of risk assessment. *See also* RISK ASSESS-MENT.

Hazardous Materials Transportation Act. Legislation, in the USA, that governs the move-ment of hazardous materials in commerce. The Act is administered by the Department of Trans-portation.

Hazardous Substances Act. *See* FEDERAL HAZ-ARDOUS SUBSTANCES ACT.

hazardous waste. Any material that, if improp-erly disposed, can harm health or the environ-ment. Hazardous wastes are defined by the Resource Conservation and Recovery Act and are divided into two groups: listed wastes and charac-teristic wastes. Over 400 specific compounds or waste streams are identified as hazardous wastes by the US EPA. These are referred to as listed wastes. If a solid waste is not a listed waste, it must be tested to determine if it is a hazardous waste. If upon testing, the waste material demonstrates the characteristic of ignitability, corrosivity, reactivity or EP toxicity, the waste is a hazardous waste. The definitions and listings of hazardous wastes can be found in the US Federal Register 40 CFR, Part 261. *See also* RESOURCE CONSERVATION AND RECOVERY ACT.

Hb. *See* HEMOGLOBIN.

HC-3. *See* HEMICHOLINIUM-3.

γ-HCH (1,2,3,4,5,6-hexachlorocyclohexane; γ-BHC; γ-benzene hexachloride; Lindane). CAS number 58-89-9. Lindane is HCH in which the γ-isomer content is more than 99%. γ-HCH is the main insecticidal component of HCH. It acts as a stomach poison, by contact and has some fumigant action. The acute oral LD50 for rats is 88–91 mg/kg; the acute dermal LD50 for rats is 900–1000 mg/kg. Rats receiving 800 mg/kg diet for long periods suffered no ill effect.

head-only exposure. *See* ADMINISTRATION OF TOXICANTS, INHALATION.

Health Advisory Level—Drinking Water. In the USA the Office of Water of the US Environmental Protection Agency promulgates Health Advisory Levels as well as Maximum Contaminant Levels (MCLs) and Maximum Contaminant Level Goals (MCLGs) for drinking water. The Health Advisory Levels are intake levels based on the Reference Dose (RfD) and are expressed as mg/kg/day while the MCL and MCLG are concentrations expressed as mg/L. *See also* REFERENCE DOSE.

Health and Safety at Work Act. Important UK legislation of 1974, resulting from the recommendations of the Robens committee in July 1972, that covers all aspects of safety at the workplace including the potential exposure of workers to toxic substances. The Act is enforced by health and safety inspectors who visit workplaces to monitor conditions.

Health and Safety Commission. A commission, consisting of employers' and union representatives, that was established under the UK Health and Safety at Work Act. The Commission, which is advised by the Advisory Committee on Toxic Substances on health hazards in the workplace from toxic chemicals and related hazards to the public, has overall powers to propose health and safety regulations and to approve codes of practice. It is directly responsible to the Secretary of State for Employment. *See also* HEALTH AND SAFETY AT WORK ACT.

Health and Safety Executive. The body that enforces the statutory duties laid down in the UK Health and Safety at Work Act. The Executive is responsible to the Health and Safety Commission. *See also* HEALTH AND SAFETY COMMISSION.

Health Effects Test Standards. Standards for proposed health effects issued by the Environmental Protection Agency under the Toxic Substances Control Act. *See also* TOXIC SUBSTANCES CONTROL ACT.

healthy worker effect. In epidemiology, refers to the fact that, in general, populations of employed persons enjoy better health than the general population since the latter includes employed and unemployed, healthy and sick. Thus in studies of working populations, other working populations, rather than a general cross-section of the population, should be used as controls. *See also* EPIDEMIOLOGICAL STUDIES; EPIDEMIOLOGY.

heart. An organ chiefly consisting of cardiac muscle that is responsible for pumping blood. It demonstrates inherent rhythmicity of contraction because of the presence of pacemaker tissue, such as the sinoatrial node. The neurotransmitter acetylcholine slows the heart and reduces the force of contraction, whereas norepinephrine quickens the heart and increases the force. Drugs and toxicants affecting cholinergic and adrenergic transmission can therefore affect cardiac function and subsequently blood pressure. Atherosclerotic agents affect coronary arteries and can result in hypertension and heart attacks.

heavy metal poisoning, therapy. Chronic lead poisoning is probably the most common form, particularly among children, although acute lead poisoning is also a hazard. In acute lead poisoning, the unabsorbed lead compound is first removed by gastric lavage with a dilute magnesium or sodium sulfate solution or by emesis. Subsequently urine flow is maintained and chelation therapy commenced. 2,3-Dimercapto-1-propanol and CaEDTA both function by chelating the lead and rendering it excretable. These two drugs are given by injection, but subsequently penicillamine can be given orally. The treatment is monitored by following blood and urine lead concentrations. It has been hypothesized that chelation therapy may actually increase toxicity by allowing greater entry of the metal into the nervous system. Inorganic mercury, particularly mercuric salts, can give rise to either acute or chronic toxicity. In acute poisoning, gastric lavage or emesis is used to remove unabsorbed material. Subsequently, 2,3-dimercapto-1-propanol is used to complex the mercury and render it excretable. Dialysis can be used to speed elimination if necessary. 2,3-Dimercapto-1-propanol is also used to treat chronic mercury poisoning. Organic compounds of heavy metals, such as tetraethyllead and methylmercury also cause serious poisoning. They differ from the inorganic ions in uptake, toxicokinetics, mode of action and therapy, and should be treated separately. *See also* CHELATING AGENTS; LEAD; MERCURY.

heavy metals. An outdated generic term referring to lead, cadmium, mercury and some other elements which are relatively toxic in nature. Recently, the term toxic elements has been used. The term also sometimes refers to compounds containing these elements. *See also* LEAD; MERCURY; METHYLMERCURY; TOXIC METALS; TRIBUTYLTIN; TRIETHYLLEAD; TRIETHYLTIN; TRIMETHYLTIN.

Heinz bodies. Dark-staining bodies found in erythrocytes that lie on the inner surface of the cell membranes. They appear to impair membrane function, and their presence may lead to hemolysis. They consist of denatured hemoglobin, possibly the ill-defined sulfhemoglobin. They are formed in individuals with certain abnormal hemoglobins, but may also occur as a result of

exposure to toxicants such as aniline, nitrobenzenes, hydroxylamine, etc. The toxicological significance of Heinz bodies is not well understood. *See also* HYPOXIA; SULFHEMOGLOBIN.

Heloderma. *See* BEARDED LIZARD; GILA MONSTER.

helper T cells. *See* T CELLS.

hemangioma. *See* ANGIOMA.

hemangiosarcoma. *See* ANGIOSARCOMA.

hematocrit value. Clinical parameter representing the percentage of erythrocytes in whole blood. It can be used as an index of anemia or polycythemia. A typical value for humans is about 44.

hematology. The study of the blood and blood-forming tissues. Hematology is important in toxicology, particularly in chronic toxicity testing, since many toxic effects are apparent in blood, either because of effects on blood-forming tissues or because of release of enzymes from damaged tissues or from direct effects on the blood cells. *See also* TOXIC ENDPOINTS.

hematology, in chronic toxicity testing. *See* TOXIC ENDPOINTS.

hematology, in subchronic toxicity testing. *See* TOXIC ENDPOINTS.

hematopoiesis. The process of blood cell formation in the red bone marrow involving the maturation of stem cells into erythrocytes or one of the several types of leukocytes. A number of drugs, as well as radiation and vitamin deficiences, can retard hematopoiesis.

hematopoietic stem cells. *See* STEM CELLS.

hematuria. The appearance of blood in the urine. This may be a result of chemical poisoning. *See also* DIAGNOSTIC FEATURES, URINARY TRACT.

heme. An iron-containing cyclic tetrapyrrole or porphyrin, based on protoporphyrin IX. It is the prosthetic group of a number of proteins involved in oxygen transport such as hemoglobin and myoglobin as well as a number of cytochromes, including cytochrome P450. Thus it is important in toxicology as the site of several toxic actions (e.g., carbon monoxide poisoning, cyanide poisoning) and in the metabolism of toxicants (e.g., monooxygenase reactions) including both activation and detoxication reactions. *See also* CYTOCHROME P450; HEMOGLOBIN; HEMOPROTEIN.

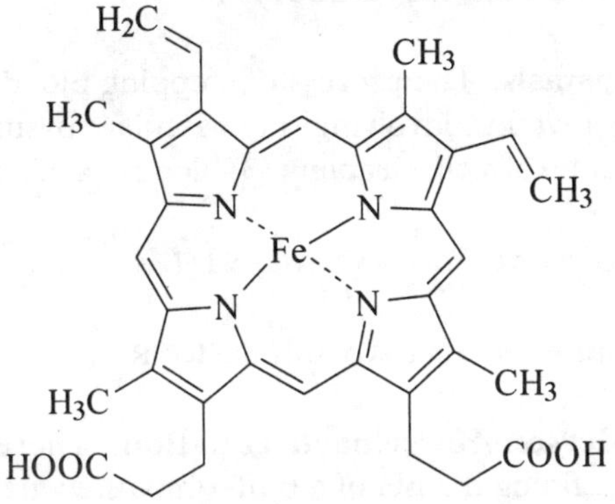

Heme

heme biosynthesis. Porphyrins are synthesized from glycine and succinyl CoA, which condense in a reaction catalyzed by Δ-aminolevulinic acid synthetase to yield Δ-aminolevulinic acid. Two molecules of Δ-aminolevulinic acid then condense to form porphobilinogen. Four porphobilinogens are combined to form a linear tetrapyrrole, which forms a cyclic tetrapyrrole with the loss of an ammonium ion. The cyclic pyrrole uroporphyrinogen III is transformed via coproporphyrin III to protoporphyrin IX. Insertion of the iron into proporphyrin IX by ferrochelatase yields the complete heme molecule. The iron is transferred from the iron-storage protein ferritin by the enzyme transferritin. Regulation of the pathway is complex and includes feedback inhibition, by heme, of Δ-aminolevulinic acid synthetase, Δ-aminolevulinate dehydratase and ferrochelatase, as well as heme depression of Δ-aminolevulinic acid synthesis. In addition to the importance of heme in energy metabolism, lead exerts its toxic effect by inhibition of Δ-aminolevulinic acid metabolism. *See also* HEME; HEMOPROTEIN.

heme degradation. *See* HEME OXYGENASE.

heme oxygenase. A microsomal oxidative enzyme, distinct from cytochrome P450, that catalyzes the oxidative cleavage of heme at the α-meso bridge to form the linear tetrapyrrole bilirubin. This is the initial, and regulated, step in heme degradation. Bilirubin is then reduced to biliverdin by the enzyme bilirubin reductase. The electrons for heme oxygenase are derived from NADPH via NADPH-cytochrome c (P450) reductase. Heme oxygenase is known to exist in the rat in at least two molecular forms, one of which is inducible by metals such as cadmium and cobalt, as well as by organic xenobiotics such as bromobenzene. *See also* BILE PIGMENTS, HEME; HEME BIOSYNTHESIS.

hemicholinium-3 (HC-3). An agent that blocks the sodium-dependent high-affinity transport of choline into nerve terminals. Since this transport system is the rate-limiting step in acetylcholine formation, the synthesis of acetylcholine is inhibited, and only limited supplies of acetylcholine are available for release from cholinergic neurons.

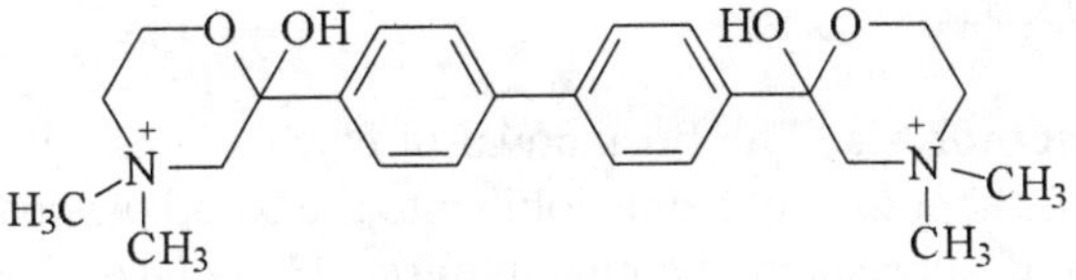

Hemicholinium-3

hemlock. Poison hemlock, *Conium maculatum*. A biennial weed that grows luxuriantly in open areas, roadsides, ditches, etc., and may be mistaken for wild carrot, the leaves for parsley or the seeds for anise. Previously used by the Greeks as a means of suicide and for executions, as in the case of Socrates. In modern times most poisonings are the result of mistaken identification. *Conium* toxicity is caused by piperidine alkaloids, including coniine. Symptoms are similar to nicotine poisoning. *See also* ALKALOIDS, CONIINE.

hemochromatosis. A disease in which excess iron is deposited within the body. Symptoms include an enlarged liver, pigmented skin, diabetes and cardiac failure. The disease is more common in males and does not usually occur before middle age.

hemodialysis. *See* DIALYSIS.

hemoglobin (Hb). The iron-containing protein capable of transporting oxygen and carbon dioxide in the blood that has an iron heme moiety, which binds reversibly to oxygen to form oxyhemoglobin, and a globin moiety, which binds reversibly to carbon dioxide to form carbaminohemoglobin. Typically 97% of the oxygen transported in the blood is bound to hemoglobin, whereas only 3% is dissolved in the plasma. Thus, when hemoglobin is bound to carbon monoxide in carboxyhemoglobin, oxygen transport in the organism is greatly compromised. The transport of carbon dioxide by hemoglobin is a considerably less-important function, with only about 20% of the transported carbon dioxide being bound to hemoglobin. *See also* CARBOXYHEMOGLOBIN; CARBOXYHEMO-GLOBINEMIA.

hemoglobinuria. The appearance of hemoglobin in the urine. It may be a result of chemical poisoning. *See also* DIAGNOSTIC FEATURES, URINARY TRACT.

hemolysis. The breakdown of erythrocytes with the liberation of hemoglobin into the blood plasma and subsequent hemoglobinuria. Hemolysis can result from bacterial toxins, snake venom and chemical poisoning. It can be caused by a direct effect of chemicals on the erythrocytes, as in the case of arsine, or indirectly in individuals deficient in glucose-6-phosphate dehydrogenase, as in the case of naphthalene, primaquine and a number of other chemicals. *See also* DIAGNOSTIC FEATURES, BLOOD.

hemolytic anemia. Anemia resulting from hemolysis, either as a result of toxic chemicals or as a congenital condition. Hemolytic anemia associated with Heinz bodies in the erythrocytes arises from oxidant stress and may occur as a result of chemicals that oxidize hemoglobin to methemoglobin such as nitrites, phenylhydroxylamine, etc. *See also* HEINZ BODIES; HEMOLYSIS.

hemolytic plaque assay. *See* JERNE PLAQUE ASSAY.

hemoprotein. A protein that contains a heme prosthetic group. Heme is an iron-containing protoporphyrin, the latter being a compound containing four pyrrole rings with two vinyl and two propionic acid side chains attached peripherally. As a result of the presence of protoporphyrin IX, this class of proteins has a characteristic visible absorption spectrum. One toxicologically important example is cytochrome P450. *See also* CYTOCHROME P450; HEMOGLOBIN.

hemostasis. The process of stopping blood flow from a wound involving: (1) vascular spasm; (2) formation of a platelet plug; (3) blood coagulation.

hemp plant. *See* CANNABIS SATIVA.

henbane. *See* HYOSCYAMUS NIGER.

Henderson–Hasselbach equation. The equation defining the pH of a buffer mixture when the pK_A of the weak acid in the buffer is known.

$$pH = pK_A + \log\left(\frac{[\text{salt}]}{[\text{acid}]}\right)$$

The equation also relates the degree of ionization of an acid or base to the pH of the medium in which it is dissolved. This value is important in studies of the uptake of ionizable toxicants. The most useful forms of the equation are as follows: for acids

$$\log\left(\frac{[\text{un-ionized form}]}{[\text{ionized form}]}\right) = pK_A - pH$$

for bases

$$\log\left(\frac{[\text{ionized form}]}{[\text{un-ionized form}]}\right) = pK_A - pH$$

See also ENTRY MECHANISMS, PASSIVE TRANSPORT; IONIZATION AND UPTAKE OF TOXICANT.

Henri–Michaelis–Menten equation. *See* MICHAELIS–MENTEN EQUATION.

heparin. **CAS number 9005-49-6**. An anticoagulant released by mast cells during type I hypersensitivity reactions.

hepatic. Referring to the liver.

hepatic clearance. *See* KINETIC EQUATIONS.

hepatic excretion. *See* EXCRETION, HEPATIC.

hepatitis. A general term for inflammation of the liver. Although the term is usually used for viral hepatitis, it is also used for the effects of chemicals (i.e., hepatotoxicants). It is often accompanied by jaundice and in some cases liver enlargement. *See also* HALOTHANE; HEPATOTOXICITY.

hepatobiliary system. The anatomical/physiological system consisting of the liver, bile duct and gall bladder (in some species). Bile (containing the bile salts to emulsify dietary fats) is produced in the liver and delivered into the small intestine via the bile duct. In species possessing a gall bladder, the bile is stored in the gall bladder until required. A number of xenobiotics and xenobiotic metabolites can be excreted by the liver into the bile and can be eliminated in the feces. Some toxicants exert a cholestatic effect, preventing bile flow.

hepatocytes. Parenchymal liver cells. Hepatocytes are the most common cell type in the liver and form the bulk of the organ. They are important sites for the metabolism of xenobiotics and the site of action of hepatotoxicants. *See also* HEPATO-CYTES, ISOLATED; HEPATOTOXICITY; LIVER.

hepatocytes, isolated. Isolated hepatocytes are liver cells that have been enzymatically separated and removed from intact tissues. Collagenase perfusion of the liver is the method most frequently used to obtain healthy, viable cells. The cells are then placed in a medium that contains the essential nutrients for cell maintenance. These cells will not divide *in vitro* and are thus a primary culture. Due to a marked decrease in enzyme levels within hepatocytes following isolation and maintenance of cells in culture, the primary cultures are used either immediately or within a few days. Hepatocytes have been used in toxicology as a system for studying xenobiotic metabolism. For example, induction of cytochrome P450 in isolated hepatocytes has been observed on incubation of cells with phenobarbital, 3-methylcholanthrene and other inducers. Hepatocytes have also been used as a tool for investigating the biochemical mechanisms involved in detoxication or activation sequences. For example, it has been found that hepatocytes depleted of glutathione due to the presence of certain xenobiotics release cellular Ca^{2+}, and this change in Ca^{2+} homeostasis results in cytotoxicity.

hepatoma. A malignant tumor of the liver.

hepatotoxicants. Chemicals that cause adverse effects on the liver. *See also* HEPATOTOXICITY.

hepatotoxicity. Adverse effects on the liver. The liver is particularly susceptible to chemical injury because of its anatomical relationship to the most important portal of entry, the gastrointestinal tract, and its high concentration of xenobiotic-metabolizing enzymes. Many of these enzymes, particularly the cytochrome P450-dependent monooxygenase system, metabolize xenobiotics to produce reactive intermediates that can react with endogenous macromolecules such as proteins and DNA to produce adverse effects. *See also* HEPATO-TOXICITY, BIOTRANSFORMATION AND REACTIVE METABOLITES.

hepatotoxicity, biotransformation and reactive metabolites. Chemically induced injury to the liver cell involves a series of events in the affected animal and in the target organ. They include the chemical agent being activated to form the initiating (toxic) agent followed by either detoxication of the toxic agent or early molecular changes in the cell. Either recovery or irreversible changes follow and finally, in the absence of recovery, there is the altered cell, culminating in cell death. Cell injury can be initiated by a number of mechanisms, such as inhibition of enzymes, depletion of cofactors or metabolites, interaction with receptors and alteration of cell membranes. All of them may include biotransformation of the toxicant to highly reactive metabolites. Many compounds, including clinically useful drugs, can cause cellular damage through metabolic activation to highly reactive compounds, such as free radicals, carbenes and nitrenes. These reactive metabolites may bind covalently to cellular macromolecules such as nucleic acids or proteins, thereby changing their biological properties. The liver is particularly vulnerable to toxicity produced by reactive metabolites since it is a major site of xenobiotic metabolism. Most activation reactions are catalyzed by the cytochrome P450-dependent monooxygenase system, and pretreatment with inducers of these enzymes, such as phenobarbital and 3-methylcholanthrene, usually increases toxicity. Conversely, pretreatment with inhibitors of cytochrome P450, such as SKF-525A and piperonyl butoxide, frequently decreases toxicity. A number of mechanisms exist within the cell for the rapid removal and inactivation of many potentially toxic compounds, such as conjugation of the reactive chemical with glutathione. Thus cellular toxicity depends primarily on the balance between the rate of formation of reactive metabolites and the rate of their removal. Frequently tissue damage is most severe in the regions of the liver containing the highest concentration of activating enzymes. For example, the centrilobular region of the liver contains the highest concentration of cytochrome P450 and is often the site of focal necrosis following toxic chemical injury. The principal manifestations of hepatotoxicity (and examples of causative agents) are: fatty liver (ethionine, cycloheximide); necrosis (bromobenzene, thioacetamide); cholestasis (chlorpromazine, thioridazine); hepatitis (phenylbutazone, isoniazid); carcinogenesis (aflatoxin B1, pyrrolizidine alkaloids). *See also* CHOLESTASIS; FATTY LIVER; HEPATITIS; HEPATOTOXICITY; NECROSIS.

hepatotoxicity, induction. *See* HEPATOTOXICITY, BIOTRANSFORMATION AND REACTIVE METABOLITES.

hepatotoxicity, inhibition. *See* HEPATOTOXICITY, BIOTRANSFORMATION AND REACTIVE METABOLITES.

heptachlor. *See* CYCLODIENE INSECTICIDES.

heptachlor epoxide. *See* CYCLODIENE INSECTICIDES.

herbicide orange. *See* AGENT ORANGE.

herbicides. Chemicals developed for the control of weeds in agricultural or horticultural crops. They include a wide variety of different chemical classes and different modes of action. For example, there are triazines (e.g., atrazine), dinitro compounds (e.g., 4,6-dinitro-*o*-cresol), phenoxy compounds (e.g., 2,4-D), substituted ureas (e.g., monuron, diuron) and dipyridyl derivatives (e.g., paraquat). In general, the mammalian toxicity of most classes of herbicides is low on either acute or chronic exposure, although there are exceptions. The toxicity of TCDD first came to public attention as a result of its presence, as a contaminant, in the herbicide 2,4,5-T.

heroin (7,8-didehydro-4,5α-epoxy-17-methylmorphinan-3,6-diol diacetate; diamorphine; diacetylmorphine). A semisynthetic opium alkaloid derived from extracts of the opium poppy, made by acetylation of morphine. Heroin is much more potent than opium, and somewhat more potent than its parent compound, morphine. Unlike morphine, heroin is not generally employed clinically, but is primarily a major drug of abuse. The pharmacological responses and the problems of tolerance to and dependence on heroin are essentially identical to those of morphine. The primary toxicological problem is one of overdose, marked by three cardinal signs: depressed respiration, coma and pinpoint pupils. Therapy consists of making sure a patent airway exists and the administration of a narcotic antagonist (e.g., naloxone or naltrexone). Indirect toxicological concerns with the illicit use of heroin are toxic or allergic responses to chemicals used to dilute ("cut") the product in street use. *See also* MORPHINE; NARCOTIC ANTAGONISTS; NARCOTICS; OPIOIDS.

Heroin

heterocyclic compounds (heterocycles). Cyclic organic compounds in which one or more of the ring carbons is replaced by another atom, often referred to as the heteroatom. The commonest heteroatoms are nitrogen, oxygen and sulfur. The double bonds in the five-membered and some of the six-membered heterocycles are conjugated as in benzene and these compounds are aromatic to a greater or lesser extent.

heterozygote. An organism possessing dissimilar alleles for a given trait or characteristic on its two homologous chromosomes. *Compare* HOMOZYGOTE.

heterozygous. Possessing dissimilar alleles for a given trait or characteristic on its two homologous chromosomes. The two gene products resulting from the heterozygous condition may give the organism added capacity (i.e., so-called "hybrid vigor") or it may reduce the organism's potential tolerance of adversity (e.g., genes for toxicant resistance). *Compare* HOMOZYGOUS.

Heubach dustmeter. A device that agitates dusty substances in a stream of air, then collects the generated dust for weighing in chambers that select the dust. This allows an estimate of respirable dust. The instrument has become standard for the Stauber–Heubach test.

hexacarbon neuropathy. An obsolete term for γ-diketone neuropathy. *See also* γ-DIKETONE NEUROPATHY.

hexachlorobenzene. CAS number 118-74-1. Formerly used as a fungicidal seed grain dressing. Has caused outbreaks of severe poisoning when treated grain was used for food. Symptoms similar to congenital porphyria cutania tarda with high mortality in young infants caused by contamination first via the placenta and, subsequently, through milk. Carcinogenic and teratogenic in experimental animals and probably so in humans. Not to be confused with the insecticide lindane, one of the isomers of hexachlorocyclohexane,

Cl
Cl   Cl
Cl   Cl
Cl

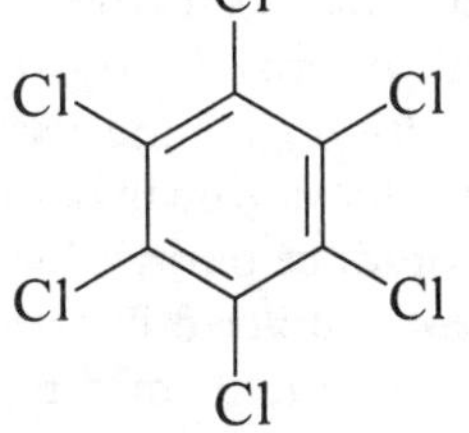

Hexachlorobenzene

commonly (but erroneously) referred to as benzene hexachloride. *See also* ATSDR DOCUMENT, AUGUST 1994; HEXACHLOROCYCLOHEXANE.

hexachlorobutadiene (HCBD, perchlorobutadiene, Dolen-Pur). CAS number 87-68-3. Chemical intermediate in rubber compounds and lubricants, by-product in the manufacture of tetrachloroethylene and other chlorohydrocarbons. Heat transfer fluid and, in countries other than the USA, a soil pesticide. Long-term inhalation affects liver function. Possible human carcinogen (EPA) but not classifiable as to human carcinogenicity (IARC). *See also* ATSDR DOCUMENT, MAY 1994; DATABASES, TOXICOLOGY; LEWIS, HCDR NUMBER HCD250.

hexachlorocyclohexane (alpha, beta and gamma). CAS number of γ-form (lindane) is 58-59-9 (benzenehexachloride). Exists as eight isomers, named according to the position of the hydrogen atoms. The gamma isomer is lindane, an insecticide, also known as γ-HCH. Inhalation may cause dizziness, headaches and hormonal changes in human; ingestion may cause seizures and death. Hepatocarcinogen in rodents. *See also* ATSDR DOCUMENT, MAY 1994; DATABASES, TOXICOLOGY; γ-HCH.

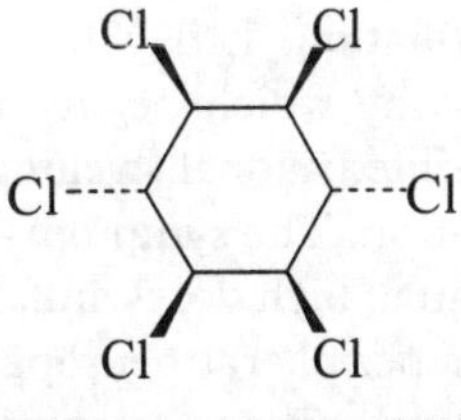

Cl   Cl
Cl   Cl
Cl   Cl

Hexachlorocyclohexane (Lindane)

hexachlorophene (2,2′-methylene *bis*[3,4,6-trichlorophenol]; 2,2-dihydroxy-3,3,5,5,6,6-hexachlorodiphenylmethane). CAS number 70-30-4. An antibacterial that is used chiefly in the manufacture of germicidal soaps (Phisohex). It is the product of 2,4,5-trichlorophenol plus formaldehyde in the presence of sulfuric acid. Hexachlorophene is a polychlorinated *bis*-phenol that in large doses is neurotoxic in animals, presumably due to its effects on brain and spinal cord myelin. Hexachlorophene exerts its antibacterial action by, at low concentrations, inhibiting the bacterial electron transport chain, and, at high concentrations, disrupting bacterial membranes. The phenol coefficient (calculated by dividing the minimal inhibitory concentration of an antiseptic against a standard bacterium by that of phenol) is about 125. Hexachlorophene has greater efficacy against gram-positive bacteria than gram-negative bacteria. Hexachlorophene can be toxic and, in some cases, fatal when applied repeatedly to the skin, particularly in infants. Confusion, lethargy and convulsions may occur, as well as diffuse status spongiosus of the reticular formation. Teratogenic effects have been reported in pregnant nurses routinely using hexachlorophene. Hexachlorophene is used by health care personnel in hand washing and in preparing the skin of surgical patients. Because of potential neurotoxicity, it is no longer commonly used in nurseries. *See also* ANTIBACTERIALS; PHENOL.

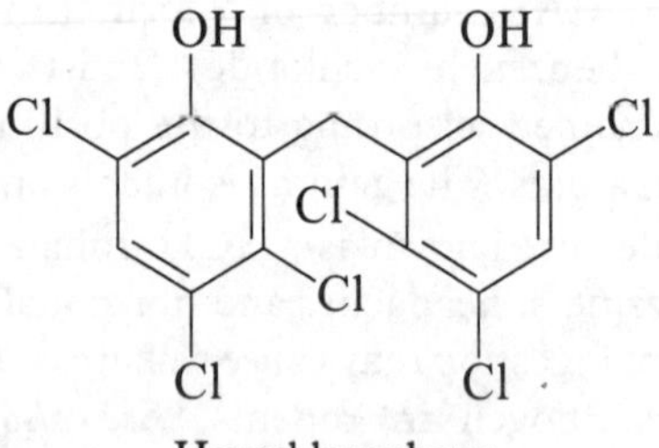

Hexachlorophene

n-hexane. CAS number 110-54-3. A product of petroleum distillation. It is a neurotoxicant that causes axonopathy which begins with paranodal neurofilament-filled axonal swellings, followed by distal degeneration. The symptoms in humans are CNS depression in high doses and, in lower doses, a sensorimotor peripheral neuropathy. The therapy for acute poisoning is to remove from exposure, and to provide ventilatory support if necessary. The CNS depression produced in humans and animals requires inhalation of high concentrations of *n*-hexane (e.g., 5000 ppm for 10 minutes). The LD50 in rats is 24–40 ml/kg by oral administration; the LC50 in rats by inhalation is 48,000 ppm in less than four hours. Chronic exposure to *n*-hexane (more than 400 ppm by inhalation for 45 days, more than 650 mg/kg orally for 90 days) results in a peripheral neuropathy. The neuropathy begins with paranodal axonal swellings filled with neurofilaments and progresses to degeneration of the distal axon. The neuropathy is reproduced by *n*-hexane metabolites, such as

methyl *n*-butyl ketone and 2,5-hexanedione. It has been hypothesized that the ultimate toxic metabolite, 2,5-hexanedione, reacts with lysyl amino groups to form 2,5-dimethylpyrrolyl derivatives and that oxidation of the pyrrole ring leads to covalent cross-linking of proteins. It has also been proposed that it is the stability of the neurofilament that leads to its progressive cross-linking and that the constrictions of axonal diameter that occur at nodes of Ranvier in large myelinated axons present points of obstruction to the anterograde transport of the masses of cross-linked neurofilaments, resulting in the paranodal axonal swellings and leading to degeneration of the axon distal to the swellings. *See also* AXONOPATHY; γ-DIKETONE NEUROPATHY; METHYL N-BUTYL KETONE.

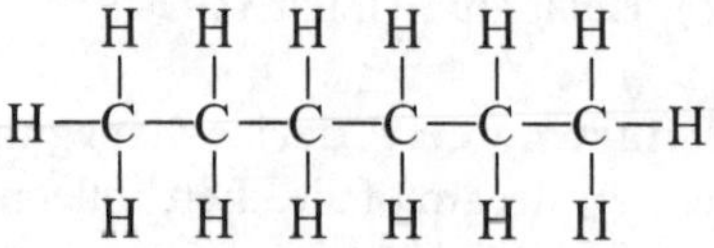

n-Hexane

2,5-hexanedione (acetonylacetone). CAS number 110-13-4. A neurotoxicant that forms protein adducts (pyrroles), leading to covalent cross-linking of neurofilaments. *See also* γ-DIKETONE NEUROPATHY; N-HEXANE.

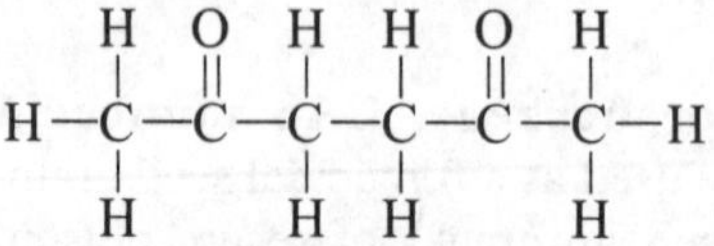

2,5-Hexanedione (Acetonylacetone)

2-hexanone. *See* METHYL N-BUTYL KETONE.

HGPRT locus (hypoxanthine guanine phosphoribosyltransferase locus). The products of the HGPRT locus allow cultured mammalian cells to incorporate purines from the medium so that these purines may be converted into nucleic acids. A mutation at this locus prevents uptake of purines, both normal and toxic, such as 8-azaguanine or 6-thioguanine; with toxic purines, such a mutation allows growth of the cultured cells since they can produce purines by *de novo* synthesis. This concept is utilized in some mutagenicity tests in which cultured mammalian cells are exposed to toxic purines in addition to possible mutagens; growth of these cells indicates that a mutation in the HGPRT locus has occurred. *See also* CHINESE HAMSTER OVARY CELLS; EUKARYOTE MUTAGENICITY TESTS; MAMMALIAN CELL MUTATION TESTS; MOUSE LYMPHOMA CELLS.

5-HIAA. *See* 5-HYDROXYINDOLEACETIC ACID.

Hifol. *See* DICOFOL.

high-performance liquid chromatography. *See* CHROMATOGRAPHY, HIGH-PERFORMANCE LIQUID.

high-pressure liquid chromatography. A term (actually of improper usage) that is synonymous with high-performance liquid chromatography. *See also* CHROMATOGRAPHY, HIGH-PERFORMANCE LIQUID.

Hill plot. A graphical representation of the equation

$$\log\left[\frac{v}{V_{max} - v}\right] = n \cdot \log[S] - \log K'$$

A plot of log $[v/(V_{max}-v)]$ versus log [S] gives a straight line with slope of n, where n is the number of substrate binding sites per molecule of enzyme. Slopes greater than 1 indicate positive or strong cooperativity, whereas slopes less than 1 indicate negative or weak cooperativity. "Pseudo-Hill" plots are also frequently used in radioreceptor assays to assess the nature and potency of the competition of a test compound for binding sites of a specific radioligand. In this case, the log of $[B/(B_{max} - B)]$ is plotted versus log [T], where B is the specific binding at [T] (a concentration of test compound) and B_{max} is the total specific binding (in the presence of no competitor). *See also* EADIE–HOFSTEE PLOT; ENZYME KINETICS; K_D; K_m; LINEWEAVER–BURK PLOT; MICHAELIS–MENTEN EQUATION; RADIORECEPTOR ASSAYS; WOOLF PLOT; XENOBIOTIC METABOLISM, INHIBITION.

histamine (**1H-imidazole-4-ethanamine; 2-(4-imidazolyl)ethylamine; β-aminoethylamidazole**). **CAS number 51-45-6**. An autocoid that is released during allergic reactions and cellular injury. Histamine is a potent vasodilator. It also stimulates the secretion of pepsin and acid by the stomach, serves as chemical transmitter or modulator in brain and contracts many smooth muscles (although it relaxes others). The H1 histamine receptor, which can be blocked by classical antihistamines, mediates such actions as bronchoconstriction and gut contraction. Gastric secretion, on the other hand, is mediated by H2 histamine receptors. Histamine is formed from histidine by *l*-histidine decarboxylase and is stored largely in mast cells or basophils. The flavoprotein diamine oxidase converts histamine to the corresponding aldehyde and ammonia, whereas histamine *N*-methyltransferase converts histamine to *N*-methylhistamine which, in turn, is converted to *N*-methylimidazoleacetic acid by monoamine oxidase. Overdosage of histamine is rare, and the symptoms are not dangerous. The LD50 in mice is about 2 g/kg, i.p. Histamine does not cross the blood–brain barrier, although when administered into the lateral ventricles it can increase heart rate, elevate blood pressure, lower body temperature, increase secretion of antidiuretic hormone and cause emesis. Histamine is useful as a diagnostic aid for gastric acid secretion or the presence of a pheochromocytoma, or for hyposensitization therapy. Histamine is produced from histidine which occurs in high levels in certain fish; when these fish are not chilled sufficiently, the accumulated histamine results in scombroid poisoning following ingestion. *See also* ANTIHISTAMINES; AUTOCOIDS; SCOMBROID POISONING.

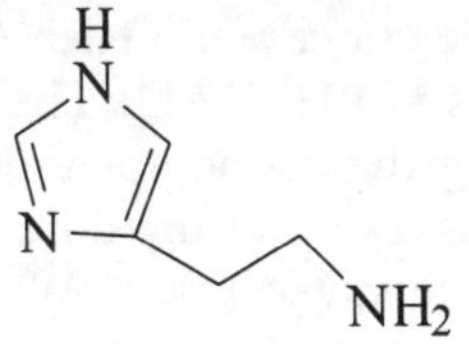

Histamine

histamine *N*-methyltransferase. *See* *N*-METHYLATION.

histamine-sensitizing factor. *See* PERTUSSIS TOXIN.

histocompatability. *See* T CELLS.

histology. The microscopic study of tissues.

histones. Basic proteins complexed with DNA in the chromosomes of eukaryotes. Histones can be one of five types of small, highly conserved proteins which are associated with nuclear DNA in eukaryotes and are involved in the folding and packaging of DNA into a compact chromosome structure. The histones must become less tightly associated with the DNA in order for the transcription of DNA to occur.

history of toxicology. Toxicology must be one of the oldest practical sciences since humans have needed, from the very beginning, to avoid the numerous toxic plants and animals in their environment. A large amount of the early history of toxicology has been lost, however, and much that has survived is of almost incidental importance in manuscripts dealing primarily with medicine. Many records dealt with the use of poisons for judicial execution, political assassination or suicide. The Ebers papyrus, an Egyptian papyrus (about 1500 BC), is the earliest surviving pharmacopeia, and the surviving medical works of Hippocrates, Aristotle and Theophrastus (published about 400–250 BC) all included some mention of poisons. The early Greek poet Nicander covers, in two poetic works, animal toxins (Therica) and antidotes to plants and animal toxins (Alexipharmica). The earliest surviving attempt to classify plants according to their toxic and therapeutic effects is that of Dioscorides, a Greek employed by the Roman emperor Nero around 50 AD. There appear to have been few advances in either medicine or toxicology between Galen (131–200 AD) and Paracelsus (1493–1541). The latter laid the groundwork for the development of modern toxicology. He was aware of the dose–response relationship, and he stated that: "All substances are poison; there is none that is not a poison. The right dose differentiates a poison and a remedy." This is properly regarded as a landmark in the development of the science. His belief in experimentation also represented a break with much earlier tradition. Orfila, a Spaniard working at the University of Paris, identified toxicology as a separate science, and in 1815 he wrote the first book devoted exclusively to it (an English translation, published in 1817, was entitled General System of Toxicology or, a Treatise on Poisons, Found in the Mineral, Vegetable and Animal Kingdoms, Considered in their Relations with Physiology, Pathology and Medical Jurisprudence). Although Orfila, writing in the early 19th century, is generally regarded as the father of modern toxicology, there had been important developments in the 18th century. The publication of Ramazzini's Diseases of Workers in 1700 lead to his recognition as the father of occupational medicine. Another noteworthy milestone was the observation in 1775 by Percival Potts, who reported the incidence of scrotal cancer in chimney sweeps. Workers of the later 19th century who produced treatises on toxicology include Christison, Kobert and Lewin. Since then numerous advances have increased our knowledge of the chemistry of poisons, the treatment of poisoning, the analysis both of toxicants and of toxicity, as well as the mode of toxic action and detoxication. During the last two or three decades, toxicology has entered a phase of rapid development and has changed from a previously almost entirely descriptive science to one in which the study of mechanisms is emphasized.

histotoxic hypoxia. *See* HYPOXIA.

histrionicotoxin. A bicyclic alkaloid neurotoxin found in frogs.

hit models. *See* LOW-DOSE EXTRAPOLATION.

HMTA. *See* HAZARDOUS MATERIALS TRANSPORTATION ACT.

HMX. An acronym for high melting explosive. Toxicity not well characterized. *See also* ATSDR DOCUMENT, JUNE 1994.

homeostasis. The dynamic steady state that organisms are adapted to in order to maintain their internal environment and to compensate for changes that would otherwise occur as a result of internal or external changes. Physiological systems, involving nervous and endocrine control, maintain homeostasis through negative feedback mechanisms. Examples of parameters under homeostatic regulation include blood pressure, blood volume, pH, glucose levels, oxygen content and body temperature.

homologous. Describing an organ or tissue that is similar in structure and origin, although not necessarily in function. At the level of the cell nucleus, homologous chromosomes are the two chromosomes, one derived from each parent, which contain the alleles for the same characteristic and which synapse during meiosis.

homozygote. An organism possessing the same allele for a given trait or characteristic on its two homologous chromosomes. *Compare* HETEROZYGOTE.

homozygous. Possessing the same allele for a given trait or characteristic on its two homologous chromosomes. The gene product may make the individual either more or less tolerant of toxicant effects (e.g., genes for resistance or xenobiotic-metabolizing enzymes). *Compare* HETEROZYGOUS.

hormesis. The concept that a higher dose of toxicant can yield a lesser toxicological response than a lower dose of toxicant.

hormones. A compound, secreted in one part of the body, that has a specific effect in another part of the body. Chemical substances are secreted by an endocrine gland and transported by the blood to target tissues where they exert a specific physiological action. They may be steroids or simple organic amines. Auxins are the plant equivalent of hormones. *See also* ANDROSTERONE; CALCITONIN; EPINEPHRINE; ESTRONE; 17α-ETHYNYLESTRADIOL; FOLLICLE-STIMULATING HORMONE; GLUCAGON; INSULIN; LUTEINIZING HORMONE; MESTRANOL; NOREPINEPHRINE; OXYTOCIN; PARATHYROID HORMONE; PROGESTERONE; PROLACTIN; TESTOSTERONE; THYROID; THYROTROPIN.

host-mediated assay. *See* HOST SUSCEPTIBILITY ASSAY.

host susceptibility assay (host-mediated assay). An assay designed to assess the effect of chemicals on the immune system of the intact animal. This is done by assessing resistance to infectious bacteria or to transplantable tumor cells. Organisms used include *Listeria mono-*

cytogenes and *Streptococcus myogenes*, and in some cases the tests are carried out with endotoxin from *Escherichia coli* followed by challenge with *Pseudomonas aeruginosa*. Resistance to these organisms is primarily T cell-dependent, with the mononuclear phagocytic system also playing a major role. An exception is *Streptococcus pyogenes*, resistance to which is largely antibody-dependent. *See also* IMMUNE SYSTEM; IMMUNOTOXICITY TESTING.

HPLC. *See* CHROMATOGRAPHY, HIGH-PERFORMANCE LIQUID.

HSC. Health and Safety Commission established under UK's Health and Safety at Work Act of 1974. *See also* COSHH.

5-HT (5-hydroxytryptamine). *See* SEROTONIN.

human equivalent dose. A dose which, when administered to humans, produces an effect equal to that produced by a given dose in another animal.

human test data. The objective of much toxicity testing is the elimination of potential risks to humans. However, because our knowledge of quantitative structure–activity relationships (QSAR) does not yet permit accurate extrapolation to new compounds and because human test data are difficult to obtain for ethical reasons, most testing is carried out on animals. Human data are necessary for effects such as irritation, nausea, allergies, odor evaluation and some higher nervous system functions. In some cases insight may be obtained from occupational exposure data, although this tends to be irregular in time and not clearly defined as to composition of the toxicant. For certain tests human test panels can be used, but clearly any experiments involving humans must be carried out under carefully defined conditions after other testing, *in vitro* or on experimental animals, is complete. Although extrapolation from experimental animals to humans presents problems due to differences in metabolic pathways, penetration and mode of action, experimental animals present numerous advantages for toxicity testing. These include clearly defined genetic constitution, controlled exposure, controlled duration of exposure and detailed examination of all tissues following necropsy.

human toxicity testing. Experimental studies on humans are difficult to carry out for both ethical and experimental reasons. As a result they are usually designed to answer specific questions, rather limited in scope, that cannot be answered by tests on experimental animals. Examples include: blood cholinesterase determinations to estimate worker re-entry periods; tests for irritancy to the nasal membranes; or tests for effects on higher nervous function. *See also* DECLARATION OF HELSINKI; HUMAN TEST DATA.

humoral immunity. *See* B CELLS; IMMUNE SYSTEM.

hyaluronidase. An enzyme that hydrolyzes hyaluronic acid (the intercellular cement), chondroitin and chondroitin sulfates A and C, and therefore tends to liquify the gel-like consistency of the interstitial space. By this action, it serves as a spreading factor for toxins. In addition to its lysosomal location in cells, it is secreted by several virulent microorganisms and a component of snake venoms.

hybridoma. *See* MONOCLONAL ANTIBODY.

hydrangea. A member of the *Saxifragaceae* family. The leaves and buds contain cyanogenic glycosides that may produce cyanide poisoning, especially if the leaves are extracted as a herbal tea.

hydraulic fluids. Numerous different chemicals from several different chemical classes are used as hydraulic fluids, i.e., they transfer pressure from one point in machinery to another. They include mineral oils, organophosphate esters and polyolefins. Toxicity is not well characterized. *See also* ATSDR DOCUMENT, JUNE 1994.

hydrazines. Organic derivatives of hydrazine. Many of those compounds such as 1,2-dimethylhydrazine or their metabolites (azomethane, azoxymethane) or derivatives (methylazoxymethanol, the aglycone of cycasin) are potent

carcinogens, hepatoxicants or are toxic to the reproductive system. *See also* CYCASIN; ATSDR DOCUMENT, JUNE 1994.

$$H \diagdown \qquad H \diagup$$
$$N-N$$
$$H \diagup \qquad H \diagdown$$

Hydrazine

hydrocarbons. Compounds composed of hydrogen and carbon primarily, either aliphatic or aromatic; a major class of pollutants. Hydrocarbons comprise about 12% of air pollutants and arise mainly from the combustion of fossil fuels or their products refined for energy generation, or in industry and transportation. They also contribute to water pollution through oil spills and other contamination by crude oil. *See also* CRUDE OIL; OIL SPILLS; POLLUTION, FOSSIL FUELS; POLLUTION, PETROLEUM PRODUCTS.

hydrocortisone. *See* CORTISOL.

hydrofluoric acid. *See* FLUORIDES.

hydrogen bonding. These bonds arise when a hydrogen atom, covalently bound to one electronegative atom, is shared to a significant degree with a second electronegative atom. As a rule, only the most electronegative atoms (oxygen, nitrogen and fluorine) form stable hydrogen bonds. Protein side chains containing hydroxyl, amino, carboxyl, imidazole and carbamyl groups can form hydrogen bonds, as can the nitrogen and oxygen atoms of peptide bonds themselves. Hydrogen bonding plays an important role in the structural configuration of proteins and nucleic acids. *See also* BINDING.

hydrogen fluoride. *See* FLUORIDES.

hydrogen sulfide (H_2S). **CAS number 7783-06-4**. A colorless gas with a characteristic odor of rotten eggs. It has been designated a hazardous substance and a hazardous waste (EPA). Hydrogen sulfide is used in the synthesis of organic and inorganic sulfides, and is generated in the decomposition of sulfur-containing organic matter and in industrial processes involving sulfur compounds. It may also be found in natural waters and in natural gas. The most common route of entry into the body is by inhalation. Hydrogen sulfide is an acutely toxic gas that may bring about immediate coma. It is an irritant to the eyes and respiratory system. The systemic action of hydrogen sulfide is due to inhibition of cytochrome oxidase and death, when it results, is due to respiratory failure. Although hydrogen sulfide is an extremely toxic gas, fatalities are less common than might be expected due to its foul odor, to which the human olfactory sense is particularly sensitive, acting as an early warning system.

hydrolases. *See* ENZYMES; HYDROLYSIS; HYDROLYTIC ENZYMES.

hydrolysis. Cleavage of a molecule by the addition of water. Hydrolysis is important in toxicology and is catalyzed by a large number of different enzymes. Enzymes with carboxylesterase and amidase activity are widely distributed occurring in most, if not all, tissues and in microsomal and soluble fractions. Carboxylesterases and amidases were formerly believed to be different enzymes. At the present time, however, these two activities are regarded as different manifestations of the same activity with specificity being dependent primarily on the nature of R, R' and R'' groups and, secondarily, on the heteroatom (oxygen, sulfur or nitrogen) adjacent to the carboxyl group. Because of the large number of esterases and the large number of substrates, it has been difficult to derive a meaningful system for their classification. The classification below is one devised by Aldridge. B-Esterases, the most important group, are inhibited by paraoxon, which phosphorylates a serine residue in their active site. It is a rather heterogeneous group of enzymes and their isozymes, which hydrolyze physiological substrates as well as xenobiotics; many have quite different substrate specificities. For example, the group contains carboxylesterase/amidases, cholinesterases, monoacylglycerol lipases and arylamidases. A-Esterases (arylesterases) are not inhibited by phosphotriesters such as paraoxon, but do hydrolyze them. C-Esterases (acetylesterases) are those esterases that prefer acetyl esters as substrates, paraoxon serving neither as a substrate nor an inhibitor. *See also* ACETYLCHOLINESTERASE; CARBOXYLESTERASES.

hydrolytic enzymes. Any enzyme capable of splitting a molecule into components by inserting water. Hydrolytic enzymes include lysosomal acid hydrolases and a number of the enzymes in protein, carbohydrate, lipid and nucleic acid catabolism. Hydrolytic enzymes exist that degrade xenobiotic esters, amides and conjugates. Acetylcholinesterase is the only hydrolytic enzyme that is a major target of acutely toxic agents. *See also* HYDROLYSIS.

hydrophiidae. The family of true sea snakes, which are venomous.

hydrophilic. Water-loving; refers to chemicals that are water-soluble or to the regions of chemicals that are polar and therefore attracted to water. Many toxicants are not hydrophilic, but are made more hydrophilic through metabolism and thus can more readily be excreted. Hydrophilic compounds do not diffuse easily through membranes.

hydrophobic binding. When two non-polar groups come together they exclude the water between them, and this mutual exclusion of water results in a hydrophobic interaction. In the aggregate they present the least possible disruption of interactions among polar water molecules, and thus can lead to stable complexes. Some authorities consider this a special case involving van der Waals' forces. The minimization of thermodynamically unfavorable contact of a polar grouping with water molecules provides the major stabilizing effect in hydrophobic interactions.

8-hydroxy-2-deoxyguanosine. An excretory product indicative of oxidative damage to DNA used as a measure of oxidative stress *in vivo*. *See also* OXIDATIVE STRESS.

5-hydroxyindoleacetic acid (5-HIAA). The primary product of the metabolism of serotonin. Formed by the oxidative deamination of serotonin by monoamine oxidase, presumably the A isozyme, 5-HIAA is subsequently cleared by an active transport mechanism. Unlike serotonin, 5-HIAA is not a neurotransmitter and thus its formation contributes to the termination of the synaptic actions of serotonin. Inhibition of monoamine oxidase activity enhances and prolongs the actions of serotonin. *See also* MONOAMINE OXIDASES; SEROTONIN.

5-Hydroxyindoleacetic acid

hydroxyindole   *O*-methyltransferase. *See O*-METHYLATION.

4-hydroxyphenyl glycine. *See* AMINOPHENOLS.

hydroxy radical. *See* ACTIVE OXYGEN.

hydroxysteroid sulfotransferase. *See* SULFATE CONJUGATION.

5-hydroxytryptamine. *See* SEROTONIN.

hymenoptera. The insect order comprised of several venomous groups, the wasps, ants, bees and hornets. In the United States, these insects are responsible for more human deaths than all other venomous animals, usually as a result of allergic reactions and anaphylaxis.

hyoscine. *See* SCOPOLAMINE.

***dl*-hyoscyamine**. *See* ATROPINE.

Hyoscyamus niger. Henbane, a poisonous plant containing *l*-hyoscamine and scopolamine.

hyperactivity. *See* ATTENTION DEFICIENT HYPERACTIVITY DISORDER.

hyperglycemia. A high concentration of blood glucose. Hyperglycemia can result from diabetes mellitus or exposure to hyperglycemic chemicals. *Compare* HYPOGLYCEMIA.

hyperkinesis. *See* ATTENTION DEFICIENT HYPERACTIVITY DISORDER.

hyperplasia. Excessive proliferation of normal cells in the normal tissue organization.

hypersensitivity. Any allergic response or only immediate and delayed-type hypersensitivity reactions. Type I allergic responses (anaphylactic) and type IV allergic responses (delayed-type hypersensitivity) are the two types of reactions most commonly produced by environmental agents and are therefore most commonly referred to as allergic responses or hypersensitivity reactions. The term immediate hypersensitivity is often used interchangeably with the term anaphylactic response (or type I reaction) although the class of immediate hypersensitivity reactions referred to as Arthus reactions are either type II reactions (cytolytic) or type III reactions (immune complex). Immediate and delayed-type hypersensitivity are distinguished primarily by the speed of onset of the reactions (within minutes to hours for immediate or within hours to days for delayed-type) as well as by the mechanism involved (antibody-mediated for all classes of immediate and T cell-mediated for delayed-type). *See also* ALLERGIC RESPONSE; IMMEDIATE HYPERSENSITIVITY.

hypertension. A condition in which the blood pressure is higher than normal. Hypertension can result from excessive sympathetic stimulation to the heart (increasing rate and force of contraction) and blood vessels (causing vasoconstriction) or by lipid or lipid/calcium plaque deposits in the arteries (atherosclerosis and arteriosclerosis, respectively), which reduce blood vessel elasticity.

hypertensive. Having a higher than normal blood pressure. *Compare* HYPOTENSIVE.

hypertriglyceridemia. High levels of triglycerides in the blood stream.

hyperventilation. Increased ventilation (breathing rate and depth of ventilation) caused primarily by an increase in blood carbon dioxide and secondarily by a decrease in blood pH, and only rarely by a decrease in blood oxygen.

hypervitaminosis A. Substantial increases in the intake of vitamin A or retinol in excess of required amounts results in the toxic syndrome of hypervitaminosis. Chronic daily ingestion of 2500–50,000 IU/kg may cause plasma concentrations of 300–2000 mg/dl, resulting in irritability, vomiting, loss of appetite, headache and dermatological conditions. The occurrence of the condition may be greater than suspected because the symptoms are similar to idiopathic benign intracranial hypertension. Excessive consumption of vitamin A by pregnant women can also result in congenital abnormalities in the offspring.

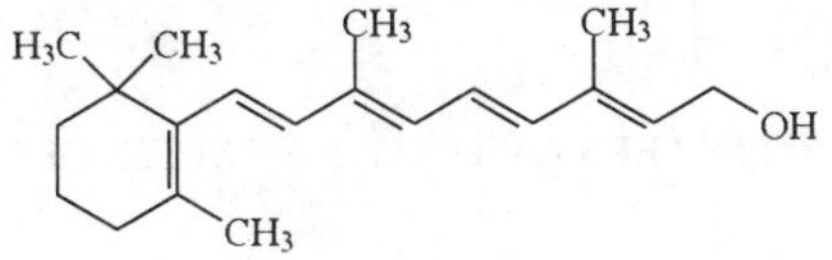

Vitamin A

hypoglycemia. A condition in which the blood sugar concentration is below the normal range. In the normal individual low blood sugar stimulates the pancreas to release glucagon, which stimulates the breakdown of glycogen and the release of glucose from the liver. The toxicity of oral hypoglycemic agents (e.g., sulfonylureas) is low, but their action may be potentiated by anti-inflammatory agents such as phenylbutazone and salicylates. *Compare* HYPERGLYCEMIA.

hypophysis. *See* PITUITARY GLAND.

hyposulfite, sodium. *See* THIOSULFATE, SODIUM.

hypotensive. Possessing lower than normal blood pressure. Since blood pressure is dependent upon heart rate and force, and blood vessel diameter, and these are both impacted by the autonomic nervous system, toxicants affecting cholinergic or adrenergic function can lead to hypotension. *Compare* HYPERTENSIVE.

hypothalamus. A portion of the vertebrate brain's diencephalon, underlying the thalamus, that exerts a major control over a variety of autonomic functions as well as the majority of endocrine functions of the body. It is extremely important in homeostasis by monitoring a variety of parameters, such as blood glucose or temperature, and it initiates a variety of negative feedback systems to keep these parameters in homeostasis. By releasing hormones (releasing factors) or inhibitory factors, it controls the secretion of the adenohypophysis (anterior pituitary) and, thereby, the function of the thyroid, the adrenal cortex and the gonads. By direct neural connections, it controls the neurohypophysis (posterior pituitary) and the adrenal medulla. It also is responsible for hunger, thirst and appetite.

hypoxanthine guanine phosphoribosyl transferase locus. *See* HGPRT LOCUS.

hypoxia. Any condition in which there is an inadequate supply of oxygen to the tissues. This condition can arise from several distinct causes, and hypoxias have been classified under several different names. Arterial or anoxic hypoxia results from pulmonary irritants or toxicants that depress respiration. Characteristically the pO_2 of the arterial blood is low even though oxygen capacity and blood flow are normal. Anemic hypoxia is characterized by a lower than normal oxygen-carrying capacity with normal arterial pO_2 and blood flow. It is due primarily to agents that affect the oxygen-carrying capacity of hemoglobin, such as carbon dioxide, or chemicals that generate methemoglobin (e.g., sodium nitrite). Stagnant hypoxia is due to decreased blood flow. Histotoxic hypoxia is not strictly speaking a hypoxia as defined above, since the oxygen supply to the tissues is normal, but the tissues are unable to utilize the oxygen. Typical examples of this last category are seen in cyanide and hydrogen sulfide poisoning. *See also* HEINZ BODIES; TOXICITY.

I

IAEA. *See* INTERNATIONAL ATOMIC ENERGY AGENCY.

IARC. *See* INTERNATIONAL AGENCY FOR RESEARCH ON CANCER.

ibotenic acid (α-amino-2,3-dihydro-3-oxo-5-isoxazoleacetic acid). CAS number 2552-55-8. An excitatory amino from the fly agaric *Amanita muscaria* and the panther amanita *A. pantherina,* both found in woodland in the western United States. Toxicity to humans involves central nervous system depression, ataxia, hysteria and hallucinations.

ibuprofen (α-methyl-4-(2-methylpropyl) benzeneacetic acid). CAS number 15687-27-1. A non-steroidal anti-inflammatory agent that produces its therapeutic effect via inhibition of prostaglandin synthetase. Several different forms of nephrotoxicity have been associated with the use of ibuprofen. Nephrotoxicity can result either from acute intake of an overdose or on chronic use.

*IC*50 **(median inhibitory concentration).** The concentration of a chemical present in an *in vitro* incubation system which is estimated to inhibit 50% of the measured parameter, such as enzyme activity or ligand binding to a receptor. It is also sometimes called I_{50}.

ICSH. *See* INTERSTITIAL CELL-STIMULATING HORMONE.

icterus. Jaundice; pigmentation of tissues with bile pigments. This is a sign of hepatic dysfunction.

ileum. The posterior of the three divisions of the small intestine, occurring anterior to the large intestine.

ILSI. *See* INTERNATIONAL LIFE SCIENCES INSTITUTE.

β,β′-iminodipropionitrile (IDPN). A neurotoxic synthetic nitrile that causes proximal axonopathies in the spinal cord and brain stem. The proximal axonal swellings are due to interruption of slow axonal transport, resulting in a large accumulation of neurofilaments. Secondary to these effects is a progressive atrophy of the distal axon, secondary demyelination and gliosis. The slow axonal transport defect appears to be selective, as little evidence for perturbations in fast axonal transport have been reported. Behaviorally, IDPN induces hyperactivity, a "waltzing syndrome", circling and head-rolling in mice and rats. IDPN intoxication has been advanced as a model for certain motor neuron degenerative diseases such as amyotropic lateral sclerosis (ALS) and hereditary canine spinal muscular atrophy (HCSMA). *See also* AMYOTROPHIC LATERAL SCLEROSIS; AXONOPATHY; LATHYRISM.

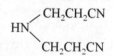

β,β′-Iminodipropionitrile

imipramine (10,11–dihydro-*N*,*N*-dimethyl-5*H*-dibenz[*b,f*]azepine-5-propanamine; 5-(3-dimethylaminopropyl)-10,11-dihydro-5*H*-dibenz[*b,f*] azepine; Tofranil). CAS number 50-49-7. A tertiary amine tricyclic antidepressant that is thought to exert its therapeutic effect by inhibiting the re-upake of serotonin and norepinephrine centrally. A major metabolite is *N*-desmethylimipramine (desipramine), also used as an antidepressant drug. Desipramine differs from imipramine in being a better blocker of norepinephrine, rather than serotonin, uptake. Side effects, including sedation and drowsiness, dry mouth, urinary retention, constipation and orthostatic hypotension, are probably due to the anticholinergic, anti-α-adrenergic and antihistaminergic receptor-blocking properties. Imipramine should not be used in conjunction with a monoamine oxidase inhibitor or other treatment that increases catecholamine concentrations (e.g., drugs containing sympathomimetic amines). Imipramine should be avoided in patients with cardiovascular disease or seizure disorder, or in those who may abuse alcohol, as imipramine lowers seizure threshold, can produce cardiovascular toxicity and may potentiate the effects of alcohol. Imipramine intoxication can include CNS abnormalities (e.g., drowsiness, stupor, coma, extrapyramidal symptoms), cardiac arrhythmia and respiratory depression. Children appear to be particularly vulnerable to the cardiotoxic and seizure-inducing effects of high doses of imipramine. The oral LD50 in female rats is 305 mg/kg. *See also* ANTIDEPRESSANTS; TRICYCLIC ANTIDEPRESSANTS.

$$CH_2CH_2CH_2N(CH_3)_2$$

Imipramine

immediate hypersensitivity. A specific immunological reaction mediated by antibodies that takes place within minutes to hours of exposure to antigen. There are two classes: (1) a complement-dependent hypersensitivity produced by IgG and IgM antibodies; (2) a complement-independent hypersensitivity produced by IgE antibodies. The IgG/IgM complement-dependent hypersensitivity is considered a type II (cytolytic) or type III (immune complex) allergic response, depending on whether the antibodies are directed against cells in the vascular lining or form complexes with an antigen which then deposit in the vascular epithelium. These reactions are the classical Arthus reactions and produce a local inflammation, vasculitis and hemorrhaging in the skin at the site of antigen deposition. The IgE-mediated hypersensitivity is a type I (anaphylactic) allergic response, and the symptoms are similar. Although both frequently cause only a local inflammation, there can be more serious manifestations such as immune complex diseases (IgG/IgM-mediated) and anaphylactic shock (IgE-mediated). *See also* ALLERGIC RESPONSE; COMPLEMENT; DELAYED HYPERSENSITIVITY; MAST CELLS/BASOPHILS.

immune function. *See* IMMUNE SYSTEM.

immune system. The complex and highly cooperative system of cells, tissues and organs whose primary function is to protect an organism from infection by foreign organisms and from newly arising neoplasms. These tasks can be accomplished in a non-specific manner, such as the ingestion of particles by phagocytes, or in a very specific manner, such as the neutralization of some bacterial endotoxins by antibodies, or in ways that have both specific and non-specific components, such as antibody-dependent cellular cytotoxicity (ADCC), where the binding of specific antibodies enables non-specific phagocytes to destroy the cells. Most organisms have some form of non-specific defense, but only vertebrates have the capability to make a specific, adaptive, anamnestic response. This is primarily due to the B and T cells. A brief summary of the interactions and functions of the immune system's cells is shown in the figure. All of these cells, as well as the erythrocytes, are derived from the pluripotent stem cell in the bone marrow. Progenitors of the lymphocytes migrate to the primary lymphoid organs, the bone marrow and the thymus, where they mature into B and T cells, respectively. From here, the lymphocytes enter the circulation and home to the secondary lymphoid organs. The lymphocytes are continually circulated through these organs, via the blood stream and lymphatic system, which serve as the major filtering organs of the lymph (lymph nodes), blood (spleen), gut (Peyer's patches, appendix) and upper respiratory tract (adenoids, tonsils). Non-specific responses to foreign material are generally initiated by phagocytic cells at the site of infection or irritation. Also, some microorganisms trigger the alternative pathway of complement activation. If this response is inadequate, the antigen load increases and the lymphocyte response is activated. It is in the lymph nodes and spleen that the humoral responses to blood- and lymph-borne antigens is initiated. The humoral immune response consists of those interactions that lead to the production of circulating antibodies. These antibodies can have a number of

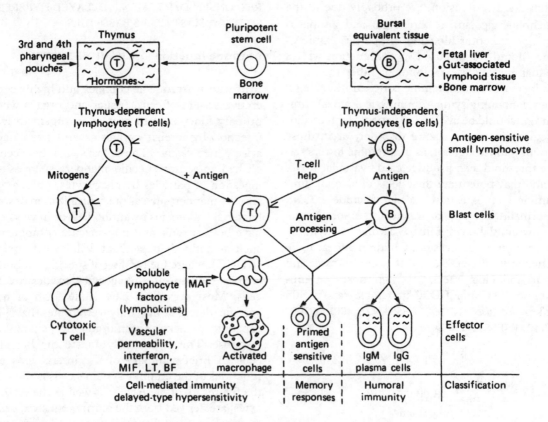

Immune system
From Klaassen, C.D., Amdur, M.O. & Doull, J. (eds) *Casarett and Doull's Toxicology.*
3rd edn (New York, Macmillan, 1986)

different roles in host defense. They can neutralize toxins by binding to the active site and can prevent mucosal attachment of gut parasites by a similar mechanism. Additionally, antibodies bound to a cell surface can activate the complement pathways, inducing inflammation and can enhance the phagocytic efficiency of macrophages. Since antibodies are multivalent they can also agglutinate viruses and bacteria into more easily removed particles. Cell-mediated immunity, the other arm of the immune response, leads to the generation of cytotoxic T cells. Cytotoxic T cells are able to destroy virally infected cells, tumor cells and foreign tissue. Typically, extracellular bacteria and viruses induce humoral immunity, whereas fungi, intracellular viruses, cancer and foreign tissue induce cell-mediated immunity, although this is by no means absolute. Environmental agents, including drugs, can affect the immune system in

several general ways. They can cause immunosuppression, either by a general decrease in cellularity or by a decrease in the numbers and/or function of particular cell types, or cause uncontrolled proliferation. Both of these can lead to substantial alterations in host defense mechanisms and therefore to increased vulnerability to pathogens and neoplasms. Additionally, environmental agents can cause the immune system to respond in a way that is detrimental to the host, as in allergic responses and autoimmunity. Screening tests to determine alteration in immune system function include complete blood cell counts, white blood cell differentials, weights and histology of lymphoid organs, lymphocyte response to nonspecific stimulators (mitogens), delayed-type hypersensitivity responses and quantitation of antibody response to standard antigens. *See also* ALLERGIC RESPONSE; AUTOIMMUNITY.

immunoassay. Any of a number of assays based on the binding of antibody to antigen. The avidity and specificity of the reaction makes it possible to quantitate amounts (in the picogram to nanogram range) of a compound, such as a hormone, tumor antigen or drug, in complex biological fluids. The most common immunoassay is the radioimmuno-assay (RIA), which is a competitive binding assay where a known amount of purified radiolabeled ligand (usually the antigen) competes with an unknown amount of unlabeled antigen for the available binding sites. The fraction of label bound to antibody (or antigen) is inversely proportional to the amount of antigen (or antibody) in the sample. The enzyme-linked immunosorbent assay (ELISA) is a variation of RIA in which the ligand (frequently an antibody) is linked to an enzyme rather than to a radioactive tracer. Often the ligand is attached to a solid matrix to facilitate separation of the bound and free fractions. Substrate is added and the amount of enzyme bound is quantitated spectrophotometrically. The radioallergosorbent (RAST) assay uses similar principles to detect IgE specific for a given allergen. After the antibody-antigen reaction, radiolabeled anti-IgE is added so that only the IgE antibodies (the antibodies responsible for allergic reactions to ingested and inhaled allergens) are quantitated. Other immuno-assays include radial immunodiffusion (RID) and immunoelectrophoresis (IEF), both of which util-ize antibody incorporated into a uniform gel matrix. In RID, a sample diffuses radially from a well in the gel until the antigen and antibody con-centrations are approximately equal and a precipi-tin ring forms; the diameter of the ring is propor-tional to the amount of antigen in the sample. In IEF, the sample is electrophoresed through the gel and a precipitin "rocket" forms, the height of which is proportional to the amount of antigen in the sample. All of these methods are limited to compounds against which antibodies of suffi-ciently high avidity and low cross-reactivity can be generated. *See also* ELISA; RADIOIMMUNOASSAY; RADIORECEPTOR ASSAYS.

immunodepressants. *See* IMMUNOSUPPRES-SION.

immunoelectrophoresis (IEF). *See* IMMUNO-ASSAY.

immunoglobin. *See* IMMUNOGLOBULIN.

immunoglobulin. Large globular proteins found in the body fluids of vertebrate animals. The basic unit of immunoglobulin structure consists of four polypeptide chains (two identical light chains and two identical heavy chains) which are disulfide-bonded to form two identical antigen-binding (variable) regions. Mammals possess five distinct classes of immunoglobulin (IgG, IgA, IgM, IgD, IgE) distinguishable by differences in the carboxy-terminal portion of the heavy chain. The concentration of each immunoglobulin class in various body fluids is relatively constant in healthy animals. Immunoglobulin is a generic term. Immunoglobulins known to bind specifically with a particular antigen are referred to as antibodies. *See also* ANTIBODY.

immunostimulants. Agents that boost the natu-ral immune response. Therapeutic immunostimu-lants have been used in cancer treatments to restore or augment the antitumor response. These include non-specific agents such as attenuated mycobacteria and therapeutic doses of interleuk-ins and interferons, as well as relatively specific agents such as non-viable tumor cells. Some immunostimulants are not truly stimulatory, but act by depressing regulatory mechanisms. In gen-eral, these therapies have serious side effects and are not widely used. It is important to note that allergy and autoimmunity are the result of a too vigorous or inappropriate immune response. A large number of environmental agents have this type of immunostimulatory effect. *See also* ALLER-GIC RESPONSE; AUTOIMMUNITY.

immunosuppression. Many environmental agents and drugs can produce alterations in the immune system that lead to impaired immune function. Some of the most severe secondary immunodeficiencies (i.e., those not due to inher-ited or congenital abnormalities) are iatrogenic. Cytotoxic drugs that inhibit cell division are pow-erful immunosuppressants since considerable rapid cell division is required to mount an effective immune response. The immunosuppressive effects of the antimetabolites, ionizing radiation and radiomimetic drugs used in cancer therapy are produced via this general mechanism. Other drugs, such as the adrenocorticosteroids used in treatment of inflammation, are more selectively toxic to the immune system, affecting lymphocyte numbers and function. In the case of organ transplant patients, immunosuppressants are necessary to prevent graft rejection. Many environmental agents can also depress immune function. Benzene is a potent bone marrow toxicant causing overall decreases in immune cell numbers, as well as alterations in function. Diethylstilbestrol, polychlorinated biphenyls, polybrominated biphenyls and metals are among the compounds that can cause immunosuppression at sublethal doses. Depression of immune function can lead to increased susceptibility to bacterial, viral and parasitic infections, and possibly increased incidence of neoplasm. Increased rates of cancers have been noted in transplant recipients, but it is not clear whether these are spontaneously arising neoplasms not eliminated by the comprised immune system or whether the neoplasms are actually produced and/or enhanced by the immune alterations. Immunosuppression must be assessed by a panel of tests since no one test can measure the many different effector functions of the immune system. These should include tests of both humoral immunity and cell-mediated immunity. Immunosuppression should not be confused with the action of suppressor T cells, which are a normal and necessary element of the immune system responsible for the suppression of unnecessary and detrimental immune responses. *See also* CELL-MEDIATED IMMUNITY; IMMUNE SYSTEM; LYMPHOCYTES; T CELLS.

immunosuppressive drugs. *See* IMMUNOSUPPRESSION.

immunosuppressor. A cell or soluble mediator that suppresses immune responses. Immunosuppressors may function to regulate immune responses, preventing excessive, potentially tissue-damaging responses. They are also involved in at least some types of immunological tolerance in which the immune system specifically fails to respond to certain substances, including all structures recognized as self. The major cell type involved in immunosuppression, the suppressor T cells (Ts), may secrete antigen-specific or non-specific soluble mediators (suppressor factors),

which suppress the functions of other cells required for the immune response. Certain naturally occurring agents (e.g., cortisol, prostaglandin E_2), as well as drugs and toxicants (e.g., cyclosporin A, cyclophosphamide), can also suppress the immune response by a variety of mechanisms.

immunotoxicity. (1) The toxic effects mediated by the immune system such as dermal sensitivity reactions to compounds like 2,4-dinitrochlorobenzene. (2) The toxic effects that impair the functioning of the immune system, for example, the ability of a toxicant to impair resistance to infection. This is the currently most acceptable definition.

immunotoxicity testing. Tests for immunotoxicity (toxic effects on the immune system rather than the immune system as a mediator of toxic effects) is an area of great interest, both in the fundamental mechanisms of immune function and in the design of tests to measure impairment of immune function. However, there is no agreement on a test or series of tests to be used. Moreover, as with the nervous system, there is considerable functional reserve in the immune system so that the demonstration *in vitro* of impairment of a particular facet of the system may not be reflected in an impairment of overall *in vivo* function. Many compounds can elicit immune reactions even though they may not be proteins or other macromolecules normally associated with antibody formation. The humoral and cell-mediated systems represent the two major parts of the overall immune system, the former involving primarily the B cells and the latter the T cells. The humoral system is involved in the production of antibodies, which react with foreign material (antigens), whereas the latter involves primarily the mobilization of phagocytic leukocytes to ingest such foreign organisms as bacteria. The two systems function together by complex feedback mechanisms. Rapid amplification of the number of cells capable of specific reaction to an antigen derives from memory cells which were specifically adapted to the antigen at the time of initial exposure. Tests of the immune system involve: (1) the weight and morphology of the lymphoid organs; (2) the capacity to respond to challenges such as those of mitogens (e.g., phytohemagglutinin, concanavalin A, lipopolysaccharide, pokeweed mitogen) or antigens (*Candida*, typhoid); (3) specific *in vitro* tests of components of the immune system. Changes in blood cells, particularly in the differential leukocyte count, may be indicative of effects on the immune system. The weight and pathology of the thymus and spleen are more important since effects noted therein are more specific, although not infallible, indications of immune impairment. Atrophy of the thymus usually indicates immunosuppression, although some non-immunosuppressive chemicals can cause thymus atrophy. Similarly, changes in the bone marrow, lymph nodes, spleen and thymus may, after treatment with a particular chemical, indicate changes in the immune system such as B- or T cell deficiency. Tests for overall immunocompetance include skin tests for antibody-mediated responses and for delayed hypersensitivity. Also included are tests that determine the predisposition of animals for disease or infection by *Streptococcus pneumoniae*. Tests that examine some narrow aspect of the immune system in great detail include tests for the production of different classes of antibodies, as well as tests of leukocyte function and differentiation: macrophage aggregation; inhibition of macrophage migration; lymphocyte transformation by antigens and mitogens; and many others. *See also* IMMUNE SYSTEM; IMMUNOTOXICITY.

implantation. *See* ADMINISTRATION OF TOXICANTS, IMPLANTATION.

indigo carmine (E132) (2-(1,3-dihydro-3-oxo-5-sulfo-2H-indol-2-ylidene)-2,3-dihydro-3-oxo-1H-indole-5-sulfonic acid disodium salt). **CAS number 860-22-0**. A compound that is used as a dye and has been approved by the FDA and the EEC for use in food and drugs. It is also used in a test of kidney function and as a reagent for the detection of nitrite and chlorate.

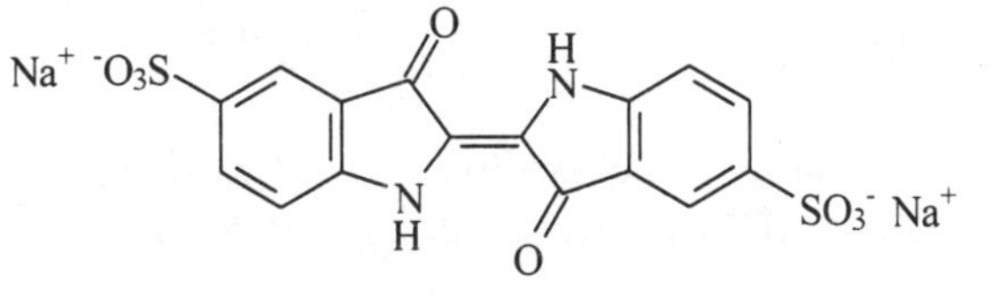

Indigo carmine

indoleethylamine N-methyltransferase. *See* N-METHYLATION.

indomethacin (1-(4-chlorobenzoyl)-5-methoxy-2-methyl-1H-indole-3-acetic acid; Indocin). **CAS number 53-86-1**. A methylated indole derivative that has anti-inflammatory, antipyretic and analgesic activity. Indomethacin is significantly more potent than salicylates and exerts its effects by potently inhibiting prostaglandin synthesis. Indomethacin is used as an antipyretic in patients refractory to other drugs (e.g., Hodgkin's disease) and in the treatment of rheumatoid arthritis. Despite its potency, however, it is not routinely used as an analgesic or antipyretic because chronic administration is associated with toxic effects in a large percentage of patients. Adverse effects include nausea, anorexia, abdominal pain, ulcers, headache, dizziness, depression, psychosis, hematopoietic reactions and hypersensitivity. The i.p. LD50 in rats is 13 mg/kg. *See also* ANALGESICS.

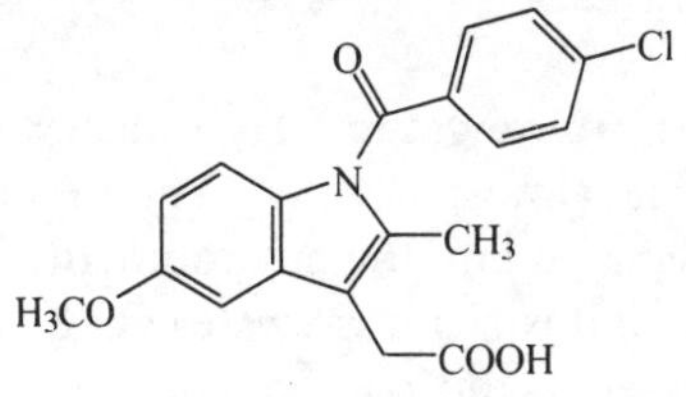

Indomethacin

indoor air pollution. The concept that the air of modern buildings, which are closed and whose air is recirculated, may be polluted with chemicals which are not allowed to escape. Examples of these pollutants would be tobacco smoke, pest control chemicals and chemicals vaporized from carpets, paints, insulation, furniture, varnishes, etc. Also known as "sick building syndrome". Similar concern also exists for the quality of air in aircraft.

induction. The process of increasing the amount of an enzyme following exposure to an inducing agent. Increasing the amount of an enzyme can occur via decreasing the degradation rate and/or increasing the synthesis rate. Increasing the synthesis rate is the most common mechanism for induction by xenobiotics. Coordinate (pleiotypic) induction refers to the induction of multiple enzymes by a single inducing agent (e.g., phenobarbital induction of several of the cytochrome P450-dependent monooxygenases). *See also* MECHANISM OF INDUCTION.

induction mechanisms. *See* MECHANISM OF INDUCTION.

industrial processes. *See* POLLUTION, INDUSTRIAL PROCESSES.

industrial toxicology. A specific area of environmental toxicology that deals with the work environment and includes risk assessment, establishment of permissible levels of exposure and worker protection. Because of the large number of industrial chemicals and the many possibilities for exposure, most industrialized nations have a significant body of laws that impact in this area and must be considered by the industrial toxicologist. *See also* HEALTH AND SAFETY AT WORK ACT; OCCUPATIONAL HEALTH AND SAFETY ACT; THRESHOLD LIMIT VALUES.

industrial wastewater. The wastewater from industry; it almost always requires treatment before discharge into the environment. The composition of industrial wastewater varies according to the industry, and consequently the treatment processes required before discharge must be designed for the specific wastewater. Unlike normal domestic sewage, some industrial wastewaters contain toxic substances, such as carcinogens, heavy metals or radioactive materials.

infrared spectrophotometry. *See* SPECTROMETRY, INFRARED.

inhalant abuse. *See* SOLVENT ABUSE.

inhalation apparatus. *See* ADMINISTRATION OF TOXICANTS, INHALATION.

inhalation reference concentration (RfC). An estimate of a continuous inhalation exposure to the human population that is likely to be without appreciable risk of deleterious noncancer lifetime health effects. Since this estimate includes sensitive population subgroups it may be considered a conservative estimate.

inhalation tests. Tests for toxicity of chemicals administered by inhalation are particularly difficult to carry out and are done only when the expected route of exposure to humans is via the respiratory tract. The engineering involved in the generation and administration of stable aerosols is complex and expensive. For this reason, subchronic studies (30–90 days) are more commonly attempted than chronic studies lasting the greater part of the lifetime of the test species. Apart from the route and duration of exposure, the testing variables and toxic endpoints are similar to those for other chronic and subchronic toxicity tests. *See also* ADMINISTRATION OF TOXICANTS, INHALATION; CHRONIC TOXICITY TESTING; SUBCHRONIC TOXICITY TESTING, INHALATION; TOXIC ENDPOINTS.

inhalation toxicology. The study of adverse effects of toxicants administered in the air entering the respiratory system. The inhaled toxicants are either volatile or are particles or droplets suspended in air. Deleterious effects on the respiratory system as well as other systems are studied.

inhibition. In its most general sense, a restraining, a holding back (from the Latin inhibere, to hold back, to restrain). More specifically, in biochemistry and biochemical toxicology, it is used in the sense of being a reduction in the rate of an enzymatic reaction, an inhibitor being any compound that causes such reduction in rate. Inhibition, by xenobiotics, of enzymes important in normal metabolism is important as a mode of toxic action, whereas inhibition of xenobiotic-metabolizing enzymes can have important consequences in the ultimate toxicity of their substrates. Inhibition is sometimes used in toxicology in a more general, and rather ill-defined, way to refer to the reduction of an overall process of toxicity, as in the inhibition of carcinogenesis by a particular chemical. *See also* XENOBIOTIC METABOLISM, INHIBITION.

inhibition, irreversible. *See* XENOBIOTIC METABOLISM, IRREVERSIBLE INHIBITION.

inhibitors, cholinesterase. *See* ANTICHOLINESTERASES.

inhibitors, electron transport. *See* ELECTRON TRANSPORT SYSTEM INHIBITORS.

inhibitors, monoamine oxidase. *See* MONOAMINE OXIDASE INHIBITORS.

inhibitors, oxidative phosphorylation. *See* OXIDATIVE PHOSPHORYLATION INHIBITORS.

inhibitory complexes. *See* METABOLITE INHIBITORY COMPLEXES.

inhibitory concentration (IC). The concentration of a compound that causes a specific magnitude of inhibition of a response in an *in vitro* system. It almost always is used with a numerical modifer relating to the percentage of response: for example, IC50 is the concentration that causes a 50% inhibition of some normal or induced response. The term provides a comparison of the potencies of various toxicants in inhibiting a specific physiological responses or drug/hormone-induced effects. *See also* ENZYME KINETICS; METABOLITE INHIBITORY COMPLEXES; RADIO-RECEPTOR ASSAYS; XENOBIOTIC METABOLISM, INHIBITION.

initiation. The conversion of a normal cell to a neoplastic cell in the process of carcinogensis. Initiation is considered to be a rapid, essentially irreversible change involving the interaction of the ultimate carcinogen with DNA; this change primes the cell for subsequent neoplastic development via the promotion process. *See also* CARCINOGENS; NEOPLASM; PROGRESSION; PROMOTION.

injection. *See* ADMINISTRATION OF TOXICANTS, INJECTION.

inorganic insecticides. Inorganic insecticides have largely been replaced by synthetic organics due primarily to their lack of specificity and their lower toxicity to insects. However, two classes of inorganic insecticides, i.e., arsenicals and lead arsenate, have been widely utilized in the past. The arsenicals included such compounds as calcium arsenate $\left[Ca_3(AsO_4)_2\right]$ and lead arsenate $(PbHAsO_4)$, sodium arsenite $(NaAsO_2)$ and

Paris Green $\left[(CH_3COO)_2 Cu \bullet 3Cu(AsO_2)_2\right]$. The inorganic fluorides used were sodium fluoride (NaF), cryolite or sodium fluoroaluminate (Na_3AlF_6) and sodium fluorosilicate (Na_2SiF_6). Boric acid (BH_3O_3) still receives some use for the control of household insects. *See also* INSECTICIDES.

insecticides. Chemicals developed and produced specifically for the control of populations of insects of agricultural or public health importance. Important classes of insecticides include: chlorinated hydrocarbons (including DDT analogs, chlorinated alicyclic compounds, cyclodienes and chlorinated terpenes); organophosphates; carbamates; thiocyanates; dinitrophenols; botanicals (including pyrethroids, rotenoids and nicotinoids); juvenile hormone analogs; growth regulators; and inorganics (including arsenicals and fluorides). *See also* CARBAMATE INSECTICIDES; CYCLODIENE INSECTICIDES; INORGANIC INSECTICIDES; ORGANOCHLORINE INSECTICIDES; ORGANOPHOSPHORUS INSECTICIDES; PYRETHROID INSECTICIDES.

in situ. In the normal or natural location. In toxicology is used primarily in two contexts. The first relates to the intact organism, for example the study of organ toxicity as expressed in the intact organism, and the second relates to environmental toxicology, for example the study of a toxic effect as expressed in the natural ecosystem.

Institute of Biology (IOB). A UK professional body, which awards the Diploma of the Institute of Biology in Toxicology (DIBT).

insulin. A protein hormone (M_r = 5800), produced by the β-cells of the pancreatic islets of Langerhans consisting of two peptide chains. The A and B chains are 21 and 30 amino acid residues, respectively, linked by disulfide bridges between cystine residues. Insulin is responsible for increasing the permeability of cells to glucose, thereby reducing blood glucose. A notable exception is the brain which is not insulin-dependent. Insulin is secreted in response to hyperglycemia, such as following a high carbohydrate meal. A lack of insulin results in diabetes mellitus. Diabetogenic chemicals (e.g., alloxan) can destroy the β-cells and cause diabetes mellitus.

integrated exposure. *See* EXPOSURE, INTE-GRATED.

Integrated Risk Information System (IRIS). A database maintained and made available by the US Environmental Protection Agency that describes the rationale for a chemical's risk status with background bibliographic information. Available since 1988, this database contains over 500 chemicals reviewed by the EPA.

interactions. In toxicology this refers to the effect of one chemical or toxicant on the toxicity of another, or the toxicity of mixtures as compared with the toxicity of their individual components, administered separately. Such interactions may be additive, synergistic (or potentiated) or antagonistic. In pharmacology the problem of toxic effects from using multiple drug regimens is important and may involve life-threatening interactions. Synergistic interactions are utilized in agrochemicals applications to increase the toxicity of insecticides and herbicides. *See also* SYNERGISM AND POTENTIATION.

Interagency Regulatory Liaison Group. A group formed in 1977 by four US regulatory agencies, the Consumer Products Safety Commission, the Environmental Protection Agency, the Food and Drug Administration and the Occupational Safety and Health Administration, in an effort to reform the regulatory process as it applies to chemicals. They were joined in 1979 by the Food Safety and Quality Service of the US Department of Agriculture. Although their efforts and those of the Organization for Economic Cooperation and Development (OECD) have brought about some consolidation of the many testing requirements and protocols, differences still exist.

Interagency Testing Committee. A committee set up in the USA under the Toxic Substances Control Act (TSCA) to recommend a priority list of chemicals for toxicity testing. Members are appointed by the Environmental Protection Agency, Occupational Safety and Health Administration, Council for Environmental Quality, National Institute for Occupational Safety and Health, National Institute for Environmental Health Sciences, National Cancer Institute,

National Science Foundation, and the Department of Commerce. Once a chemical has been placed on the priority testing list the Environmental Protection Agency must either initiate appropriate tests or make public its reasons for not initiating such tests. *See also* TOXIC SUBSTANCE CONTROL ACT.

intercalating agent. In toxicology, a chemical that exerts its action by interposing between two substituents of a macromolecule, specifically between two base pairs of DNA. For example, actinomycin D binds tightly, but not covalently, to double-helical DNA. It does not bind to single-stranded DNA or RNA or double-stranded RNA or DNA-RNA hybrids. At low concentrations, an intercalating agent inhibits transcription without affecting replication or protein synthesis. Certain flat aromatic molecules such as the acridines appear to be mutagenic by intercalation rather than by covalent adduct formation. *See also* ACRIDINE ORANGE.

interleukin I (IL1). A 17,000-dalton protein produced by macrophages. It exhibits a wide range of biological activities including induction of T-cell proliferation, bone resorption, fibroblast proliferation, release of acute-phase proteins from hepatocytes, cartilage breakdown and fever. These activities are consistent with a role for IL1 as a mediator of inflammatory responses. There are at least two distinct molecules with IL1 activity (IL1a and IL1b). However, these molecules apparently bind to the same receptor on target cells. *Compare* INTERLEUKIN II.

interleukin II (IL2). A small protein produced by T cells that apparently plays an important role in at least immune responses. It can sustain T-cell proliferation, induce release of other immunologically active molecules and stimulate B-cell proliferation and differentiation. The capacity of mitogen-activated peripheral blood lymphocytes to produce interleukin II in culture might be a useful indicator of immunocompetence in animals exposed to drugs or toxicants. *Compare* INTERLEUKIN I.

intermediates. *See* METABOLITES.

International Agency for Research on Cancer (IARC). An agency of the United Nations located in Lyon, France; IARC was established by the World Health Organization. It provides expert committees to evaluate the carcinogenicity of chemicals based on information in the published literature. In addition, it publishes reports on individual chemicals and groups of chemicals, as well as summary compilations classifying chemicals according to their potential as human carcinogens.

International Atomic Energy Agency (IAEA). An agency headquartered in Vienna formed initially to exchange information among those working with radioactive materials. Later, with the advent of civil nuclear power, it was adopted by the United Nations. It is concerned with all aspects of atomic energy and the commercial and scientific uses of radioisotopes. It is a partner with the Food and Agricultural Organization of the United Nations in the Division of Atomic Energy in Food and Agriculture.

International Life Sciences Institute (ILSI). A Washington DC based institute, supported by industry, particularly the food industry of the USA. Conducts studies, prepares reports and supports research in the life sciences, particularly studies concerning the interaction of synthetic chemicals with living organisms and the way in which studies may be related to food safety.

International Program on Chemical Safety (IPCS). A joint venture of the United Nations Environment Program, the International Labor Organization, and the World Health Organization. The main objective of the IPCS is to carry out and disseminate evaluations of the effects of chemicals on human health and the quality of the environment.

International Register of Potentially Toxic Chemicals (IRPTC) (WHO). Created in 1972 by the World Health Organization, the IRPTC is designed to facilitate access to data on chemical effects on humans and the environment, to identify important knowledge in the above and to provide information on national, regional and global policies, recommendations and regulations for the control of potentially hazardous chemicals. Publishes the IRPTC bulletin, maintains a computer database on chemicals and publishes chemical profiles.

International Society for the Study of Xenobiotics (ISSX). An international society with over 2400 members from 50 countries dedicated to the study of xenobiotics of all types, including drugs, agricultural chemicals, environmental chemicals and industrial chemicals. While all aspects are considered, the metabolism of xenobiotics and the molecular biology of xenobiotic-metabolizing enzymes are of particular interest as is the role of these aspects in drug development, regulation and safety. Headquarters are in Bethesda, Maryland, USA.

International Union of Toxicology (IUTOX). A group with both member societies and individual members that fosters international cooperation in toxicology primarily through the organization of International Congresses of Toxicology.

interspecies extrapolation. *See* SPECIES, EXTRAPOLATION.

interstitial cell-stimulating hormone (ICSH). A gonadotropin from the adenohypophysis that stimulates the testicular interstitial cells (cells of Leydig) to produce androgens. It is equivalent to luteinizing hormone (LH) in the female. Its secretion is stimulated by hypothalamic gonadotropin-releasing hormone (GnRH).

intestinal lavage. The washing of the lumen of the intestine by introduction of fluid, usually saline, sorbitol or mannitol solution, through a lavage tube. This procedure is carried out to remove unabsorbed poisons or excreted poisons. Neither intestinal lavage nor catharsis are appropriate when there is imbalance of fluid or electrolytes or poisoning by corrosive materials. *See also* POISONING, LIFE SUPPORT.

intestinal perfusion techniques. *See* PENETRATION ROUTES, GASTROINTESTINAL; PERFUSION STUDIES, INTESTINE.

intestine. The major segment of the digestive tract of the mammal, comprising the small intestine distal to the stomach and the large intestine (colon). The small intestine is the longest section of the gut and is composed of the duodenum, the jejunum and the ileum, and is separated from the stomach by the pyloric sphincter. The small intestine, primarily the duodenum, is responsible for most of the digestion and absorption of nutrients. It is also the site of the enterohepatic circulation in which bile salts and xenobiotics excreted in the bile into the duodenum are reabsorbed into the circulation more distally. The ileocecal sphincter separates the small and large intestine. The latter comprises the cecum, ascending colon, transverse colon, descending colon and sigmoid colon which then merges with the rectum. *See also* COLON.

intoxication. (1) In the general sense, primarily inebriation with ethanol and secondarily the causing of excitement or delirium by other means, including other chemicals. In the clinical sense, intoxication refers to poisoning or becoming poisoned. (2) In toxicology, a synonym for activation or the production of a more toxic metabolite from a less toxic parent compound. This use of the term is ambiguous and should be abandoned in favor of the aforementioned general meanings.

intradermal injection. *See* ADMINISTRATION OF TOXICANTS, INJECTION.

intragastric. *See* ADMINISTRATION OF TOXICANTS, ORAL.

intramuscular injection. *See* ADMINISTRATION OF TOXICANTS, INJECTION.

intraperitoneal injection. *See* ADMINISTRATION OF TOXICANTS, INJECTION.

intrapleural pressure. The pressure within the pleural cavity or the space between the pleural membrane covering the lungs (visceral pleura) and that covering the inner surface of the thoracic cage (parietal pleura). This pressure is usually 4–5 cm H_2O less than atmospheric pressure (760 mm Hg). It should be referred to as subatmospheric rather than "negative."

intratracheal. Introduced into the lumen of the trachea, a term used in respiratory toxicology.

intravenous infusion. *See* ADMINISTRATION OF TOXICANTS, INJECTION.

intravenous injection. *See* ADMINISTRATION OF TOXICANTS, INJECTION.

intron. *See* GENE.

in utero. Within the uterus; in toxicology usually used in connection with toxic effects consequent upon exposure of the embryo or fetus during development. Such exposure can be accidental or during reproductive toxicity tests.

invermectins. *See* IVERMECTINS.

inversions. *See* CHROMOSOME ABERRATIONS.

in vitro. Literally in glass, or in the test tube, taking place outside the body of the organism, as in *in vitro* tests or in studies involving isolated perfused organs, isolated cells or subcellular preparations. *Compare* IN VIVO. *See also* IN VITRO TOXICITY TESTS.

in vitro **toxicity tests**. Literally, tests conducted outside the body of the organism. In toxicity testing, they include studies using isolated enzymes, subcellular organelles or cultured cells. Although technically it does not include tests involving intact eukaryotes (e.g., the Ames test), the term is frequently used by toxicologists to include all short-term tests for mutagenicity that are normally used as indicators of potential carcinogenicity. As an example, *in vitro* tests of the genotoxicity of chemicals are typically conducted with cell cultures (prokaryotic or eukaryotic) to estimate the carcinogenic or teratogenic potential of the chemical without the time, expense and large number of animals required for traditional *in vivo* tests. These test systems include assays to detect mutagenicity in prokaryotic and eukaryotic cells, chromosomal aberrations and mammalian cell transformation ability. Although *in vitro* tests cannot substitute for *in vivo* tests, they can screen chemicals under development that are most likely to display chronic toxicity and also can quickly indicate which chemicals in the environment are of the greatest potential long-term hazard. *Compare* IN VIVO TOXICITY TEST. *See also* AMES TEST; EUKARYOTE MUTAGENICITY TEST; FETAX; PROKARYOTE MUTAGENICITY TEST.

in vivo. In the living organism; in toxicology usually used in connection with toxicity tests carried out on intact animals. *Compare* IN VITRO. *See also* IN VIVO TOXICITY TESTS.

in vivo **toxicity tests**. Traditionally the basis for the determination of toxicity has been administration of the suspected compound *in vivo* to one or more species of experimental animal, followed by examination for mortality in acute tests or by pathological examination for tissue abnormalities in chronic tests. Such results are then used, by a variety of extrapolation techniques, to estimate hazard to humans. Although these techniques offer many advantages and are still widely used, it should be mentioned that they suffer from a number of disadvantages. They require large numbers of animals, numbers deemed unnecessary by both animal rights and animal welfare advocates, they are expensive to conduct and they are time consuming. More recently they have been supplemented by many specialized *in vitro* tests. *Compare* IN VITRO TOXICITY TESTS. *See also* BEHAVIORAL TOXICITY TESTING; CARCINOGENICITY TESTING; CHRONIC TOXICITY TESTING; COVALENT BINDING TESTS; DELAYED NEUROPATHY TESTS; DERMAL IRRITATION TESTS; DERMAL SENSITIZATION TESTS; EYE IRRITATION TEST; LC50; LD50; POTENTIATION TESTS; REPRODUCTION TOXICITY TESTING; SUBCHRONIC TOXICITY TESTS; TERATOLOGY TESTING; TOXICITY TESTING; TOXICOKINETICS.

IOB. *See* INSTITUTE OF BIOLOGY.

ion channel toxins. The importance of ion channels in the function of excitable tissue in mammals makes them an important target for natural toxins. Various scorpion toxins block K^+ channels, toxins from the tropical sponge *Agelas conifera* act on Na^+ channels, and polyamine toxins from spiders and wasps target ligand gated ion channels, especially glutamate receptors which mediate neuromsuscular transmission in the invertebrate prey of these species. Funnel web spider toxins preferentially block P-type calcium channels and prevent presynaptic calcium currents and transmitter release. *See also* MAMBA TOXINS; CONUS; TETRODOTOXIN; SAXITOXIN.

ionic binding. Electrostatic attraction that occurs between two oppositely charged ions, e.g., proteins binding with metal ions. The degree of binding varies with the chemical nature of each compound and the net charge. Dissociation of ionic bonds usually occurs readily, but some members of the transition group of metals exhibit high association constants (i.e., low Kd values) and exchange is slow. Ionic interactions may also contribute to binding of alkaloids and other ionizable toxicants with ionizable nitrogenous groups. *See also* BINDING.

ionization and uptake of toxicants. Membranes are much less permeable to compounds in the ionized state than those in the non-ionized form. This is not important for the majority of toxicants as they are not in an ionizable form and are unaffected by pH. However, a small number of toxicants (e.g., alkaloids and organic acids) are ionizable, and their penetration may be appreciably altered by pH. The amount in the ionized or un-ionized form depends upon the pK_a (negative logarithm of the acidic dissociation constant) of the potential toxicant and the pH of the bathing medium. When the pH of a solution is equal to the pK_a of the dissolved compounds, one-half exists in the ionized form and one-half exists in the un-ionized (free) form. The degree of ionization is given by the Henderson–Hasselbach equation. As the un-ionized form of a weak electrolyte is the diffusible molecule, weak organic acids diffuse most readily in acid and organic bases in alkaline environments. There are exceptions to the generalizations concerning ionization; such compounds as pralidoxime (2-PAM), paraquat and diquat are absorbed to an appreciable extent in the ionized forms. *See also* ENTRY MECHANISMS, PASSIVE TRANSPORT; HENDERSON–HASSELBACH EQUATION; MEMBRANES.

ionizing radiation. Radiation of sufficiently high energy to produce ions in the medium through which it passes, for example, high-energy particles (electrons, protons, α-particles) or short-wave radiation (UV, X-, γ-rays). Extensive damage to the molecular structure of the medium occurs either as a result of direct transfer of energy or of secondary electrons released. Toxic effects occur particularly because of the formation of free radicals that can have powerful oxidizing or reducing properties.

IPCS. *See* INTERNATIONAL PROGRAM ON CHEMICAL SAFETY.

ipecac, syrup of. A syrup prepared from the dried roots and rhizome of *Uragoga ipecacuanha*. The syrup contains a number of alkaloids, of which emetine is the most common. It is used in the treatment of poisoning as an emetic, to induce vomiting in those cases in which emesis is not contraindicated. The fluid extract is not used because of its greater potency and potential for hazardous side effects. *See also* EMESIS; POISONING, EMERGENCY TREATMENT.

ipomeanol (1-(3-furyl)-4-hydroxypentanone). The most important member of a group of furan derivatives responsible for the lung edema found in cattle fed moldy sweet potatoes infected with the fungus *Fusarium solani* and known collectively as the "LE factor." It causes edema and thickening of the alveolar septum associated with extensive damage to the bronchiolar epithelium. It appears that these furans are produced by the fungus from a precursor produced by the plant in response to fungal infection. Ipomeanol is the best known example of a toxic compound activated in the lung. Pulmonary injury by 4-ipomeanol is caused by a highly reactive, alkylating metabolite, probably an epoxide, produced by cytochrome P450 isozymes. The two major lung cytochrome P450 isozymes both readily metabolize 4-ipomeanol. Consequently, activation by the lung is much greater than that in the liver, which contains significantly lower levels of these two isozymes. In addition, these isozymes are highly concentrated in the Clara cells, which are most affected by

4-ipomeanol toxicity. *See also* PULMONARY TOXICITY, BIOTRANSFORMATION AND REACTIVE METABOLITES.

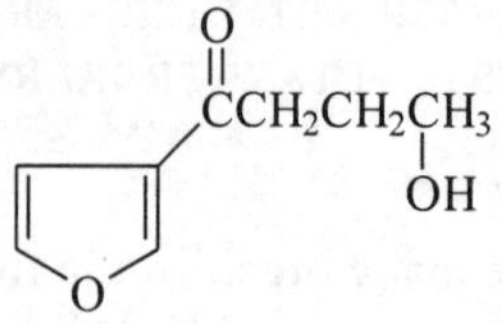

Ipomeanol

iproniazid (4-pyridinecarboxylic acid 2-(1-methylethyl)hydrazide; isonicotinic acid 2-isopropylhydrazide). CAS number 54-92-2. An isopropyl derivative of isoniazid that was found to have mood-elevating effects in tuberculosis patients. It was later found to be a monoamine oxidase (MAO) inhibitor and, although not currently approved for clinical use as an antidepressant, it led to the development of other MAO inhibitors. In addition to hepatotoxic effects, iproniazid is a hypotensive agent and can cause potentially hazardous reactions with other drugs and amine-rich foods. *See also* ANTIDEPRESSANTS; MONOAMINE OXIDASE INHIBITORS.

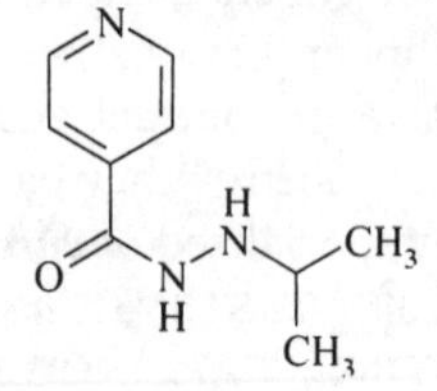

Iproniazid

IR. *See* SPECTROPHOTOMETRY, INFRARED.

Irene Serenade. *See* ENVIRONMENTAL DISASTERS.

IRIS. *See* INTEGRATED RISK INFORMATION SYSTEM.

IRPTC. *See* INTERNATIONAL REGISTER OF POTENTIALLY TOXIC CHEMICALS.

irreversible effect. In toxicology, an effect of a toxicant that the body cannot repair or reverse. *See also* REVERSIBLE EFFECT.

irreversible inhibition. *See* XENOBIOTIC METABOLISM, IRREVERSIBLE INHIBITION.

irritants. Any non-corrosive substance that, on immediate, prolonged or repeated contact with normal living tissue produces a local inflammatory reaction. Toxicants that exert their deleterious effects by causing inflammation of mucous membranes with which they come into contact. Irritants principally act on the respiratory system and can cause death from asphyxiation due to lung edema. Other mucous membranes that may be affected by irritants are those of the eyes. Respiratory irritants differ not only in the severity of their effects, but also in the region of the respiratory system affected. Aldehydes, such as acetaldehyde, formaldehyde and acrolein, primarily affect the upper respiratory tract as do ammonia, hydrogen chloride and other acids and bases. Cyanogen bromide, chlorine oxides and phosphorus trichloride are examples of irritants that primarily affect lung tissue, as well as the upper respiratory tract, whereas phosgene and nitrogen dioxide primarily affect the terminal airways and alveoli. *See also* ASPHYXIANTS.

irritation assays. *See* DERMAL IRRITATION TESTS.

isoamyl nitrite. *See* AMYL NITRITE.

isochromosome. A chromosome aberration in which one of the arms of a particular chromosome is duplicated because the centromere divided transversely and not longitudinally during cell division.

isocyanates. Organic compounds containing the -NCO group. Alkyl- and arylisocyanates are used as chemical intermediates, particularly in the manufacture of plastics. Acute exposure may cause airway irritation, cough and dyspnea while chronic exposure may lead to asthma and reduced lung function.

isoelectric focusing. A method used to separate mixtures containing proteins of different pI. The migration of ampholytes (e.g., proteins) occurs through a pH gradient under an applied electric field. Molecules possessing an electric charge migrate towards a region in which they are isoelectric. *See also* ISOELECTRIC POINT.

isoelectric point (pI). pH at which a species (amino acid, protein or colloid) does not move in an electric field. *See also* ISOELECTRIC FOCUSING.

isoenzymes. *See* ISOZYMES.

isoflurane (1-chloro-2,2,2-trifluoroethyl difluoromethyl ether; Forane). CAS number 26675-46-7. An isomer of enflurane with similar anesthetic properties. Isoflurane has less effect on myocardial function, leaving the cardiovascular system normally responsive to epinephrine or hypercarbia, and it does not cause a marked increase in seizure susceptibility. It was not widely used because of reports that it caused increases in liver neoplasms in mice, but this observation has been challenged and the compound reintroduced. *See also* ANESTHETICS; ENFLURANE.

$$\underset{\displaystyle \overset{|}{F}}{\overset{\displaystyle \overset{|}{F}}{F-C}}-\underset{\displaystyle \overset{|}{H}}{\overset{\displaystyle \overset{|}{Cl}}{C}}-O-\underset{\displaystyle \overset{|}{F}}{\overset{\displaystyle \overset{|}{H}}{C}}-F$$

Isoflurane

isolated organ techniques. *See* PERFUSION STUDIES.

isolated perfused tubule. A method used in investigations of kidney tubule function in which a segment of tubule is dissected out and suspended between two micropipettes, the perfusion pipette and the collection pipette. Although clearly applicable, this technique has not yet been applied to the study of the effects of chemicals on renal function, presumably because it is technically difficult to carry out and has been developed primarily with tubules from one species, the rabbit. *See also* NEPHRON.

isomerases. *See* ENZYMES.

isoniazid (4-pyridinecarboxylic acid hydrazide; isonicotinic acid hydrazide). CAS number 54-85-3. An antibacterial drug used in the treatment of tuberculosis. Adverse effects, although relatively uncommon, may include rash, fever, jaundice and peripheral neuritis. Co-administration of pyridoxine prevents the development of peripheral neuritis. The LD50 in mice is 151 mg/kg i.p., and 149 mg/kg i.v. *See also* ANTIBAC-TERIALS; ANTIBIOTICS; FAST AND SLOW ACETY-LATORS.

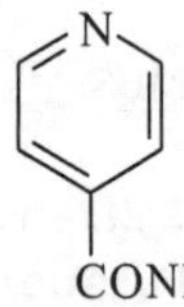

CONHNH$_2$

Isoniazid

isopropanol (2-propanol, isopropyl alcohol, (CH$_3$)$_2$CHOH). CAS number 67-63-0. A typical secondary alcohol, it is used in the preparation of propanone, esters, amines and glycerol. Common household and industrial solvent. On acute dosing is a CNS depressant that can also cause cardiovascular depression in large doses. Cancer of the paranasal sinuses has been established as an effect of workplace exposure during isopropanol manufacture. *See also* DATABASES, TOXICOLOGY; LEWIS HCDR NUMBER INJ000.

isoquinolines. *See* TETRAHYDROISOQUINOLINES.

isosafrole (5-(1-propenyl)-1,3-benzodioxole). CAS number 120-58-1. A compound isolated from the root of sassafras. Before being banned because of its carcinogenicity in the 1960s, it was used in perfumes, soaps and as a flavor in root beer and toothpaste. Its oral LD50 in mice is 2.47 g/kg and in rats is 1.34 g/kg. It is carcinogenic, producing DNA adducts following oxidation at the side chain; it causes hepatic adenomas and carcinomas. It is an insecticide synergist by virtue of its inhibition of cytochrome P450; a carbene produced by oxidation of the methylene carbon forms a stable adduct with the heme iron of the cytochrome. *See also* METHYLENEDIOXYPHENYL RING CLEAVAGE; SAFROLE.

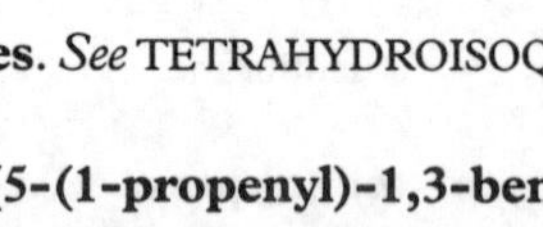

Isosafrole

isotopes. Atoms housing the same atomic (proton) number (Z) but different numbers of neutrons (N) and hence different atomic mass numbers (A). The most precise way of denoting the isotopes is as $^A_Z X$ (e.g., $^1_1$H, $^2_1$H, $^3_1$H). The atomic mass of an element is the average mass percentage of all its isotopes. Isotopes have similar chemical properties, but slight differences in physical properties. There are three kinds of isotopes: natural non-radioactive, natural radioactive and artificially radioactive (prepared by neutron bombardment).

isotopic footpad assay. A method for the investigation of delayed hypersensitivity reactions that involves the use of ^{125}I-labeled serum albumin as an indicator of changes due to increased capillary permeability and edema at the reaction site. *See also* DELAYED HYPERSENSITIVITY.

isozymes (isoenzymes). Multiple forms of a given enzyme that occur within a single species or even a single cell and catalyze the same general reaction, but are coded for by different genes. Such multiple forms can usually be separated by gel electrophoresis since they differ in amino acid composition and isoelectric points. Different isozymes may occur at different life stages and/or in different organs and tissues. Isozymes usually differ in their K_m and V_{max} toward the substrate. The first well-characterized isozymes were those of lactic dehydrogenase (LDH). Mammalian tissue makes two electrophoretically distinguishable subunits (A and B), which combine in a tetramer to form the active enzyme. Five distinct isozymes of LDH occur: A$_4$, A$_3$B$_1$, A$_2$B$_2$, A$_1$B$_3$ and B$_4$. These forms display different K_m and V_{max} values and can be separated electrophoretically. Several xenobiotic-metabolizing enzymes exist as multiple isozymes, including cytochrome P450 and glucuronosyltransferase.

ISSX. *See* INTERNATIONAL SOCIETY FOR THE STUDY OF XENOBIOTICS.

itai-itai disease. A case of human environmental toxicity, resulting from the ingestion of cadmium-contaminated rice, characterized in Japan. The cadmium was from industrial sources. The syndrome includes damage to both the renal and skeletoarticular systems; the latter is very painful (itai means pain).

IUTOX. *See* INTERNATIONAL UNION OF TOXICOLOGY.

ivermectins. A mixture of semisynthetic derivatives of abamectin, primarily 22,23-dihydroavermectin B_{1a} used as an anthelminthic and as an insecticide. Abamectin is a microbial insecticide and anthelminic isolated from *Streptomyces avermitilus*.

Ixtox 1. *See* ENVIRONMENTAL DISASTERS.

J

James River. *See* CHLORDECONE, ENVIRONMENTAL DISASTERS.

jasmine. *See* ESSENTIAL OILS.

jaundice. A condition characterized by a yellow appearance of the whites of the eyes, the skin and mucous membranes. This discoloration is due to the presence of excess bilirubin in the blood. Although jaundice can be a symptom of a number of diseases or of biliary obstruction by gallstones, it can also occur in both acute and chronic hepatotoxicity, for example, that caused by carbon tetrachloride. *See also* DIAGNOSTIC FEATURES, SKIN; HEPATOTOXICITY.

JECFA. *See* JOINT FAO/WHO EXPERT COMMITTEE ON FOOD ADDITIVES.

jejunum. *See* INTESTINE.

jequirity bean. Black and scarlet beans of the plant *Abrus precatorius* sometimes used in "folk-art" necklaces. Contain toxic lectins similar to those found in castor beans. Abrin-a, consisting of an A chain of 250 amino acids and a B chain of 267 amino acids is the most effective protein synthesis inhibitor of several abrins found in this species. LD50 to mouse is less than 0.1 µg/kg, thus abrin is one of the most acutely toxic compounds known. *See also* CASTOR BEAN; RICIN; RICININE.

Jerne plaque assay (hemolytic plaque assay; plaque-forming cell assay). A method of quantitating antibody-producing cells, developed in 1963 by Niels K. Jerne. Cells from an immunized animal or a culture are mixed with sufficient red blood cells (RBCs) to form a homogeneous lawn of RBCs in an agar matrix. The antibody secreted by the antibody-producing cell diffuses radially in the gel, binding RBCs directly (if it is an anti-RBC antibody) or binding any protein or hapten of interest that has been attached to the RBC. A source of complement is then added. This causes lysis of any RBC bound to an antibody of IgM or some particular subclasses of IgG, and a clear plaque forms around each cell producing antibodies of the correct specificity and complement-fixing class. Antibodies of other classes can be quantitated by adding an anti-immunoglobin antibody (itself an IgM) to the mixture before adding complement. Cells to be assayed should be sufficiently diluted to assure each plaque is formed by only one cell. Results are usually expressed as plaque-forming cells (PFC) per spleen (the spleen is the primary location of these cells), PFC per culture or PFC per 10^6 cells. Since many proteins and compounds can be conjugated to RBC, this test has a very wide applicability. It is often used to assess the health of the T cell-dependent antibody-producing cell response (e.g., after exposure to chemicals) since the generation of differentiated antibody-producing cells (i.e., plasma cells) requires the functional cooperation of B cells, T cells and macrophages. It can also be used as a direct quantitative assay for complement since the hemolysis of sensitized RBC is also dependent on an intact complement system. *See also* B CELLS; COMPLEMENT.

jimsonweed. *Datura* spp. (including *D. stramonium, D. sanguinea, D. aurea*). Jimsonweed is also known as thorn apple, datura, devil's apple, locoweed, etc. Its toxic, mind-altering properties have been known for millennia and it is frequently abused for its hallucinogenic properties. Toxic properties are due to tropane belladonna alkaloids such as atropine, hyoscyamine and scopolamine. Related plants include *Atropa belladonna* or deadly nightshade, *Hyoscyamus niger* or henbane, and

Mandragora officinarum or mandrake, all containing hyoscamine and scopolamine. *See also* ATROPINE; HYOSCAMINE; SCOPOLAMINE.

Joint FAO/WHO Expert Committee on Food Additives (JEFCA). JEFCA serves as a scientific advisory body to FAO, WHO, their member states and the Codex Alimentarius Commission regarding the safety of food additives, residues of veterinary drugs, and contaminants in food.

K

karyotype. The particular chromosome constitution of an individual or species, as determined by the number and morphology of (usually) the somatic chromosomes at metaphase of mitosis. Karyotypes are usually prepared by treating the mitotic cells with a spindle poison, which increases the ease with which the chromosomes can be distinguished. Recently, various methods of banding the chromosomes have greatly increased the degree of precision with which the karyotype can be analyzed. A diagrammatic representation of the karyotype is called an idiogram; the two terms are not synonymous.

Kastenbaum–Bowman test. A test of statistical significance used in calculation of mutation frequencies.

K_D **(dissociation constant).** In the interaction of ligands with binding sites, a frequently derived constant originating (like the Michaelis constant, K_M) from the law of mass action. Experimentally, it is usually presented as Scatchard, Woolf, Eadie–Hofstee or, less frequently, Lineweaver–Burk plots although analyses are now commonly done by nonlinear regression. The K_D is inversely proportional to the affinity of a ligand for its recognition site and often reflects the importance of the binding of a particular toxicant to a recognition site. *See also* DISSOCIATION CONSTANT; EADIE–HOFSTEE PLOT; K_M; LINEWEAVER–BURK PLOT; MICHAELIS–MENTEN EQUATION; RADIORECEPTOR ASSAYS; WOOLF PLOT; XENOBIOTIC METABOLISM, INHIBITION.

Kelthane. *See* DICOFOL.

Kepone. *See* CHLORDECONE.

kerosene (kerosine; paraffin). CAS number 8008-20-6. A petroleum distillate that contains mainly C10–C16 aliphatic hydrocarbons, as well as aromatics such as benzene and naphthalene. Its boiling point range is 175–325 °C. The oral LD50 in rabbits is 28 g/kg. It is used in kerosene lamps, stoves and flares, in insecticides and as a degreaser and cleaner. Its toxicological effects are similar to gasoline with dermatitis, resulting from the defatting of the skin, vomiting, pneumonitis, headache, drowsiness and coma.

Ketaject. *See* KETAMINE.

Ketalar. *See* KETAMINE.

Ketamine (2-(2-chlorophenyl)-2-(methylamino) cyclohexanone; Ketaject; Ketalar). CAS number 6740-88-1. An anesthetic that causes a sensation of dissociation, followed rapidly by unconsciousness. Intense analgesia and amnesia are also rapidly established, and the analgesia and amnesia persist after the anesthesia ceases. Muscle relaxation is generally poor, and purposeless movements or exaggerated responses to stimuli are occasionally observed. Awakening after ketamine anesthesia is often delayed and may be characterized by disagreeable dreams or hallucinations. These adverse psychological symptoms occur less frequently in young adults or children; almost half of adults over 30 years of age exhibit psychological symptoms. Its LD50 in rats or mice is about 225 mg/kg i.p. The drug phencyclidine ("angel dust") is a compound of similar structure. *See also* PHENCYCLIDINE.

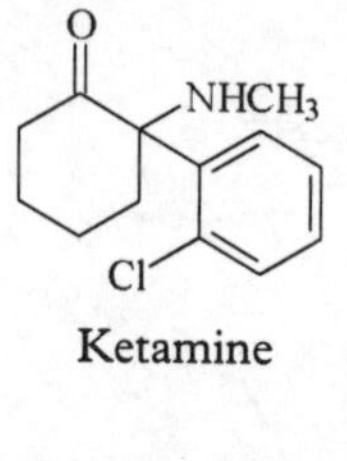

Ketamine

ketone reduction. *See* ALDEHYDE AND KETONE REDUCTION.

ketonuria. An excess of ketone bodies in the urine, resulting from an excessive metabolism of fatty acids. Ketonuria usually indicates starvation, injudicious dieting or uncontrolled diabetes mellitus.

K_I **(inhibition constant).** In the interaction of ligands with binding sites, this is a frequently derived constant originating (like the Michaelis constant, K_M) from the law of mass action. For competitive inhibitors, it can be derived from the IC_{50} using one of the Cheng–Prusoff relationships

$$K_I = \frac{IC_{50}}{\left(1 + \dfrac{K_D}{L}\right)}$$

Like K_D, K_I provides a measure of the affinity of a toxicant for a specific site. However, it is derived indirectly from competition studies, rather than directly from saturation studies. *See also* ENZYME KINETICS; K_D; K_M; RADIORECEPTOR ASSAYS; XENOBIOTIC METABOLISM, INHIBITION.

kidney dropsy. *See* RENAL FAILURE.

kidneys. Major organs of excretion in vertebrates. The kidneys are also critical in regulation of the pH, ionic balance and osmolarity of the blood. In toxicology, kidneys are important in several respects: they excrete the products of xenobiotic metabolism, and they are important sites of toxic action. *See also* NEPHRON; NEPHROTOXICITY.

killer cells. *See* NATURAL KILLER CELLS.

killer T cells. *See* T CELLS.

kinetic equations. In toxicology, mathematical expressions describing the time course of a substance in the body. Typically, a set of linear differential equations is obtained, which represents the compartmental or physiological kinetic model. These equations are used in differential or, in most cases, integrated form and are used to obtain parameter estimates by mathematical regression techniques. *See also* CLEARANCE; COMPARTMENT;

FIRST-ORDER KINETICS; FIRST-PASS EFFECT; KINETIC EQUATIONS, ELIMINATION; KINETIC EQUATIONS, HEPATIC CLEARANCE; KINETIC EQUATIONS, NONLINEAR; KINETIC EQUATIONS, PLASMA PROTEIN BINDING; KINETIC EQUATIONS, RENAL CLEARANCE; KINETIC EQUATIONS, UPTAKE; MULTI-COMPARTMENT MODELS; ONE-COMPARTMENT MODEL; PHARMACOKINETICS; PROBIT/LOG TRANSFORMS; TOXICOKINETICS; TWO-COMPARTMENT MODEL; VOLUME OF DISTRIBUTION.

kinetic equations, elimination. First-order or Michaelis–Menten expressions that describe the removal of a substance from the body. The first-order equations contain a rate constant for elimination from which a half-life can be calculated. The Michaelis–Menten equations contain values for the maximum rate of the process and the concentration at which the rate is one-half maximum. This permits the concentration-dependent rate of elimination (or clearance) to be calculated. *See also* CLEARANCE; PHARMACOKINETICS; TOXICOKINETICS.

kinetic equations, hepatic clearance. Expressions that quantify the ability of the liver to remove a substance by biliary excretion and hepatic metabolism. From a physiological perspective, hepatic clearance is equal to the product of hepatic blood flow and the hepatic extraction ratio. This implies that the hepatic clearance of substances that are highly extracted by the liver is limited by blood flow to the liver. Due to the complexity of the hepatic clearance processes, it is rarely possible to estimate hepatic clearance from a compartmental pharmacokinetic analysis. *See also* CLEARANCE; PHARMACOKINETICS; TOXICOKINETICS.

kinetic equations, nonlinear. Michaelis–Menten expressions that quantify the maximum rate of elimination of a substance and the concentration at which the rate is one-half maximum. The pharmacokinetic implications of nonlinear processes include an increasing apparent half-life with increasing concentration (dose) and decreasing clearance with increasing concentration (dose). The occurrence of nonlinear kinetics has important ramifications in toxicological studies where large doses are often administered. *See also* CLEARANCE; PHARMACOKINETICS; TOXICOKINETICS.

kinetic equations, plasma protein binding. Expressions that describe the reversible binding of substances to constituents in plasma. The identity of the binding protein, the affinity of binding to the protein and the capacity of the binding sites can influence the disposition of the substance. Also, expressions for the concentration of the substance unbound to plasma protein (and the free clearance) exist, and these relationships can frequently be used to predict pharmacological or toxic effects. *See also* PHARMACOKINETICS; TOXICOKINETICS.

kinetic equations, renal clearance. Mathematical expressions that quantify the removal of a substance by the kidneys via the processes of filtration and secretion. Clearance is calculated by relating the rate of renal excretion to the plasma concentration. Factors that influence renal clearance include urine pH, urine flow and protein binding. *See also* CLEARANCE; PHARMACOKINETICS; TOXICOKINETICS.

kinetic equations, uptake. Expressions describing the rate of appearance and the amount of a substance in a tissue. The rate of appearance is dependent upon the rate of tissue perfusion and the concentrations entering and leaving the tissue. The ultimate amount appearing in the tissue is dependent upon the partition coefficient between blood and tissue, the volume of the tissue and the concentration entering the tissue. *See also* PHARMACOKINETICS; TOXICOKINETICS.

K_M **(Michaelis constant)**. In enzyme kinetics, a constant derived from the Michaelis–Menten equation; it is equal to the substrate concentration

at half-maximal velocity. Experimentally K_M can be derived from one of several forms that linearize the Michaelis–Menten equation, such as the Lineweaver–Burk, Eadie–Hofstee, Scatchard or Woolf plot. The K_M is a valuable concept in toxicology, as well as in enzyme kinetics, since it reflects the affinity of the enzyme for the substrate. Also the effect or lack of effect of inhibitors on K_M provides valuable clues to the mode of action and, in some cases, the role in toxic action. *See also* EADIE–HOFSTEE PLOT; ENZYME KINETICS; LINEWEAVER–BURK PLOT; METABOLITE INHIBITORY COMPLEXES; MICHAELIS–MENTEN EQUATION; RADIORECEPTOR ASSAYS; SCATCHARD PLOT; WOOLF PLOT; XENOBIOTIC METABOLISM, INHIBITION.

Kruskall–Wallis H test. A non-parametric or distribution-free test for use with ranked data. Differences between group means are tested in a manner analogous to a single-factor ANOVA without repeated measures. If the sample size is greater than five, the sampling distribution of this statistic is approximated by a chi-square distribution with degrees of freedom equal to the number of treatments minus one. For small values of n, special tables for the H statistic are available. *See also* ANALYSIS OF VARIANCE; NON-PARAMETRIC; STATISTICS, FUNCTION IN TOXICOLOGY.

K_s **(spectral binding constant)**. Analogous to K_M (the Michaelis constant), in enzyme kinetics, the K_s is the ligand concentration at half-maximum spectral size for ligands that bind to other molecules to give rise to spectral changes. In the case of cytochrome P450, it is often used as a measure of the affinity of the cytochrome for xenobiotic ligands. *See also* CYTOCHROME P450, OPTICAL DIFFERENCE SPECTRA; OPTICAL DIFFERENCE SPECTRA.

L

label. An isotope (radioactive or stable) that replaces a stable atom in a compound. The course of a chemical or biochemical reaction or physical process can be followed by tracing the radioactivity using a counter or, in the case of stable isotopes, a mass spectrometer. The exact position of the isotope in the molecule must be known for mechanistic studies. *See also* ISOTOPES.

Laboratory Animal Science Association (LASA). A UK body for the promotion of laboratory animal science.

laboratory tests, for ecological effects. *See* ECOLOGICAL EFFECTS, LABORATORY TESTS.

lacrimation. Tearing, often in response to an irritant to the eyes. It results from exposure to irritating fumes, air pollutants, smog, aromatic compounds from plants, etc. Very strong effects result from military-style lacrimators.

lacrimator. A chemical causing lacrimation (tearing of the eyes). Some powerful lacrimators have been used in military situations or in personal protection devices.

lactation. The secretion of milk in mammals. It can be important as a source of toxicants to the neonate, since a number of lipophilic xenobiotics (e.g., mirex, chlordecone, DDT, PCBs, etc.) are known to appear in milk. Under experimental conditions (often using high doses), xenobiotics in the milk may sometimes cause pharmacological or toxicological effects in the young. However, such effects are less common in human populations under normal conditions of dose or exposure.

lactic dehydrogenase (LDH). An enzyme that catalyzes the reduction of pyruvate to lactate in the following reaction.

$$\text{pyruvate} + \text{NADH} + \text{H}^+ \rightarrow \text{lactate} + \text{NAD}^+$$

The enzyme is found in all cells capable of glycolysis. LDH exists as several different isozymes, and different tissues have either different isozymes or different sets of isozymes. Release of LDH into the blood is a sign of tissue damage and can occur under many circumstances (e.g., myocardial infarction, hepatotoxicity, nephrotoxicity, etc.). Identification of the particular isozyme can be used to identify the organ involved. For example, the serum concentration of LDH_5 is increased in liver injury, whereas LDH_1 and LDH_2 are increased in kidney injury. *See also* HEPATOTOXICITY; ISOZYMES; LIVER ENZYMES, IN BLOOD; LIVER FUNCTION TESTS.

laetrile. *See* AMYGDALIN.

lanosterol (isocholesterol, $C_{30}H_{50}O$). CAS number 79-63-0. Trimethyl sterol or triterpenoid found in the non-saponifiable fraction of wool wax. Formed by oxidative cyclization of squalene, followed by rearrangement of the methyl group; the precursor of sterols such as cholesterol in animals and fungi.

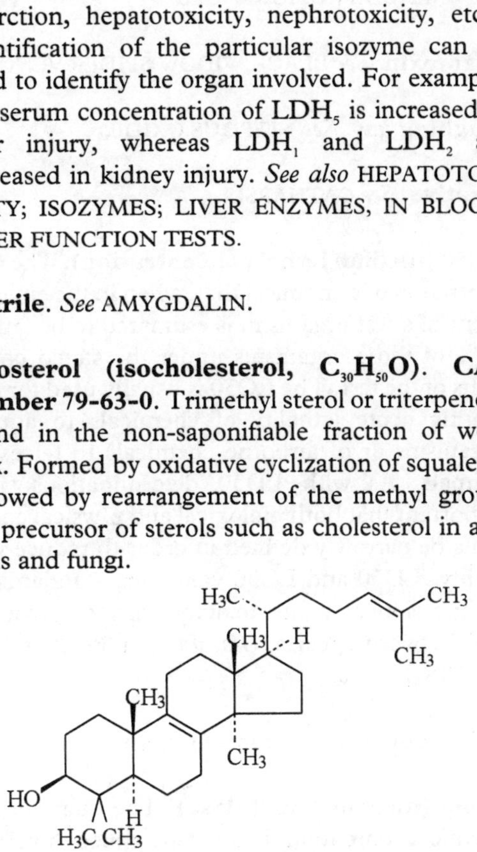

Lanosterol

large intestine. *See* COLON.

laser spectroscopy. *See* SPECTROMETRY, LASER.

latency period. The period of time between the application of an agent to a living organism and a demonstrable effect of such application.

lathyrism. A neurological disorder involving spastic paraplegia, pain and parathesia that results from ingestion of *Lathyrus* plant seeds. Osteolathyrism is a related skeletal disorder produced in animals by the sweet pea *Lathyrus odoratus* or its active constituent, β-aminoproprionitrile or other aminonitriles. This disorder is characterized by skeletal and connective tissue damage, dissecting aneurysm, hemorrhaging and growth retardation. An important mechanism underlying such effects is reduced tensile strength in collagen due to impaired cross-linking of its subunits. *See also* β,β′-IMINODIPROPIONITRILE.

latrotoxin. *See* BLACK WIDOW SPIDER VENOM.

laughing gas. *See* NITROUS OXIDE.

laxative. *See* CATHARSIS.

LC50 (median lethal concentration). The concentration of a chemical that, when in the environment of a test organism, is estimated to be fatal to 50% of those organisms under the stated conditions of the test. The LC50 is usually used for estimating acute lethality of chemicals to aquatic organisms or of airborne chemicals to terrestrial animals. As with LD50 determinations, it is important that both biological and physical conditions be narrowly defined in order to reduce variability. LD50 and LC50 values are standards for comparison of acute toxicity between toxicants and between species. *See also* ACUTE TOXICITY TESTING; LD50.

LCL₀. Lowest lethal concentration.

LD50 (median lethal dose). The quantity of a chemical compound that, when applied directly to test organisms, is estimated to be fatal to 50% of those organisms under the stated conditions of the test. The LD50 value is the standard for compa-

rison of acute toxicity between toxicants and between species. Since the results of LD50 determinations may vary widely, it is important that both biological and physical conditions be narrowly defined (e.g., strain, sex and age of test organism, time and route of exposure, environmental conditions). The value may be determined graphically from a plot of log dose against mortality expressed in probability units (probits) or, more recently, by using one of several computer programs available. The LD50 test has been criticized on a number of grounds, including the following: as generally carried out, it is an expression of lethality only; large numbers of experimental animals are required to obtain statistically acceptable values, but despite this the values are seldom closely similar from one laboratory to another; since regulation is concerned primarily with chronic toxicity, the LD50 test provides little useful information. Such information could, in any case, be acquired from an approximation requiring only a small number of animals; extrapolation to humans is difficult. Continued use of the LD50 test has, however, been advocated on the following grounds: acute toxicity tests can yield additional information on other acute effects; the mode of action and likelihood of metabolic detoxication can sometimes be inferred from the slope of the mortality curve; the results can form the basis for the design of subsequent subchronic studies; the LD50 is a useful first approximation of hazards to workers. As a result of this controversy, there has been a concerted effort to modify the concept of acute toxicity testing and to substitute methods that utilize fewer experimental animals. For example, it has been suggested that LD50 tests on large animals be abandoned and comprehensive acute toxicity tests using small numbers of animals be substituted, including detailed observations of symptoms, physiological measurements such as blood pressure, body temperature, reflex activity, electrocardiogram, electroencephalogram, food and water intake, respiration and behavior. Blood chemistry, urinalysis and the measurement of excretion of the parent compound and metabolites, as well as gross and microscopic pathology, could also be a part of these tests. Alternatives to the classical LD50 tests, including the approximate lethal dose method of Deichman and Le Blanc, the moving average method of Thompson, the up and down method of Dixon and Mood, or the method recently proposed by Molinengo based on the relationship between dose and survival time should be employed. All of these methods use small numbers of animals. For many regulatory purposes classification of chemicals into toxicity classes is adequate, and when the compound is pharmacologically inert the test is unnecessary. *See also* ACUTE TOXICITY TESTING; LC50.

LDH. *See* LACTIC DEHYDROGENASE.

LDL$_0$. Lowest lethal dose.

LDLP (low-density lipoprotein). *See* LIPOPROTEINS.

lead (Pb; plumbic; plumbous). An element that causes a variety of dose-dependent toxic changes. Lead and its salts are used in industry in the manufacture of lead-based paints, solder, batteries, linings of equipment for handling corrosive gases and liquids, fuel additives (organoleads) and other organic and inorganic lead compounds. Acute toxicity is most common in children who have ingested leaded paint chips (pica). Lead poisoning in adults is usually occupational, but food and air are the primary routes of exposure for the general populace. LD50 varies considerably between lead compounds and is dependent on the route of exposure. Acute lead intoxication presents clinically as an encephalopathic syndrome (i.e., gross ataxia, repeated vomiting, lethargy, stupor, convulsions, headache, hallucinations, tremors and coma). Chronic intoxication leads to weight loss, central and peripheral nervous system effects and anemia. Disturbance of renal function may also occur. Lead can induce kidney tumors in rodents, but has not been shown to be a human carcinogen to date. Recently, even very low doses have been shown to cause subtle and persistent changes in the development of the CNS. Inorganic lead is absorbed from the respiratory and gastrointestinal systems and is poorly absorbed through the skin, unlike the organoleads. Significant lead accumulation occurs mainly in the bones and teeth; stored lead can be released from this compartment if physiological changes lead to hydroxyapatite breakdown. The number of organs affected by lead reflects the ability of lead to bind to a number of cellular ligands and interfere with cellular homeostasis and some calcium-regulated functions. Lead has affinity for sulfhydryl groups, many of which are required for enzymatic activity. Chelatable blood lead, rather than absolute blood or tissue lead levels, is used as an index of the toxic fraction of lead. Even when chelatable lead concentrations return to close to normal, however, there remain very high concentrations in skeletal matrix that may be mobilized if physiological events lead to mobilization of the bone matrix. One effect usually seen after exposure to lead is changes in heme synthesis due to inhibition of Δ-aminolevulinic acid dehydratase and other heme biosynthetic enzymes. This has made increases in free erythrocyte protoporphyrins (FEP) a sensitive indicator of lead exposure. Removal from exposure and use of chelating agents (e.g., CaEDTA or penicillamine) are the primary treatments of intoxication. *See also* CHELATING AGENTS; FREE ERYTHROCYTE PROTOPORPHYRIN; HEAVY METALS; LEAD OXIDES; POLLUTION, METALS; TRIETHYLLEAD; ATSDR DOCUMENT, APRIL 1993.

lead arsenate (PbHAsO$_4$). **CAS number 10102-48-4**. An inorganic lead salt that occurs in nature as the mineral schultenite. It has been used as a constituent of insecticides for control of the larvae of gypsy moths, boll weevils, etc., and in veterinary medicine as an anthelmintic agent in cattle, goats and sheep. Poisoning by this inorganic pentavalent arsenic compound has primarily been in connection with its use as an insecticide. Occupational exposures may occur during the manufacture of arsenates. Arsenate-contaminated wine from vineyards treated with arsenical pesticides has also been a source of human exposure. In 1972 the EPA stopped the registration of lead arsenate, with the result that its use as a pesticide has decreased. The oral LD50 in rats is 800 mg/kg. An exposure to lead arsenate results in exposure to two toxicants: lead and arsenic. The symptoms of poisoning reflect this dual nature; gastrointestinal irritation, vertigo, lower limb weakness and jaundice may occur. Combination therapy with CaEDTA and British Anti-Lewisite is required. *See also* ARSENIC; LEAD.

lead oxides. Lead monoxide (PbO; lead oxide yellow) is used in pigments for pottery, leaded glass and for coloring sulfur-containing substances such as wool and horn. The i.p. LD50 in rats is 400 mg/kg. Lead dioxide (PbO_2, lead oxide brown) occurs in nature as the mineral plattnerite and is used as electrodes in batteries, as an oxidizing agent in the manufacture of dyes and in the manufacture of rubber substitutes. The i.p. LD50 in guinea pigs is 200 mg/kg. The acute toxicity of lead oxides is characterized by anorexia, vomiting, malaise, convulsions and increases in intracranial pressure. Chronic intoxication results in weight loss, weakness and anemia. *See also* LEAD.

LE factors. *See* IPOMEANOL.

lectins. A general term for proteins or glycoproteins of non-immune origin that have multiple highly specific carbohydrate-binding sites. The carbohydrate specificity is often assayed by. the ability of monosaccharides (in some cases a di-, tri- or polysaccharide is required) to inhibit lectin-induced cell agglutination. Many different lectins have been purified from diverse natural sources. The specific affinity of purified lectins makes them a widely used biochemical tool to characterize blood groupings, lymphocyte subpopulations, immunohistochemical distribution of particular carbohydrate-containing molecules, fractionation of different cell types, etc. Examples of common, commercially available lectins used as biochemical tools include concanavalin A (specific for α-D-mannose and α-D-glucose) and eel lectin (*Anguilla anguilla*, specific for α-L-fucose). Some of the purified lectins are extremely toxic (e.g., a 60,000-dalton lectin, ricin, from castor bean *Ricinus communis* strongly inhibits protein synthesis). Another toxic effect of certain lectins can be demonstrated by parenteral application, leading to lymphocyte stimulation and inhibition of the ability to make antibodies to unrelated antigens. Toxic effects have been associated with diets high in vegetables containing certain lectins. For example, lectins in kidney beans affect the morphology of the small intestine; at high dietary levels, the ability of the lectins to combine with receptors in cells of the wall of the small intestine leads to non-specific inhibition of utilization of certain nutrients. *See also* ABRIN; RICIN.

leptophos (*O*-methyl *O*-2,5-dichloro-4-bromophenyl phenylphosphonothioate; Phosvel). **CAS number 21609-90-5**. A pesticide registered only briefly for the control of crop pests and certain animal ectoparasites. Registration of leptophos was cancelled following an episode of delayed neuropathy in water buffalo in Egypt. Acute toxicity is via acetylcholinesterase inhibition. The oral LD50 in rats is 52 mg/kg. *See also* DELAYED NEUROPATHY; ORGANOPHOSPHORUS INSECTICIDES.

Leptophos

lethal synthesis. The process by which a toxicant similar in structure to an endogenous substrate is incorporated into the same metabolic pathway as the endogenous substrate, ultimately being transformed into a toxic or lethal product. For example, fluoroacetate simulates acetate in intermediary metabolism, being transformed via the tricarboxylic acid (TCA) cycle to fluorocitrate, which then inhibits aconitase, resulting in disruption of the TCA cycle and energy metabolism.

leukemia. A disease characterized by excess formation of leukocytes and their precursors. Leukemias are classified according to the dominant cell type increased, and the severity and time course of the disease (e.g., acute granulocytic leukemia, chronic granulocytic leukemia, acute lymphocytic anemia). Although the causes or causative agents are generally unknown, ionizing radiation has been established as one possible cause.

Leukerin. *See* 6-MERCAPTOPURINE.

leukocytes (**white blood cells; white blood corpuscles**). *See* LYMPHOCYTES; MACROPHAGES/MONOCYTES; MAST CELLS/BASOPHILS.

leukocytopenia. *See* LEUKOPENIA.

leukopenia (leukocytopenia). An abnormal decrease of circulating white blood cells (leukocytes), usually below 5000/mm³. Leukopenia can result from the effect of toxicants (e.g., benzene) on the bone marrow stem cells or from the interaction of cytolytic antibody with leukocytes or their progenitors.

Leydig cells. The interstitial cells in the testes surrounding the seminiferous tubules that secrete androgens, primarily testosterone. This secretion is stimulated by interstitial cell-stimulating hormone (ICSH) from the adenohypophysis.

lidocaine (2-(diethylamino)-N-(2,6-dimethylphenyl)acetamide). CAS number 137-58-6. Used in veterinary and medical practice as a local anesthetic. Acts as a sodium channel inhibitor. Few undesirable side effects.

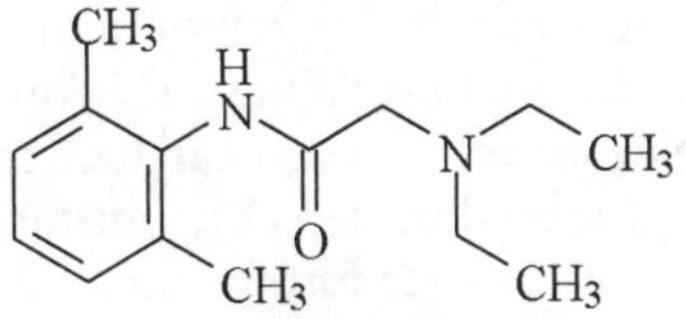

Lidocaine

Life Sciences Research Office (LSRO). See FEDERATION OF ASSOCIATED SOCIETIES FOR EXPERIMENTAL BIOLOGY.

life support. See MAINTENANCE THERAPY; POISONING, EMERGENCY TREATMENT; POISONING, LIFE SUPPORT.

life tables. Normative values that indicate age-specific probabilities of death or survival based upon current health and mortality data. Life tables are used to calculate the average number of years that people of a certain age would live if current mortality trends continue to apply. This estimate is crucial in comparing mortality rates, either spatially or geographically and/or temporally. Life tables can be of great utility to the toxicologist assessing the impact of proximity to hazardous waste dumps or to the investigator following workers potentially exposed to a toxicant in the workplace. See also STATISTICS, FUNCTION IN TOXICOLOGY.

ligand. A small organic molecule that is bound to a macromolecule in a stable, but not covalent, bond. It is used in toxicology particularly to describe molecules being transported by blood proteins or molecules binding to the heme iron of heme proteins. In the latter case, these compounds may or may not be substrates. The nature of ligand binding and the strength of the bonds involved are important. See also AFFINITY CONSTANT; BINDING; TRANSPORT OF TOXICANTS.

ligases. See ENZYMES.

lily of the valley. *Convallaria majalis* contains in its bulbs convallatoxin, a cardioactive glycoside resembling digitalis.

limited evidence, for carcinogenicity. See CARCINOGENS, CLASSIFICATION.

lindane. See γ-HCH.

linear extrapolation. A method used to predict that the effects of a dose of toxicant outside the range of available test data will produce responses directly proportional to those doses within the test range. This assumption may be invalidated by many factors, including saturable repair systems, dose-dependent pharmacokinetics, different mechanisms of toxicity at different doses, etc. Therefore, its use in systems that are not well characterized must be undertaken with great caution. See also LOW-DOSE EXTRAPOLATION.

linear regression. A method for finding the line of best fit between an independent variable X, the values of which are fixed, and a dependent variable Y, the values of which are subject to random variation. The regression line is obtained from the regression equation:

$$Y = a + bX$$

where a equals the Y intercept (the value of Y where the regression line intercepts the Y-axis) and b, the regression coefficient, is the slope of the line (i.e., the change in Y for each unit change in X). The regression coefficient b is solved by summing the product of the X deviations multiplied by the Y deviations and dividing this result by the squared deviations of X. The regression line is referred to as the line of best fit, as the solution of the regression equation yields a line around which the sum of the squared deviations is at a minimum. *Compare* NONLINEAR REGRESSION. *See also* CORRELATION COEFFICIENT.

Lineweaver–Burk plot. One of several ways of linearizing enzyme- or receptor-binding data, based on derivations of the law of mass action (with appropriate assumptions). Based on rearrangement of the Michaelis–Menten equation, the equation for the Lineweaver–Burk plot is:

$$\frac{1}{v} = \left(\frac{K_M}{V_{max}}\right) \cdot \left(\frac{1}{[S]}\right) + \frac{1}{V_{max}}$$

Experimentally, if $1/v$ is plotted versus $1/[S]$ (where v is the initial velocity of the enzyme reaction in the presence of a given concentration of substrate [S]), the intercept on the ordinate is $1/V_{max}$, and the slope of the line is K_M/V_{max}. This permits the apparent K_M and the apparent maximum velocity (V_{max}) to be estimated. The equation is essentially identical for radioreceptor assays, except that B (amount bound) is equivalent to v (the initial velocity), [F] (concentration of free ligand) to [S] (concentration of substrate), K_D (dissociation constant) to K_M (Michaelis constant) and B_{max} (theoretical number of sites) to V_{max} (maximal theoretical velocity). *See also* EADIE–HOFSTEE PLOT; ENZYME KINETICS; K_D; K_M; METABOLITE INHIBITORY COMPLEXES; MICHAELIS–MENTEN EQUATION; RADIORECEPTOR ASSAYS; WOOLF PLOT; XENOBIOTIC METABOLISM, INHIBITION.

linuron. *See* UREA HERBICIDES.

lipemia. Abnormally high lipid level in the blood.

lipid. A general term for constituents of living organisms soluble in organic solvents such as chloroform; methanol, ether, etc. Includes such categories as neutral fats, phospholipids, sterols, etc.

lipid hydroperoxides. *See* LIPID PEROXIDATION.

lipid peroxidation. A form of cellular injury implicated in the liver necrosis evoked by hepatotoxicants such as carbon tetrachloride and yellow phosphorus. It involves initiation, propagation and termination reactions. The hydrogen atoms on methylene carbons separating double bonds in polyenoic fatty acids are highly susceptible to free radical attack. The abstraction of hydrogen from unsaturated fatty acids during this attack yields free radicals of lipids, and this represents the initiation of lipid peroxidation. Initiation of lipid peroxidation is still not fully understood. Its promotion by oxygen, singlet oxygen, hydroxyl radical, superoxide anion or some form of perferryl ion has been proposed. Free radicals generated during the metabolism of various chemicals have also been suggested as initiators. The free radicals generated from fatty acids are unstable and undergo a series of transformations, including shifting of double bonds to give the diene configuration. The fatty acid free radicals react rapidly with molecular oxygen to form organic peroxy free radicals. The peroxy free radicals from one fatty acid chain abstract methylene hydrogen of a neighboring unsaturated fatty acid, yielding one hydroperoxide and one new radical. This autocatalytic chain reaction is the propagation step. The unstable hydroperoxides decompose to form additional free radicals. When substrate is depleted, termination reactions are initiated, yielding non-radical products, thus stopping the lipid peroxidation process. Subcellular membranes rich in unsaturated fatty acids are targets of lipid peroxidation, resulting in the loss of structural integrity and function in the affected organelles. In addition, breakdown products of lipid peroxides, such as aldehydes, may migrate far from the production site and cause damage at distant loci. Several lipid peroxides are known for their extremely high toxicity.

lipid solubility. The ability of a compound to dissolve in lipids or in lipid solvents. Relative lipid solubility is indicated by the partition coefficient. High lipid solubility compounds (with high partition coefficients) penetrate biological membranes readily, although the correlation between high partition coefficient and rapid penetration may be more generally accepted than is warranted. Early studies in particular showed good correlations between high partition coefficients and rapid penetration, and the relationship has been generally accepted. Recent studies, however, have indicated that this generalization may be obscured by other factors. Lipid solubility is clearly necessary for initial uptake, but once the toxicant has entered the membrane other factors may complicate further penetration. For example, very high lipid solubility may reduce penetration through the highly lipid membrane by restricting exit. *See also* ENTRY MECHANISM, PASSIVE TRANSPORT; ENTRY MECHANISMS, SPECIAL TRANSPORT.

lipophilicity. The physical property of chemical compounds that causes them to be soluble in non-polar solvents (e.g., chloroform and benzene) and, generally, relatively insoluble in polar solvents such as water. This property is important toxicologically since lipophilic compounds tend to enter an organism easily and to be excretable only when they have been rendered less lipophilic by metabolic action.

lipoproteins. Proteins that exist in combination with lipids, primarily phospholipids and cholesterol. The density of such proteins varies with the lipid content, those with higher lipid content having the lowest density. Lipoproteins are divided into classes based on their buoyant density (e.g., low-density lipoprotein, LDLP; very-low-density lipoproteins, VLDLP). Lipoproteins exist both intra- and extracellularally, and their normal function includes the transport of lipid-soluble metabolites, such as glycerides, fat-soluble vitamins and steroid hormones. In toxicology, they are important for the transport of toxicants from the portal of entry and their distribution to the tissues. Toxic effects may also be mediated by defects of lipoprotein function (e.g., in carbon tetrachloride-induced hepatotoxicity. *See also* DISTRIBUTION OF TOXICANTS; HEPATOTOXICITY; LIPID SOLUBILITY; TRANSPORT OF TOXICANTS.

liposomes. A term first coined in 1965 to describe lipid droplets in the endoplasmic reticulum that occur during the formation of a fatty liver. They are, presumably, primarily triglyceride in composition. More recently, the term has been used for artificially formed lipid droplets small enough to form relatively stable suspensions in water, buffer or other aqueous media. These are spherical, microscopic, membrane-enclosed vesicles (20–30 nm diameter); prepared by the addition of an aqueous solution to a phospholipid gel. It is similar to a cell organelle, and the membrane resembles a cell membrane. Their use has been suggested for drug delivery, administration of lipophilic substrates to membrane-bound enzymes and other experimental uses, such as the behavior of membranes (e.g., during anesthesia) with respect to permeability changes.

liquid scintillation counting. *See* SPECTROMETRY, LIQUID SCINTILLATION.

Listeria. A genus of bacteria associated with food poisoning, *L. monocytogenes* being a member of this genus. The sources of the organism include tissues, urine and milk of infected animals and the foods commonly associated with outbreaks include milk and milk products, eggs, meat and poultry.

lithium (Li). An element used clinically as one of its salts. It is effective against both mania and depression. Despite its effectiveness, there are no clear mechanisms that have been directly related to its therapeutic effectiveness although its inhibition of the formation of inositol from inositol phosphate is thought to be important. At therapeutic concentrations, lithium causes almost no discernible psychotropic effects in healthy humans. The major complaints when the serum concentrations of the drug are carefully monitored include slight muscular weakness, thirst and excessive urination. The major difficulty with lithium is that a fairly high concentration of the ion is needed in the blood (0.5–1.0 mmol/l) for maintenance, higher for acute mania. Toxic symptoms (which can involve many physiological symptoms) may occur, however, at doses of 1.5 mmol/l or higher. This low therapeutic index is indicative of the need for regular monitoring of lithium concentrations in the serum.

liver. The largest organ and the largest gland in the body of vertebrates. Its glandular secretion is known as bile, and it is secreted into the small intestine via the common bile duct. In those species having a gallbladder (including humans), the common bile duct originates at the point at which the hepatic duct, draining the intrahepatic bile passages, and comes together with the cystic duct that connects the gallbladder to the common duct.

Bile salts function in the digestion of fats in the small intestine. The liver is supplied with blood via the hepatic artery and the hepatic portal vein, and drains into the inferior vena cava via hepatic veins. The liver receives blood, via the hepatic portal vein, from the small intestine, thus receiving the products of digestion and absorption of food. It forms glycogen from glucose, proteins from amino acids and glycerides from fatty acids. It also carries out many reactions of intermediary metabolism. It is responsible for the excretion of bilirubin and biliverdin, products formed by degradation of heme. The liver is important in toxicology for many reasons. It receives, from the hepatic portal vein, essentially all xenobiotics absorbed in the small intestine. As the richest source of both phase I and phase II xenobiotic-metabolizing enzymes, it is important in the detoxication and activation of these xenobiotics. Because of the high concentration of both xenobiotics and xenobiotic-activating enzymes, hepatotoxicity is a common form of toxic action. The liver is also an important organ for excretion of toxic compounds since conjugation products, particularly those of high molecular weight, are secreted into the bile and excreted via the alimentary canal. In pharmacokinetics or toxicokinetics, the liver is important because of so-called "first-pass" effects. *See also* BILE; BILE ACIDS; BILE PIGMENTS; BILE SAMPLING; HEPATOTOXICITY; XENOBIOTIC METABOLISM.

liver damage. *See* HEPATOTOXICITY.

liver enzymes, in blood (serum enzymes). The measurement of hepatic enzymes released into the blood as a consequence of injury has proven to be a sensitive indicator of hepatotoxicity. Since the enzymes may be of cytoplasmic or organelle origin, such measurements may also help define the subcellular site of damage. One or more of the following enzymes are measured: alkaline phosphatase; 5-nucleotidase; leucine aminopeptidase; glutamyl transpeptidase; lactic dehydrogenase isozymes; isocitrate dehydrogenase; alcohol dehydrogenase; fructose mono- or diphosphate aldolase; arginase; quinine oxidase; β-hydroxybutyrate dehydrogenase; glutamic-pyruvic transaminase; glutamic-oxaloacetic transaminase; sorbitol dehydrogenase. Some of these are measured only rarely; the ones utilized most commonly being the two transaminases, lactic dehydrogenase and alkaline phosphatase. *See also* HEPATOTOXICITY; LIVER FUNCTION TESTS.

liver function tests. There are numerous types of toxicant-induced liver injuries and many tests of liver function designed for these diagnoses. Some are sufficiently non-invasive to be used routinely on humans, others are suitable only for experimental studies. The different types of liver injuries are summarized under hepatotoxicity. The principal type of test for liver function of use in toxicology is that based on serum enzymes, specifically on the release of hepatic enzymes into the blood. The particular enzymes released may be indicative of the particular type of injury; for example, elevated serum alkaline phosphatase may reflect cholestatic rather than parenchymal injury, whereas other enzymes reflect cytotoxicity. These enzymes may be quite specific for the liver, but not exclusively hepatic (e.g., glutamic-pyruvic transaminase), they may be highly specific for the liver (e.g., ornithine carbamyl transferase) or they may be relatively non-specific (e.g., lactic dehydrogenase), sometimes reflecting injury to extrahepatic tissues. Another type of test examines the ability of the liver to excrete chemicals via the bile: for example, the ability of the liver to remove bromosulfophthalein from the plasma and secrete it into the bile, since bromosulfophthalein clearance is delayed following hepatic injury. Since the entire process involves several steps (uptake into the cells, metabolic transformation (conjugation) and secretion into the bile), the interpretation of a positive result may present problems. Analysis of the lipid triglyceride content of the liver may be indicative of fatty liver, a condition that may result from poisoning by such hepatotoxicants as carbon tetrachloride, ethionine, phosphorus and many others. There are a number of chemical methods for the determination of lipid peroxidation in the liver, including the determination of malondialdehyde, a degradation product of lipid peroxides, using thiobarbituric acid and the determination of conjugated dienes by ultraviolet spectrometry. In addition to these highly invasive methods, the appearance of exhaled ethane and pentane has also been used as a measure of lipid peroxidation, although this method cannot indicate the tissue from which these products arise and therefore cannot localize the site of lipid peroxidation. Biochemical techniques may demonstrate injury to particular cells, organelles or liver functions. Such tests include measurement of glucose-6-phosphate or assessment of effects on hepatic xenobiotic-metabolizing enzymes. A less invasive approach to the latter is the use of the hexobarbital sleeping time or zoxazolamine paralysis time as a measure of the effect. Finally, the structure of the liver tissue can be examined either by light or electron microscopy either after necropsy in the case of experimental animals or following biopsy in humans. *See also* HEPATOTOXOCITY; LIVER ENZYMES, IN BLOOD.

liver perfusion. *See* PERFUSION STUDIES, LIVER.

liver toxicity. *See* HEPATOTOXICITY.

LOAEL. *See* LOWEST OBSERVED ADVERSE EFFECT LEVEL.

local anesthetics. *See* LIDOCAINE.

local effect. A toxic response occurring at the site of contact between the toxicant and the organism.

locomotor behavior. A frequently used measure of motor activity in toxicological studies. In rodents this behavior involves movement of all four paws in a horizontal direction, resulting in a change in the animal's location in the test chamber. Operational definitions vary with the testing apparatus being used and how the behavior is being transduced. If automated apparatus is used, definitions vary from the number of photocell interruptions per unit of time to fluctuations in a magnetic field. If observers are used, the behavior is usually defined as the number of discrete locations in which an animal moves or the number of scoring intervals during which locomotion was observed to occur. *See also* HYPERACTIVITY; NEUROBEHAVIORAL TERATOLOGY; NEUROBEHAVIORAL TOXICOLOGY; POSTNATAL BEHAVIORAL TESTS.

locus. A particular site. Usually the term is used to refer to a particular sequence of chromosomal DNA that serves as a gene.

LOEL. *See* LOWEST OBSERVED EFFECT LEVEL.

logarithmic transformation. Transforming data into their logarithms has several important features for the toxicologist. (1) Any process that may be modeled by a first-order mechanism can be linearized by a logarithmic transformation. (2) Such a transformation may be used for stabilizing the variance, thereby avoiding departures from the assumptions inherent in parametric tests of statistical significance. This transformation is particularly useful with proportional data as the magnitude of the variance tends to vary with the magnitude of the mean. Expressing each observation as its log reduces this correlation. *See also* STATISTICS, FUNCTION IN TOXICOLOGY.

logistic curve. A function, often applied to growth curves, fitting the general equation

$$y = \frac{k'}{1 + e^{a + bt}}$$

where t represents time, y the population size and a and b are derived constants with b always greater than 0. k' is the maximum carrying capacity for that population or species. The resulting curve continually increases, slowly at first, more rapidly in the middle phase and slowly again near the end of growth.

logit transformation. A transformation that relates the response to a given concentration or dose of toxicant to the reponse in the absence of the toxicant using the following formula

$$logit = log\left[\frac{B}{B_0 - B}\right]$$

where B is the response to a given concentration of toxicant and B_0 the response in the absence of toxicant. Usually the logit function is plotted versus the log of the concentration of toxicant to give a linear function; the function can be used when the toxicant either elicits or inhibits the response being measured. A common analysis that uses the equivalent of a logit transformation is the Hill plot, but logit transformations are also used to linearize various types of *in vitro* assays such as radioimmunoassays. *See also* HILL PLOT.

log/logit plot. *See* HILL PLOT; LOGIT TRANSFORMATION.

lomustine. *See* 1-(2-CHLOROETHYL)-3-CYCLOHEXYL-1-NITROSOUREA.

London. *See* ENVIRONMENTAL DISASTERS.

long-range transport. *See* POLLUTION, LONG-RANGE TRANSPORT.

Loo–Riegelman method. *See* BIOAVAILABILITY.

lophotoxin. A naturally occurring cyclic diterpene that was isolated from the marine coral *Lophogorgia*. It reacts covalently with tyrosine residues in subunits of the *Torpedo* nicotinic receptor.

Lou Gehrig disease. *See* AMYOTROPHIC LATERAL SCLEROSIS.

Love Canal. An area in Niagara Falls, New York where industrial wastes were buried in drums in the 1940s and early 1950s. The drums corroded, leaking substances that included suspected carcinogens. In 1978, Love Canal was declared a disaster area, and about 240 families were evacuated. Medical examinations revealed that 11 people had chromosome damage, but this observation was not confirmed by further investigation. In 1982, the Centers for Disease Control declared part of the evacuated areas fit for habitation, and it was not believed that any of the residents would suffer permanent injury. *See also* ENVIRONMENTAL DISASTERS.

low-dose extrapolation. The prediction of the effects of low concentrations expected in the environment from results of tests using high-dose levels. This is complicated by many factors, but basically because the shape of the dose–response curve at lower doses cannot be predicted with certainty. The extremely high doses (maximum tolerated dose) used in carcinogenesis assays are unrealistic in that they may cause metabolic and pharmacokinetic effects not seen at lower doses, and thus they may not even lie on an upward extrapolation from intermediate doses. They are valuable for demonstrating carcinogenic potential, but it may not be appropriate to use them in extrapolations for risk assessment. Models used for low-dose extrapolation fall into the following classes: tolerance distribution; simple linear extrapolation; hit models, such as one-hit and multi-hit; time-to-tumor models. The tolerance distribution model assumes a lower threshold for each individual below which they would not be affected and further assumes that the variation in this threshold can be described by a probability distribution function. The Mantel–Bryan model is a log/probit extrapolation in which a straight line is extrapolated from the measured values to an acceptable level of risk (e.g., 10^{-6}). This model has been criticized in that it often does not fit the observed values, and various corrective factors have been proposed. Despite the attempted corrections, this type of simple extrapolation is still subject to criticism, and most risk assessment involves more complex models. The Weibull model is a further development of the distribution models. The various mechanistic models assume either a one-hit hypothesis (i.e., there is a finite probability of tumor formation if a single target interacts with an effective unit of dose) or a multi-hit hypothesis, which does not make the single-hit assumption, but assumes a more complex set of events prior to tumor formation. This last is probably the most rational, but it is still not without problems. The most complex of the models based on tumor frequency at different dose levels over the time of the study is the gamma multi-hit model of Cornfield and Van Ryzin. This assumes a multi-hit mechanism and can be corrected for spontaneous tumor formation. Currently attempts are being made to incorporate time-to-tumor occurrence into predictive models, and this shows promise as an improvement in predictability. Even more assurance of accuracy of low-dose predictions should come from the incorporation of pharmacokinetic and metabolic parameters into the model, and currently efforts are being made in this direction. *See also* DOSE–RESPONSE CURVE; MAXIMUM TOLERATED DOSE.

low-dose extrapolation models. *See* LOW-DOSE EXTRAPOLATION.

lowest observed adverse effect level (LOAEL). The lowest dose or concentration of a toxicant that causes a significant increase in the frequency or severity of an adverse effect when compared with the frequency or severity of the same biological endpoint in an appropriate unexposed control population.

lowest observed effect level (LOEL). The lowest dose or concentration of a chemical that causes a significant increase in the frequency or severity of any effect, whether adverse or not, when compared with the frequency or severity of the same effect in an appropriate unexposed control population.

low-level wastes. Radioactive wastes such as of clothing and equipment from hospitals and laboratories where radioactive substances have been used, or slightly contaminated soil and rubble from demolished buildings in which radioactive substances were stored or used. Low-level waste primarily contains radionuclides with short half--lives. It presents no serious hazard to the public and is suitable for disposal by shallow burial in trenches.

LSD   ((5R,8R)-(+)-9,10-didehydro-N,N diethyl-6-methylergoline-8-β-carboxamide; D-lysergic acid diethylamide; N,N-diethyl-D-lysergamide; LSD-25; lysergide). CAS number 50-37-3. A hallucinogenic (psychedelic) agent that has been a drug of abuse as well as being used experimentally as an adjunct to psychotherapy. Its LD50 in rabbits is 0.3 mg/kg, i.v., in rats is 16 mg/kg, i.p., and in mice is 46 mg/kg, i.p. LSD may catalyze the onset of severe emotional problems or psychosis in predisposed individuals. Although this compound has actions as an agonist (or in some cases antagonist) at serotonin 5-HT$_1$ and 5-HT$_2$ and dopamine receptors, how these actions produce intoxication is not understood at the present time. The cardinal symptom is pupillary dilation, but hyperreflexia, restlessness and some degree of peripheral vasoconstriction are also usually observed. Perceptual alterations and illusions are characteristics, including changes in touch, taste and odor; synesthesia also is common. The thinking process is substantially altered, and at high doses there are hallucinations and loss of contact with reality. There have been no overdose deaths attributed to the direct effects of LSD. Acute panic reactions can usually be treated in a quiet, supportive

environment. Diazepam has also been used for management of severe anxiety, and antipsychotic drugs are also sometime used. *See also* HALLUCINOGENS.

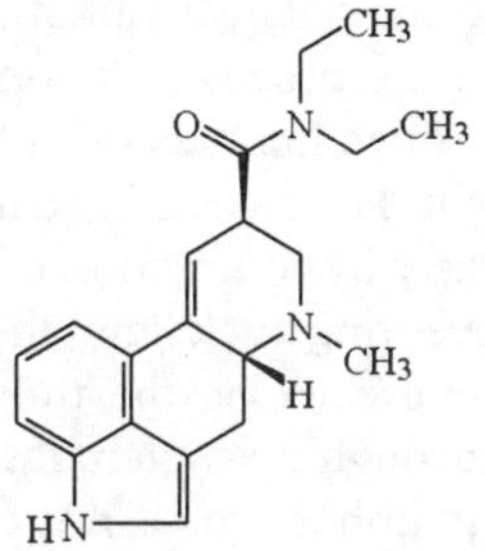

LSD (Lysergic acid diethylamide)

lung. The principal organ of respiratory gas exchange in mammals. The lung consists of conducting airways and an extensive exchange system, the alveoli. It is a complex of as many as 40 different cell types, some of which, such as the Clara cells, are important sites of xenobiotic metabolism. Many inhaled toxicants such as ozone and chlorine are directly toxic to the lung; others are activated by metabolism in the lung. Some systemic pulmonary toxicants, such as methylfuran are also activated in the lung. Chemical toxicity can have many different manifestations both acute and chronic and inhalation or pulmonary toxicology is an important branch of toxicology.

lung toxicity. *See* PULMONARY TOXICITY.

luteinizing hormone (LH). A glycoprotein gonadotropin from the adenohypophysis that stimulates the mature ovarian follicle to ovulate and the subsequent luteinization of the ruptured follicle to convert it into the corpus luteum, which produces estrogen and progesterone. It is equivalent to interstitial cell-stimulating hormone (ICSH) in the male. Its secretion is stimulated by hypothalamic gonadotropin-releasing hormone (GnRH).

lyases. *See* ENZYMES.

lymph. *See* B CELLS; LYMPHATIC SYSTEM; T CELLS.

lymphangioma. *See* ANGIOMA.

lymphatic system. Tissue fluid, consisting mainly of fluid forced out of the capillaries by the pressure of circulating blood, is known as lymph, and is in part recirculated by a system known as the lymphatic system. The lymphatic system arises as capillaries in the tissues that come together to form an interconnecting network of progressively larger vessels, similar to veins in structure. Flow is maintained largely by contraction of body muscles with valves preventing back flow; the system empties into the vena cava via the thoracic duct. As lymph moves through the system it passes through lymph nodes (lymph glands is not correct usage). Lymph nodes contain T and B cells derived from the bone marrow stem cells and remove foreign particles by phagocytosis. The spleen and the thymus are both largely composed of lymphoid tissue. *See also* B CELLS; SPLEEN; THYMUS.

lymphocytes. The primary nucleated cells of the lymphatic system. Resting lymphocytes are small, densely staining and have little cytoplasm. Activated lymphocytes enlarge and have increased cytoplasm. Lymphocytes comprise 20–80% of the nucleated blood cells and more than 99% of the cells in the lymphatic system. Lymphocytes originate from stem cells in the bone marrow and migrate to secondary lymphoid organs for further maturation. The two major classes of lymphocytes, which are morphologically indistinguishable, are the B cells, the effector cells of the humoral immune response, and T cells, the effector cells of the cellular immune response. Lymphocytes circulate through the blood stream and lymphatic vessels, passing through the spleen and lymph nodes, which have filtered and retained antigen for presentation to the B and T cells. They enter the lymph nodes from the bloodstream via high endothelial venules (HEV) in the node, percolate through the lymph node and exit via the efferent lymphatics that drain into the venous system at the thoracic duct. The spleen is primarily a blood-filtering organ, and lymphocytes enter and exit via the capillaries. *See also* B CELLS; T CELLS.

lymphokines. Biologically active molecules produced by lymphocytes that have diverse effects on many different cell types. They can be produced in response to stimulation by antigen, cell contact or other lymphokines. The majority of lymphokines have been defined only functionally, although the structures of a few, such as interleukin I, are now known. Most lymphokines have a variety of actions on several different target cells, and many of these activities overlap with those of other lymphokines. Some lymphokines, such as macrophage chemotactic factor (MCF), macrophage inhibitory factor (MIF) and macrophage activation factor (MAF), primarily affect the movement and actions of macrophages. Others, such as β-interferon, can enhance natural killer cell activity and can interfere with viral replication. Many others, such as IL2 and B-cell-replacing factor (BCRF), are necessary for the growth and differentiation of B and T cells. The lymphokines used in *in vitro* assays for toxicity are generally derived from partially purified tissue culture supernatants of appropriately stimulated cells. These complex mixtures of lymphokines can be added to other cell cultures to promote development of specific activities, expression of particular receptors or differentiation markers, etc. Often such assays are used to determine which phase of growth or differentiation of a cell type is most vulnerable to a given toxicant, as well as the phase in which the toxicity is manifest. *See also* INTERLEUKIN I; INTERLEUKIN II.

lymphoma. A tumor, almost always malignant, of the lymphatic tissues. Examples include Hodgkin's disease, diffuse histocytic lymphoma, etc.

lysergic acid (9,10-didehydro-6-methylergoline-8-β-carboxylic acid). CAS number 82-58-6. A precursor of the semisynthetic ergot derivatives, but having no biological activity itself. It is subject to controls under the Controlled Substances Act of 1970 in the USA, since it is the immediate precursor for the synthesis of LSD. Lysergic acid is obtained by hydrolysis of ergot

Lysergic acid

alkaloids, either obtained from grains infected with *Claviceps* or, more commonly, by fermentation in submerged culture. *See also* LSD.

lysergide. *See* LSD.

lysosome. A cellular organelle bounded by a single membrane that contains numerous acid hydrolases. Its normal function is the destruction of ingested exogenous material (heterophagy) or cellular components (autophagy). Lysosomes can be damaged by rigid xenobiotics such as asbestos or silica, leading to unwarranted cellular destruction. Lysosomes can be stabilized by anti-inflammatory agents such as aspirin.

M

mAb. *See* MONOCLONAL ANTIBODY.

MAC. *See* MAXIMUM ALLOWABLE CONCENTRA-TION.

macrolides. *See* ANTIBIOTICS.

macrophages/monocytes. Monocytes are the blood-borne phagocytic precursors of most tissue macrophages. They are derived from bone marrow stem cells, enter the circulation and eventually migrate into various tissues and differentiate into macrophages. They can be found in the pleural and peritoneal cavities, the lungs (alveolar macrophages), the liver (Kupffer cells), connective tissue (histiocytes), the lymph nodes and other tissues. Macrophages are highly phagocytic and serve in the first line of defense against microorganisms and foreign toxins. Their phagocytic ability is greatly enhanced if the target is coated with antibody. In addition, macrophages can trigger the immune response cascade by serving as antigen-presenting cells. Helper T cells, which must be activated to induce most antibody production, can respond to antigen only when it is presented in conjunction with certain "recognition" glycoproteins (class II histocompatability molecules) expressed by certain cell types of the immune system, including macrophages and B cells. Macrophages also participate in the cell-mediated immune response both as lymphomodulatory cells and as effector cells capable of specific and non-specific tumoricidal activity. They secrete various lysosomal enzymes, interferons, prostaglandins, and many lymphoregulatory molecules, especially when activated. Since macrophages participate in the initiation of the humoral immune response, and in several aspects of the cell-mediated immune response toxicity to macrophages can have far-reaching consequences, the evaluation of the number and functional status of both resident (naive) and activated macrophages is essential. There are a large number of *in vivo* and *in vitro* assays for quantifying different aspects of macrophage function, including uptake of radiolabeled compounds, clearance and killing of intracellular microorganisms, tumoricidal activity and monitoring of metabolic changes related to phagocytic ability. The route of exposure usually determines which tissue macrophages should be tested (e.g., airborne pollutants will generally affect the alveolar macrophages). *See also* T CELLS.

MAFF. *See* MINISTRY OF AGRICULTURE, FISHERIES AND FOOD.

Magnussen–Kligman maximization test. A test for contact sensitization by chemicals (i.e., a test to determine the allergenic potential of the test substance). Although this is one of several such tests, it is regarded as one of the most discriminating for most allergens. Carried out with guinea pigs, it includes pretreatment, by injection, of the test substance and Freund's adjuvant, followed by challenge in topical application patch tests. *See also* DERMAL SENSITIZATION TESTS.

main-stream smoke. Tobacco smoke that is drawn through the cigarette and inhaled by the smoker. *See also* SECONDHAND SMOKE; SIDE-STREAM SMOKE.

maintenance therapy. Following first aid and the initiation of life support procedures to poisoning victims, maintenance therapy is initiated. This is non-specific in that it is usually not designed to counteract the effects of a specific toxicant; rather it is designed to maintain vital signs on a long-term basis. During this phase of treatment nutrition is important. This is done i.v. or by stomach tube if necessary, but p.o. is preferable. In general, energy metabolism is most important, and excess fat and protein should be avoided to reduce stress on the liver and kidneys. Pain can also contribute to functional difficulties, particularly in the case of shock. The treating physician may elect to relieve pain with Demerol since morphine is often contraindicated, particularly in the case of CNS depression, respiratory difficulties or liver involvement. *See also* MAINTENANCE THERAPY, BLOOD; MAINTENANCE THERAPY, CIRCULATORY SYSTEM; MAINTENANCE THERAPY, GASTROINTESTINAL TRACT; MAINTENANCE THERAPY, HEPATIC INVOLVEMENT; MAINTENANCE THERAPY, NERVOUS SYSTEM; MAINTENANCE THERAPY, RESPIRATION; MAINTENANCE THERAPY, URINARY TRACT; MAINTENANCE THERAPY, WATER AND ELECTROLYTE BALANCE.

maintenance therapy, blood. Methemoglobinemia is caused by the oxidation of ferrous (Fe^{2+}) hemoglobin to ferric (Fe^{3+}) hemoglobin and may result from poisoning by such toxicants as nitrites and chlorates. The reaction can be reversed by methylene blue, whereas oxygen may be administered on an emergency basis. Hemolytic reactions may also occur, particularly in people with glucose-6-phosphate dehydrogenase deficiency. In such cases urine flow must be maintained and, if renal failure is imminent (high serum hemoglobin), an exchange transfusion may be necessary.

maintenance therapy, body temperature. Neither hyperthermia nor hypothermia are desirable in the poisoned patient. Hyperthermia increases metabolic rate and oxygen requirements, as well as requirements for food and water. Hypothermia, although reducing the metabolic rate, may also reduce the rate of detoxication and elimination of the toxicant and/or its metabolites. Chemical intervention in the case of hyperthermia would place additional stress on the detoxication and excretory systems and is not generally recommended. Wet towels, cooling blankets and air circulation are more appropriate. Similarly, in hypothermia, total or partial immersion in warm water is recommended, but not local heating because of its effect on skin capillaries.

maintenance therapy, circulatory system. Congestive heart failure, which may result from poisons causing myocardial damage, is treated with rest, sodium restriction and, in serious cases, digitalis. Emergency treatment resulting from asphyxiation, carbon monoxide, etc., consists of chest massage and artificial respiration. If this is not successful, 0.9% saline may be given i.v., epinephrine injected, or defibrillation attempted. Thus any of the techniques available to the physician for the treatment of cardiac arrest, whatever the cause, may be attempted. *See also* SHOCK.

maintenance therapy, gastrointestinal tract. Problems due to toxicants can include vomiting, diarrhea and distension of the abdomen. Although vomiting may be beneficial initially, it eventually causes excessive fluid loss. It can be treated by i.v. glucose in saline until vomiting stops, followed by dry foods in small quantity, followed by fluids. If not contraindicated by the nature of the poison, or by other medical considerations, drugs such as chlorpromazine or promethazine that can be given orally or by suppositories may be prescribed. Diarrhea may also affect fluid balance, which must be corrected by i.v. glucose administration, whereas food intake is restricted to liquids or low-residue foods. Drugs that may be used include codeine or atropine, although pectin-kaolin mixtures may also be effective. Distension of the abdomen is usually due to gas that can be released by proper use of a rectal or colonic tube or intestinal intubation. *See also* DIARRHEA; MAINTENANCE THERAPY; VOMITING.

maintenance therapy, hepatic involvement. Liver damage can be acute, for example following ingestion of chloroform or carbon tetrachloride, or chronic, as with continued excessive ingestion of ethanol. Characteristically, liver enzymes such as glutamic-oxaloacetic transaminase, glutamic-pyruvic transaminases, lactic dehydrogenase and alkaline phosphatase are found at elevated levels in the serum. Blood bilirubin levels are also increased, and bilirubin and urobilinogen are found in the urine. In general, all drugs are discontinued, and the patient is maintained under complete bed rest. Other symptoms, such as vomiting, are controlled and, when feeding can be resumed, the diet is one with low protein, low fat, and high carbohydrate content.

maintenance therapy, nervous system. Stimulation by toxic chemicals of peripheral receptors that affect the CNS can cause convulsions due to oxygen lack (hypoxia) or low blood glucose (hypoglycemia). Such convulsions can be life-threatening due to respiratory failure caused by spasms of the respiratory muscles or due to post-convulsion depression. Treatment may include artificial respiration in the post-convulsion period and restraint to prevent injury. Neither emesis nor gastric lavage is attempted unless failure to do so might cause death. Maintenance of fluid balance, an adequate airway and glucose to treat hypoglycemia are important. Although anticonvulsants can be given, none should be used that cause coma or respiratory depression. Coma caused by poisons generally results from effects on brain cell function. Emergency measures include maintaining an adequate airway, artificial respiration and treatment for shock. Subsequently, attention is given to fluid balance and renal function. In any case, it is important to remove the toxicant by gastric lavage, activated charcoal, or dialysis. Treatment for CNS symptoms and signs (e.g., delirium or psychoses) caused by toxicants must be undertaken carefully to avoid exacerbation of the underlying intoxication. Hypoglycemic convulsions and coma are treated by administration of glucose, using the most appropriate route. *See also* COMA; CONVULSIONS; DELIRIUM; HYPERACTIVITY; HYPOGLYCEMIA; SHOCK.

maintenance therapy, respiration. Many poisons affect respiration, directly or indirectly; the effects including hypoxia, respiratory depression and pulmonary edema. All respiratory problems involve certain common principles, including maintaining an adequate airway, adequate pulmonary ventilation and an adequate oxygen supply. An adequate airway is maintained either by the oropharyngeal method using a metal or plastic airway or the tracheal method using a catheter, tracheotomy or cricopharyngeal puncture, a procedure creating an opening in the cricopharyngeal cartilage that can be carried out by a physician when other methods are not immediately possible. Adequate pulmonary ventilation can be assured by artificial respiration or a respirator, whereas oxygen can be administered directly. Pulmonary edema is treated first with morphine sulfate, oxygen and aminophylline, and subsequently with diuretics and corticoid anti-inflammatory agents if necessary. *See also* HYPOXIA; PULMONARY EDEMA; RESPIRATORY DEPRESSION.

maintenance therapy, urinary tract. Renal failure is treated by methods designed to restrict fluid retention until function can be restored, including fluid restriction and oral administration of salts. If recovery does not occur within a few days, however, or if blood creatine rises, dialysis is carried out. Urine retention can be treated by catheterization. *See also* FLUID RETENTION; RENAL FAILURE.

maintenance therapy, water and electrolyte balance. Although water and electrolytes must be replaced, the means are usually not critical if kidney function is not impaired. Electrolytes and/or water lost in urine, feces, expired air, sweat and vomiting must be replaced either orally or i.v. The amount necessary can be calculated based on body weight and serum ion analysis. In addition, glucose may also be given to provide an energy source. *See also* ACIDOSIS.

major tranquilizers (antipsychotic drugs). A class of drugs used to treat schizophrenia and other psychoses. The term is now considered archaic since "major tranquilizers" and "minor tranquilizers" refer to drugs with different modes of actions, and effects that are not simply graded responses. *Compare* MINOR TRANQUILIZERS. *See also* ANTIPSYCHOTIC DRUGS.

malaoxon (*O,O*-dimethyl *S*-(1,2-dicarbethoxyethyl)phosphoroate). A neurotoxicant that inhibits acetylcholinesterase and carboxylesterase. It is formed on activation of malathion by cytochrome P450. Its oral LD50 in rats is 158 mg/kg. *See also* ANTICHOLINESTERASES; MALATHION; ORGANOPHOSPHATE POISONING, SYMPTOMS AND THERAPY.

$$(CH_3O)_2P\overset{\displaystyle O}{\overset{\|}{-}}S-CH-\overset{\displaystyle O}{\overset{\|}{C}}-OC_2H_5$$

$$CH_2-\overset{\displaystyle O}{\overset{\|}{C}}-OC_2H_5$$

Malaoxon

malathion (*O*,*O*-dimethyl *S*-(1,2-dicarb-ethoxyethyl)phosphorodithioate; Cythion; Celthion). CAS number 121-75-5. An insecticide used in the control of sucking and chewing insects attacking fruits, vegetables, ornamentals and stored products. Malathion is used inside homes and particularly where a high degree of safety to mammals is desired. The oral LD50 in rats is 1375 mg/kg for males and 1000 mg/kg for females, whereas the dermal LD50 is greater than 4444 mg/kg for both sexes. Malathion is a neurotoxicant, after activation to its oxygen analog, malaoxon, by cytochrome P450, by virtue of the ability of malaoxon to act as an acetylcholinesterase inhibitor. *See also* INSECTICIDES; MALAOXON; ORGANOPHOSPHATE POISONING, SYMPTOMS AND THERAPY; ORGANOPHOSPHORUS INSECTICIDES.

$$(CH_3O)_2P\overset{\displaystyle S}{\overset{\|}{-}}S-CH-\overset{\displaystyle O}{\overset{\|}{C}}-OC_2H_5$$

$$CH_2-\overset{\displaystyle O}{\overset{\|}{C}}-OC_2H_5$$

Malathion

malformation. A permanent structural change arising during development.

malignancy (cancer). A state of tumor characterized by its non-encapsulation, invasiveness, poor differentiation, possessing common cell division and rapid growth characteristics that are anaplastic to various degrees giving rise to metastases. *See also* NEOPLASM.

malignant hemangioendothelioma. *See* ANGIOSARCOMA.

malignant hyperpyrexia. *See* HALOTHANE.

malignant hyperthermia. Malignant hyperthermia ia a lethal complication related to anesthesia. This syndrome is a chain reaction of abnormalities triggered in susceptible individuals by commonly used general anesthetics. The signs include greatly increased body metabolism, muscle rigidity, and eventual hyperthermia that may exceed 44 °C. Death can result from cardiac arrest, brain damage, internal hemorrhaging or failure of other body systems. Susceptibility is inherited, although the basis varies from a single defective gene from one parent to more complex genetic patterns. Volatile gaseous inhalation anesthetics (e.g., halothane, enflurane, isoflurane, sevoflurane and desflurane), as well as the muscle relaxant succinylcholine, can trigger it, whereas injectable local anesthetics, barbiturates, opioids, other sedative-hypnotics, and nitrous oxide, are safe for persons susceptible to this disorder. While the cause is not known, research suggests a generalized derangement of the processes that regulate muscle contraction, possibly initiated when the drug toxicity induces increased concentrations of calcium in the muscle cells. This results in hyperthermia and muscle cell breakdown. Dantrolene has been effectively and has contributed greatly to a dramatic decline in death and disability. *See also* ANESTHETICS.

mallard ducks. A standard avian test species for wildlife toxicology tests.

MAM. *See* METHYLAZOMETHANOL.

Mamba toxins. The venom of the green mamba (*Dendroaspis augusticeps*) is the source of α-dendrotoxin (α-DTX), a specific blocker of certain voltage-gated K$^+$ channels. In the brain, intracerebral injection of α-DTX causes convulsions by precipitating neurotransmitter release, probably largely of glutamate. Dendroaspis venom also contains fasciculin, a natural peptide inhibitor of acetylcholinesterase (AChE). Finally, mamba venom contains protein toxins that are agonists for the muscarinic acetycholine receptor. *See also* SNAKE VENOM.

mammalian cell mutation tests. The mutagenicity of chemicals is tested in cultured mammalian cells, such as Chinese hamster ovary cells or mouse lymphoma cells, by observing the ability of mutagens to confer resistance within these cell lines to normally toxic agents, such as toxic purines (HGPRT locus), toxic pyrimidines (TK locus) or ouabain (Na^+/K^+-ATPase locus). Mutations at these loci allow the cells to grow in the presence of these toxic agents. The S-9 fraction from induced rat liver is sometimes added to ensure metabolic activation of promutagens. *See also* CHINESE HAMSTER OVARY CELLS; EUKARYOTE MUTAGENICITY TESTS; HGPRT LOCUS; MOUSE LYMPHOMA CELLS; NA^+/K^+-ATPASE; S-9 FRACTION; TK LOCUS.

mammalian cell transformation tests. These *in vitro* tests, usually utilizing BABL/3T3 and C3H/10T1/2 fibroblast cultures from mouse embryos, estimate the ability of chemicals to cause carcinogenic transformation of cells. Normally these cells will form a monolayer in culture with very few, if any, foci of cellular growth. In the presence of a carcinogen, numerous foci develop, which, if injected into an animal, would produce malignant tumors. The occurrence of a significant number of foci in the cultures exposed to the test chemical compared with the numbers developing spontaneously in the negative controls indicates the carcinogenic potential of the chemical. Positive controls are run concurrently.

Mandragora officinarum. Mandrake, a poisonous plant containing 1-hyoscamine and scopalamine. *See also* ATROPINE; SCOPOLAMINE.

mandrake. *See* MANDRAGORA OFFICINARUM.

Manganese (Mn). An element that is essential as a cofactor for many enzymes, including hexokinase, xanthine oxidase and superoxide dismutase. Excessive exposure, first noted in manganese miners, can, however, produce CNS disorders. The first phase has been termed "manganese madness" and is marked by aggressive behavior and signs of mania. Within several weeks, this is followed by a second phase with marked parkinsonism, including cogwheel rigidity, mask-like faces and stooped postures. It has been shown that the primary cause of these signs is manganese-induced alterations in dopamine neurotransmission in the brain, and available data suggest an initial

hyperactivity, followed by hypoactivity due to the death of dopamine neurons. The pseudoparkinsonism of the latter phase has been successfully treated with L-dopa *See also* L-DOPA; DOPAMINE; PARKINSONISM.

MANOVA (multivariate analysis of variance). A procedure for testing differences among means. This procedure is similar to the univariate ANOVA, except that MANOVA is designed to test the significance of an independent variable or variables on more than one dependent variable. The MANOVA procedure protects against an inflated alpha (increased probability of a type I error) by controlling for the intercorrelation among dependent variables. The various main effects and interaction effects generated by a MANOVA are typically tested for by Hotelling's T^2 or Wilk's Lambda. *See also* ANALYSIS OF VARIANCE; MULTIVARIATE STATISTICAL ANALYSIS; STATISTICS, FUNCTION IN TOXICOLOGY.

Mantel–Bryan model. *See* LOW-DOSE EXTRAPOLATION.

MAO. *See* MONOAMINE OXIDASES.

MAO-I. *See* MONOAMINE OXIDASE INHIBITORS.

margin of exposure (MOE). The ratio of the no observed adverse effect level (NOAEL) to the estimated human exposure. Formerly referred to as the margin of safety (MOS).

margin of safety (MOS). *See* MARGIN OF EXPOSURE.

marihuana (marijuana) The term is derived from the indigenous Mexican or Central American word maraguango, a general term meaning any intoxicating substance. Marihuana is not a simple drug, but is a complex mixture of over 400 individual chemicals. For self-administration purposes, the leaves and flowering tops of *Cannabis sativa* are finely chopped, rolled in cigarette paper or placed in the bowl of pipes of various configurations for smoking. It can also be ingested by incorporation into salads or baked foods (i.e., brownies). Marihuana is widely used for the purpose of obtaining a temporary euphoric effect with diversely perceived sensory, somatic, affective and cognitive changes that are commonly described as a "high". The intensity and duration of the pharmacological effects are dose-dependent and vary with the route of administration. Thus, after oral ingestion, the effects appear slowly, but last longer than after smoke inhalation. Figures from the National Household Drug Use Survey (1985) show that nearly one-third (62 million) of all Americans had tried marihuana at least once in their lives. Even though the number of regular marihuana users declined from 20 million to 18.2 million between 1982 and 1985, 6 million people reported that they use marihuana almost every day. *See also* CANNABINOIDS; *CANNABIS SATIVA*; Δ^9-*TRANS*-TETRAHYDROCANNABINOL.

marijuana. *See* MARIHUANA.

marker enzymes. Enzymes used either as an indicator of organelle function or cellular or organ toxicity. *See also* LIVER ENZYMES, IN BLOOD; ORGANELLE EVALUATION.

marketing authorization. The authorization required from the regulatory authority before a medicine may be placed on the market in the European Community.

mass spectrometry. *See* SPECTROMETRY, MASS.

mass spectroscopy. *See* SPECTROMETRY, MASS.

mast cells/basophils. A mast cell is a mononuclear granular cell found in connective tissue. It has receptors for the constant non-antigen-binding portion of the IgE antibody molecule. The mast cell passively acquires IgE of various specificities from the circulation. When the IgE molecules are cross-linked by a multivalent antigen, or an anti-IgE antibody, the mast cell is triggered to degranulate, releasing a number of potent biological mediators into the intracellular space. The primary compounds are already present in these granules and include: (1) vasoactive amines (e.g., histamine in humans) that cause contractions of smooth muscle, increased vascular permeability,

vasodilation of some vessels and vasoconstriction of other vessels; (2) chemotactic factors for granulocytes—primarily for eosinophils in humans; (3) a large array of enzymes whose function is unclear; (4) a proteoglycan, heparin, that has anticoagulant properties. Basophils are granulocytes that circulate in the blood and are also triggered to degranulate by cross-linking of surface-bound IgE. Their granules contain a similar array of chemicals. Secondary biological mediators are also produced by degranulation. These are not stored in the granules, but are synthesized following antigen triggering. These are primarily products of arachidonic acid breakdown, itself a product of membrane phospholipid breakdown. Three of the leukotrienes produced—C4, D4 and E4—formerly called the slow-reacting substance of anaphylaxis (SRS-A) cause slow smooth muscle contractions and are a major cause of lung changes in anaphylactic reactions. Release of granule contents and synthesis of secondary mediators results in an anaphylactic reaction. The reaction may be local, as when mast cells in the lung are triggered by an inhaled allergen and produce an asthmatic reaction, or systemic, as when large numbers of mast cells and/or basophils degranulate in response to an i.v. dose of a drug or venom and anaphylactic shock ensues. The location and severity of the anaphylactic response are dependent on the location and number of mast cells/basophils that degranulate, that is, in turn, dependent on both the magnitude of the initial IgE response to the allergen and the concentration of the allergen in the subsequent exposure. Although the role of the mast cell and basophil are fairly well established in allergic reactions, their role in normal functioning is still poorly understood. They are thought to be active in protection against parasites since IgE levels on intestinal mast cells are often elevated in people with parasitic infections, and the eosinophil chemotactic factor binds to parasites. Additionally, it is thought that the smooth muscle contractions brought about by the histamine and the leukotrienes might help to expel parasites. *See also* ALLERGIC RESPONSE; IMMEDIATE HYPERSENSITIVITY.

Material Safety Data Sheet (MSDS). First required as a Hazard Communication standard by the US OSHA, the MSDS that accompanies each hazardous chemical provides detailed hazard and safety information to employees on all hazardous chemicals used in the workplace. Since most chemicals sold are ultimately used in a workplace, vendors of chemicals are required to provide an MSDS with each hazardous chemical sold. Numerous databases are available that contain hundreds to thousands of MSDSs.

maternal toxicity. It is important, in teratogenicity testing, to distinguish developmental effects from effects due to maternal toxicity. In routine teratogenicity testing, maternal toxicity is evaluated from a relatively small number of parameters, including body weight, food consumption, clinical signs and necropsy data such as organ weights. It is useful in assessing the validity of the high-dose level and the possibility that maternal toxicity is involved in subsequent events. Since exposure starts after implantation, conception and implantation rates should be the same in controls and all treatment levels. If this is not the case, the test is suspect, perhaps due to an error in the timing of the dose. *See also* REPRODUCTIVE TOXICITY TESTING; TERATOLOGY TESTING.

mathematical models. *See* MODEL.

maximum allowable concentration (MAC). The upper limit of concentration of certain atmospheric contaminants allowed in the ambient air of the workplace. *See also* THRESHOLD LIMIT VALUES.

maximum individual risk (MIR). Increased risk for an individual exposed to the highest measured or predicted concentration of a toxicant.

maximum residue level. A special case of the maximum residue limit. The maximum amount of a veterinary pharmaceutical that should be present as a residue in food of animal origin. The EC is to set MRLs for all veterinary pharmaceuticals used in food-producing animals by 1997. *See also* MAXIMUM RESIDUE LIMIT.

maximum residue limit (MRL). The limit on the amount of an "additive" that may be present in food. The limit is based either on: the limit considered to be without hazard to human health based on an ADI (MRL_T); or on residues achieved in practice for veterinary drugs when used according to good practice (MRL_U); or based on the availability of a validated practical analytical method for measuring residues (MRL_M). The MRL must always be equal or lower than the MRL_T. But if practicable the MRL_U will be used instead, except where a suitable analytical technique is unavailable —in which case a MRL_M intermediate in value between the MRL_U and the MRL_T will be used. The use of MRL_M ensures compliance can be checked.

maximum tolerated dose (MTD). The highest dose of a toxicant that causes toxic effects without significant mortality during a chronic toxicity study and that does not decrease the body weight by more than 10% compared with an appropriate control group. Although mandated by some regulatory agencies, the use of the maximum tolerated dose in chronic toxicity tests is one of the most controversial issues in regulatory toxicology.

maximum velocity. *See* K_M; V_{MAX}.

MDA (methylenedioxyamphetamine; 1-(1,3-benzodioxol-5-yl)-2-aminopropane; 1-(3,4-methylenedioxyphenyl)-2-aminopropane). CAS number 4764-17-4. A hallucinogenic (psychedelic) agent that has also been used experimentally as an adjunct to psychotherapy. It is obtained by direct chemical synthesis. Its LD50 is 68 mg/kg, i.p., 27 mg/kg, i.p., 7 mg/kg, i.v. and 6 mg/kg, i.v. in mice, rats, dogs and monkeys, respectively. It may catalyze severe emotional problems or psychosis in predisposed individuals, and a number of deaths have been attributed to MDA overdose. The hallucinogenic effects of MDA may be due to an agonist effect at $5-HT_2$ receptors. The toxic and life-threatening action, however, may be related to a powerful sympathomimetic action of MDA, principally the release of norepinephrine from nerve terminals. Symptoms include mydriasis, hyperreflexia, restlessness, perceptual alterations

Methylenedioxyamphetamine

and illusions. There is a marked enhancement in emotion and affect, leading MDA to have been called the "love drug", these actions also possibly involving activation of dopamine receptors. At toxic doses, MDA causes agitation, hallucinations, delirium, convulsions, coma, elevated blood pressure, heart rate, diarrhea, diaphoresis and marked hyperthermia. In dogs, the toxic effects of a sublethal dose of MDA is blocked by phenoxybenzamine or phentolamine. In dogs, death due to potentially lethal doses of MDA (20 mg/kg, i.v.) has been prevented by subsequent administration of chlorpromazine (10 mg/kg, i.v.). *See also* AMPHETAMINES; HALLUCINOGENS; METHYL-ENEDIOXY RING CLEAVAGE.

MDD. *See* MEDICAL DEVICES DIRECTORATE.

MDI. *See* TOLUENE DIISOCYANATE.

MDK. *See* METHYL N-BUTYL KETONE.

MDM. *See* MDMA.

MDMA (*N*-methyl-1-(1,3-benzodioxol-5-yl)-2-aminopropane; *N*-methyl-3,4-methylene-dioxyamphetamine; 3,4-methylenedioxy-methamphetamine; MDM; ADAM; Ecstasy). CAS number 42542-10-9. A novel psychoactive drug chemically related to the hallucinogenic agent MDA, but reported to be non-hallucinogenic. Obtained by direct synthesis, at high doses it is reported to show a stimulant-like effect in animals. Its LD50 is 97 mg/kg, i.p., 49 mg/kg, i.p., 14 mg/kg, i.v., and 22 mg/kg, i.v. in mice, rats, dogs and monkeys, respectively. At higher doses, MDMA has pressor effects and produces tachycardia, and causes damage to serotonin neurons in both rats and monkeys. The (S)-(+)-enantiomer is more active than the (R)-(i)-enantiomer and, like amphetamine, the pharmacological effects may be due to a release of endogenous monoamine neurotransmitter, probably serotonin and/or norepinephrine. MDMA is also an inhibitor of monoamine uptake into brain synaptosomes. Symptoms include pronounced mydriasis, with nystagmus and jaw clenching, and nausea also is often reported. This substance produces a feeling of well-being and euphoria, and is similar in some

respects to MDA, in that it seems to enhance a sense of empathy and emotional openness in users. Toxic reactions would appear to occur as a result of the pressor action, and sympathomimetic effects of the drug. No appropriate therapeutic intervention has been reported. Peripheral adrenergic blocking agents, or chlorpromazine, have been used, however, to prevent death in dogs following a lethal i.v. dose of the chemically related agent MDA. *See also* AMPHETAMINES; HALLUCINOGENS; METHYLENEDIOXY RING CLEAVAGE.

MDMA

mean corpuscular hemoglobin. A measure of the hemoglobin content of red blood cells derived from the formula:

$$MCH = \frac{\text{hemoglobin} \left(g \text{ per } 100 \text{ ml blood} \right)}{\text{red cell count in } 10^6 \text{ per mm}^2} \times 100$$

It is a standard hematological parameter typical of those used in chronic toxicity tests.

mean corpuscular volume. A measure of the volume of red blood cells derived from the formula:

$$MCV = \frac{\text{volume of packed red cells per } 100 \text{ ml blood}}{\text{red cell count in } 10^6 \text{ per mm}^2} \times 100$$

It is a standard hematological parameter typical of those used in chronic toxicity tests. *See also* TOXIC ENDPOINTS.

measurement of toxicants. *See* ANALYTICAL TOXICOLOGY.

mechanism of action. *See* MODE OF ACTION.

mechanism of induction. Most induction by xenobiotics involves *de novo* protein synthesis. Induction of xenobiotic-metabolizing enzymes is not understood, except for aromatic hydrocarbon (Ah) induction of the cytochrome P450-dependent monooxygenase. In this model, the aromatic hydrocarbon moves passively across the cell membrane; once inside it binds to a cytosolic receptor protein (designated the Ah receptor) coded for by a putative regulatory gene. Translocation of the ligand-Ah receptor complex into the nucleus and its interactions with structural genes stimulate transcription of those genes, resulting in augmented enzyme levels. *See also* AH RECEPTOR; INDUCTION.

median effective dose (ED50). *See* EFFECTIVE DOSE.

median lethal concentration. *See* LC50.

median lethal dose. *See* LD50.

Medical Devices Directorate (MDD). The UK regulatory body for medical devices.

Medical Research Council (MRC). A government organization that supports MRC research institutes in the UK, as well as providing funds for research projects carried out at universities. Research is concerned with all medical topics including pharmacology and toxicology.

Medicines Act. UK legislation, passed in 1968, that restricts the supply and manufacture of all medicines to license-holders. Product licenses are only granted by the Medicines Division of the Department of Health and Social Security after the submission of the results of toxicological and clinical trials.

meiosis. Process of cell division in which the diploid number ($2n$) of chromosomes is reduced to the haploid (n). It is characteristic of cells in the male and female germ lines of eukaryotes. The process of fertilization results in a fusion nucleus with chromosomes of both gametes, restoring the diploid number.

MEL. Maximum exposure limit (usually expressed in air in ppm or mg/m^3), for long-term exposure (8-hour TWA reference period) or short-term exposure (10-minute reference period) under COSHH regulations.

melanoma. A tumor, almost always malignant, of melanocytes, the pigment-containing cells of the iris, skin, retina, etc. These tumors are nearly always darkly pigmented, reflecting their origin, but melanomas may also be non-pigmented.

Mellaril. *See* THIORIDAZINE.

melphalan (4-[bis(2-chloroethyl)amino]-l-phenylalanine; Alkeran; l-phenylalanine mustard; l-PAM; L-sarcolysine). CAS number 148-82-3. An antineoplastic primarily. Both the effectiveness of the drug and its toxicity probably result from the ability of melphalan to cross-link DNA strands, thus preventing DNA replication. Its oral LD50 in mice is 21 mg/kg. The principal toxicity of melphalan is to the bone marrow, although hypersensitivity, gastrointestinal toxicity, pulmonary toxicity and infertility have also been observed. The drug is also probably leukemogenic. Melphalan shows highly variable uptake after oral dosage, is not extensively metabolized in man, but is unstable in aqueous solution breaking down to monohydroxy- and 2-dihydroxyethyl derivatives. The stability of melphalan is enhanced by acid pH, taurocholic acid and chloride ions. Up to one-half of the administered dose of melphalan can be recovered in urine after six days as either the parent form or one of the metabolites. Melphalan is transported via a carrier-mediated high-affinity amino acid transport system of the leucine type. Thus, not unexpectedly, melphalan toxicity can be prevented by leucine or glutamine administration. *In vitro* studies suggest that resistance can result from an increased glutathione content.

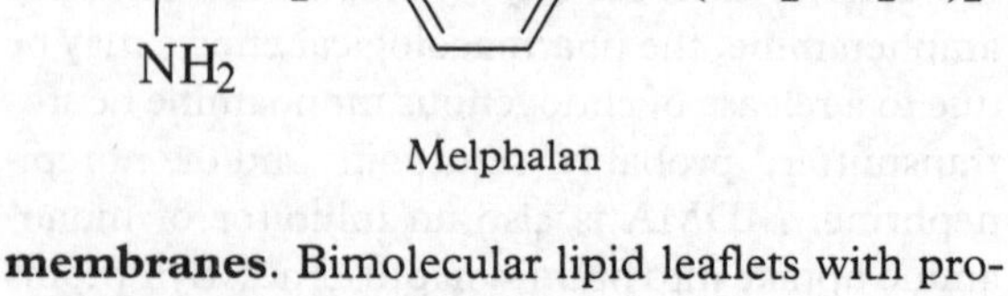

$$HOC\overset{\overset{\displaystyle O}{\|}}{C}HCH_2 \underset{NH_2}{\underset{|}{}} \!\!\!—\!\!\! \langle \rangle \!\!\!—\!\!\! N(CH_2CH_2Cl)_2$$

Melphalan

membranes. Bimolecular lipid leaflets with proteins embedded in the matrix and also arranged on the inner and outer polar surfaces. Membranes of tissues, cells and cell organelles are all basically similar in structure. This basic plan is present despite many variations, and it is important in toxicological studies of uptake of toxicants by passive diffusion and active transport.

memory cells. Memory, or the ability to mount a quantitatively and qualitatively different response upon secondary exposure to a specific antigen, is one of the hallmarks of the vertebrate immune response. In the humoral, or antibody, secondary response, antibody is produced more quickly, in larger quantities, for a longer period of time, and of different classes and affinities than in a primary response. The secondary response in cell-mediated immunity produces faster elimination of viral antigens, faster and more severe delayed-type hypersensitivity reactions and decreased graft rejection time. The ability to mount a secondary immune response is due to the generation of antigen-specific memory cells during the primary response. Memory B cells and probably memory T cells, as well as effector B cells (plasma cells) and effector T cells (cytotoxic T cells) are produced from naive B and T cells during the primary response to that antigen. The effector cells are generally short-lived, but a clone of long-lived antigen-primed memory cells is thought to survive and provide for the heightened secondary response by bypassing the early stages of clonal expansion. *See also* CLONAL EXPANSION; IMMUNE SYSTEM.

menstrual cycle. The uterine changes that occur as a result of the cyclic secretion of the hypophyseal gonadotropins and consequently the ovarian hormones in primates. The average cycle length in humans is 28 days. Events during the menstrual cycle occur in three major phases: (1) menstruation (days 1–5), the shedding of the endometrium developed during the previous cycle because of a lack of estrogen and progesterone; (2) proliferative phase (days 6–14), the proliferation and vascularization of the endometrium under the influence of estrogen; (3) secretory phase (days 15–28), the further development of endometrial thickness and glandular complexity under the influence of progesterone and estrogen.

mental retardation. A biobehavioral condition, the classification of which is made on the basis of three criteria: (1) an intelligence quotient (IQ) that is greater than two standard deviations below the mean (i.e., less than 70); (2) deficits in adaptive behavior; (3) onset before age 18. This disorder may be due to any of a number of etiologies, including genetic and chromosomal disorders, infections, inborn errors of metabolism, toxic agents or other pre- or postnatal factors. Traditionally, mild mental retardation, a category that includes about 80% of persons classified as mentally retarded, was associated with a psychosocial etiology. More recently, brain maldevelopment or dysfunction is thought to play a causative role. Prevalence data indicate that about 3% of the population are classified as mentally retarded. Mental retardation can be the result of pre- or postnatal exposure to toxicants or teratogens such as methylmercury or alcohol. *See also* HYPERACTIVITY; NEUROBEHAVIORAL TERATOLOGY; NEUROBEHAVIORAL TOXICOLOGY; POSTNATAL BEHAVIORAL TESTS; TREMORS.

Mepergan. *See* MEPERIDINE.

meperidine (ethyl 1-methyl-4-phenyl-4-piperidinecarboxylate; ethyl 1-methyl-4-phenylisonipecotate; Demerol; Mepergan; pethidine). CAS number 57-42-1. A narcotic analgesic that is used as a preoperative medication, for supporting anesthesia and during obstetrical anesthesia. Its oral LD50 in rats is 170 mg/kg. It has multiple actions qualitatively similar to those of morphine, and therapy is similar to that for morphine. *See also* MORPHINE; NARCOTIC ANTAGONISTS; NARCOTICS.

Meperidine

mephenesin (3-(2-methylphenoxy)-1,2-propanediol). CAS number 59-47-2. A muscle relaxant that is no longer used, primarily because of its short duration of action and toxic side effects. It is believed to depress transmission through a number of spinal and supraspinal polysynaptic (intraneural) pathways. Administration of high i.v. doses of mephenesin has resulted in serious blood disorders that occasionally have caused death. The oral LD50 in mice and rats is 990 and 945 mg/kg, respectively.

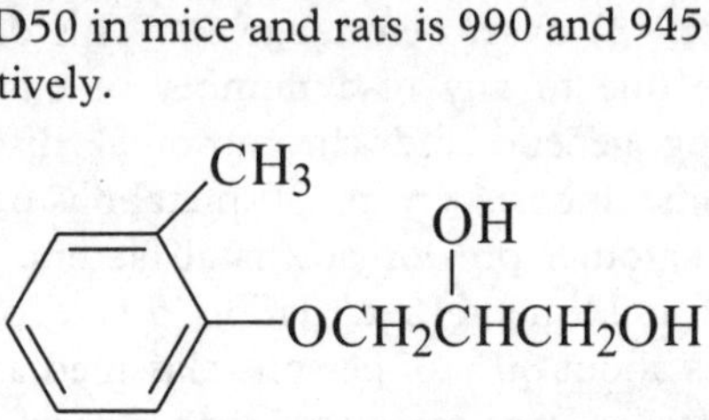

Mephenesin

meprobamate   (2-methyl-2-propyl-1,3-pro-panediol   dicarbamate;   carbamic   acid 2-methyl-2-propyltrimethylene ester; Equanil; Miltown). CAS number 57-53-4. The first of the modern antianxiety/sedative drugs; first introduced on the market in 1955. Its i.p. LD50 in mice is 800 mg/kg. Animal studies showing multiple CNS sites of action, including the thalamus and limbic system. It causes drowsiness and ataxia, and may cause allergic skin reactions, hypotension, respiratory depression, shock, pulmonary edema and heart failure. Therapy for overdosage is to empty the stomach by lavage or induce vomiting while monitoring respiration, kidney function and blood pressure. Respiratory assistance, stimulants, pressor agents, diuresis or dialysis may be required. *See also* ANTIANXIETY DRUGS.

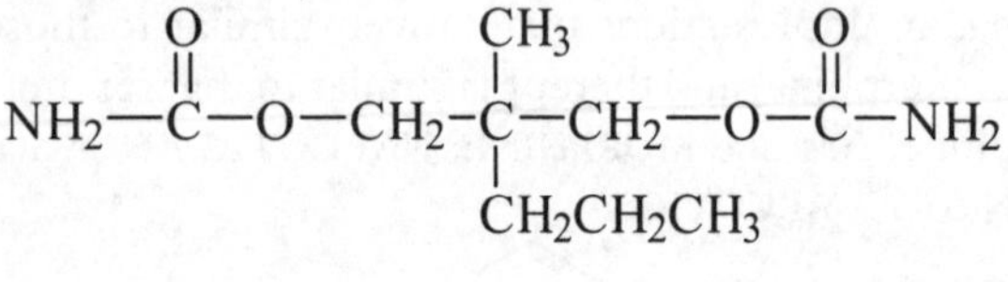

Meprobamate

Meractinomycin. *See* ACTINOMYCIN D.

mercaptans. Organic compounds with the general formula R-SH, meaning that the thiol group (-SH) is attached to a radical (e.g., CH_3 or C_2H_5). The simpler mercaptans have strong, repulsive odors, but these become less pronounced with increasing molecular weights and higher boiling points. Mercaptans may be produced in oil refinery feed preparation units.

6-mercaptopurine   (6-MP;   1,7-dihydro-6*H*-purine-6-thione; Leukerin; Purinethol). CAS number 50-44-2. An antineoplastic metabolic

antagonist with an i.p. LD50 in mice of 240 mg/kg. It inhibits DNA and RNA synthesis, by being metabolically converted to 6-thioinosine-5′-phosphate, that inhibits purine biosynthesis at multiple steps. In humans, it causes acute nausea and vomiting, followed by bone marrow depression, predominantly due to effects on white cells, and liver damage. *See also* ABNORMAL BASE ANALOGS.

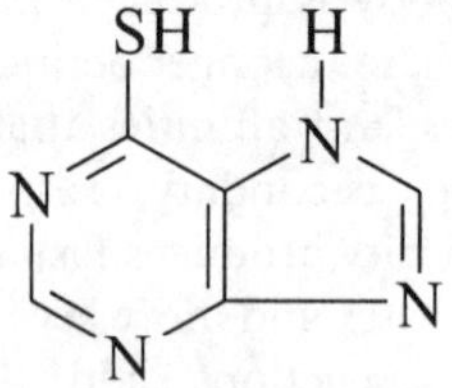

6-Mercaptopurine

mercapturic acids (*N*-acetylcysteine conjugates). The final product in an important detoxication sequence for potentially harmful electrophiles. The initial stage in mercapturic acid biosynthesis involves conjugation of the electrophile with endogenous glutathione by the glutathione *S*-transferases. The glutathione conjugates are converted in separate steps to the mercapturic acid by removal of the γ-glutamyl moiety, removal of the glycine moiety and *N*-acetylation of the cysteine conjugate. Mercapturic acids are excreted in either the bile or urine. *See also* ACETYLATION; GLUTATHIONE TRANSFERASES; β-GLUTAMYLTRANSPEPTIDASES.

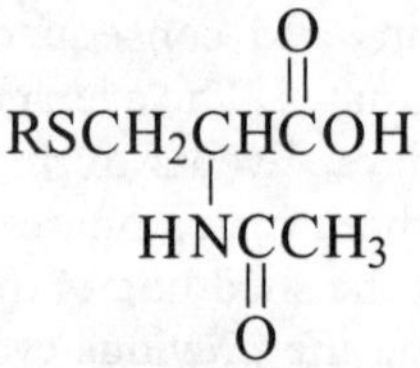

Mercapturic acid

mercury (Hg; quicksilver). An element that is used in thermometers, lamps, manufacture of all mercury salts, as a chemical catalyst, in pharmaceuticals, dentistry, agriculture, as a cathode and elsewhere. Although the major source of mercury in the environment is the natural degassing of the Earth's crust, mining, smelting and industrial wastes contribute to environmental contamination. There are three general forms of mercury that require different toxicological considerations:

elemental; inorganic compounds; and organic compounds. Elemental mercury is volatile at ambient temperatures, is readily absorbed in the lung, and has affinity for erythrocytes and the CNS due to its lipophilicity. Inhalation of vapor causes acute bronchitis, pneumonitis and CNS effects, including tremor and excitability. The CNS is the major target in chronic elemental mercury exposure that results in a syndrome termed micromercurialism (neurasthenia, tremor, gingivitis, memory loss, excitability, etc.). Acute intoxication with inorganic mercury is usually due to the ingestion of mercury salts resulting in gastrointestinal disturbances and renal failure due to tubular necrosis. In contrast to elemental and organic mercury, mercuric ions do not readily cross the blood–brain barrier. Chronic intoxication leads to inflammation of mouth and gums, salivation, loose teeth, glomerulonephropathy, muscle tremors, jerky gait, spasms in extremities, depression, irritability and nervousness. The lethal dose in man is about 1 g of a mercuric salt. Human exposure to organomercurials is primarily via the gastrointestinal system. Methylmercury, the major organomercurial of toxicological importance, may be formed environmentally in the aquatic environment by biomethylation and is also used as a fungicide. Several epidemics of methylmercury poisoning have been reported, the most notable in Japan and Iraq. Because of its lipophilic nature, the target of methylmercury is the CNS. Symptoms include tunnel vision, paresthesias, ataxia, dysarthria and deafness. Phenyl and alkoxyalkyl mercurials are also absorbed through the skin, and can cause skin burns and nephrotic syndrome. The LD50 for mercury is dependent upon route of exposure and the specific compound. The mechanism of Hg^{2+} or RHg^+ toxicity may be due to the ability to bind to macromolecules and thiol groups, forming mercaptides that thereby result in enzyme inhibition. Therapy of severe mercury intoxication may require hemodialysis, along with chelators such as cysteine or penicillamine. In less severe cases, 2,3-dimercapto-1-propanol (BAL) may be effective. Chelation therapy is not very helpful in alkylmercury poisoning. Surgical gallbladder drainage or the administration of a nonabsorbable thiol mercury-binding resin can be used to interrupt the enterohepatic cycling of the alkyl compound. *See also* 2,3-DIMERCAPTO-1-PROPANOL; METHYLMERCURY; MINAMATA DISEASE; POLLUTION, METALS; ATSDR DOCUMENT, MAY 1994.

mescaline (2-(3,4,5-trimethoxyphenyl)ethanamine; 3,4,5-trimethoxy-β-phenethylamine). CAS number 54-04-6. A hallucinogenic (psychedelic) agent that has been used experimentally as an adjunct to psychotherapy. It can be obtained by direct synthesis, but it also occurs naturally in the "peyote" cactus *Lophophora williamsii* (Lemaire) Coulter, the latter being used ceremonially by the Native American Church. Its LD50 is 212 mg/kg, i.p., 132 mg/kg, i.p., 54 mg/kg, i.v., and 130 mg/kg, i.v., in mice, rats, dogs and monkeys, respectively. Mescaline may catalyze the onset of severe emotional problems or psychosis in predisposed individuals. Although the underlying mechanisms of action for hallucinogens are not understood at the present time, mescaline may act, at least in part, as a serotonin 5-HT_2 agonist. It typically causes pupillary dilation, hyperreflexia and restlessness; perceptual alterations and illusions (including changes in touch, taste and odor) are characteristic. Synethesia is common, and the thinking process is substantially altered. At high doses, mescaline causes hallucinations and loss of contact with reality. There have been no overdose deaths attributed to the direct effects of mescaline. Acute panic reactions can usually be treated in a quiet, supportive environment; diazepam has also been used for management of anxiety. *See also* HALLUCINOGENS.

Mescaline

mesocosm. An experimental system used in the field of environmental toxicology in which a limited artificial ecosystem is set up in an artificial container, such as an aquarium or a vat. The mesocosm is stocked with representative plants, animals and microbes such that all trophic levels are represented. The mesocosm will give more environmentally representative information, yet is still controlled in time, space and experimental conditions.

mesothelioma. A tumor, either benign or malignant, arising from cells lining the abdominal, pericardial or pleural spaces; archaic synonyms (celioma and celothelioma) reflect the origin of these tumors from cells lining the embryonic coelom or primitive body cavity. Pleural mesotheliomas are most common. These tumors are causally linked to exposure to asbestos. *See also* ASBESTOS.

mesothelium. The layer of cells of mesodermal origin that lines the early body cavity. In the adult it is the epithelium of the serous membranes. *See also* MESOTHELIOMA.

mestranol **((17*a*)-3-methoxy-19-norpregna-1,3,5,(10)-trien-20-yn-17-ol)**. **CAS number 72-33-3**. The 3-methyl ether of ethynylestradiol; it is inactive as an estrogen until it is metabolized to ethynylestradiol. This is frequently a component of the combination-type oral contraceptives, which have additional uses in dysmenorrhea, amenorrhea, habitual or threatened abortion and other gynecological problems. *See also* ESTROGENS.

Mestranol

metabolic acidosis. *See* ACIDOSIS, METABOLIC.

metabolic alkalosis. *See* ALKALOSIS, METABOLIC.

metabolic inhibitors. Although technically used to describe any inhibition of any metabolic reaction or process, in toxicology, metabolic inhibitors inhibit energy metabolism and thus cause a generalized effect on overall function in the organism. Metabolic inhibitors reduce ATP production by inhibiting specific enzymes in the energy metabolism pathways, or by interfering with oxidative phosphorylation. Important metabolic inhibitors with their targets include: sodium fluoroacetate (compound 1080), aconitase; arsenite, pyruvate oxidase complex and ketoglutarate oxidase complex; rotenone, NADH dehydrogenase; antimycin A, b-c complex; cyanide and carbon monoxide, cytochrome oxidase; oligomycin, ATP synthetase; 2,4-dinitrophenol, valinomycin and gramicidin, oxidative phosphorylation. *See also* ELECTRON TRANSPORT SYSTEM INHIBITORS; OXIDATIVE PHOSPHORYLATION INHIBITORS.

metabolic tolerance (dispositional tolerance). A situation in which repeated exposure of an agent results in a decreased response to the same dose of the agent, with the smaller effect being caused by decreased availability of the agent. The change in availability may be due to alterations in any one of several toxicokinetic or pharmacokinetic properties. *See also* ADAPTATION TO TOXICANTS; PHYSIOLOGICAL TOLERANCE; TOLERANCE; TOXICOKINETICS.

metabolism. In biochemistry and physiology, the total of all chemical transformations of normal body constituents taking place in a living organism, whether they are synthetic (anabolic) or degradative (catabolic) reactions. The great majority, but not all, of these reactions are catalyzed by enzymes. In this sense it does not include the chemical transformations of xenobiotics, but rather is a normal function that may be adversely affected by those xenobiotics that are toxicants. *See also* XENOBIOTIC METABOLISM.

metabolism tests. In toxicology, the metabolism of a potential toxicant rather than a measure of some parameter of endogenous metabolism. The metabolic study, considered separately from toxicodynamics, usually consists of treatment of the animal with a radiolabeled compound followed by chemical analysis of all metabolites formed *in vivo* and excreted via the lungs, kidneys or bile. Although reactive intermediates are unlikely to be isolated, the chemical structure of the end products may provide clues to the nature of the intermediates involved in their formation. The use of tissue homogenates, subcellular fractions and purified enzymes may serve to clarify events occurring during metabolic sequences leading to the end products, although they are not generally part of the routine metabolism test. Information of importance in test animal selection is the similarity in toxicodynamics and metabolism to humans. Dose selection may be influenced by a knowledge of whether a particular dose saturates a physiological process such as excretion or whether it accumulates in a particular tissue, since these factors become increasingly important the longer a chronic study continues. *See also* TOXICODYNAMICS, IN TOXICITY TESTING.

metabolite. Any product of the metabolic processes of a living organism. In toxicology, it is usually used to refer to the products of metabolism of xenobiotics, products that may be less toxic than the parent compound or more toxic than the parent compound.

metabolite inhibitory complexes. The inhibition of enzymes may be caused by the parent compound being metabolized by the enzyme in question to a reactive metabolite, that then interacts with the enzyme in such a way as to cause inhibition of further activity. Although reversible inhibition (product inhibition) is known, it is less important in toxicology. Irreversible inhibition due to the formation of stable complexes (metabolite inhibitory complexes) with the enzyme is more important. Such complexes may involve covalent binding or may result in degradation of the enzyme. In the case of synergists such as piperonyl butoxide, it is probable that the metabolite is a carbene formed spontaneously by elimination of water following hydroxylation of the methylene carbon by cytochrome P450. Piperonyl butoxide inhibits the *in vitro* metabolism of many substrates of the cytochrome P450-dependent monooxygenase system, including ethylmorphine, aniline and *p*-nitroanisole. Other cytochrome P450 inhibition, such as amphetamine derivatives and SKF-525A, also form metabolite inhibitory complexes. Allylisopropylacetamide, on the other hand, is an example of a "suicide substrate," inasmuch as the metabolite inhibitory complex brings about the destruction of the heme of cytochrome P450 and its release as a pigment. *See also* INHIBITION; XENOBIOTIC METABOLISM, IRREVERSIBLE INHIBITION.

metabolites, reactive. *See* REACTIVE METABOLITES.

metallothionein (MT). A low-molecular-weight (6500–7000 daltons) cytosolic protein found in many eukaryotic species. It has a high metal content, usually containing bound zinc, cadmium or copper. Of the total amino acid composition, 30% consists of cysteinyl residues. The metal ions are bound to the sulfhydryl groups of the protein by mercaptide bonds. *De novo* synthesis of MT is induced by dietary or parenteral administration of Cd, Zn, Cu, Hg or Au. While little is known about the mechanisms of MT induction by nonmetallic inducers (e.g., growth factors), MT is highly expressed during liver regeneration. The possibility that the MT could participate in a DNA synsthesis-related process through donation or abstraction of Zn to and from transcription factors has been inferred from *in vitro* studies. Overexpression of MT is often accompanied by increased resistance towards a variety of alkylating agents and chemotherapeutic drugs, involving several mechanisms that are dependent on the metal composition of MT. *See also* METALLOTHIONEIN GENES.

metallothionein genes. A small gene family of some 11 separate sequences in the mammal, including human; the number of genes in the family is less in lower eukaryotes. The genes code for the metal-binding protein metallothionein, and are inducible by heavy metals such as cadmium and zinc, and corticosteroid hormones. The genes are generally 900 bases in length, with two introns of 400 and 200 base pairs, although some of the genes in the family are pseudogenes and lack introns. There are two particular features of interest. In the mouse these genes are subject to amplification when induced with heavy metals. Also the sequence involved in heavy metal induction, upstream from the coding sequence, shows evidence of being palindromic, thus having a dyad symmetry and capable of adopting a unique tertiary configuration. *See also* METALLOTHIONEIN.

metaphase. *See* MITOSIS.

metaplasia. Alterations in adult cells to a form that is abnormal for that tissue.

metastasis. The transfer of abnormal cells or pathogenic microorganisms from one organ to another in the body. The term frequently refers to the implantation of malignant tumor cells at a site distant from the primary tumor site. Transportation of detached tumor cells is typically accomplished through blood or lymph channels.

metestrus. *See* ESTRUS CYCLE.

methadone (6-dimethylamino-4,4-diphenylheptan-3-one hydrochloride). CAS number 1095-90-5. A narcotic analgesic whose effects approximate those of morphine, but which unlike morphine, is very effective orally. Although methadone produces drug dependence similar to that seen with morphine, withdrawal from methadone is somewhat less traumatic because active compounds are slowly released from binding sites in the body. Methadone is used as an analgesic, for detoxification of narcotic addiction and for temporary maintenance programs of addicts. The s.c. LD50 in rats is 44 mg/kg. Like morphine, it acts as an agonist at opioid receptors. Therapy for overdosage (antagonists and gavage) is similar to that of other narcotics, but with consideration given to the long half-life of this drug. *See also* MORPHINE; NARCOTIC ANTAGONISTS; NARCOTICS; OPIOIDS.

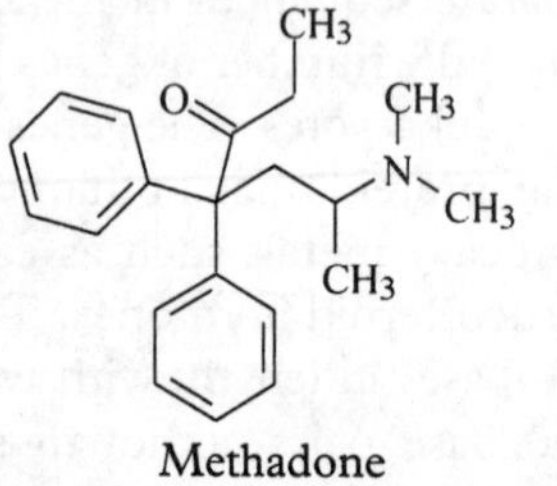

Methadone

methamphetamine   (1-phenyl-2-(methylamino)propane;   *d*-N^α-dimethylphenethylamine;   *d*-deoxyephedrine;   "speed"). CAS number 537-46-2. A widely abused drug; a sympathomimetic and central stimulant that has been used clinically as an anorectic agent. The use of methamphetamine and related drugs in treating obesity is, however, now generally discredited. It may cause elevation of blood pressure, palpitation and tachycardia, as well as various CNS effects, including psychotic effects at higher doses. Chronic use of methamphetamine and related compounds, especially at high doses as often

occurs with drug abuse, can cause a condition often indistinguishable from schizophrenia. Abrupt withdrawal may cause fatigue, depression and sleep changes. Methamphetamine is an indirect-acting adrenergic and dopamine agonist that acts principally to release endogenous catecholamines, thereby increasing their synaptic availability. Many of its actions can be blocked by adrenergic and dopamine antagonists. The i.p. LD50 in mice is 70 mg/kg. *See also* AMPHETAMINES; HALLUCINOGENS; STIMULANTS.

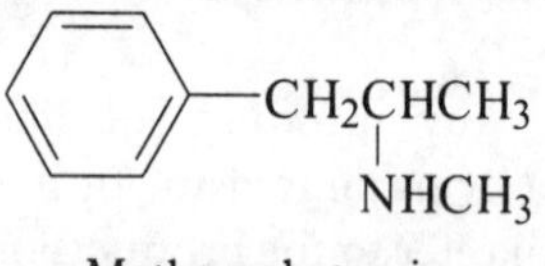

Methamphetamine

methanesulfonic acid. CAS number 75-75-2. A catalyst in polymerization, alkylation and esterification reactions. It is also used as a solvent and as a salt form for basic drugs. Both ethyl and methyl esters are known carcinogens. *See also* METHYL METHANESULFONATE.

$$CH_3SO_2OH$$

Methanesulfonic acid

methanethiol. *See* S-METHYLATION.

methanol (CH$_3$OH; methyl alcohol; wood alcohol). CAS number 67-56-1. The simplest member of the series of primary aliphatic alcohols (C$_n$H$_{2n+1}$OH). It is known as wood alcohol because of the earlier method of industrial synthesis, destructive distillation of wood. Methanol is used as an industrial solvent and synthetic intermediate, and is synthesized for these purposes from hydrogen and carbon monoxide or carbon dioxide. Methanol is a colorless, flammable liquid that is miscible in all proportions with water. It is highly toxic and may be absorbed from the gastrointestinal tract, the skin or, as a vapor, from the lungs. Its importance in toxicology is due to its toxicity to humans, in whom it can cause blindness and death. *See also* METHANOL POISONING, THERAPY.

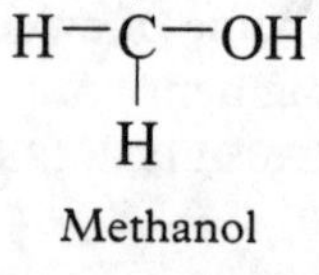

Methanol

methanol poisoning, therapy. The acute effects of methanol poisoning appear to be due to the formation of formaldehyde by the action of alcohol dehydrogenase and, subsequently, formic acid by the action of aldehyde oxidase. Formaldehyde has been shown to affect the retina, and is probably the cause of the blindness associated with methanol poisoning, whereas formic acid causes the characteristic acute acidosis. Non-specific treatment includes induction of vomiting with syrup of ipecac and the use of gastric lavage, whereas acidosis is countered by the administration of sodium bicarbonate, and urine flow is maintained by oral or i.v. fluids. Dialysis is carried out upon failure to respond to specific or non-specific therapy. The specific therapy for methanol poisoning is the administration of ethanol, initially orally and subsequently i.v. The ethanol acts by competition for alcohol-metabolizing enzymes, thus permitting the excretion of methanol before it is activated to formaldehyde and formic acid. The toxicity of the acetaldehyde and acetic acid formed from ethanol is low compared with that of formaldehyde and formic acid. Methanol in its unmetabolized form is also teratogenic in experimental animals. *See also* METHANOL.

methapyrilene (*N,N*-dimethyl-*N'*-2-pyridinyl-*N'*-(2-thienylmethyl)-1,2-ethanediamine). CAS number 91-81-5. A commonly used hypnotic and antihistaminic drug that was removed from non-prescription sleep aids in the USA in 1979 because of potential carcinogenic properties.

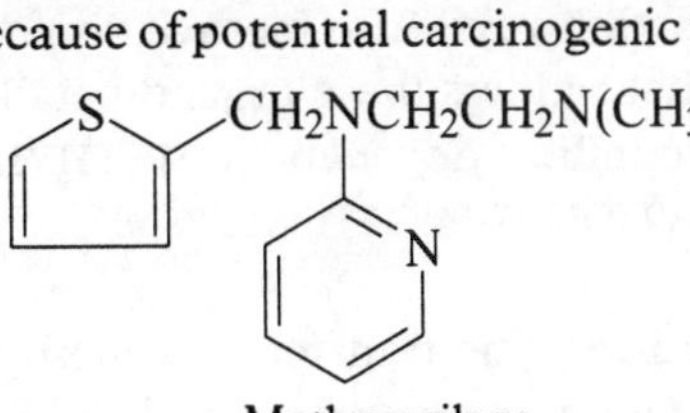

Methapyrilene

methaqualone (2-methyl-3-(2-methylphenyl)-4(3H)-quinazolinone; Quaalude). CAS number 72-44-6. A sedative-hypnotic that has been frequently abused. Its abuse potential is apparently increased by the fact that it causes a "high" (i.e., loss of normal contact with reality) without the concomitant drowsiness caused by the barbiturates. Like the barbiturates, however, rapid withdrawal from chronic high-dose administration

of methaqualone may result in severe grand mal convulsions. The oral LD50 in rats is 255 mg/kg. *See also* SEDATIVE-HYPNOTICS.

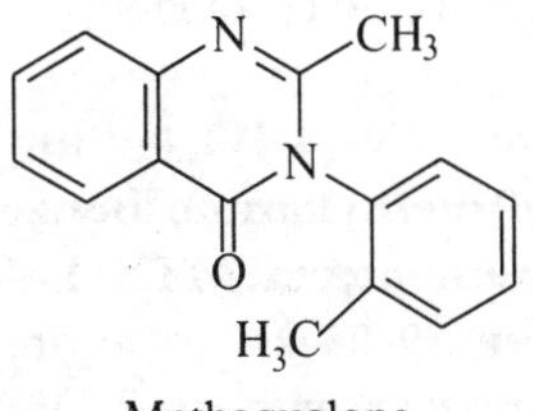

Methaqualone

methemoglobin. Oxidized hemoglobin, with the iron existing in the ferric instead of the ferrous state. Methemoglobin is incapable of binding reversibly with oxygen or carbon monoxide. *See also* HEMOGLOBIN; METHEMOGLOBINEMIA.

methemoglobinemia. The condition arising from the presence of methemoglobin that, because of its inability to bind oxygen, results in hypoxia. Chemicals that can generate methemoglobin *in vivo* include nitrite and some aminophenols, *N*-hydroxyarylamines, aromatic amines and aryl-nitro compounds. Methemoglobin can be reduced to hemoglobin, and therefore restored to normal function, by erythrocyte NADH-dependent methemoglobin reductase. Administration of methylene blue and sometimes hyperbaric oxygen exposure can assist survival of the poisoning victim. *See also* HEMOGLOBIN; METHEMOGLOBIN; MAINTENANCE THERAPY, BLOOD.

Methergine. *See* METHYLERGOVINE.

methohexital (1-methyl-5-(1-methyl-2-pentynyl)-5-(2-propenyl)-2,4,6(1*H*,3*H*,5*H*)-pyrimidinetrione sodium salt; Brevital). CAS number 22151-68-4. An ultra-short-acting i.v. anesthetic. Because its use causes respiratory depression, apnea and hypotension, establishment

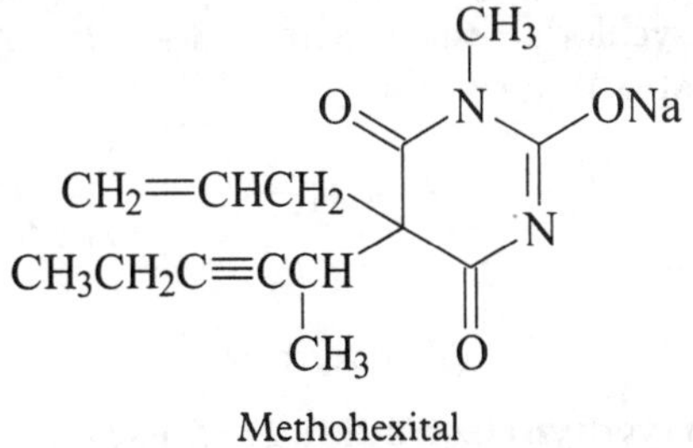

Methohexital

and maintenance of airways, oxygen administration, etc. are required. Various allergic responses have sometimes been reported with its use. *See also* ANESTHETICS; BARBITURATES.

methotrexate   (N-[4-[[2,4-diamino-6-pteridinyl]methyl]methylamino]benzoyl-L-glutamic acid; amethopterin; MTX; Folex; Mexate). **CAS number 59-05-2.** An antineoplastic and immunosuppressant with an LD50 in mice of 94.0 mg/kg, i.p. It is a carcinogen and teratogen that inhibits one-carbon metabolism. As a folic acid analog, it inhibits the enzyme dihydrofolate reductase, thus blocking synthesis of the substrates for nucleic acid and protein synthesis. It causes bone marrow depression, hepatotoxicity, ulcerative stomatitis and renal toxicity. Therapy consists of Leucovorin "rescue".

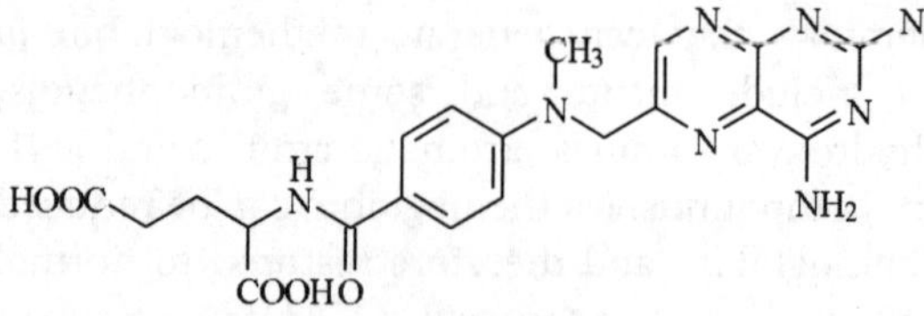

Methotrexate

methoxychlor (1,1,1-trichloro-2,2-bis(4-methoxyphenyl)ethane). CAS number 72-43-5. A biodegradable, low-toxicity DDT analog. Because of its relative safety and rapid degradation to innocuous metabolites, methoxychlor is still widely used in the USA, although almost all other organochlorine insecticides have been banned or severely restricted. The mode of toxic action is the same as that of DDT. The oral LD50 in rats is 6000 mg/kg. Methoxychlor is estrogenic *in vivo*, but not *in vitro*. The demethylated metabolite binds to estrogen receptors and mediates methoxychlor's estrogencity. *See also* ATSDR DOCUMENT, MAY 1994.

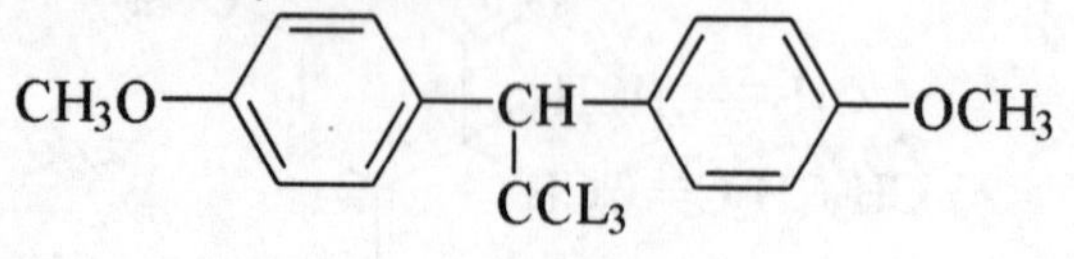

Methoxychlor

methoxyethynylestradiol. *See* MESTRANOL.

methoxyflurane   (2,2-dichloro-1,1-difluoro-1-methoxyethane; Penthrane; Metafane). CAS number 76-38-0. One of the most potent of the inhalational anesthetics, having a very high blood-gas partition coefficient and low vapor pressure at room temperature. Methoxyflurane is metabolized to a great extent (about 50–70%) in the liver and, as a consequence, there may be release of high concentrations of fluoride, sufficient to exceed the threshold for renal damage. Its use for sustained anesthesia is limited because of this renal toxicity. *See also* ANESTHETICS.

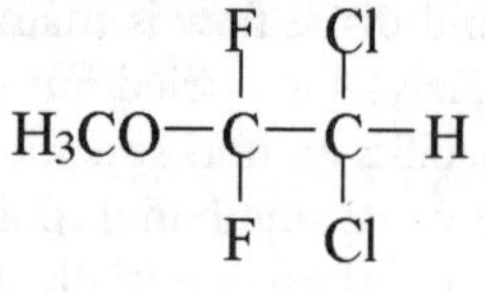

Methoxyflurane

4-methylaminophenol. *See* AMINOPHENOLS.

4-methylaminophenol sulfate. *See* AMINOPHENOLS.

o-methylaniline. *See* O-TOLUIDINE.

methylation. The transfer of a methyl group to a heteroatom in an organic compound. This can be non-enzymatic, as in the case of methylation of amino groups using methyl iodide. In toxicology, enzymatic methylation from *S*-adenosylmethionine by a variety of methyltransferases is more important as such reactions occur in a variety of detoxication pathways. Also methylation of metals can occur that renders these organometallic compounds lipophilic. *See also* N-METHYLATION; O-METHYLATION; S-METHYLATION.

N-methylation. The transfer of a methyl group to a nitrogen atom in an organic molecule. Several enzymes are known that catalyze N-methylation reactions. Histamine N-methyltransferase, a highly specific enzyme, occurs in the soluble fraction of the cell. Phenylethanolamine N-methyltransferase catalyzes the methylation of norepinephrine to epinephrine, as well as the methylation of other phenylethanolamine derivatives. Indoethylamine N-methyltransferase, or non-specific N-methyltransferase, has been isolated from rabbit lung and also occurs in other tissues. It catalyzes the methylation of endogenous compounds such as serotonin and tryptamine and exogenous compounds such as nornicotine and norcodeine. *See also* METHYLTRANSFERASES.

O-methylation. The transfer of a methyl group to the oxygen atom of an organic hydroxyl substituent. Catechol *O*-methyltransferase occurs as multiple isozymes in the soluble fraction of several tissues and has been purified from rat liver. The purified enzyme has a molecular weight of 23,000 daltons, requires *S*-adenosylmethionine and Mg^{2+} and catalyzes the methylation of epinephrine, norepinephrine and other catechol derivatives. A microsomal *O*-methyltransferase that methylates a number of alkyl-, methoxy- and halophenols has been described from rabbit liver and lungs. A hydroxyindole *O*-methyltransferase, that methylates *N*-acetylserotonin to melatonin, has been described from the pineal gland of mammals, birds, reptiles, amphibians and fish. *See also* METHYLTRANSFERASES.

S-methylation. The transfer of a methyl group to the thiol group of an organic compound, including some xenobiotics, the reaction being catalyzed by the enzyme thiol *S*-methyltransferase. This enzyme is microsomal and utilizes *S*-adenosylmethionine, the purified form from rat liver being a monomer of about 28,000 daltons. Substrates methylated include thioacetanilide, mercaptoethanol and phenylsulfide. This enzyme may be important in the detoxication of hydrogen sulfide, which is methylated first to methanethiol and then to dimethylsulfide, although the intermediate, methanethiol, is itself highly toxic. *See also* METHYLTRANSFERASES.

methylazoxymethanol (MAM). A naturally occurring alkylating agent that is produced by the cycad. It was found originally as the active agent formed from cycasin (methylazoxymethanol-β-D-glucoside). Ingestion of this plant by animals or humans has been associated with hepatotoxicity, carcinogenicity and teratogenesis. MAM is an alkylating agent that is probably metabolized to diazomethane, that subsequently forms active methyl groups that methylate nucleotide bases and impair DNA and RNA synthesis. Administration of MAM during fetal life causes a microcephaly that is associated with extensive necrosis in the area normally occupied by differentiating cells, and seems to result from the disruption of cell replication. Administration restricted to postnatal life has selective effects on areas that mature postnatally. Marked cerebellar lesions characterize the neuropathology observed following postnatal administration to experimental animals, with measurable but less dramatic effects on the hippocampus and olfactory bulb, two regions that undergo a significant part of their development postnatally. Behaviorally, the animals show fairly specific neurological signs related to disruption of motor function. Anatomical findings are characterized by decreased cerebellar mass, diminished numbers of cells that can be attributed to a deficit in the number of granule cells. In contrast, postnatal MAM effects on developing spinal cord are characterized by fairly specific decreases in indices of glia and myelin formation, again consistent with the mainly prenatal differentiation of this region, that is therefore spared. *See also* CYCAD; CYCASIN; NEUROTOXICITY.

MAM

methylbenzene. *See* TOLUENE.

methyl bromide (CH_3Br; bromomethane). **CAS number 74-83-9**. Used for its insecticidal properties as a fumigant of food supplies, warehouses, barges, buildings, furniture and even in quarantine situations. It exists as a gas at normal temperatures (b.p. = 4.5 °C), has a density three times as great as air and is extremely penetrating, yet is rapidly air-washed. In both acute and chronic intoxication, there is damage to the pulmonary tract (e.g., pulmonary edema) and both neurological and psychiatric symptoms, including headache, dizziness, loss of coordination and gait, difficulty in focusing, speech impairment, delirium, hallucinations, depression and psychoses. Many of these changes in the CNS may involve alterations in catecholamine systems. Although the mechanism of action of methyl bromide is unknown, covalent alteration (methylation) of important biological macromolecules is probably more important than debromination. *See also* ATSDR DOCUMENT, SEPTEMBER 1992; DATABASES, TOXICOLOGY; LEWIS HCDR, NUMBER MHR200; CATECHOLAMINES; FUMIGANTS.

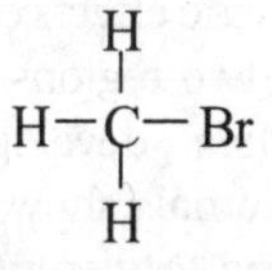

$$H-\underset{\underset{H}{|}}{\overset{\overset{H}{|}}{C}}-Br$$

Methyl bromide

methyl *t*-butyl ether (MTBE). CAS number 1634-04-4. Gasoline additive. Acute inhalation effects include dizziness, nausea, headaches, confusion and irritation of mucus membranes. Some chronic effects in long-term high-dose inhalation studies in rats including kidney disease and, in males only, kidney failure. Carcinogenicity in humans is not classified. *See also* ATSDR DOCUMENT, AUGUST 1994.

methyl *n*-butyl ketone (MBK; 2-hexanone). CAS number 591-78-6. A colorless liquid used as a solvent, in paints and in the printing industry. It enters the body primarily by inhalation or skin absorption. MBK causes irritation of the skin and mucous membranes and, on continued exposure, peripheral axonopathy; the latter is due to its metabolic conversion to 2,5-hexanedione. It is known to potentiate the hepatotoxicity of haloalkanes. *See also* γ-DIKETONE NEUROPATHY; *N*-HEXANE; ATSDR DOCUMENT (HEXANONE), SEPTEMBER 1992.

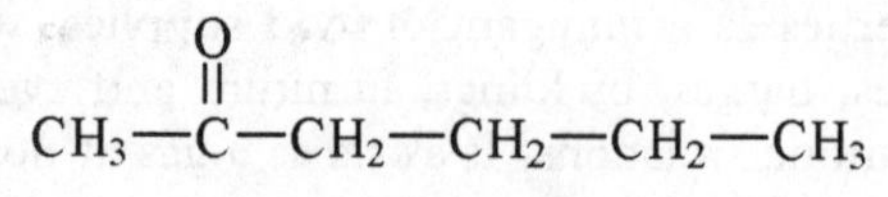

$$CH_3-\overset{\overset{O}{\|}}{C}-CH_2-CH_2-CH_2-CH_3$$

Methyl *n*-butyl ketone

methyl-CCNU. *See* 1-(2-CHLOROETHYL)-3-CYCLOHEXYL-1-NITROSOUREA.

methyl chloride (CH_3Cl; chloromethane). CAS number 74-87-3. Used as a refrigerant and local anesthetic. Little toxicity at low doses but overexposure may cause dizziness, nausea, vomiting, convulsions, liver and kidney damage, and

may be fatal. Potential occupational carcinogen, although human carcinogenicity is not well established. *See also* DATABASES, TOXICOLOGY; LEWIS, HCDR, NUMBER MIF765.

methylchloroform (1,1,1-trichloroethane). CAS number 71-55-6. A colorless liquid that has been used as a substitute for carbon tetrachloride in degreasing and dry-cleaning operations. It has been designated a hazardous waste and a priority toxic pollutant (EPA). The principal route of entry into the body is by inhalation or skin absorption. Methylchloroform acts as a CNS depressant, causing dizziness, incoordination and, in severe cases, death. Methylchloroform has proved negative in chronic tests for carcinogenesis. *See also* ATSDR DOCUMENT ON 1,1,1-TRICHLOROETHANE, OCTOBER 1993.

$$Cl_3C-CH_3$$

Methylchloroform (1,1,1-trichloroethane)

3-methylcholanthrene. *See* POLYCYCLIC AROMATIC HYDROCARBONS.

methyldopa (L-3(3,4-dihydroxyphenyl)-2-methylalanine). CAS number 300-48-1. An analog of levodopa that inhibits biosynthesis of all catecholamines. Used as an antihypertensive. *See also* CATECHOLAMINES.

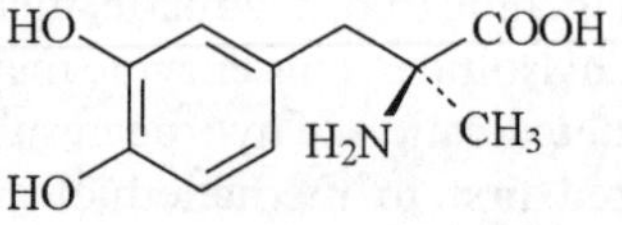

Methyldopa

4,4′-methylenebis(2-chloroaniline) (4,4′-methylenebis(2-chlorobenzenamine)); MBOCA). CAS number 101-14-4. Used as a curing agent in the manufacture of polyurethane foam and epoxy resins. Known mutagen and animal carcinogen and may reasonably be expected to be a human carcinogen. *See also* LEWIS, HCDR NUMBER MJM200; DATABASES, TOXICOLOGY.

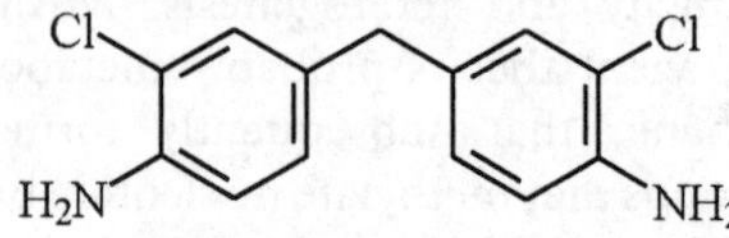

4,4′-Methylenebis(2-chloroaniline)

methylene blue (3,7-bis(dimethylamino) phenothiazin-5-ium chloride). CAS number 61-73-4. Used as a stain in microbiology and as an oxidation–reduction indicator. As an antimethemoglobinemic agent is used as an antidote in cyanide poisoning. *See also* CYANIDE.

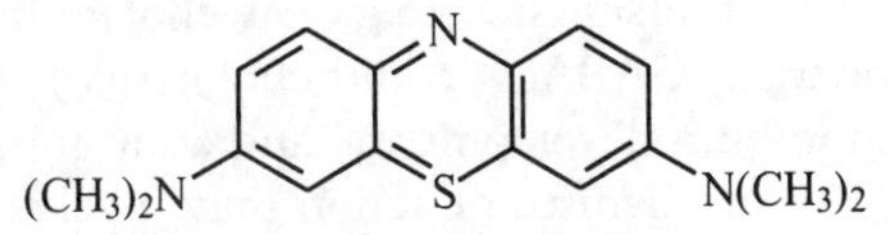

Methylene blue

methylene bromide (dibromethane, CH$_2$Br$_2$). CAS number 74-95-3. Methylene bromide is not an important toxicant and should not be confused with methyl bromide (CH$_3$Br), a highly toxic fumigant. *See also* METHYL BROMIDE; DATABASES, TOXICOLOGY.

methylene chloride. CAS number 75-09-2. A volatile, colorless liquid that has been designated a potential carcinogen, a hazardous waste and a primary toxic pollutant. It is a common ingredient in paint removers and is a solvent in aerosol products. Due to its extreme volatility, high concentrations may occur readily in poorly ventilated areas. Following inhalation, methylene chloride is metabolized by the cytochrome P450 monooxygenase system to carbon dioxide and carbon monoxide. Significant levels of carboxyhemoglobin may occur due to carbon monoxide binding to hemoglobin in the blood. In common with other low-molecular-weight halogenated hydrocarbons, methylene chloride is a CNS depressant. Initial signs of inhalation are dizziness and numbness; other symptoms are tingling of the extremities, fatigue and nausea. Severe or prolonged exposure may lead to respiratory depression and death. If high carboxyhemoglobin levels are present, the symptoms of acute carbon monoxide poisoning also occur. It is possibly carcinogenic to humans (IARC) and a probable human carcinogen (US EPA). *See also* ATSDR DOCUMENT, APRIL 1993; DATABASES, TOXICOLOGY; LEWIS HCDR NUMBER MJP450.

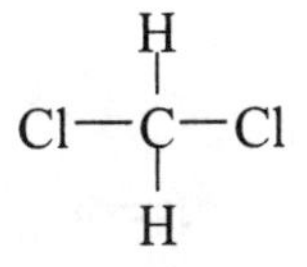

Methylene chloride

methylenedioxyamphetamine. *See* MDA.

3,4-methylenedioxymethamphetamine. *See* MDMA.

methylenedioxyphenyl synergists. *See* METHYLENEDIOXY RING CLEAVAGE.

methylenedioxy ring cleavage (benzodioxole ring cleavage). An oxidative attack on the methylenedioxy ring that results in ring-opening and the formation of a catechol or dihydroxy compound. Naturally occurring methylenedioxyphenyl compounds, including safrole and isosafrole as well as insecticide synergists such as piperonyl butoxide, are effective inhibitors of cytochrome P450 and are themselves metabolized to catechols. The probable mechanism is an attack on the methylene carbon, followed by elimination of water to yield a carbene. The highly reactive carbene either reacts with the heme iron to form an inhibitory complex or breaks down to yield the catechol. *See also* CYTOCHROME P450-DEPENDENT MONOOXYGENASE SYSTEM; ISOSAFROLE; PIPERONYL BUTOXIDE; SYNERGISM AND POTENTIATION.

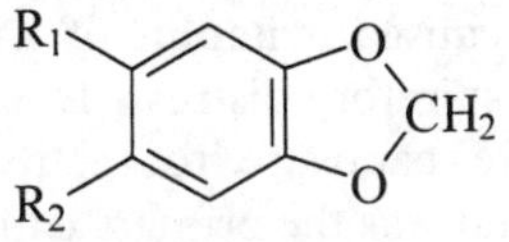

General structure of methylenedioxyphenyl compounds

methylergonovine (9,10-didehydro-N-[1-(hydroxymethyl)propyl]-6-methylergoline-8-carboxamide; N-α-(hydroxymethyl)-propyl]-d-lysergamide; d-lysergic acid (+)-butanolamide-(2); Methergine). CAS number 113-42-8. A semisynthetic ergot alkaloid used for the prevention and control of postpartum hemorrhaging. Methylergonovine has a rapid onset of action, and shortens the third stage of labor and prevents blood loss. Hypertensive or cerebrovascular accidents may result following i.v. administration. Adverse effects include nausea, vomiting, hypertension and dizziness. The effects of methylergonovine on the uterus are thought to be mediated by interactions with monoamine receptors. *See also* ERGOT ALKALOIDS.

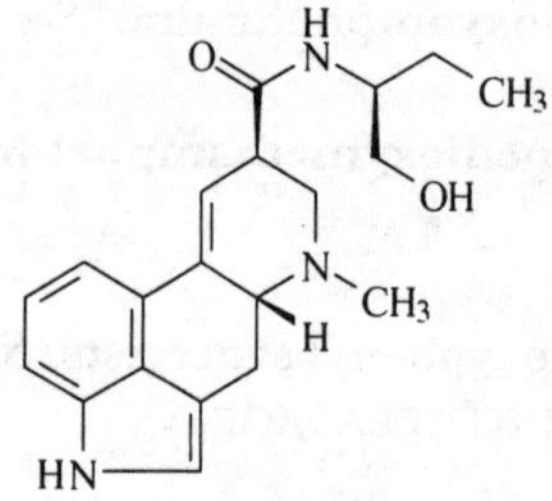

Methylergonovine

methyl ethyl ketone (2-butanone). CAS number 78-93-3. Used as a solvent and in resin manufacture. Irritant, with neurotoxic effects at high acute doses. Does not appear to be mutagenic or carcinogenic. *See also* DATABASES, TOXICOLOGY.

3-methylfentanyl (α-methylfentanyl). CAS number 79704-88-4. Controlled opiate substance, erroneously referred to as "China White." *See also* NARCOTICS; OPIOIDS.

methyl isocyanate (CH_3NCO). A colorless, low-boiling liquid that has been designated a hazardous waste (EPA). It is used in the manufacture of polyurethane and plastics and in the synthesis of pesticides, primarily *N*-methyl carbamates. Entry may be via inhalation, percutaneous absorption or ingestion. It causes irritation of mucous membranes and respiratory distress. Death may result from excessive exposure to methyl isocyanate. This compound was the primary cause of death in the Bhopal (India) poisoning incident. *See also* BHOPAL; ENVIRONMENTAL DISASTERS.

$$CH_3—N=C=O$$

Methyl isocyanate

methyl mercaptan. (CH_3SH; methanethiol). CAS number 74-93-1. Very malodorous, acutely poisonous chemical. *See* ATSDR DOCUMENT, SEPTEMBER 1992; LEWIS, HCDR, NUMBER MLE650.

methylmercury (monomethylmercury). An organomercurial of major toxicological importance; it has been used as a fungicide and also may be formed in anaerobic aquatic environments by microbial biomethylation. Several epidemics of methylmercury poisoning have been reported, the most notable being in Japan and Iraq. Methylmercury is lipophilic and readily passes across biological membranes, thereby reaching the CNS.

Symptoms of intoxication include tunnel vision, paresthesias, ataxia, dysarthria and deafness. This compound profoundly affects CNS development, possibly by inhibiting protein synthesis through effects on aminoacylation of tRNA or by inhibiting incorporation of sulfate into the myelin-lipid sulfatide. Neurotransmission (e.g., catecholaminergic, serotonergic, GABAergic and cholinergic) is also altered in both developmental and adult intoxication. The mechanism of action may involve conversion of methylmercury to inorganic mercury *in situ*, where the binding to thiol groups on macromolecules via mercaptide may cause functional changes. Chelation therapy is largely ineffective, although surgical gallbladder drainage or the administration of a non-absorbable thiol mercury-binding resin can be used to interrupt the enterohepatic cycling of the alkyl compound. *See also* MERCURY; MINAMATA DISEASE.

methylmercury neurotoxicity. *See* MINAMATA DISEASE.

methyl methanesulfonate (MMS). CAS number 66-27-3. A direct-acting carcinogen that yields the alkylating methyl carbonium ion in solution. Its carcinogenic potential is reduced by the fact that it can be detoxified by nucleophiles such as proteins, by water, by sulfhydryl compounds or by esterases.

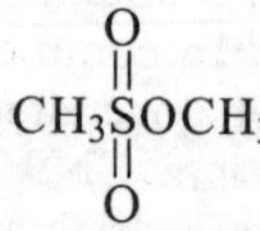

$$CH_3SOCH_3$$

Methylmethane sulfonate (MMS)

methylmorphine. *See* CODEINE.

***N*-methyl-*N*-nitrosourea (MNU).** An alkylating agent that is carcinogenic by alkylating guanylic acid in DNA by its *O*-methyl carbonium ion. It is effective in producing gastric tumors. Since it is a direct-acting carcinogen, it is very effective transplacentally. *See also* NITROSOUREAS.

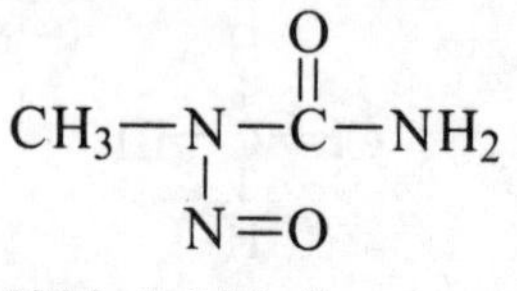

$$CH_3—N—C—NH_2$$
$$N=O$$

N-Methyl-*N*-nitrosourea

methyl parathion (*O,O*-dimethyl *O*-4-nitrophenyl phosphorothioate). CAS number 298-00-0. An organophosphorous insecticide. Once the major insecticide used in cotton and soybeans in the USA, it has been replaced largely by the synthetic pyrethroids. The oral LD50 is 14 and 24 mg/kg in male and female rats, respectively. A neurotoxicant after activation to methyl paraoxon by cytochrome P450, it exerts its toxic effects as a cholinesterase inhibitor. In humans it causes lachrimation, pupillary constriction, muscle twitches, vomiting and diarrhea, tonic and clonic convulsions and respiratory collapse. The therapy for acute poisoning is supportive therapy: artificial respiration as required, atropine sulfate (acetylcholine antagonist) and 2-PAM (cholinesterase reactivator). *See also* ANTICHOLINESTERASES; INSECTICIDES; ORGANOPHOSPHORUS INSECTICIDES; ATSDR DOCUMENT, SEPTEMBER 1992; DATABASES, TOXICOLOGY; LEWIS, HCDR, NUMBER MNH000.

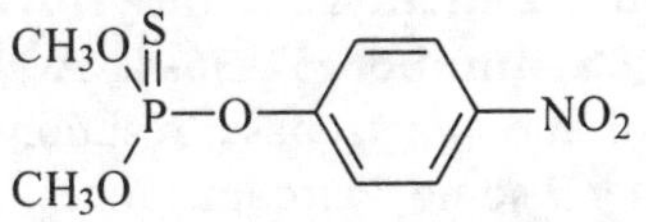

Methyl parathion

1-methyl-4-phenylpyridinium (MPP⁺). The proximal toxicant formed when MPTP (1-methyl-4-phenyl-1,2,3,6-tetrahydropyridine) is metabolized by monoamine oxidase B. Unlike MPTP, this compound will not pass the blood–brain barrier, but it is a substrate for the dopamine neurotransporter, and thus is able to enter dopamine neurons. It is believed to destroy dopamine neurons by mechanisms involving both free radical production and inhibition of mitochondrial electron transport. *See also* 1-METHYL-4-PHENYL-1,2,3,6-TETRAHYDROPYRIDINE.

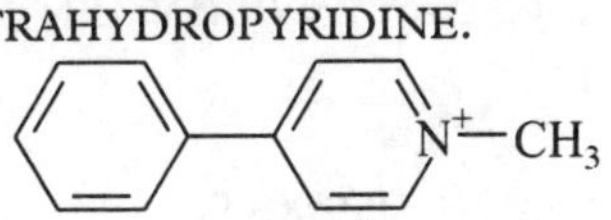

MPP⁺

1-methyl-4-phenyl-1,2,3,6-tetrahydropyridine (MPTP). CAS number 28289-54-4. Human toxicity originally discovered when it was an unexpected by-product from the illicit synthesis of a heroin substitute (i.e., meperidine analog). Currently used experimentally as the primary animal model for the study of Parkinson's disease.

MPTP is a neurotoxicant that is activated to 1-methyl-4-phenylpyridinium ion (MPP⁺) by the actions of monoamine oxidase B located in the mitochondria of brain astrocytes. The MPP⁺ is then transported into dopamine, and to a lesser extent, other monoaminergic neurons. Once inside these dopamine neurons in the substantia nigra, it destroys these neurons by mechanisms that may involve an oxidative cascade and/or inhibition of electron transport. Intoxication causes a parkinsonism syndrome almost identical in signs and symptoms to Parkinson's disease, including rigidity, bradykinesia, tremor, and postural instability. In the event of known ingestion, immediate (but not delayed) administration of a monoamine oxidase inhibitor (especially one selective for MAO-B like deprenyl) and dopamine uptake inhibitor can be therapeutic. *See also* DOPAMINE; NEUROTOXICITY; PARKINSON'S DISEASE.

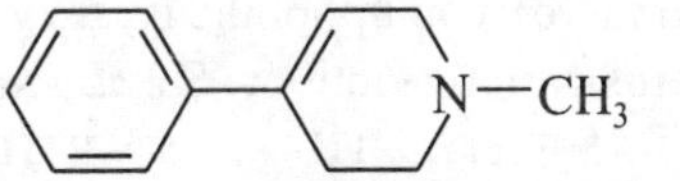

MPTP

***N*-methylpyridinium-2-aldoxime (2-PAM; pralidoxime; 2[(hydroxyimino)methyl]-1-methylpyridinium chloride). CAS number 51-15-0.** A pyridine oxime reactivator of phosphorylated acetylcholinesterase that is used therapeutically in cases of acute organophosphate poisoning in combination with atropine sulfate. 2-PAM is of little or no use in carbamate poisoning. The i.v. LD50 in rats is 96 mg/kg and the oral LD50 in mice is 4100 mg/kg. *See also* ORGANOPHOSPHATE POISONING, SYMPTOMS AND THERAPY; OXIMES.

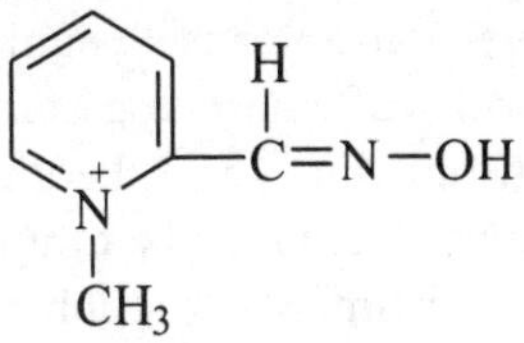

N-Methylpyridium-2-aldoxime (2-PAM)

methylsulfonate. *See* METHANESULFONIC ACID.

methylthiolation. The apparent transfer of a methylthio (CH₃S-) group to a foreign compound may actually occur through the action of a recently discovered enzyme, cysteine conjugate β-lyase. This enzyme acts on cysteine conjugates of xenobiotics by the following reaction:

$$RSCH_2CH(NH_2)COOH \longrightarrow RSH + NH_3 + CH_3C(O)COOH$$

after which the thiol group can be methylated to yield the methylthio derivative of the original xenobiotic. *See also* CYSTEINE CONJUGATE β-LYASE; METHYLTRANSFERASES.

methyltransferases. Enzymes that catalyze the transfer of a methyl group to a heteroatom in an organic molecule. Both endogenous and exogenous compounds can be methylated by *N*-, *O*- or *S*-methyltransferases. The methyl donor is *S*-adenosylmethionine, formed from methionine and ATP. Although most of these reactions involve an increase in lipophilicity, they are nevertheless detoxication reactions. *See also* *N*-METHYLATION; *O*-METHYLATION; *S*-METHYLATION; METHYLTHIOLATION .

methylxanthines. Central stimulants that are methylated derivatives of 3,7-dihydro-1*H*-purine-2,6-dione. They include caffeine, theophylline and theobromine. The primary source of these compounds is dietary, although caffeine and theophylline are in several over-the-counter and prescription drugs. Coffee contains significant quantities of caffeine, whereas tea contains theophylline and caffeine as well as theobromine. Cocoa, chocolate and cola drinks are some of the other dietary sources for these compounds. In addition to their actions in the periphery, the methylxanthines also cause significant CNS stimulation, with caffeine being somewhat more potent than theophylline, and theobromine being relatively inactive. The methylxanthines were once believed to act primarily via inhibition of the enzyme phosphodiesterase (PDE), that hydrolyzes cyclic nucleotides. Although these compounds are effective PDE inhibitors *in vitro*, this is probably not of significance *in vivo*. The most important mechanism of action is via adenosine and other purine receptors. *See also* CAFFEINE; THEOBROMINE; THEOPHYLLINE.

methyprylon   (3,3-diethyl-5-methyl-2,4-piperidinedione; Noludar). CAS number 125-64-4. Used occasionally as a sedative-hypnotic, although its use for longer than seven days is not recommended. Like many other sedative-hypnotics, abrupt withdrawal after chronic use or abuse resembles that of ethanol or the barbiturates, and must be managed accordingly. *See also* GLUTETHIMIDE; SEDATIVE-HYPNOTICS.

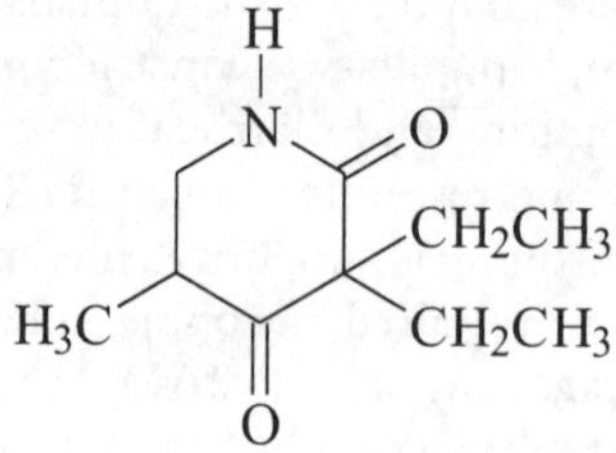

Methylprylon

metolachlor. *See* PHENOXYACETIC ACIDS.

metyrapone (2-methyl-1,2-dipyridyl-1-propanone). CAS number 54-36-4. A well-known inhibitor of monooxygenase reactions and can also, under some circumstances, stimulate metabolism of xenobiotics *in vitro*. In either case, the effect is non-competitive, in that the K_m does not change whereas V_{max} does, decreasing in the case of inhibition and increasing in the case of stimulation. *See also* XENOBIOTIC METABOLISM, REVERSIBLE INHIBITION.

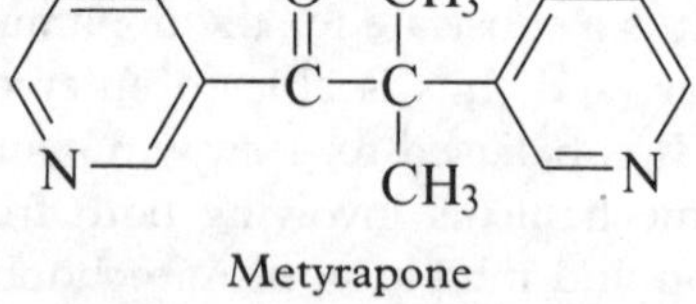

Metyrapone

Meuse Valley. *See* ENVIRONMENTAL DISASTERS.

Mexate. *See* METHOTREXATE.

MF. *See* MODIFYING FACTOR.

MFP (sodium monofluorophosphate). *See* FLUORIDES.

Michaelis constant. *See* K_m; MICHAELIS–MENTEN EQUATION.

Michaelis–Menten equation (Henri–Michaelis–Menten equation). One of the earliest theoretical descriptions of the kinetics of enzyme reactions based on several assumptions of initial velocity and rapid equilibrium. The actual equation

$$\frac{v}{V_{max}} = \frac{[S]}{K_m + [S]}$$

is usually transformed to equivalent algebraic forms that yield straight lines in orthogonal plots. The equation is essentially identical for radioreceptor assays, except that B (amount bound) is equivalent to v (the initial velocity), [F] (concentration of free ligand) to [S] (concentration of substrate), K_d (dissociation constant) to K_m (Michaelis constant) and B_{max} (theoretical number of sites) to V_{max} (maximal theoretical velocity). *See also* EADIE–HOFSTEE PLOT; ENZYME KINETICS; K_D; K_M; LINEWEAVER–BURK PLOT; METABOLITE INHIBITORY COMPLEXES; RADIORECEPTOR ASSAYS; WOOLF PLOT; XENOBIOTIC METABOLISM, INHIBITION.

Mickey Finn. A potent sedative-hypnotic consisting of a combination of ethanol and chloral hydrate. In addition to the individual depressant effect of each drug, chloral hydrate appears to inhibit the metabolism of ethanol, and ethanol enhances the generation of trichloroethanol, the principal pharmacologically active metabolite of chloral hydrate. *See also* CHLORAL HYDRATE; ETHANOL; SEDATIVE-HYPNOTICS.

microbial toxins. Pathogenic microorganisms generally inflict damage to a host organism through the synthesis of toxins rather than by massive cell invasion. Virulence is a measure of the capacity of these toxins to harm host cells. Bacterial toxins can be categorized as follows. Exotoxins are generally released from the progenitor, and these include neurotoxins that cause paralysis (botulinium toxin has an LD50 of 0.000025 µg/mouse), hemolysins, cardiotoxins, diphtheria toxin, plague toxin and various cell-disrupting enzymes (e.g., lecithinase and collagenase). Endotoxins are associated with the outer cell envelope of gram-negative bacteria. Generally lipopolysaccharide in nature with an approximate LD50 of 400 µg/mouse. Among the effects of endotoxins are fever, hemorrhagic shock, gastroenteritis and tissue necrosis. The endotoxins of food and water-borne enteric bacteria are designated enterotoxins. Often these toxins act on the small intestine, causing a massive secretion of fluid into the intestinal lumen resulting in severe diarrhea. Cholera, shigellosis and salmonellosis are manifestations of enterotoxin damage.

microcystins. *See* MICROCYSTIS.

microcystis. Blooms of toxic cyanobacteria (blue-green algae) were first reported in 1878, and are becoming increasingly common in fresh waters receiving nutrients (phosphates and nitrates) from agricultural fertilizers or treated domestic sewage. Deaths of livestock and other domestic animals are well known, and the hazard to humans is now receiving attention. Recently, an epidemiological study has been done of hepatic enzymes in the blood of people drinking from a water supply containing a bloom of microcystis compared with those of other consumers on different water supplies at the same time. This showed a significant rise in γ-glutamyl transferase in the blood of people whose water supply contained microcystis. A highly toxic cyanobacterium has been isolated from a drinking water supply reservoir that was the origin of a severe outbreak of hepatoenteritis. *Microcystis aeurginosa* is the most common of all toxin-forming cyanobacteria. There are reports of toxic blooms of this species from all continents except Antarctica. Microcystis has been shown to be hepatotoxic. The hepatotoxicity is due to a family of closely related hepatapeptides, called microcystins [structure: cyclo-D-Ala-L-X-erythro-beta-methyl-D-isoAsp-L-Y-Adda-D-isoGlu-*N*-methyldehydroAla; where Adda is 3-amino-9-methoxy-2,6,8-trimethyl-10-phenyldeca-4,6-dienoic acid, and the amino acids X and Y are variable]. The microcystins are very stable, with little loss of toxicity in boiling or from typical water treatment. The liver is the target organ with many reports detailing the observed pathology. Although the liver lesions caused by microcystin are well documented, the mode of action of microcystin is not known. Microcystins are toxic orally, by i.p., or i.v. injection. Following a lethal dose of microcystin (LD50 in mice i.p. 0.1 mg/kg) death can occur in as little as one hour. Circulatory shock, brought on by a massive liver hemorrhage is the cause of death. However, no direct cardiovascular toxicity has been seen. Hepatocyte necrosis, disruption of endothelial cells, and of the Space of Disse has been shown, by electron microscopy, to occur as early as 15 minutes following toxin injection. There is no explanation as to the mechanism by which microcystin causes these lethal changes, and whether liver injury is due to a direct effect on hepatocytes or whether other cells and/or the microcirculation of the organ are directly or indirectly involved. The hepatic lesion in rats following i.p. injection of microcystin is initially centrilobular; with increasing time it spreads to involve the rest of the lobule. In mice, the reverse was found; the initial lesion in the liver is perilobular, and only later extends to the central vein.

microenvironment. The immediate environment in contact with, or close to, an organism.

microfilament. Intracellular fiber of polymerized actin, between 5 and 7 nm in diameter. Many cellular extensions have cores of such cross-linked actin filaments, as for example the microvillus brush border of many intestinal cells, and the hair cells of the cochlea of the ear. Dynamic actin filament structures are also found on the surfaces of many cells, and appear to act as sensory devices, enabling the cell to detect particular features of its immediate environment. Belt desmosomes, the constituents of many epithelial cells, are also composed of microfilaments, as are the stress fibers. Actin filaments are often anchored in cell membranes, at least at one end, and these are known as adhesion plaques.

micromercurialism. *See* MERCURY.

micronucleus test. An *in vivo* test, usually performed with mice, for chemicals causing chromosome breaks (clastogenic agents) or interfering with mitosis (including spindle fiber function) and cytokinesis. Following treatment with the test chemical, erythrocyte stem cells are removed from the bone marrow and are observed for the presence of micronuclei, that indicate chromosome fragments or chromosomes failing to migrate properly in anaphase. This is not among the most

sensitive tests for chromosome aberrations. *See also* CHROMOSOME ABERRATION TESTS; EUKARYOTE MUTAGENICITY TESTS.

microorganisms, co-metabolism. The catabolic phenomenon wherein a compound is transformed by a microorganism even though the organism does not derive energy or nutritive value from the process or product. In the environment, the product may be attacked by other microbial species that are unable to attack the parent compound. Thus co-metabolism contributes to the recycling of some recalcitrant compounds in nature. *See also* MICROORGANISMS, HYDROCARBON METABOLISM; MICROORGANISMS, PESTICIDE METABOLISM.

microorganisms, hydrocarbon metabolism. Normally the utilization of hydrocarbons by microorganisms, although microorganisms produce a wide array of hydrocarbons. The microbial utilization of hydrocarbons was first reported around the turn of the century. Microorganisms vary from species to species in their ability to utilize hydrocarbons; some species can utilize a single hydrocarbon as a sole source of carbon and energy, whereas other species can utilize a multiplicity of hydrocarbons. Still other microorganisms only degrade hydrocarbons co-metabolically. Hydrocarbon-utilizing ability is constitutive in some species, whereas in others it is an adaptive phenomenon. In mixtures of hydrocarbons, straight-chain alkanes are utilized more readily than branched-chain or aromatic hydrocarbons. Anaerobic utilization of hydrocarbons is extremely slow to nonexistent. *See also* MICROORGANISMS, CO-METABOLISM; MICROORGANISMS, PESTICIDE METABOLISM.

microorganisms, pesticide metabolism. Normally the utilization of pesticides by microorganisms, although some microorganisms produce substances that kill other organisms. Microorganisms vary from species to species in their ability to utilize pesticides; some species can utilize pesticides as the sole source of carbon and energy, whereas other species only degrade pesticides co-metabolically. Although some pesticide molecules are recalcitrant, very few, if any, are completely resistant to microbial attack. *See also* MICRO-

ORGANISM, CO-METABOLISM; MICROORGAN-ISMS, HYDROCARBON METABOLISM; MICROORGANISMS.

micropuncture, in renal toxicity studies. A technique used in the study of nephron function and in the study of toxic effects on the nephron. It involves collection of fluid directly from the lumen of the nephron in intact anesthetized animals. *See also* NEPHROTOXICITY.

microsomal. Pertaining to, or present in, microsomes. *See also* MICROSOMES.

microsomes. Small closed vesicles (about 100 nm in diameter), representing membrane fragments formed from the endoplasmic reticulum (ER) when cells are disrupted by homogenization. Microsomes are easily separated from other cell organelles by differential centrifugation. The cell homogenate contains rough microsomes that are studded with ribosomes and are derived from rough ER (RER), and smooth microsomes that are devoid of ribosomes and are derived from smooth ER (SER). Rough microsomes are more dense than smooth microsomes, and the two can be separated by sucrose density gradient centrifugation. Because they can be purified with the structural and functional integrity of the ER intact, microsomes represent a specially useful preparation for studying the many processes carried out by the ER, such as protein biosynthesis and xenobiotic metabolism. *See also* ENDOPLASMIC RETICULUM.

microsomes, preparation. The method of choice for preparation of microsomes, or microsomal fractions, is tissue homogenization followed by differential centrifugation. Following homogenization by one of several techniques (e.g., Potter–Elvejhem or Dounce rotating pestle-type homogenizers, blenders, etc.) in a suitable medium (e.g., tris buffer, phosphate buffer, 0.25 M sucrose or combinations of these) the homogenate is centrifuged at low speed to remove whole cells, nuclei and debris, at an intermediate speed to remove mitochondria and finally at a high speed to sediment the microsomal fraction. Homogenization method and speeds are varied to suit the particular tissue; the speeds for liver would typically be 600 g

for 5 minutes, 9000 g for 10 minutes and 105,000 g for 60 minutes. Rough and smooth microsomes can be separated by further centrifugation on a continuous or step-wise density gradient. Other methods have been developed for preparation of microsomes, including sedimentation by the addition of calcium chloride, but none of these have been accepted as routine. *See also* MICROSOMES.

millipedes. Arthropods of the class Myriapoda that can produce toxic secretions containing hydrocyanic acid, capable of irritating the skin. Millipedes are not considered dangerous to humans.

Miltown. *See* MEPROBAMATE.

Minamata disease (methylmercury neurotoxicity). A neurological condition caused by methylmercury intoxication. Clinical findings include concentrically constricted visual fields, paresthesias and cerebellar ataxia. The principal morphological alteration is loss of neurons, mainly from the cerebral cortex and cerebellar cortex. The disease is so named because of an epidemic of methylmercury neurotoxicity that occurred in the 1950s in Japan due to ingestion of contaminated seafood from Minamata Bay, which was polluted by mercury from industrial sources. The mercury was converted to methylmercury by bacteria and subsequently contaminated the higher trophic levels. The mercury toxicity resulted in nervous system damage, as well as more than 100 deaths. *See also* ENVIRONMENTAL DISASTERS; MERCURY; METHYLMERCURY.

mineral based crankcase oil. General term used for motor oil or engine oil. Used mineral based crankcase oil has been suspected as a health hazard but there is little definitive evidence for any significant acute or chronic human toxic effects. *See also* ATSDR DOCUMENT, JUNE 1994.

mineralocorticoids. Corticosteroids produced by the adrenal cortex and involved primarily in Na^+ and K^+ balance and secondarily in water balance. The most important of these is aldosterone, which causes Na^+ retention by the kidneys (and thereby water retention) and concurrently K^+ excretion. Aldosterone secretion is controlled by levels of blood K^+ and angiotensin II, and not by ACTH. *Compare* GLUCOCORTICOIDS. *See also* ADRENAL GLAND TOXICOLOGY.

Ministry of Agriculture, Fisheries and Food (MAFF). A government department that, in England and Wales, provides advice on the composition of foods, food microbiology, food irradiation, food additives and contaminants, and food surveillance. The activities of the Veterinary Services Division include the licensing of veterinary pharmaceutical products. In Scotland similar activities are undertaken by the Scottish Home and Health Department and in Northern Ireland by the Department of Health and Social Services.

minor tranquilizers. Antianxiety (anxiolytic) drugs like the benzodiazepines. The term is now considered archaic since "major tranquilizers" and "minor tranquilizers" refer to drugs with different modes of action, and effects that are not simply graded responses. *Compare* MAJOR TRANQUILIZERS. *See also* ANTIANXIETY DRUGS; BENZODIAZEPINES.

minute volume. In respiratory physiology, indicates the total tidal volumes inhaled per minute (i.e., tidal volume × respiration rate). *See also* TIDAL VOLUME.

miosis. Constriction of the pupil of the eye. Pupillary diameter is controlled by the pupillary sphincter and pupillary dilator muscles of the iris. Pupilloconstrictor fibers are parasympathetic and innervate the sphincter muscle. Pupillodilator fibers are sympathetic and innervate the dilator muscle. Miosis has numerous causes, including intoxication with chemicals that cause parasympathomimetic activation (cholinesterase inhibitors or muscarinic agonists) or opiate agonists like morphine. *Compare with* MYDRIASIS.

mipafox (*N*,*N'*-diisopropylphosphorodiamidic **fluoride**). **CAS number 371-86-8**. Formerly used as a systemic insecticide. Its use was discontinued because of severe delayed neuropathy hazard in humans. The oral LD50/LC50 in rabbits is 100 mg/kg. Toxic action is as a neurotoxicant with both acute and delayed actions, acting as

a cholinesterase inhibitor (acute toxicity) and as a neurotoxic esterase inhibitor (possibly linked to delayed toxicity). Symptoms in humans are typical anticholinesterase symptoms. Therapy is supportive as well as atropine sulfate and 2-PAM. *See also* DELAYED NEUROPATHY; NEUROTOXIC ESTERASE; ORGANOPHOSPHATE POISONING, SYMPTOMS AND THERAPY; TOCP.

$$(CH_3)_2CHNH$$
$$\overset{O}{\underset{\parallel}{P}}-F$$
$$(CH_3)_2CHNH$$

Mipafox

MIR. *See* MAXIMUM INDIVIDUAL RISK.

mirex (**1,1a,2,2,3,3a,4,5,5,5a,5b,6-dodecachlorooctahydro-1,3,4-metheno-1H-cyclobuta[*cd*]pentalene**). **CAS number 2385-85-5**. A chlorinated hydrocarbon insecticide and fire retardant, formerly used extensively against the imported fire ant. It is not acutely toxic since the oral LD50 in rats is 360–740 mg/kg. and the dermal LD50 in rabbits is 850 mg/kg. However, it is teratogenic to rats, producing cataracts in the young when 25 ppm is fed in the diet of the dams. It causes reproductive toxicity in mice and is carcinogenic to rats. Mirex has been shown to be a tumor promotor in skin carcinogenesis. There is some, but not extensive, evidence that mirex affects the immune system. Mirex is a potent inducer of cytochrome P450 isozymes in rats and mice and is transmitted to the young via the milk, causing induction in the offspring. It is not metabolized by animals and is stable in the environment.

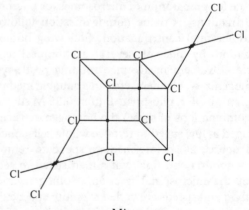

Mirex

mist. Small liquid particles contributing to air pollution, with particle diameters of less than 2 μm. An example is sulfuric acid mist. *See also* AIR POLLUTION.

mistletoe. Parasitic plants that produce toxins. In the USA, mistletoe is *Phoradendron tomentosum* and produces phoratoxin, a peptide of molecular weight of about 13,000. In Europe, mistletoe is *Viscum album* and produces viscotoxin, a peptide of molecular weight about 5000. The American plant is about one fifth as potent as the European plant. Signs of intoxication include gastrointestinal distress and hypotension.

Misuse of Drugs (Notification of and Supply to Addicts) Act. UK legislation of 1973 that requires that a medical practitioner must be licensed by the Home Office to administer, supply or authorize any person to administer, supply or prescribe certain listed drugs unless for the relief of pain due to organic disease or injury. The controlled drugs covered under this act are: amphetamine, cocaine, dexamphetamine, diamorphine, dihydrocodeine, levorphanol, mephentermine, methadone, methaqualone, methylphenidate, morphine, opium, pethidine and phenmetrazine.

Mitigan. *See* DICOFOL.

mitochondria. Organelles of eukaryotic cells bounded by a double membrane that contains the enzymes of the tricarboxylic acid cycle and electron transport system, as well as a number of other metabolic pathways. By oxidative phosphorylation, they generate the majority of the ATP produced in the cell. Their enzymes are the targets of such metabolic inhibitors as rotenone and cyanide. *See also* ELECTRON TRANSPORT SYSTEM; METABOLIC INHIBITORS; OXIDATIVE PHOSPHORYLATION.

mitogenic. A property of some chemicals enabling them to stimulate mitosis. Lectins such as phytohemagglutinin and concanavalin A are mitogenic. Mitogens can be used to stimulate cell growth in culture.

mitogens. *See* MITOGENIC.

mitomycin C. CAS number 50-07-7. The mitomycins are antibiotics produced by *Streptomyces caespitosus* (griseovinaceseus) from soil. Mitomycin C is used as an antineoplastic agent against carcinomas of the stomach, cervix, colon, breast, pancreas, bladder, head and neck. The i.v. LD50 in mice is 5 mg/kg. Its action is by a bioreductive alkylation reaction that may be selective to hypoxic cells. It inhibits DNA synthesis, cross-links DNA and causes single-strand breaks. It is carcinogenic and teratogenic in rodents. Toxicity observed includes myelosuppression, nausea, dermatitis, fever, malaise, pneumonia and glomerular damage.

Mitomycin C

mitosis. The process of chromosome separation and the formation of two nuclei during cell division. Although the process is continuous, mitosis is generally said to consist of four phases. (1) Prophase involves the condensation of the chromatin into chromosomes, migration of the centrioles and dissolution of the nuclear envelope. (2) Metaphase involves the arrangement of the chromosomes in the center of the microtubule-based spindle. (3) Anaphase involves the migration of the chromosomes toward the poles. (4) Telophase involves the decondensation of the chromosomes once they have reached the poles and the reformation of the nuclear envelope. Mitosis is usually followed by cytokinesis, the division of the cytoplasm. Mitosis is inhibited by spindle poisons. *See also* SPINDLE POISONS.

mitotic interference. Many genotoxic agents exert their toxic effects by adversely affecting mitosis, usually by preventing spindle formation. Probably the best-known genotoxic agent is colchicine, a compound that combines with tubulin, a protein component of the microtubules, that associates to form the mitotic spindle fibers. Combination with colchicine results in an inability of tubulin to polymerize. Podophyllotoxin binds to the same site on tubulin as colchicine and has the same effects. *See also* CHROMOSOME ABERRATIONS; COLCHICINE; PODOPHYLLOTOXIN.

mitotic recombination. Both reciprocal and non-reciprocal recombination of genetic material can occur at mitosis. The former is the exchange of genetic material between two non-sister chromatids, whereas the latter is the exchange of material between sister chromatids. Such recombinations can be deleterious and can be caused by exogenous chemicals. Tests have been devised, using the D5 strain of *Saccharomyces cerevisiae*, to measure the potential of chemicals, with or without activation by the S-9 fraction of mammalian liver, to bring about mitotic recombination. *See also* CHROMATID; S-9 FRACTION.

mixed function oxidase. *See* MONOOXYGENASES.

MMS. *See* METHYL METHANESULFONATE.

MNU. *See* N-METHYL-N-NITROSOUREA.

model. An idealized mathematical description, usually computer based, of a natural system. Ideally, models should permit prediction of changes in the system that would result from variations in those factors known to modify the system.

model ecosystems. Artificial test systems set up in the laboratory to monitor the fate of toxicants in a controlled situation that has many of the characteristics of the environment. The most widely used system has an aquatic phase with vertebrates, invertebrates and plankton, and a terrestrial phase with substrate, plants and herbivores. The bioconcentration of a radiolabeled test compound can be determined, as can its degradation. More elaborate models involving such aspects as drainage, rainfall and tides, as well as strictly terrestrial model ecosystems, have also been devised. *See also* AQUATIC ECOSYSTEMS; ECOLOGICAL EFFECTS, SIMULATED ECOSYSTEMS; TERRESTRIAL-AQUATIC ECOSYSTEMS.

modeling. The development and testing of mathematical models of natural systems. In toxicology, modeling is probably most important in pharmacokinetics. *See also* MODEL.

mode of action. The cellular or molecular actions by which a toxicant exerts its adverse effects. Examples include enzyme inhibition, ion channel effects, oxidative damage, DNA adduct formation, and membrane solubilization. This term is used more frequently than mechanism of action with respect to the mechanism responsible for lethal action of a toxicant.

modification of metabolism. Summation of all of those factors that change the overall ability of organisms to metabolize xenobiotics. Such changes may affect the overall rate at which metabolites are excreted or may affect the ratio of different metabolites produced from a single xenobiotic. Such effects may be physiological, genetic, nutritional, chemical or environmental, and entries appear under all of these headings. The alternate meaning, that of effects on endogenous metabolism, is less common in toxicology than in biology or medicine, but may be encountered in discussions on the effect of xenobiotics on endogenous metabolism.

modifying factor (MF). A factor, from 1 to 10, that is used in the derivation of the reference dose. Its magnitude depends upon the assessment of uncertainties not explicitly treated with standard uncertainty factors.

MOE. *See* MARGIN OF EXPOSURE.

molecular dosimetry. An approach to extrapolation between species (based on sensitive detection methods such as radioactive-labeling or mass spectroscopy) that permit the determination of the relationship between external exposure (e.g., mg/kg) and effective target dose (e.g., alkylations per nucleotide or alkylations per haploid genome). Such an approach can be used in a species such as *Drosophila* (the doubling dose can then be calculated), or by using conversion factors from radiation research on the mouse, the equivalent doubling dose for a given species can be estimated. This value can then be used to calculate the effect of known human exposure. The system has obvious problems, requiring labeled compounds and more knowledge of specific mechanisms in different species than is currently available. It is, however, regarded as a significant development. *See also* SPECIES EXTRAPOLATION.

molluscicides. Pesticides designed to kill snails and slugs, with primary uses on terrestrial molluscs that feed on ornamental plants or on aquatic molluscs that serve as intermediate hosts for parasitic flukes. Common examples include methiocarb and clonitralid.

Molybdenum (Mo). An element, a silvery white metal used primarily in various alloys and in electronics applications. Molybdenum compounds are used as lubricants, in the petroleum and printing industries, and in fertilizers. Molybdenum trioxide may produce irritation of the eyes and mucous membranes. Molybdenum is the prosthetic group of some enzymes, including xanthine oxidase and aldehyde oxidase, and for this reason is considered an essential nutrient. Excessive molybdenum may, however, cause anemia, diarrhea and reduced growth in sheep and cattle.

monitoring. Measuring, usually over time, the concentration of substances in either environmental media or living organisms.

Monkshood. *See* ACONITINE.

monoamine oxidase, type A. *See* MONOAMINE OXIDASES.

monoamine oxidase, type B. *See* MONOAMINE OXIDASES.

monoamine oxidase inhibitors (MAO-I). A heterogeneous group of drugs that have in common the ability, via the inhibition of the enzyme monoamine oxidase, to block the oxidative deamination of endogenous and exogenous monoamines. The first MAO-I drug was the hydrazine derivative isoniazid, which was discovered accidently. Iproniazid, a close structural relative of isoniazid, came to have wide clinical use as an antidepressant. The treatment of major depressive disorders represents the major medical use of

MAO-I. In animals and in normal humans, MAO-I antidepressants do not have marked behavioral effects, yet they elevate mood and increase adaptive responding in depressed patients. The pharmacological actions of these drugs are generally attributed to a potentiation of the actions of monoamine neurotransmitters and trace amines by inhibiting their metabolic inactivation. Selective inhibitors of the MAO isozymes have been developed, although the selectivity of action is dependent upon the inhibitor and substrate concentration. MAO-Is have the potential to interact with many drugs or food constituents, and also have been shown to damage the liver parenchyma (especially with the MAO-Is that are hydrazine derivatives). Because of their biochemical action, contraindications for MAO-I include pheochromocytomas, concomitant use of other drugs that have sympathomimetic actions and consumption of foods like cheeses that contain certain monoamines. The major toxicoses associated with the administration of MAO-Is is the hypertensive crisis associated with the inhibited metabolic inactivation of pressor substances such as tyramine contained in foods such as cheese, yeast, coffee, some wines, pickled herring and broad beans. MAO-Is are of further toxicological interest as they interfere with the detoxication mechanisms for concurrently administered drugs such as general anesthetics, sedatives, antihistamines and alcohol, as well as enhancing greatly the actions of tricyclic antidepressant drugs. *See also* MONOAMINE OXIDASES; TYRAMINE.

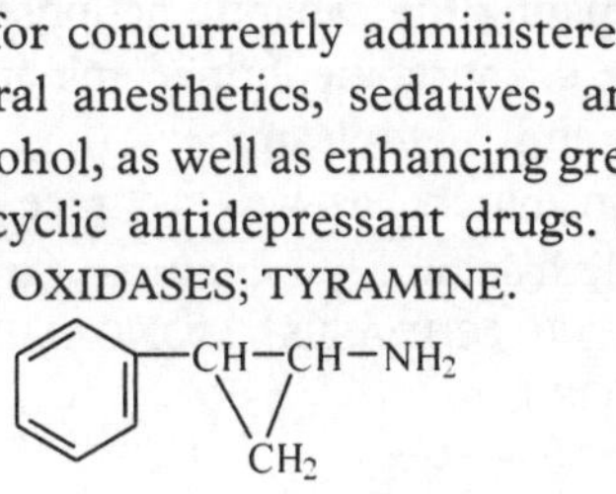

Tranylcypromine

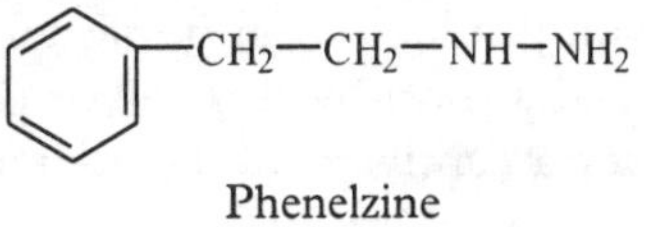

Phenelzine

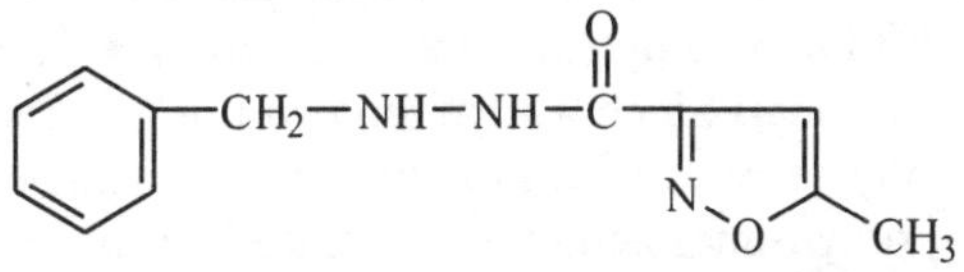

Isocarboxazid

Monoamine oxidase inhibitors

monoamine oxidases (MAO; monoamine:O₂ oxidoreductases). A family of flavoproteins found largely in the outer membranes of mitochrondria of many tissues. MAOs catalyze the oxidative deamination of a variety of monoamines to their corresponding aldehydes. Although the enzyme in the CNS is concerned primarily with neurotransmitter turnover, those in the liver will deaminate aliphatic amines, with primary amines being the preferred substrates. MAO is present in at least two different forms or isozymes, designated type A and type B based on their substrate specificity, sensitivity to inhibition by selected inhibitors and demonstrated physical separation. MAO-type A preferentially oxidizes norepinephrine and serotonin and is preferentially inhibited by clorgyline. MAO-type B preferentially oxidizes β-phenethylamine and benzylamine and is preferentially inhibited by deprenyl. The clinically used MAO inhibitors include hydrazine derivatives, that bind irreversibly to MAO (phenelzine, isocarboxazid), and reversible inhibitors like tranylcypromine. The physiological and toxicological significance of MAOs results from the role of monoamines in synaptic transmission in the central and peripheral nervous systems and in cardiovascular function. MAO represents one of several enzymes involved in terminating the synaptic actions of catecholamines (e.g., norepinephrine, epinephrine, dopamine) and indoleamine (e.g., serotonin) neurotransmitters, as well as trace amines (e.g., β-phenylethylamine, tryptamine, tyramine). *See also* AMINE OXIDASES; MONOAMINE OXIDASE INHIBITORS.

monoclonal antibody (mAb). A homogeneous antibody produced by a hybridoma. Hybridomas are the fusion product of an immortal myeloma tumor cell and a short-lived B cell or plasma cell that is making an antibody of the desired specificity. Such antibodies are referred to as "monoclonal" because they are the product of only one B cell and its progeny (i.e., its clone) and are therefore identical. Since a myeloma tumor cell itself generally secretes an antibody of unknown specificity, only tumor cell lines that have lost this ability are suitable for hybridoma production. The successful hybridomas possess both genomes and therefore retain the immortality of the myeloma and the desired antibody production of the original B cell. These hybridomas can then be propagated in tissue culture or *in vivo* as solid tumors. Although the monoclonal antibody is produced against only one epitope on the antigen molecule, a very small portion of the antigen molecule, there can be significant cross-reaction with structurally related epitopes on otherwise unrelated proteins. Frequently, a panel of monoclonal antibodies is used for positive identification. Monoclonal antibodies have had an enormous impact in a wide variety of areas. The technique is used to produce the large quantities of specific antibodies needed for standardized immunoassays for therapeutic use and for purification by immunoabsorption of antigens such as membrane proteins. Monoclonal antibodies have also been used to identify large numbers of cells by their cell surface markers (e.g., fluorescence-activated cell sorting; FACS), and to characterize closely related proteins such as the isozymes of xenobiotic-metabolizing enzymes. *See also* B CELLS; CLONAL EXPANSION; IMMUNOASSAY.

monocrotaline. *See* PYROLLIZIDINE ALKALOIDS.

monocytes. *See* MACROPHAGES/MONOCYTES.

monooxygenases (mixed function oxidases). Enzymes for which the cosubstrates are an organic compound and molecular oxygen. The distinguishing characteristic of the reaction catalyzed by monooxygenases is that one atom of a molecule of oxygen is incorporated into the substrate whereas the other is reduced to water. Monooxygenases of importance in toxicology include cytochromes P450 and the FAD-containing monooxygenase, both of which initiate the metabolism of lipophilic xenobiotics by the introduction of a reactive polar group into the molecule. Although usually part of a detoxication sequence, such reactions may generate reactive intermediates of importance in toxic action. *See also* CYTOCHROME P450; FAD-CONTAINING MONOOXYGENASE; PHASE I REACTIONS.

monooxygenations. *See* MONOOXYGENASES.

monosodium glutamate. *See* CHINESE RESTAURANT SYNDROME; GLUTAMATE.

monosomy. A special case of aneuploidy, the condition in which the chromosome number (e.g., in humans 46) is increased or decreased. Aneuploids lacking a chromosome (e.g., in humans 45) are said to be monosomic, those with an extra chromosome are said to be trisomic. An example of monosomy is monosomy X or Turner syndrome. If the whole chromosome set is replicated (e.g., in humans 69) the condition is known as polyploidy.

monuron (3-(4-chlorophenyl)-1,1-dimethyl-urea; N'-(4-chlorophenyl)-N,N-dimethylurea). **CAS number 150-68-5**. A herbicide that functions as an inhibitor of photosynthesis. The acute oral LD50 for rats is 3600 mg/kg. The "no effect" level for rats and dogs is 250–500 mg/kg of diet.

Monuron

morbidity. The number, or proportion, of sick or impaired individuals in a population.

morning glory. Plants of the family Convolvulaceae. The seeds of several, but by no means all, species of this family contain psychomimetic compounds structurally related to LSD. Seeds of several species including *Ipomoea violacea* and *Turbina corymbosa* have been used in religious rites in Mexico since the Aztec era. Compounds found in the above species include elymoclavine, lysergol, ergometrine, ergine, isoergine and chanoclavine. Effects are similar to those of LSD, including the effects of toxic overdose.

morphine (7,8-didehydro-4,5α-epoxy-17-methylmorphinan-3,6α-diol; morphium; morphia). **CAS number 57-27-2**. An alkaloid of the opium poppy that makes up between 9 to 14% of good grades of opium. Morphine is usually used clinically as an analgesic in the form of the sulfate or hydrochloride salt. The most important acute toxic effect of large doses of morphine is depression of the respiratory centers in the medulla and pons. Morphine and related drugs also cause somnolence, coma, cold clammy skin, bradycardia and hypotension. Initial doses of morphine seem to stimulate the chemoreceptor trigger zone to induce emesis, with subsequent doses blocking the vomiting center, hence blocking emesis. Morphine also has profound effects on the gastrointestinal tract, increasing the tone of the intestinal tract, but decreasing the propulsive or spasmodic reflexes, thus resulting in constipation. Morphine stimulates the nucleus of the third cranial nerve to produce miosis, making pinpoint pupil a diagnostic sign both in morphine overdose and morphine addiction. Morphine causes a variety of effects on the CNS and is highly addictive. Many behavioral changes are seen, ranging from euphoria to sedation. These behavioral effects contribute to the problem of abuse with all of the opiates. Tolerance and dependence occur with repeated dosing, with increasingly larger doses being needed to obtain the original effect. Abrupt withdrawal after chronic use can lead to physiological rebound in these same systems. Therapy for acute overdosage involves physiological support (establishment of adequate respiratory exchange), gastric lavage and use of narcotic antagonists. Morphine and related compounds act by binding to specific high-affinity receptors concentrated in the nervous system, but also located elsewhere in the body. In the nervous system, the endogenous ligands for these morphine receptors are the opioid peptides, that include the enkephalins, endorphins and dynorphins. The multiple and complex actions of morphine are due, in part, to the fact that it acts as an agonist at many of these classes of receptors. Paregoric (camphorated tincture of opium) is used as an antidiarrheal. Paregoric is a schedule III drug under the US Controlled Substances Act and may produce physical dependence. *See also* ANALGESICS; CODEINE; HEROIN; NARCOTIC ANTAGONISTS; NARCOTICS; OPIOIDS; OPIUM.

Morphine

mortality. The number, or proportion, of deaths in a population.

MOS. *See* MARGIN OF EXPOSURE.

mouse lymphoma cells. The L5178Y TK+/– mouse lymphoma cell line is used to test for the ability of chemicals to induce forward mutations at the thymidine kinase (TK) locus. The heterozygous cell line produces TK, that incorporates the toxic thymidine analogs 5-bromo-2′-deoxyuridine (BrdU) or 5-trifluorothymidine (TFT) into DNA, and the cells die in the presence of these analogs. A forward mutation to the homozygous TK–/– genotype allows the cells to live in the presence of the toxic analogs. The mutagenic potential of a test chemical can be assessed if cell survival in the presence of these toxic thymidine analogs is enhanced following exposure (either non-activated or activated with S-9) to the test chemical. *See also* MAMMALIAN CELL MUTATION TESTS.

mouse lymphoma test. *See* MAMMALIAN CELL MUTATION TESTS.

mouse mutation spot tests. *See* SPECIFIC LOCUS TEST.

mouth. In general the opening of any cavity; specifically the opening of the gastrointestinal tract. Synonymous with buccal cavity and oral cavity, it is the space between the cheeks, containing the tongue and teeth and leading into the pharynx. In toxicology, it is important as a portal of entry of ingested toxicants, some of which (e.g., nicotine) are not only passed through to the gastrointestinal tract, but are readily absorbed by the buccal membrane. The condition of the mouth is also useful in the diagnosis of poisoning. *See also* DIAGNOSTIC FEATURES, MOUTH.

movement of pollutants. The movement of pollutants in the environment by atmospheric, aquatic and biological transport. Pollutants are carried different distances by the winds, depending on their chemical state (gaseous, vapor or particulate), before deposition onto land or water. Movement in the aquatic environment may include coastal and river transport. Transport of pollutants by living organisms also plays a role in total movement. *See also* POLLUTION, LONG-RANGE TRANSPORT.

moving average. *See* AUTOREGRESSIVE INTEGRATED MOVING AVERAGE.

6-MP. *See* 6-MERCAPTOPURINE.

MPP⁺. *See* 1-METHYL-4-PHENYL-PYRIDINIUM.

MPTP. *See* 1-METHYL-4-PHENYL-1,2,3,6-TETRA-HYDROPYRIDINE.

MRL. *See* MAXIMUM RESIDUE LIMIT.

MS. *See* SPECTROMETRY, MASS.

MSDS. *See* MATERIALS SAFETY DATA SHEETS.

MSG (monosodium glutamate). *See* GLUTAMATE.

MT. *See* METALLOTHIONEIN.

MTBE. *See* METHYL *T*-BUTYL ETHER.

MTD. *See* MAXIMUM TOLERATED DOSE.

MTX. *See* METHOTREXATE.

mucin. A glycoprotein found in mucus, in secretions such as saliva and bile, and also in the skin and connective tissue.

mucous. An adjective used to describe a tissue or cell that secretes mucus or something that resembles mucus.

mucus. A viscous fluid secreted by mucous membranes and certain glands. It contains mucin, leukocytes, inorganic ions and epithelial cells. Mucus often serves a protective or lubricating function. Mucous membranes are, however, often sensitive to xenobiotics.

multi-compartment models. A pharmacokinetic term describing the disposition of exogenously administered substances when a finite time is required for distribution to occur. The concentration-time profile is multiexponential. The model typically consists of a central compartment that is in rapid distribution equilibrium with the blood and one or more peripheral compartments in which distribution occurs more slowly. The compartments usually do not have anatomical significance. However, the central compartment is frequently associated with highly perfused tissues such as lung, heart and liver, and the peripheral compartments may consist of poorly perfused tissues such as fat and muscle. *See also* COMPARTMENT; KINETIC EQUATIONS; ONE-COMPARTMENT MODEL; PHARMACOKINETICS; TOXICOKINETICS; TWO-COMPARTMENT MODEL.

multidrug resistance protein. *See* P-GLYCOPROTEIN.

multi-hit model. *See* LOW-DOSE EXTRAPOLATION.

multiple chemical sensitivity syndrome (MCS). A term used to describe hypersensitivity, in the same individual, to a broad range of chemicals, representing several to many chemical classes and frequently without a history of prior exposure. Commonly described symptoms include headache, lack of concentration, fatigue, memory loss and congestion of nasal and other membranes. It is not clear whether this represents a true chemical toxicity; there is frequently a psychological component and a significant percentage of patients reporting MCS can be cured by psychiatric methods. Self-styled "clinical ecologists," the principal protagonists of this syndrome, frequently claim dramatic cures by the use of untested "detoxication" procedures. Whether or not this syndrome exists is highly controversial with many authorities stating that it is a psychological dysfunction with no relation to the toxicity of chemicals, others recognizing it as a valid response to chemicals that follows serious acute poisoning incidents.

multiplicity, of enzymes. *See* ISOZYMES.

multipotent stem cell. *See* STEM CELL.

multistage model. *See* CARCINOGENESIS.

multivariate analysis of variance. *See* MANOVA.

multivariate statistical analysis. Tests of significance or descriptive statistical analysis that are appropriately applied when more than one dependent variable is being measured on all subjects. *See also* MANOVA; STATISTICS, FUNCTION IN TOXICOLOGY.

municipal wastes. *See* POLLUTION, DOMESTIC AND MUNICIPAL WASTES.

muscarine **([2S-(2α,4β,5α)]-tetrahydro-4-hydroxy-N,N,N-5-tetramethyl-2-furanmethanaminium**. **CAS number 300-54-9**. A toxic alkaloid of the mushroom *Amanita muscaria* and certain other fungi. Although useful as a pharmacological tool, muscarine has no clinical or pesticidal applications. The compound is a potent and selective mimic of acetylcholine at parasympathetic neuromuscular junctions and at central muscarinic acetylcholine receptors. Symptoms of poisoning are primarily those attributable to peripheral parasympathetic stimulation (i.e., miosis, vomiting, diarrhea, bradycardia and cardiovascular collapse). The i.v. LD50 in mice is 0.23 mg/kg. *See also* ACETYLCHOLINE RECEPTORS, MUSCARINIC AND NICOTINIC.

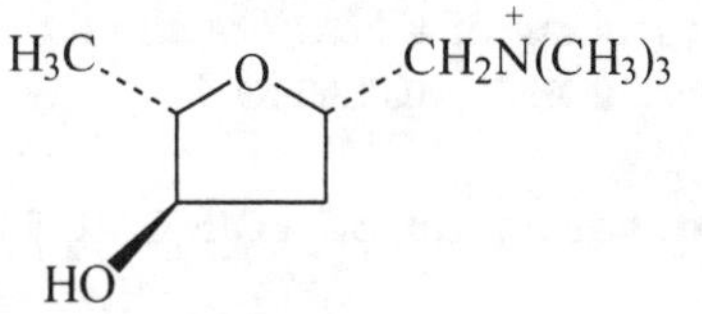

Muscarine

muscarinic receptors. *See* ACETYLCHOLINE RECEPTORS, MUSCARINIC AND NICOTINIC.

mushrooms. Fungi which produce a variety of toxic and/or hallucinogenic chemicals. *See also* FUNGI.

musk tetralin. *See* ACETYLETHYLTETRAMETHYLTETRALIN.

mustard gas (bis(2-chloroethyl)sulfide). **CAS number 505-60-2**. An oily liquid that is used as a chemical warfare agent, with an i.v. LD50 in rats of 3.3 mg/kg and in mice of 8.6 mg/kg. This is a severe vesicant that results in conjunctivitis, blindness, cough, erythema of skin, edema, ulceration and necrosis of respiratory tract and exposed skin. Permanent eye damage and respiratory impairment may result. Ingestion can lead to nausea. Mustard gas forms the highly reactive sulfonium derivative in solution that alkylates functional

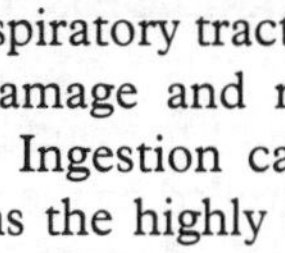

Mustard gas

groups of macromolecules. This property makes mustard gas a direct-acting carcinogen as well. Little therapy is possible.

mutagen. *See* MUTATION.

mutagenesis. *See* MUTATION.

mutation. Gene mutations are changes in the DNA sequence of a gene. Also called point mutations due to their restriction to a particular site in the DNA molecule, distinct from changes in large sequences of DNA molecules characteristic of chromosome aberrations. The two principal types of gene mutations are base-pair substitutions and frameshift mutations. In the past, mutations were detected by genetic analysis of unusual phenotypes; in addition they may now be detected by direct sequencing of DNA. *See also* FRAMESHIFT MUTATION; POINT MUTATION.

mutation, base-pair. *See* POINT MUTATION.

mutation, dominant visible. Mutations in visible characteristics of the phenotype that are inherited as Mendelian dominants. Mutant genes regulating coat color in mice form the basis of one of the tests for chemical mutagens.

mutation, forward. *See* FORWARD MUTATION.

mutation, frameshift. *See* FRAMESHIFT MUTATION.

mutation, reverse. *See* REVERSE MUTATION.

mycotoxins. Toxins produced by fungi. Many, such as aflatoxins, are particularly important in toxicology. *See also* AFLATOXINS; CYCLOPIAZONIC ACID; ERGOT ALKALOIDS; TRICOTHECENES.

mydriasis. Dilation of the pupil of the eye. Pupillary diameter is controlled by the pupillary sphincter and pupillary dilator muscles of the iris. Pupilloconstrictor fibers are parasympathetic and innervate the sphincter muscle. Pupillodilator fibers are sympathetic and innervate the dilator muscle. Mydriasis has numerous causes, and is a sign of intoxication with certain chemicals including muscarinic cholingeric antagonists, and sympathomimetic drugs such as amphetamine and its derivatives. *Compare* MIOSIS.

myelin sheath. Multilayered lipoprotein membrane that surrounds the axon of some nerves (myelinated nerve) of higher organisms. The myelin sheath is formed by the Schwann cells in peripheral nerves and by oligodendrocytes in central nerves. The sheath is not continuous along the length of the nerve; the gaps between the sheaths formed by adjacent cells are the nodes of Ranvier. During the conduction of a nerve impulse the myelin sheath acts as an insulator, preventing the local depolarization of the axonal membrane. The depolarization of the membrane, with a reduction in the membrane potential (i.e., the action potential) is thus propagated from node to node. This allows the action potential to be conducted faster in myelinated than in non-myelinated nerves. *See also* DEMYELINATION; PERIPHERAL NEUROPATHY.

Myleran. *See* BUSULFAN.

myoglobinuria. The appearance of myoglobin in the urine. This may be a result of chemical poisoning. *See also* DIAGNOSTIC FEATURES, URINARY TRACT.

myristicin. **CAS number 607-91-0**. A naturally occurring methylenedioxyphenyl compound found in nutmeg. It has been suggested that myristicin may be responsible, in whole or in part, for the toxicity of nutmeg. The spice (5–15 g) causes symptoms similar to atropine poisoning: flushing of the skin, tachycardia, absence of salivation and excitation of the CNS. Euphoria and hallucinations have given rise to abuse of this material. As a methylenedioxyphenyl compound, myristicin gives rise to a type III spectrum with reduced cytochrome P450 and can inhibit monooxygenations catalyzed by this cytochrome. *See also* AMPHETAMINES; CYTOCHROME P450, OPTICAL DIFFERENCE SPECTRA; HALLUCINOGENS; METHYLENEDIOXY RING CLEAVAGE.

$H_2C{=}CHCH_2$

OCH_3

Myristicin

N

Na⁺/K⁺-ATPase (Na⁺/K⁺ pump). The active transport system in cell membranes responsible for the simultaneous influx of K^+ and efflux of Na^+ that contributes greatly to the normal electrochemical gradient that exists across the cell plasmalemma. This is a critical site in excitable cells such as in neurons and various muscle cells. This enzyme is inhibited by the cardiac glycoside ouabain, in the presence of which cultured mammalian cells cannot grow. If a mutagen causes a mutation at the Na⁺/K⁺-ATPase locus such that ouabain no longer binds, then the cultured cells can grow in the presence of ouabain. This concept provides the basis for some mutagenicity tests in which resistance of the cells to ouabain indicates the presence of a mutagen. *See also* CHINESE HAMSTER OVARY CELLS; EUKARYOTE MUTAGENICITY TESTS; MAMMALIAN CELL MUTATION TESTS; MOUSE LYMPHOMA CELLS.

NADH (reduced nicotine adenine dinucleotide). CAS number 58-68-4. A reduced pyridine nucleotide important in energy metabolism. It is considerably less effective than NADPH in supporting monooxygenation of xenobiotics, but is involved, via NADH-cytochrome b_5 reductase, in the functioning of cytochrome b_5, a cytochrome that appears to be involved in some cytochrome P450-dependent monooxygenases.

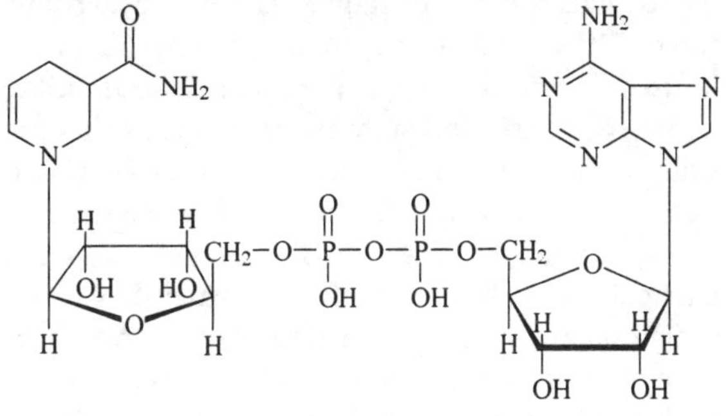

NADH oxidase. An enzyme found in polymorphonuclear leukocytes that is believed to be involved in the production of active oxygen species by this cell type when the cell is triggered by inflammatory stimuli. The active oxygen species have potent microbiocidal and inflammatory properties and include the superoxide anion (O_2^-), hydrogen peroxide (H_2O_2) and the hydroxyl radical (OH). NADH oxidase, associated with the cell membrane, is believed to be dormant until activated, for example, by inflammatory stimuli. The tumor promoter phorbol myristate acetate is also a potent activator of this enzyme. Carcinogens such as methylaminoazobenzene can be activated by the active oxygen products of this enzyme to intermediates that bind covalently to DNA. This activation can be inhibited by antioxidants and sulfhydryl inhibitors. *See also* PHORBOL ESTERS.

NADPH (reduced nicotine adenine dinucleotide phosphate). CAS number 53-57-6. The reduced form of the cofactor nicotine adenine dinucleotide phosphate. NADPH is the principal electron donor for the monooxygenation reactions important in xenobiotic oxidations, the FAD-containing monooxygenase and the cytochrome P450-dependent monooxygenase system. *See also* MONOOXYGENASES; NADPH-CYTOCHROME P450 REDUCTASE.

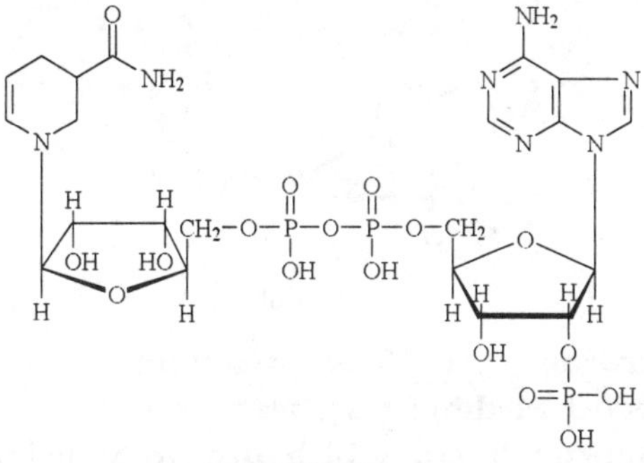

NADH

NADPH

NADPH-cytochrome *c* reductase. *See* NADPH-CYTOCHROME P450 REDUCTASE.

NADPH-cytochrome P450 reductase. A flavoprotein that transfers electrons from NADPH to cytochrome P450 in the microsomal cytochrome P450-dependent monooxygenase system. This enzyme has been purified from liver microsomes of several mammals. It is a flavoprotein of about 80,000 daltons, containing one mole of flavin mononucleotide (FMN) and one of flavin adenine dinucleotide (FAD) per mole of protein. Since cytochrome *c* can also accept electrons, this enzyme is also known as NADPH-cytochrome *c* reductase, although its reduction of cytochrome *c* is not important *in vivo*. *See also* MONOOXYGENATIONS; NADPH.

naloxone   (4,5α-epoxy-3,14-dihydroxy-17-(2-propenyl)morphinan-6-one; 1-*N*-allyl-7,8-dihydro-14-hydroxynormorphinone; Narcan). CAS number 465-65-6. An opiate antagonist devoid of agonist activity except for mild, specific effects at very high doses. Naloxone displays a high affinity for the μ-opioid receptor, a lesser affinity for the k-opioid receptor and has some affinity for δ-opioid receptor subtypes. Naloxone produces a rapid and profound reversal of the effects of opioid administration (e.g., 1 mg, i.v., blocks the effects of 25 mg of heroin). Naloxone also antagonizes the analgesia induced by placebo, acupuncture and stress, and in animals the hypotension due to hypovolemia or spinal cord injury. Naloxone has a short half-life (about 1 hour in plasma) and is not administered orally because of rapid, "first-pass" metabolism. *See also* NALTREXONE; NARCOTIC ANTAGONISTS; OPIOIDS.

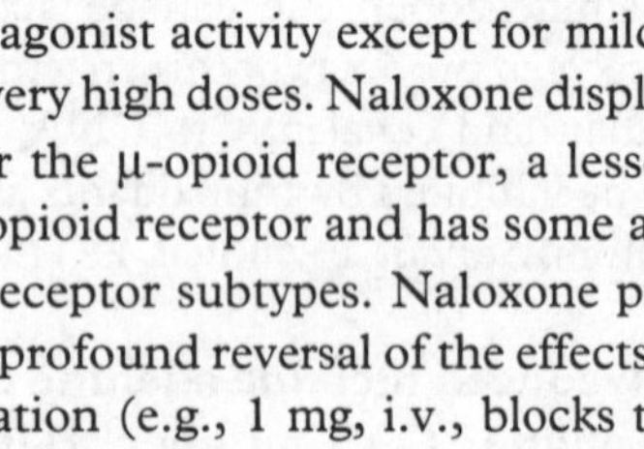

Naloxone

naltrexone   (17(cyclopropylmethyl)-4,5-epoxy-3,14-dihydroxymorphinan-6-one; *N*-cyclopropylmethyl-14-hydroxydihydromorphinone; Trexan). CAS number 16590-41-3.

An opiate antagonist, structurally similar to naloxone, that is efficacious when administered orally and also has a longer half-life (10 hours) than naloxone. Naltrexone is largely devoid of agonist actions and is metabolized to 6-β-naltrexol, a less potent antagonist that has a longer half-life than its parent drug. The s.c. LD50 in mice is 586 mg/kg. *See also* NALOXONE; NARCOTIC ANTAGONISTS; OPIOIDS.

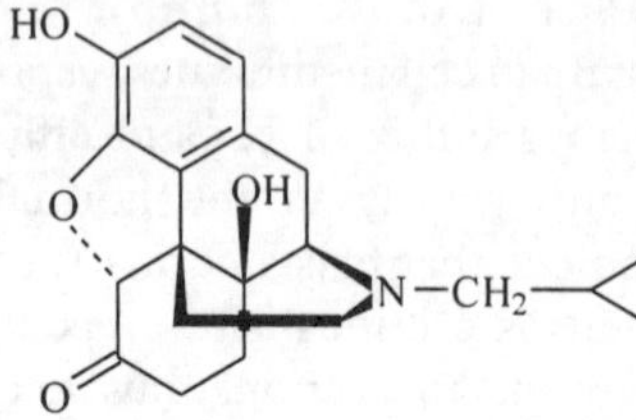

Naltrexone

naphtha. Petroleum naphthas consist mainly of aliphatic hydrocarbons; different fractions containing different proportions of aliphatic hydrocarbons, naphthenic hydrocarbons and aromatic hydrocarbons. Coal tar naphthas are primarily aromatic hydrocarbons such as toluene, xylene, cumene and benzene. Naphthas are used as organic solvents for oils, greases, paints, etc., or in the formulation of insecticides. They are irritating to the skin and mucous membranes. At high concentrations naphthas can cause CNS depression. One constituent, hexane, causes peripheral neuropathy whereas another, benzene, causes anemia. Aromatic hydrocarbons have been associated with a variety of forms of cancer. Naphthas can be taken up by inhalation, percutaneous absorption and ingestion. *See also* BENZENE; *N*-HEXANE.

naphthalene. CAS number 91-20-3. A designated hazardous substance (EPA), hazardous waste (EPA), and priority toxic pollutant (EPA). It is used in the synthesis of phthalic, anthranilic, hydroxyl, amino and sulfonic compounds that are utilized in dye manufacture. It has also been used as an insect repellent. The most serious toxic effect of naphthalene appears to be hemolytic anemia, particularly in the case of newborn infants and individuals with glucose-6-phosphate dehydrogenase deficiency, a condition that increases susceptibility. This condition is rare in Caucasians, but is more common in certain Negro and Jewish populations. Locally naphthalene is an irritant and an allergen. Systemically it causes intravascular hemolysis. The initial symptoms include nausea, abdominal pain and bladder irritation, subsequently leading to jaundice, hematuria, hemoglobinuria, renal tubule damage and renal failure. Examination of the blood reveals red cell fragments, nucleated red cells and severe anemia. *See also* ATSDR DOCUMENT, OCTOBER 1993; DATABASES, TOXICOLOGY; LEWIS, HCDR, NUMBER NAJ500.

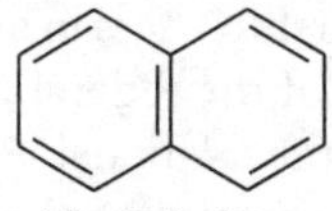

Naphthalene

α-naphthoflavone. An inhibitor of aryl hydrocarbon hydroxylase activity catalyzed by polycyclic aromatic hydrocarbon-induced isozymes of cytochrome P450.

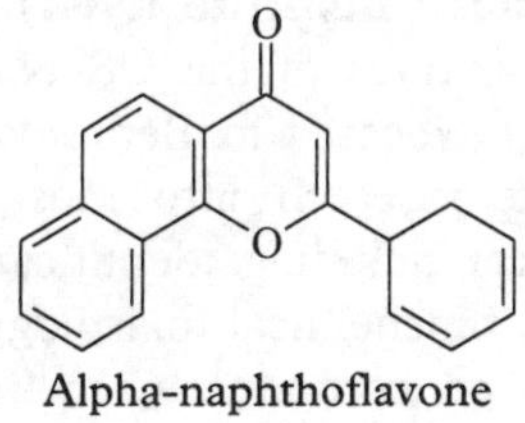

Alpha-naphthoflavone

β-naphthoflavone. An inducer of cytochrome P450 isozymes similar, if not identical, in its specificity to 3-methylcholanthrene and TCDD. *See also* INDUCTION; MECHANISM OF INDUCTION.

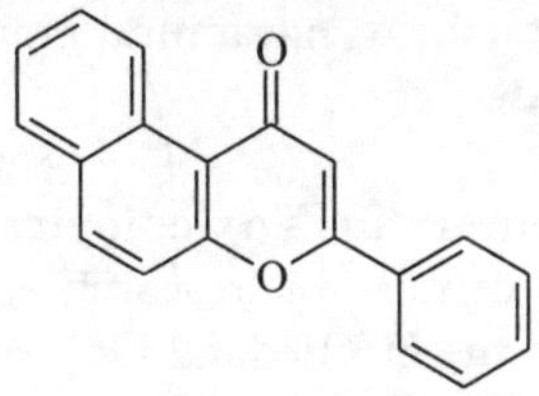

Beta-naphthoflavone

1,4-naphthoquinone. CAS number 130-15-4. A designated hazardous waste (EPA). It is used as a polymerization agent in rubber and plastics manufacture and in the synthesis of dyes and drugs. It has also been used as a fungicide. Although the toxicology *in vivo* of 1,4-naphthoquinone is not well understood, it is a potent inhibitor of electron transport *in vitro*. Only one study has found naphthoquinone to be oncogenic. *See also* ELECTRON TRANSPORT.

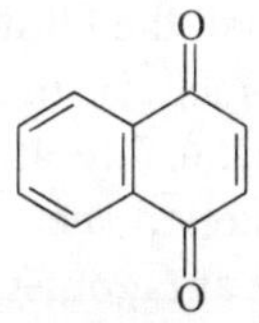

1,4-Naphthoquinone

α-naphthothiourea (ANTU). CAS number 86-88-4. Rodenticide, toxicity in humans may lead to death caused by pulmonary edema. *See also* DATABASES, TOXICOLOGY.

β-naphthylamine (2-aminonaphthalene). CAS number 91-59-8. A designated human carcinogen (IARC) and hazardous waste (EPA). α-Naphthylamine has also been described as an animal carcinogen. It is not currently in commercial use, although it may be present as an impurity in β-naphthylamine. It was formerly used as a rubber antioxidant and in dye manufacture. As shown by epidemiological studies, β-naphthylamine is a confirmed human bladder carcinogen with a latent period of about 16 years. Acute poisoning causes methemoglobinemia or hemorrhagic cystitis.

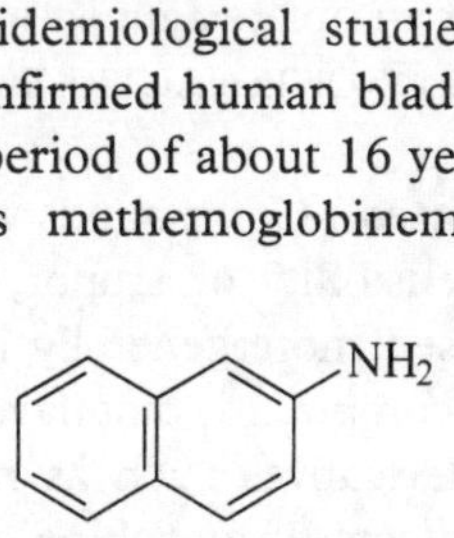

Beta-naphthylamine

α-naphthylisothiocyanate (1-isothiocyanato-naphthalene). CAS number 551-06-4. A hepatotoxicant that causes separation of the extracellular tight junctions that seal bile canaliculi, thus impairing biliary secretion and causing retention of bile acids.

Naprosyn. *See* PHENYLBUTAZONE.

Narcan. *See* NALOXONE.

narcosis. An impairment characterized by drowsiness or unconsciousness and resulting from the action of a toxicant on the central nervous system.

narcotic antagonists (opiate antagonists). A class of drugs that can occupy opioid receptors, but do not cause the physiological responses that agonists do. A major use of these compounds in toxicology is to reverse the clinical effects of over-doses of narcotics such as morphine or metha-done. An important consideration in their clinical use is pharmacokinetic, seen as differences in half-life between the antagonist and the agonist(s) whose effects are to be blocked. In general, a pure antagonist is devoid of pharmacological activity, but the actions of such drugs are evident not only in blockading the actions of opioid agonists, but also in reversing effects caused by activation of endogenous opioid systems (e.g., by pain or stress). The prototypical opiate antagonist drug is naloxone, a compound almost entirely devoid of agonist activities, but one that causes prompt reversal of the effects of morphine-like opioid ago-nists. Like naloxone, naltrexone is also a relatively pure antagonist, except that it has a longer dura-tion of action and is more potent orally. Replace-ment of the methyl group on the nitrogen by an allyl group or methylcyclopropyl group can result in conversion of an opiate agonist into an antago-nist. *See also* NALOXONE; NALTREXONE; OPIOIDS.

narcotics (opiates). Compounds with the ability to produce insensibility or stupor, although the term is often used more generally in referring to those classes of compounds that have actions simi-lar to opium derivatives such as morphine and codeine. The effects of morphine, the prototype narcotic, can be divided into effects on the gastro-intestinal tract and the CNS. The principal CNS effects include analgesia, euphoria and/or seda-tion, respiratory depression, antitussive action and effects on miosis; consequences with respect to the gastrointestinal tract include effects on emesis. With chronic usage, tolerance and physical dependence develop. There are also a number of synthetic narcotic analgesics, the best known of which are meperidine and methadone. All mem-bers of this class act by binding to specific high-affinity receptors, whose endogenous ligands are various opioid peptides. The differences in phar-macological and toxicological properties can often be explained by the relative actions at these various subpopulations. *See also* ANALGESICS; CODEINE; MEPERIDINE; METHADONE; MORPHINE; NAR-COTIC ANTAGONISTS; OPIOIDS.

NAS. *See* NATIONAL ACADEMY OF SCIENCE.

nasopharyngeal clearance. Particles are removed from the respiratory tract primarily by the mucociliary process. The beating of the cilia of ciliated cells causes a mucous coat within which the particles are trapped to move upward through the respiratory system to the buccal cavity where ingestion occurs. *See also* ALVEOLAR CLEARANCE.

National Academy of Science (NAS). A US body, chartered by the federal government, that recognizes distinction in all branches of science by election to membership. Acts in an advisory capac-ity to all branches of the federal government, par-ticularly through the National Research Council. The National Academy of Science, the National Academy of Engineering and the Institute of Medi-cine are the most prestigious representative bodies in the USA in their fields. *See also* NATIONAL RESEARCH COUNCIL.

National Cancer Institute (NCI). One of the constitutive institutes of the US National Insti-tutes of Health, located in Bethesda, Maryland. NCI conducts research into most, if not all, aspects of cancer including: identification of popu-lations at risk; biochemical toxicology of carcino-gens and related compounds; methodology for identification and measurement of carcinogens; experimental and clinical study of anticancer agents; molecular biology of cancer. NCI not only conducts an extensive intramural research pro-gram, but also supports extensive studies related to cancer through its extramural grants and con-tract programs.

National Center for Toxicological Research (NCTR). A center for research in toxicology established by the US Federal Government under the auspices of the Food and Drug Administration and located near Little Rock, Arkansas.

National Environmental Policy Act (NEPA). A US act that covers only US government agen-cies, requiring them all to prepare environmental impact statements for any federal action that might affect the quality of the human environ-ment. Such environmental impact statements must include not only an assessment of the effect of the proposed action on the environment, but also alternatives to the proposed action, the relationship between local short-term use and enhancements of long-term productivity, and a statement of irreversible commitment of resources. The Council on Environmental Quality, a group that acts in an advisory capacity to the President on matters affecting or promoting environmental quality, was also created under this act. *See also* ENVIRONMENTAL IMPACT STATEMENT.

National Institute for Environmental Health Sciences (NIEHS). A constitutive institute of the US National Institutes of Health located in Research Triangle Park, North Carolina. NIEHS conducts research into many aspects of the effect of environmental contaminants on human health. It supports biomedical research and training on the effects of environmental agents on human health through its extramural grants program. It is one of the most important US government agencies for research into fundamental aspects of toxicology and toxicology methods development.

National Institute for Occupational Safety and Health (NIOSH). *See* OCCUPATIONAL SAFETY AND HEALTH ACT.

National Institutes of Health (NIH). Principal US public agency for research in the health and related sciences through its intramural and through extramural grants. NIH consists of numerous institutes; those of most importance to toxicology are the National Institute of Environmental Health Science (NIEHS) and the National Cancer Institute (NCI).

National Library of Medicine (NLM). A division of US Health and Human Services, located in Bethesda, Maryland. As well as serving as a central library for such government organizations as the National Institutes of Health and the Armed Services Medical School, also located in Bethesda, the National Library of Medicine maintains and makes available computer databases, several of which are of importance to toxicology. They include the Toxicology Data Base, Toxline, Medline and others.

National Office of Animal Health (NOAH). A UK trade association for manufacturers of veterinary pharmaceuticals. Publishes the Veterinary Data Sheet Compendium. *See also* ASSOCIATION OF BRITISH PHARMACEUTICAL INDUSTRY.

National Poisons Information Service. A UK information service that gives details on the contents of domestic and industrial products, as well as providing laboratory analyses. Regional centers are to be found in England, Wales, Scotland and Northern Ireland.

National Research Council (NRC). A US organization that serves as an independent advisor to the federal government and is the principal operating arm of the National Academy of Science and the National Academy of Engineering. It is administered by the two academies and the Institute of Medicine. The NRC has established the Board on Environmental Studies and Toxicology to carry out studies of pollution, exposure, health effects and pollution control techniques, including risk assessment and environmental regulation and law.

National Research Council Food Chemicals Codex. *See* FOOD CHEMICALS CODEX.

National Toxicology Program (NTP). A US interagency group set up by the Department of Health and Human Services in 1978 to integrate activities and resources utilized in determining the toxicological potential of chemicals. It was granted permanent status in 1981. Member agencies include the National Cancer Institute, the Food and Drug Administration and the National Institute of Environmental Health Science. Most of the studies are carried out under the auspices of the latter organization.

natural cytotoxic cells. *See* NATURAL KILLER CELLS.

natural killer cells (NK cells). One of several possibly related groups of cells important in tumor resistance, destruction of some virally infected cells and cells modified by some bacteria and chemicals; NK cells are active in naive (unimmunized) animals. Killer cells, natural killer cells and natural cytotoxic cells have all been identified as cytotoxic cells that do not have the fine antigen specificity or histocompatability restrictions of cytotoxic T cells. These cell types have been characterized primarily functionally, with a number of overlapping functions and characteristics ascribed to each of them. The natural killer cells are perhaps the best characterized. They are large, granular lymphocytes bearing a characteristic cell surface marker (LCU 19 or CD 16) and are able to lyse a broad, although not unlimited, range of tumor cells in the absence of antibody, accessory cells or lymphokines. None of these cell types produce antibodies, nor do they undergo clonal expansion or exhibit memory after antigen exposure in the fashion of T and B cells. They are, however, responsive to interferon and some prostaglandins. *See also* CLONAL EXPANSION; T CELLS.

natural pollutant. A substance of natural origin that may be regarded as a pollutant when present in excess. Examples include volcanic dust, particles of sea salt, ozone formed photochemically or by lightning, and products of forest fires.

Natural Resources Defense Council (NRDC). A non-governmental organization in the USA that is concerned with natural resources and environmental pollution. The NRDC is especially concerned with human health effects from chemical pollutants, e.g., possible health effects from traces of pesticides on foods.

NCAS. New chemical active substance. *See also* NEW CHEMICAL ENTITY.

NCE. *See* NEW CHEMICAL ENTITY.

NCI. *See* NATIONAL CANCER INSTITUTE.

NCTR. *See* NATIONAL CENTER FOR TOXICOLOGICAL RESEARCH.

necropsy (autopsy). The examination of the organs and body tissues of a dead animal to determine the cause of death or pathological conditions.

necrosis. Death of areas of tissue, usually indicating that the affected tissue is surrounded by healthy tissue. Necrosis may be due to chemical agents acting locally, or secondary to physiological insult, infection or loss of circulation.

negative control. *See* CONTROLS, IN TESTING.

NEL. *See* NO EFFECT LEVEL.

nematocides. Pesticides designed to kill parasitic nematodes. Some of the insecticidal organophosphates, carbamates and fumigants (short-chain halogenated hydrocarbons) are used as nematocides. A common example is fenamiphos.

neonatal. Describing the developmental period immediately after birth. Neonatal toxicity may be due to toxic events initiated *in utero* or to toxicants transmitted in milk.

neoplasm. A heritably altered, relatively autonomous growth of tissue. A neoplasm is composed of abnormal cells, the growth of which is more rapid than that of other tissues and is not coordinated with the growth of other tissues. Neoplasms can be formed in any tissue and are classified or named according to their microscopic structures and original cells or tissues from which the tumor cells are derived. The suffix "-oma" is commonly used to denote malignant neoplasms; carcinoma is used to denote malignant tumors of epithelial cells and sarcoma malignant tumors of mesodermal tissue origin, such as of muscle or bone. Pitot, H.C. Fundamentals of Oncology, 3rd edn (Marcel Dekker, New York, 1986). James, R.C. & Teaf, C.M. in Industrial Toxicology (eds Williams, P.L. & Burson, J., Van Nostrand, New York, 1985). *See also* CARCINOMA; SARCOMA.

neoplastic transformation. The conversion of a normal cell to a neoplastic cell. Neoplasms can undergo qualitative changes in their phenotypic properties including transition from benign to malignant behavior. *See also* CARCINOGENISIS.

neostigmine (3-[[(dimethylamino)carbonyl]oxy]-N,N,N-trimethylbenzenaminium; Prostigmine). **CAS number 59-99-4**. An inhibitor of acetylcholinesterase that was the first synthetic carbamate to have clinical applications. Neostigmine is still the standard of comparison for new drugs developed for treatment of glaucoma and myasthenia gravis. Synthesized as an eserine mimic, neostigmine differs in that it contains a quaternary ammonium group which limits its penetration into the CNS. Also, it is a dimethylcarbamate which yields a more persistent inhibition of acetylcholinesterase than does the monomethylcarbamate eserine. The oral LD50 in mice is 7.5 mg/kg. *See also* ANTICHOLINESTERASES; ESERINE.

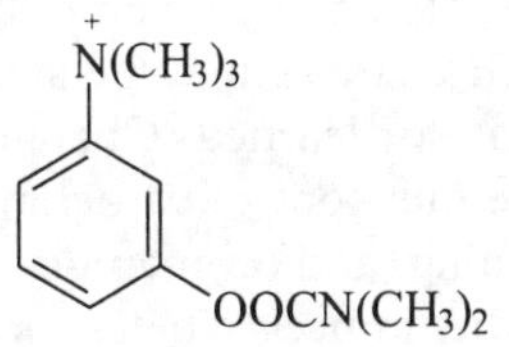

Neostigmine

NEPA. *See* NATIONAL ENVIRONMENTAL POLICY ACT.

nephritis. Inflammation of the kidney.

nephron. The kidney nephron consists of the glomerulus, which functions to filter the blood, the proximal tubule, the loop of Henle and the distal tubule. The proximal tubule is the site of much reabsorption of glucose, amino acids, water and electrolytes, but in addition is the site of secretion, by separate secretory mechanisms, of organic anions and organic cations. The loop of Henle is primarily concerned with urine concentration, whereas the distal tubule is adapted for Na^+/K^+ exchange. *See also* EXCRETION, RENAL; NEPHROTOXICITY.

nephrotoxicants. Chemicals that cause deleterious effects on the kidney. *See also* NEPHROTOXINS.

nephrotoxicity. A pathological state induced by a variety of chemicals wherein the normal homeostatic functioning of the kidney is disrupted. It is usually associated with necrosis of one or more segments of the proximal tubule. The disruption of renal function may present itself either with the excretion of large volumes of very dilute urine (high-output renal failure) or with the excretion of minimal amounts of urine. Mechanisms by which chemicals may induce this event vary widely, but renal metabolism may be involved. Brenner, B.M. & Lazarus, J.M. Acute Renal Failure (W.B. Saunders, Philadelphia, 1983). *See also* NEPHROTOXICITY, BIOTRANSFORMATION.

nephrotoxicity, biotransformation. Biotransformation of the parent compound to a toxic metabolite is a factor in nephrotoxicity. Although the kidney does not have levels of xenobiotic-metabolizing enzymes (e.g., cytochrome P450-dependent monooxygenase system) as high as those in the liver, some of the same enzymatic reactions have been shown to occur in the kidney. The concentration of cytochrome P450 is highest in the cells of the pars recta of the proximal tubule, an area that is particularly susceptible to toxic damage. Considering the unstable nature of many reactive metabolites, it is probable that covalent binding to tissue macromolecules occurs in close proximity to the site of activation. Thus chemicals that act via a reactive intermediate are probably activated in the kidney rather than being activated in the liver and transported to the kidney. As with hepatotoxicity, an important determinant in kidney toxicity is the balance between the rate of generation of reactive metabolites and the rate of their removal. For this reason glutathione concentration in renal tissue may also be important in detoxication. Thus nephrotoxins are activated in the kidney by the cytochrome P450 monooxygenase system to produce strong electrophiles or free radicals which can cause cell necrosis by binding to cell macromolecules or initiating lipid peroxidation. Many of these toxicants (e.g., acetaminophen, bromobenzene, chloroform and carbon tetrachloride) are the same as those that are activated in the liver and cause hepatoxicity. *See also* METABOLISM; REACTIVE INTERMEDIATES.

nephrotoxins. Chemicals that cause a deleterious effect on the kidney. Since the term is used to describe chemicals of both biological and synthetic origin causing kidney toxicity, it should, more properly, be nephrotoxicants, the term toxin and its derivatives being reserved for chemicals of biological origin. *See also* NEPHROTOXICITY; POISON; TOXIN.

nerve agents. *See* NERVE GASES; ORGANOPHOSPHORUS INSECTICIDES.

nerve cell. *See* NERVOUS SYSTEM.

nerve gases (nerve agents). Organophosphate chemical warfare agents that are potent anticholinesterases. Although not gases at room temperature, they are volatile liquids. Those of greatest concern are soman, sarin, tabun and VX. *See also* ORGANOPHOSPHORUS INSECTICIDES; SARIN; SOMAN; TABUN.

nervous system. The interlaced collection of neurons and glia, including the CNS (the brain and spinal cord) and the peripheral nervous system (including all other neural elements, such as spinal nerves, autonomic ganglia and ganglionated trunks and nerves). *See also* NEUROTOXICOLOGY.

neural. Pertaining to nerve cells or neurons, or pertaining to the nervous system. *See also* NEUROTOXICITY; NEUROTOXICOLOGY.

neural tube. A tissue from which the brain and spinal cord arise. It is formed during development from the fusion of the neural folds. During this period of development, toxic insult to the neural tube that either causes cell death, or affects cell division or maturation, can lead to embryotoxicity or malformations.

neurobehavioral teratology. A field of study that seeks to identify behavioral abnormalities or differences in organisms exposed pre-natally to a potentially toxic agent. Prenatal or *in utero* exposure to a toxicant may not result in demonstrable structural malformations in the brain, but rather subtle functional biochemical adaptations that are manifest in the developing organism as behavioral differences. The developing nervous system, with its cells that are undergoing mitosis or migration, may be especially vulnerable to toxic insult. The lack of an effective "blood–brain barrier" as well as the relative inability to metabolize toxicants increases the vulnerability of the developing organism. *See also* AUDITORY STARTLE; CONDITIONED AVOIDANCE; HYPERACTIVITY, LOCOMOTOR BEHAVIOR; MENTAL RETARDATION; NEUROBEHAVIORAL TOXICOLOGY; PASSIVE AVOIDANCE; PAVLOVIAN CONDITIONING; POSTNATAL BEHAVIORAL TESTS; TREMORS.

neurobehavioral toxicology. A field of study that uses methods developed in the behavioral sciences to detect, predict, measure or study toxicity. Behavioral changes are assessed by observational methods, operant techniques, learning and memory tasks, etc., or by a combination of these methods. Such changes may be simple or highly complex, innate or learned. Changes in reflexive behavior, schedule-controlled behavior, performance on learning and/or memory tasks, motor activity and other indices of behavioral functioning are thought to be potentially sensitive indicators of exposure to substances that result in CNS toxicity since these behaviors represent a final integrated expression of nervous system and motor function. Behavioral changes will occur that not only reflect gross pathological changes, but also more subtle toxicant effects such as perturbations of specific neurochemical systems or receptor cellular supersensitivity. *See also* AUDITORY STARTLE; CONDITIONED AVOIDANCE; HYPERACTIVITY; LOCOMOTOR BEHAVIOR; MENTAL RETARDATION; NEUROBEHAVIORAL TERATOLOGY; PASSIVE AVOIDANCE; PAVLOVIAN CONDITIONING; POSTNATAL BEHAVIORAL TESTS; TREMORS.

neuroblastoma. A malignant hemorrhagic tumor consisting mostly of neuroblast-like cells, giving rise to cells of the sympathetic system.

neurogenic. Originating from the nervous system, or due to or resulting from neural impulses.

neurohypophysis (posterior pituitary). The posterior portion of the pituitary (hypophysis) that has a direct neural connection with the hypothalamus. Two hormones are synthesized in cell bodies within the hypothalamus, migrate down axons to be released via nervous stimulation from the neurohypophysis. The two hormones are oxytocin, which controls uterine contractions and milk letdown, and vasopressin (antidiuretic hormone, ADH), which controls renal water reabsorption and vasoconstriction. *Compare* ADENOHYPOPHYSIS.

neuroleptic malignant syndrome. A condition marked primarily by hyperpyrexia, but also muscle rigidity, altered mental state (including catatonia) and autonomic instability. Acute renal failure, myoglobinuria and elevated blood creatine phosphokinase (CPK) levels may also occur. It is seen rarely with almost all antipsychotic drugs and requires immediate discontinuation of the drug with symptomatic treatment. The specific mechanism underlying the condition is unknown. *See also* ANTIPSYCHOTIC DRUGS.

neuromodulators. *See* NEUROTRANSMITTERS.

neuromuscular junction (myoneural junction). Junction between the motor endplate of a nerve and the muscle cell that it stimulates. Arrival of an action potential at the endplate induces the release of a chemical transmitter (neurotransmitter) which diffuses across the gap between the nerve and muscle cell membranes. The transmitter then binds to receptors on the muscle cell membrane, causing its depolarization. This in turn precipitates a cascade of events which culminates in the contraction of the muscle.

neuromuscular system. *See* DIAGNOSTIC FEATURES, NEUROMUSCULAR SYSTEM.

neuron (nerve cell). *See* NERVOUS SYSTEM.

neuropathology. The branch of pathology that is concerned with diseases of the nervous system. The term is also used to denote the constellation of macroscopic and microscopic morphological alterations in the nervous system associated with a particular disease.

neuropathy. *See* AXONOPATHY; DELAYED NEUROPATHY; γ-KETONE NEUROPATHY; PERIPHERAL NEUROPATHY.

neuropathy target enzyme. *See* NEUROTOXIC ESTERASE.

neurotoxic esterase (NTE; neuropathy target enzyme). A putative target enzyme of organophosphates that elicit delayed neuropathy. NTE is defined as the paraoxon-resistant, mipafox-sensitive component of esterases hydrolyzing phenyl valerate or phenyl phenylacetate. NTE activity is highest in nervous tissue and is also relatively high in lymphocytes, but is very low in other tissues examined. The role of NTE inhibition in the initiation of delayed neuropathy is unknown, but it is well established that it is the aging of phosphorylated NTE, rather than the phosphorylation per se, that correlates with its development of delayed neuropathy. *See also* DELAYED NEUROPATHY; MIPAFOX; TOCP.

neurotoxicity. Any toxic effect on any aspect of the central or peripheral nervous system. Such changes can be expressed as functional changes (such as behavioral or neurological abnormalities) or as neurochemical, biochemical, physiological or morphological perturbations. The complex nature of the nervous system has made detection and evaluation of neurotoxicity a more multi-disciplinary endeavor than most other branches of toxicology. *See also* NERVOUS SYSTEM; NEUROPATHOLOGY; NEUROTOXICITY TESTS; PERIPHERAL NEUROTOXICITY.

neurotoxicity tests. Endpoints that have been devised to reflect toxicant-induced changes in the nervous system. Testing for neurotoxicity is difficult due to the complexity of the nervous system and the fact that toxicants may have selective action or cause widespread effects. Thus, unless a well-characterized compound is being studied, neurotoxicity testing involves several endpoints that reflect overall function. Neurotoxicity is frequently revealed by the acute, subchronic or chronic effects on behavioral, physiological or pharmacological endpoints. Because neurotoxicity is of great potential significance in toxicology, the type of tests that may be useful is an active area of research. Some of these include direct behavioral observation (either clinically or in the laboratory). These signs may include changes in awareness, mood, motor activity, CNS excitation, posture, motor incoordination, muscle tone, reflexes and autonomic functions. More specialized tests can also be carried out that evaluate spontaneous motor activity, conditioned avoidance responses, operant conditioning and tests for motor incoordination such as the inclined plane or rotorod tests. A major problem in neurotoxicity evaluation (especially in the CNS) is the functional plasticity of the nervous system, where even observable damage may not initially affect overall function. Damage to the nervous system is often classified by the predominant affected aspect (e.g., axonopathy, myelinopathy, etc.). Once there is global evidence of effects on the nervous system, more specific approaches may be used to provide an indication of specific biochemical and anatomical loci. Such tests may include the examination of how aspects of synaptic transmission are altered (neurotransmitter uptake, degradation or turnover, receptor function, cyclic nucleotide metabolism, etc.) or specific structural or cellular elements (e.g., membrane composition or fluidity, cellular morphology, etc.). In such cases, the studies should be directed at specific hypotheses formulated from structure–activity data or from available data in the intact organism. *See also* DELAYED NEUROPATHY TESTS; NEUROBEHAVIORAL TOXICOLOGY; NEUROTOXICOLOGY.

neurotoxicology. The branch of toxicology that deals with toxicants affecting the central and/or peripheral nervous system and with the nature and mechanisms of the process of toxic insult and recovery of these aspects of the nervous system. Recent studies have demonstrated that many actions of the nervous system are endocrine-like and have also shown a close relationship between the nervous and immune systems. These advances therefore have broadened the limits and nature of neurotoxicology. *See also* POISON; TOXICOLOGY.

neurotoxin. Toxin that affects the nervous system specifically. Neurotoxins can be products of many species of bacteria (e.g., botulinum toxin, pertussis toxin, tetanus toxin), animals (e.g., snake venom toxins like cobratoxin and α-bungarotoxin, batrachotoxin, curare, ciguatera toxins), and plants and fungi (e.g., amanitin). *See also* AMANITIN; BATRACHOTOXIN; BOTULINUM TOXIN; α-BUNGAROTOXIN; β-BUNGAROTOXIN; CURARIZATION; CIGUATERA; PERTUSSIS TOXIN; TETANUS TOXIN.

neurotransmitters. Intercellular chemical messengers that are secreted by neurons across specialized structures (synapses) to transmit chemical information to one or more target cells. Historically, for a compound to be accepted as a neurotransmitter, evidence is required for localized synthesis in the neuron, release upon depolarization,

the presence of specific recognition sites (receptors) localized on the target cells close to the site of release and mechanisms of rapid inactivation (uptake or degradation). Some of the compounds generally accepted as fitting these rigid criteria include acetylcholine, norepinephrine, dopamine, glutamate and GABA. Since the middle of the 1970s, it has become clear that there are dozens of compounds which do not meet all of these criteria, yet which serve important roles in chemical message transmission in the nervous system. A compound in this class is sometimes called a neuromodulator; it differs in that rates of synthesis, release and degradation may be slower, and that action may occur over larger distances from the site of release. Examples of neuromodulators include various opioid peptides (e.g., enkephalins, endorphins, dynorphins), vasoactive intestinal polypeptide (VIP) and nearly all of the peripheral endocrine hormones and related gene products. A major mechanism of neurotoxicity can be direct or indirect effects on neurotransmitter/neuromodulator function. However, the plethora of possible chemical messages has made elucidation of specific effects a much more challenging neurotoxicology problem. *See also* ACETYLCHOLINE; CATECHOLAMINES; NEUROTOXICOLOGY; RECEPTORS.

neutropenia. *See* AGRANULOCYTOSIS.

new chemical entity (NCE). A chemical with an application for authorization to market that has not been previously considered by the regulatory agency processing the application. For pharmaceuticals this may be a New Chemical Active Substance (NCAS) or more generally any chemical entity (active or excipient).

niacin (nicotinic acid, 3-pyridinecarboxylic acid). **CAS number 59-67-6**. A water soluble vitamin, deficiency of which has been associated with pellagra. The term niacin has also been used for nicotinamide.

Niacin

nick translation. Method for uniform radioactive labeling of DNA *in vitro*. DNA in solution is mixed with trace amounts of DNase I, to generate nicks, DNA polymerase I and deoxyribonucleotide substrates, one or more of which may be radioactive. DNA polymerase binds at the randomly generated nicks, excises existing nucleotides and substitutes for them the radioactive ones provided. The polymerase accurately copies the unnicked second strand and at the end of the reaction highly radioactive DNA (10^7–10^9 counts per minute per microgram) with unchanged base sequence is produced. Nick translation is widely used to prepare probe DNA for molecular hybridization.

5'...-G-T-A-C-C-A-T-G...3' Unlabelled
3'...-C-A-T-G-G-T-A-C...5' DNA molecule

↓ *Introduce single-strand breaks ('nicks')*
(e.g. by alkali)

5'...-G T-A-C-C-A-T-G...3' 'Nicked'
3'...-C-A-T-G-G-T-A-C...5' DNA

↓ *Nuclease action of DNA polymerase I*

...-G   A-C-C-A-T-G...
... C-A-T-G-G   A-C...

↓ *Repair action of DNA polymerase I*
+ labeled nucleoside triphosphates

... -G-T* A-C-C-A-T-G...
...-C-A-T-G-G T*-A-C...

↓ *Repeat last two steps as the 'nicks' move*
along the DNA until all DNA contains
labeled nucleotides

Nick translation

Nickel (Ni). An element that is used in electroplating, in coinage, in alloys with a number of other metals such as copper, manganese, zinc and iron. It is present in stainless steel, magnetic tapes, surgical and dental instruments, batteries, crankcase oils and ceramics. It is also used as a catalyst. Nickel and several of its salts (nickel ammonium sulfate, nickel chloride, nickel hydroxide, nickel nitrate, nickel phosphate, nickel sulfate) are of toxicological importance. Occupational exposures may occur in its mining, smelting and refining.

The general population ingests nickel in food. Skin sensitization and dermatitis leading to chronic eczema, called "nickel itch," frequently occurs, especially in wearers of pierced earrings. Nickel can also irritate the conjunctiva and respiratory tract mucous membranes. Absorption from the digestive tract is poor, so systemic poisoning is rare, but since it is an irritant it acts as an emetic. Systemic effects include hyperglycemia, capillary damage, CNS depression, myocardial weakness and kidney damage. Nickel and its compounds are carcinogenic following inhalation, but not following ingestion or skin contact. Cancer of the lung and nasal passages results, with a latent period of about 25 years; smokers are at greater risk. In addition to irritation and carcinogenesis, nickel carbonyl (nickel tetracarbonyl, $Ni(CO)_4$) exerts relatively mild, transient initial symptoms including headache, giddiness, nausea and shortness of breath. These symptoms are followed by very serious symptoms hours to days later, consisting of tightness in the chest, shortnesss of breath, rapid respiration, pulmonary edema, cyanosis and extreme weakness; this can be fatal. Heat decomposition of nickel carbonyl yields carbon monoxide. Chelating agents can be used to remove nickel from the body. *See also* ATSDR DOCUMENT, APRIL 1993; DATABASES, TOXICOLOGY; LEWIS, HCDR, NUMBER NCW500.

nickel carbonyl ($Ni(CO)_4$). A very toxic, explosive, respiratory irritant and possibly a carcinogen. *See also* NICKEL.

nicotine (black leaf 40; (*S*)-3-(1-methyl-2-pyrrolidinyl)pyridine). **CAS number 54-11-5.** Constituent of *Nicotiana tabacum*. A colorless liquid produced from tobacco extracts, nicotine is a contact insecticide and greenhouse fumigant. Used as either the technical alkaloid or as nicotine sulfate, it has now been largely superceded by organophosphorus insecticides. Nicotine is a neurotoxicant acting on ganglial synapses of insect CNS and stimulates nicotinic receptors of mammalian autonomic ganglia and neuromuscular junctions. Symptoms in humans include salivation, vomiting, muscular weakness, fibrillation and, ultimately, chronic convulsions and cessation of respiration. Chronic use of tobacco-containing products is now thought to have addictive properties because of the indirect effects of nicotine on brain dopamine neurotransmission. The acute oral LD50 in rats is 50–60 mg/kg, and the acute dermal LD50 in rabbits is 50 mg/kg. Treatment of nicotine poisoning is by the use of anticonvulsants. Parpanit (20–30 mg/kg, i.v.) suppresses toxic action. Pipancol (15–30 mg/kg, i.v.) protects against lethal doses. It is also a source of nicotonic acid. In cigarettes, nicotine is both a transient stimulant and a sedative to the central nervous system. Nicotine is physically and psychologically addictive. The ingestion of nicotine results in a rapid physiological effect because of discharge of epinephrine from the adrenal cortex, that indirectly stimulates the central nervous system, as well as other endocrine glands.

Nicotine

nicotinic acid. *See* NIACIN.

nicotinic receptors. *See* ACETYLCHOLINE RECEPTORS, MUSCARINIC AND NICOTINIC.

NIEHS. *See* NATIONAL INSTITUTE FOR ENVIRONMENTAL HEALTH SCIENCES.

NIH. *See* NATIONAL INSTITUTES OF HEALTH.

nikethamide (*N,N*-**diethyl-3-pyridine-carboxamide;** *N,N*-**diethylnicotinamide; nicotinic acid diethylamide; Coramine). CAS number 59-26-7.** A CNS stimulant that increases respiration and was once thought to be useful as an analeptic agent in the management of sedative-hypnotic poisoning. The respiratory stimulation effect is brief, and repeated doses may induce seizures. Adverse effects include tachycardia, arrhythmias, increased blood pressure, sneezing, vomiting, itching, tremors, muscular rigidity, sweating and, in higher doses, seizures. Although analeptic effects are essentially absent in subconvulsive doses, limited use is made of nikethamide in the management of acute respiratory depression or insufficiency. The LD50 in rats is 272 mg/kg, i.p. *See also* ANALEPTICS; STIMULANTS.

Nikethamide

NIOSH. *See* NATIONAL INSTITUTE OF OCCUPATIONAL SAFETY & HEALTH.

nitrates (MNO$_3$, where M = Na, K, etc.). Nitrates occur in low concentrations as natural constituents in foods and are a common food additive, especially in cured meat and fish. In such products, they help prevent botulism by inhibiting the growth of *Clostridium botulinum* and also impart the desired flavor and pink color. Nitrate may be reduced microbially in the gut, as well as under poor food storage conditions, to nitrite. This, in turn, may lead to the formation of mutagenic and potentially carcinogenic *N*-nitrosamines. Nitrates, as well as nitrites and their organic derivatives, may have direct vasodilatory properties. *See also* NITRITES.

nitric acid (HNO$_3$). A colorless liquid, with a choking odor, that fumes in moist air. Fuming nitric acid contains an excess of nitrogen dioxide (NO$_2$) and is yellow in color. Nitric acid is an important industrial chemical, and its manufacture represents one of the most important chemical industries worldwide. Nitric acid is used largely in the production of fertilizers, with a significant proportion being used in the manufacture of explosives. A smaller proportion of the total nitric acid production is used in etching, engraving and the manufacture of rocket fuels and pesticides. Toxic effects arise mainly from skin contact, but may also result from inhalation or ingestion. These toxic effects consist mainly of corrosion of the skin due to contact or pulmonary edema due to inhalation.

nitric oxide (NO). A colorless gas used in the manufacture of nitric acid. On inhalation it causes cyanosis, ataxia, tachycardia and other symptoms that may lead to respiratory arrest. It may be important in air pollution. NO is also currently recognized as an important biological mediator in animals and humans. It is synthesized by constitutive (c) and inducible (i) isoforms of the enzyme NO synthase (NOS), and it can react with other biological molecules such as reactive oxygen species. NO modulates pulmonary and systemic vascular tone, has antithrombotic functions, mediates consequences of inflammatory responses, and plays important roles in neural functions. In lung, a diminution of NO production is implicated in pathological states associated with pulmonary hypertension, such as acute respiratory distress syndrome. See also NITROGEN OXIDES.

nitrites (MNO$_2$, where M = Na, K, etc.). Nitrites are important in toxicology for several distinct reasons. Nitrites can cause the oxidation of hemoglobin to methemoglobin under physiological conditions, with some individuals having an idiosyncratic sensitivity to this effect. However, the ability of nitrites to cause the formation of methemoglobin makes it useful as a first step in therapy for cyanide poisoning, where the newly generated ferric heme groups can act as a cyanide "trap" or "sink," preventing the inhibition of cytochrome oxidase. In the gut, some bacteria (e.g., *Escherichia coli*) may form nitrite from nitrate. In an acidic environment, the nitrite may lead to the formation of toxic *N*-nitrosoamines if secondary amines are present. This reaction can be inhibited by antioxidants, and the use of ascorbate, erythrobate, butylated hydroxyanisole or butylated hydroxytoluene in foods in which nitrates or nitrites are used to minimize the production of nitrosoamines. Nitrites, as well as nitrates and their organic derivatives, may have direct vasodilatory properties, and this may be a cause of toxicity in certain people. See also *N*-DIMETHYLNITROSAMINE; NITRATES; NITROSAMINES.

nitrobenzene. CAS number 98-95-3. A designated hazardous substance (EPA), hazardous waste (EPA) and priority toxic pollutant (EPA). It is a yellow/brown liquid with a characteristic odor of bitter almonds. Nitrobenzene is used in the manufacture of explosives, dyes, paints, shoe and

$$NO_2$$

Nitrobenzene

other polishes, and as an intermediate in chemical synthesis. The routes of entry of nitrobenzene are inhalation of the vapor and ingestion or percutaneous absorption of the liquid. Nitrobenzene is toxic due to the formation of methemoglobin, producing cyanosis. Symptoms include nausea, fatigue, depression and coma due to effects on the CNS. Chronic exposure can lead to spleen and liver damage, jaundice, etc. Pregnant women, individuals consuming ethanol and those with glucose-6-phosphate dehydrogenase deficiency are particularly at risk.

nitrogen mustard (2-chloro-*N*-(2-chloroethyl)-*N*-methylanamine; mechlorethamine). CAS number 51-75-2. A vesicant and an irritant; it causes necrosis. It has been used as a chemical warfare agent and as an antineoplastic agent. It is an alkylating agent and, as a consequence, a direct-acting carcinogen.

$$ClCH_2CH_2 \diagdown \!\!\!\!\!\diagup NCH_3 \atop ClCH_2CH_2$$

Nitrogen mustard

nitrogen oxides (NOx). A mixture of oxides of nitrogen, including nitric oxide and nitrogen dioxide, that is involved in air pollution. Nitrogen oxides are formed by the thermal decomposition of atmospheric nitrogen and thus can be formed by almost any combustion process. See also AIR POLLUTION.

nitro reduction. The reduction of aromatic amines by either bacterial or mammalian nitroreductase systems. There is convincing evidence that this reaction sequence is catalyzed by cytochrome P450. Although NADPH is consumed, the reaction is inhibited by oxygen. Earlier experiments had suggested that a flavoprotein reductase was involved, and it is not clear whether or not both of these mechanisms occur. However, high concentrations of FAD or FMN catalyze the nonenzymatic reduction of nitro groups. See also REDUCTION.

nitrosamides. Some nitrosamides are carcinogenic. In an aqueous environment, they release active intermediates spontaneously, making them potentially more dangerous than the nitrosamines, which require enzymatic activation. *See also* NITROSAMINES.

nitrosamines. Numerous alkyl- or alkylarylnitrosamines are carcinogenic in animal systems. Examples include dimethyl-, diethyl- and dibutylnitrosamines, methylphenylnitrosamine and the antibiotic streptozotocin. Target organs include liver, lung, kidney, bladder, esophagus and pancreas. Several carcinogenic nitrosamines are derivatives of alkaloids, such as nicotine, and are found in cigarette smoke. Nitrosamines are activated to reactive electrophiles by oxidation. Nitrosamines are potent carcinogens in animals, but their precise role in the etiology of human cancers is still unknown. Nitrites, used as preservatives in foods, can lead to the formation of nitrosamines; the concurrent presence of vitamins C or E or other antioxidants inhibits nitrosamine formation. Nitrate, which is common in foods, can be reduced to nitrite microbially. These reactions have led to recent concern over the potential danger of the use of nitrites and nitrates as food preservatives. *See also* N-DIMETHYLNITROSAMINE; NITRITES.

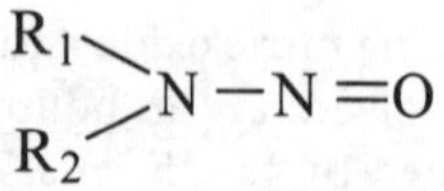

$$R_1 \atop R_2 \!\!\diagdown\!\! N - N = O$$

General structure of nitrosamines

nitrosoureas. Some nitrosoureas are carcinogens, and like nitrosamides, can be activated in aqueous solution spontaneously and do not require enzymatic activation as do the nitrosamines. Some are useful model compounds, since they produce cancers of the glandular stomach or the brain, which are difficult to induce experimentally. Some are carcinogenic transplacentally. *See also* NITROSAMINES.

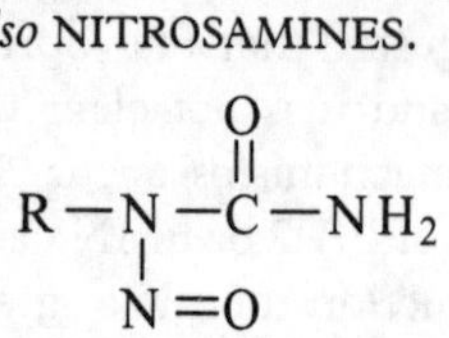

$$R - N - \overset{\displaystyle O}{\overset{\|}{C}} - NH_2 \atop N = O$$

General structure of nitrosoureas

nitrous oxide (dinitrogen oxide; N_2O; laughing gas). The only inorganic gas used for clinical anesthesia. It has both anesthetic and analgesic actions, and equilibrates with blood much more rapidly than halothane or ether. Although it cannot produce surgical anesthesia alone unless a hyperbaric chamber is used, it is frequently used as an adjuvant in general anesthetic procedures. Nitrous oxide produces analgesia equivalent to morphine when inspired at concentrations of 20%. Alone, nitrous oxide is used primarily to provide analgesia during dental procedures and during the first stage of parturition. Because of its analgesic effects and the moderate loss of inhibitions, it has been frequently abused. Such chronic problems may cause long-term toxicity not seen with appropriate use, including possible effects on the male reproductive system. *See also* ANESTHETICS.

NK cells. *See* NATURAL KILLER CELLS.

NLM. *See* NATIONAL LIBRARY OF MEDICINE.

NMR. *See* SPECTROMETRY, NUCLEAR MAGNETIC RESONANCE.

NOAEL. *See* NO OBSERVED ADVERSE EFFECT LEVEL.

NOAH. *See* NATIONAL OFFICE OF ANIMAL HEALTH.

Noctec. *See* CHLORAL HYDRATE.

Nodular. *See* METHYPRYLON.

no effect level (NEL). A term used in the UK and Europe rather than the no observed effect level. It is used to mean that no toxicologically significant effect has been detected. For example, a local, freely reversible, irritant effect might be adjudged adverse, but not toxicologically significant and would not, therefore, be used in the establishment of a no effect level for dermal exposure. *Compare* NO OBSERVED EFFECT LEVEL.

NOEL. *See* NO OBSERVED EFFECT LEVEL.

non-disjunction. *See* CHROMOSOME ABERRATIONS.

non-genotoxic carcinogen. *See* CARCINOGEN, EPIGENETIC.

nonlinear regression. Before the age of micro-computers, scientists transformed their data to force curved relationships into straight lines, thus permitting the transformed data to be analyzed with linear regression. Examples include Lineweaver–Burke plots of enzyme kinetic data, Scatchard plots of binding data, and logarithmic plots of kinetic data. Linear regression assumes that X and Y are measured independently, and that the variability among replicate Y values follows a Gaussian distribution with a standard deviation that does not depend on the value of X. These assumptions are rarely true with trans-formed data. Moreover, the X and Y variables sometimes (e.g., Scatchard plot) are intertwined during the transformation, invalidating linear regression. To use nonlinear regression, a mathe-matical model based on theory must first be defined (e.g., the interaction of a toxicant with a target site may be explained by the law of mass action). The next step is to express the model as an equation that defines Y as a function of X and one or more variables. Choosing a model is a scientific decision, not a statistical one, and each model needs to have a valid scientific basis. Then, every nonlinear regression program starts with an initial estimated value for each variable in the equation, and generates a curve defined by the initial values. It then calculates the sum-of-squares (the sum of the squares of the vertical distances of the points from the curve), and adjusts the variables to make the curve come closer to the data points. There are several algorithms for adjusting the variables, with the most common called the Marquardt method. The variables are adjusted again so that the curve comes even closer to the points and this is repeated until the adjustments make virtually no difference in the sum-of-squares. This results in values for each of the constants in the model equation, as well as information about how well the model fits the equation. Although nonlinear regression is the preferred method of data analysis, it is often quite useful to combine with figures generated by linear transformations, as the latter often make visual relationship more readily apparent. *See also* LINEAR REGRESSION; LINEWEAVER–BURKE PLOT; SCATCHARD PLOT; STATISTICS, FUNC-TION IN TOXICOLOGY.

non-microsomal oxidations. Although micro-somal enzymes are responsible for most of the oxi-dations in the metabolism of xenobiotics, non-microsomal enzymes, located in the mitochondria or soluble cytoplasm of the cell, may also be involved. The most important are alcohol dehy-drogenase, aldehyde dehydrogenase, and the amine oxidases, monoamine oxidase and diamine oxidase. *See also* ALCOHOL DEHYDROGENASE; ALDEHYDE DEHYDROGENASE; AMINE OXI-DASES; MONOAMINE OXIDASES.

non-parametric. Describing significance tests that do not involve the assumptions of normality or homogeneity of variance. In such tests, no assumptions are made about the distribution or parameters of the population from which the observations were sampled. Mann–Whitney U test, signed ranks test and chi-square test are examples of commonly employed non-parametric or distribution-free tests. *See also* PARAMETRIC; STATISTICS, FUNCTION IN TOXICOLOGY.

non-proliferative dust. *See* DUST, NON-PROLIFERATIVE.

non-steroidal anti-inflammatory drugs (NSAID). *See* ANTI-INFLAMMATORY AGENTS.

non-threshold effects. Although it is generally assumed that there is some dose of a toxicant (the threshold dose) below which it will not cause a deleterious effect (i.e., "the dose makes the poison"), for regulatory purposes it is assumed that carcinogenic chemicals and cancer-causing radiation do not have a threshold dose. This assumes that there is a finite risk of cancer from any dose. Presumably this assumption, which often does not appear to hold, makes regulation of such chemicals and radiation easier.

no observed adverse effect level (NOAEL). A variant of the no observed effect level (NOEL) that specifies that the effect in question be adverse. *Compare* NO OBSERVED EFFECT LEVEL.

no observed effect level (NOEL). The highest dose level of a chemical that, in a given toxicity test, causes no observable adverse effect in the test animals. The NOEL for a given chemical varies with the route and duration of exposure and the nature of the adverse effect (i.e., the indicator of toxicity) considered. The NOEL for the most sensitive test species and the most sensitive indicator of toxicity is usually employed for regulatory purposes (e.g., for pesticides). The NOEL is not an absolute no effect level and may require modification as new information becomes available. *Compare* NO EFFECT LEVEL; NO OBSERVED ADVERSE EFFECT LEVEL.

noradrenaline. *See* NOREPINEPHRINE.

norepinephrine (4-(2-amino-1-hydroxyethyl)-1,2-benzenediol; 2-amino-1-(3,4-dihydroxyphenyl)ethanol; noradrenaline). CAS number 51-41-2. A catecholamine formed by the action of the enzyme dopamine β-hydroxylase on the immediate precursor dopamine. Like the other catecholamines epinephrine and dopamine, it has both neurotransmitter and hormonal functions. As a neurotransmitter, it is the major transmitter of peripheral sympathetic nerve endings, as well as innervating important pathways in the brain and spinal cord. As a hormone, it is released from chromaffin granules in the adrenal medulla in response to hypotension or after splanchic stimulation. The oral LD50 in mice is 50 mg/kg. *Compare* DOPAMINE; EPINEPHRINE. *See also* BIOGENIC AMINES; CATECHOLAMINES; TYROSINE HYDROXYLASE.

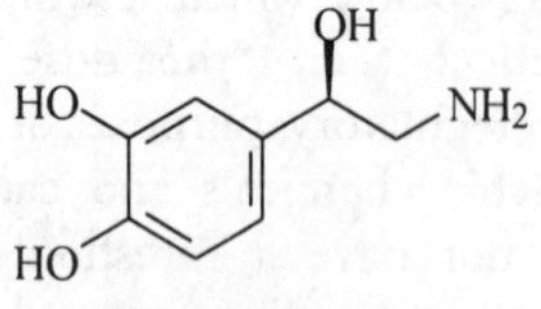

Norepinephrine

Northern blotting. Procedure, analogous to Southern blotting, except that the nucleic acid being transferred is RNA and not DNA. Nucleic acids, previously resolved by agarose gel electrophoresis, are transferred to a nitrocellulose filter by capillary action. They are then bound to the sheet by heating and can be probed with radioactive labeled nucleic acids followed by autoradiography. Note that although Southern blotting was so called after its inventor, E. Southern, Northern blotting was adopted simply as a contrasting name. *See also* WESTERN BLOTTING.

nortriptyline. *See* TRICYCLIC ANTIDEPRESSANTS.

NRC. *See* NATIONAL RESEARCH COUNCIL.

NRDC. *See* NATIONAL RESOURCES DEFENSE COUNCIL.

NSAID (non-steroidal anti-inflammatory drugs). *See* ANTI-INFLAMMATORY AGENTS.

NTE. *See* NEUROTOXIC ESTERASE.

NTP. *See* NATIONAL TOXICOLOGY PROGRAM.

nuclear envelope. *See* NUCLEAR MEMBRANE.

nuclear magnetic resonance spectrometry (NMR). *See* SPECTROMETRY, NUCLEAR MAGNETIC RESONANCE.

nuclear membrane (nuclear envelope). A lipoprotein membrane that encloses the nucleus, delimiting it from the remainder of the cell. It may be important in chemical carcinogenesis as it contains the enzymes of the cytochrome P450-dependent monooxygenase system. This system is known to activate chemical carcinogens (e.g., benzo[a]pyrene) to highly reactive electrophilic intermediates capable of reacting with cellular macromolecules, including DNA.

nucleic acids. Polynucleotides consist of a long, unbranched chain with a backbone of sugar (ribose or deoxyribose) and phosphate units with heterocyclic bases protruding from the chain at regular intervals. There are two main types: deoxyribonucleic acid (DNA), the genetic material of most living cells and a major constituent of chromosomes within the cell nucleus, and ribonucleic acid (RNA) concerned with protein synthesis found mainly in the cytoplasm (although synthesized in the nucleus). On hydrolysis nucleic acids are broken down first to nucleotides, then nucleosides

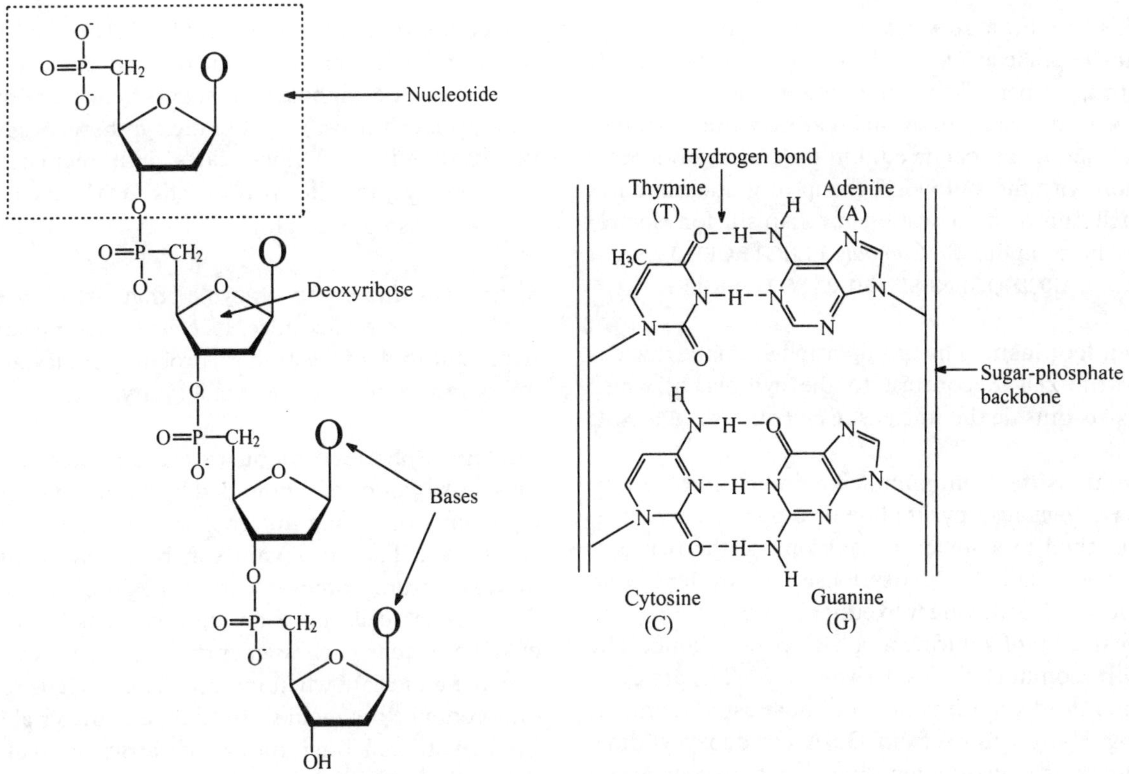

Nucleic acids

and finally purines, pyrimidines, sugar and phosphate.

The DNA molecule consists of two helical chains coiled round the same axis in which alternate deoxyribose molecules are connected through C-3 and C-5 by phosphate groups, with bases attached to the sugars (see Figure). Hydrogen bonds between the bases hold the chains together. Spatial considerations require that one of the bases in a pair be a purine and the other a pyrimidine, a condition satisfied by the pairing of thymine with adenine and cytosine with guanine. As a consequence, the sequence of bases in one chain determines that in the other. DNA replicates on cell division so that the two daughter molecules are identical to the parent molecule. In the presence of polymerases, the hydrogen bonds break, the strands unwind and each strand directs the synthesis of a complementary strand from nucleotides.

In the RNA molecule, the sugar is ribose and uracil replaces thymine. Messenger RNA (mRNA) conveys information in the form of base sequence from DNA to RNA on ribosomes where protein synthesis occurs from amino acids associated with the RNA template. A specific sequence of three bases – a codon – codes for each amino acid residue; thus the amino acid sequence is ultimately based on the order of the nucleotides in the DNA molecule (see GENETIC CODE). Ribosomal RNA (rRNA) together with ribosomal protein form the ribosomes. Transfer RNA (tRNA) is responsible for transporting specific amino acid molecules to mRNA or the ribosome during protein synthesis. See also DNA; RNA.

nucleophilic. Describing electron-rich substituents on organic molecules which react readily with electrophiles to form covalent bonds. Many of the reactive metabolites produced by oxidative metabolism of xenobiotics are potent electrophiles (e.g., epoxides) and thus the nature of their reaction with nucleophiles in the cell is critical in determining the ultimate toxicity of the parent xenobiotic. If they react with nucleophilic groups on proteins, as does the trichloromethyl radical produced from carbon tetrachloride, organ toxicity, in this case hepatotoxicity, results. If they react with nucleophilic groups on DNA, as does the epoxide group of benzo[a]pyrene-diol-epoxide, the initial event in a chain of events that may lead to tumor formation has occurred. On the other hand, reaction with the sulfhydryl group of glutathione is a well-known detoxication mechanism for electrophilic compounds. *Compare* ELECTROPHILES. *See also* CARCINOGENESIS; HEPATOTOXICITY.

nucleoplasm. The protoplasm within the nucleus of the cell in contrast to the cytoplasm, which exists outside the nucleus. *Compare* CYTOPLASM.

nucleoside. Compound containing a nitrogenous base (usually a pyrimidine or a purine derivative) attached to a sugar (usually one of the pentoses D-ribose and D-2-deoxyribose). A covalent bond joins C-1 of the sugar to either N-1 or a pyrimidine or to N-9 of a purine in a β-glycosidic bond. The common nucleosides derived from RNA are cytosine, uridine, adenosine and guanosine (containing ribose); those from DNA are deoxycytidine, thymidine, deoxyadenosine and deoxyguanosine (containing deoxyribose). Other nucleosides (naturally occurring or synthetic) act as cytotoxic drugs (e.g., cytosine arabinoside), or have antibiotic (e.g., puromycin, cordycepin) or antiviral (e.g., adenine arabinoside, 5-iododeoxyuridine, acycloguanosine, 3′-azidothymidine) properties. *See also* NUCLEOTIDE.

nucleotide. Phosphate or pyrophosphate ester of a nucleoside. Phosphorylation at the 5′-carbon or the pentose is usually implied, although 2′- and 3′-phosphates and 3′,5′-cyclic phosphates occur. Nucleotides are the monomeric units of DNA and RNA, those in DNA being deoxycytidylic acid (deoxycytidine monophosphate, dCMP), thymidylic acid (thymidine monophosphate, TMP), deoxyadenylic acid (deoxyadenosine monophosphate, dAMP) and deoxyguanylic acid (deoxyguanosine monophosphate, dGMP). Nucleotides commonly found in RNA are cytidylic acid (cytidine monophosphate, CMP), uridylic acid (uridine monophosphate, UMP), adenylic acid (adenosine monophosphate, AMP) and guanylic acid (guanosine monophosphate, GMP). The nucleotide structure is present also in the nucleotide coenzymes (e.g., NAD,$^+$ FAD), and in coenzyme A. Other nucleotide derivatives include the nucleoside diphosphate sugars (e.g., uridine diphosphate glucose) used in the synthesis of glycosidic bonds, and nucleotides with regulatory functions (e.g., cyclic AMP, cyclic GMP, guanosine 3′,5′-bisdiphosphate).

5′-nucleotidase. An enzyme that hydrolyzes nucleotides to nucleosides. Its elevation in plasma is an indication of liver injury, probably cholestatic injury rather than parenchymal injury.

nucleus. Spherical or lobular structure present in most eukaryotic cells, bounded by a nuclear envelope, and containing nucleoplasm, nucleolus and chromatin. The chromatin can be resolved into discrete chromosomes at certain stages of the cell cycle. Most cells have a single nucleus. A few eukaryotic cells such as mammalian erythrocytes become anucleate when mature. The nucleus not only contains the main store of genetic material in a eukaryotic cell, but is the site of transcription and the synthesis of RNA. Translation of the RNA into protein is exclusively cytoplasmic, however, necessitating the constant passage of messenger RNA from nucleus to cytoplasm. In non-nucleated cells such as bacteria, translation and transcription are closely linked in space and time.

null cells. Lymphocytes that do not bear the cell surface markers associated with B cells (primarily immunoglobin) or T cells (Thy-1, T4, T8). These cells may represent several different cell types, possibly in various stages of differentiation and include natural killer cells. *See also* LYMPHOCYTES; NATURAL KILLER CELLS.

null hypothesis. Used in statistics as the hypothesis that there is no difference between the two (or more) populations (or conditions) that are being studied. Commonly in pure science it is desired to show that the null hypothesis is false, and that some effect exists. In toxicological screening of compounds for mutagenicity, carcinogenicity, etc. the lack of toxicity is demonstrated by proving the null hypothesis. Incorrectly rejecting the null hypothesis is termed a "type I error" and the probability of such an error is denoted by α. It is common to require α to be 0.05 or 0.01, also referred to as being significant at the 5% or 1% level respectively. Incorrectly accepting the null hypothesis is termed a "type II error", and the probability of this happening is denoted by β. (The probability of correctly rejecting the null hypothesis is $1-\beta$, and is termed the "power" of the test.) For toxicity screening the principal desire is to avoid a type II error being made, and a toxic compound being incorrectly accepted as non-toxic; whereas pure science wishes to avoid false positive results. For this reason type I errors have been referred to as "the producer's risk" (novel compound mis-classified as hazardous) and type II errors as "the consumer's risk" (novel compound mis-classified as "safe").

nutmeg. Derived from the seed of *Myristica fragens* and used as a spice in food and also for medicinal purposes. Nutmeg poisoning (rarely, if ever, fatal) involves a variety of psychological reactions and may be due to myristin elemicin derivitives found in the volatile oil fraction. The most likely are 3-methoxy-4,5-methylenedioxyamphetamine and *p*-methoxyamphetamine Contains several compounds such as myristicin that can both affect xenobiotic metabolism and have CNS effects. *See also* MYRISTICIN.

Nutrasweet. *See* ASPARTAME.

nutritional deficiencies. Diets containing a suboptimal concentration of one or more nutrients have direct deleterious effects on function and may ultimately be fatal. They may also affect the toxicity of xenobiotics to the organism. For example, thiamine deficiency sensitizes animals to the cardiotoxicity of cobalt and of arsenicals. Nutritional deficiences may also play a role in teratogenesis. *See also* NUTRITIONAL EFFECTS ON XENOBIOTIC METABOLISM; NUTRITIONAL EFFECTS ON TOXICITY; TERATOGENIC MECHANISMS.

nutritional effects on xenobiotic metabolism. Although numerous effects on xenobiotic metabolism brought about by changes in diet have been noted, they are not well understood and to date no systematic explanation can be' attempted. Frequently one xenobiotic enzyme is suppressed by a particular deficiency, whereas another is increased and at the same time the magnitude and direction of these changes vary with species, sex, age and other variables. *See also* NUTRITIONAL EFFECTS ON XENOBIOTIC METABOLISM, CARBOHYDRATE; NUTRITIONAL EFFECTS ON XENOBIOTIC METABOLISM, LIPIDS; NUTRITIONAL EFFECTS ON XENOBIOTIC METABOLISM, MICRONUTRIENTS; NUTRITION EFFECTS ON XENOBIOTIC METABOLISM, PROTEIN; NUTRITIONAL EFFECTS ON XENOBIOTIC METABOLISM, STARVATION AND DEHYDRATION.

nutritional effects on xenobiotic metabolism, carbohydrate. Little is known of the effects of high or low carbohydrate levels on xenobiotic metabolism, although in the rat, high dietary carbohydrate tends to have much the same effect as low dietary protein, reducing such activities as aminopyrine *N*-demethylase and pentobarbital hydroxylation along with a reduction in the enzymes of the cytochrome P450-dependent monooxygenase system. This may reflect the tendency of rats to regulate total calorie intake and results from low protein intake. *See also* NUTRITIONAL EFFECTS ON XENOBIOTIC METABOLISM, PROTEIN.

nutritional effects on toxicity. Changes in toxicity mediated by changes in diet are not well understood, but are probably most often the result of changes in the ability to activate or detoxify the toxicant. For example, a change in the level of azoreductase activity in rat liver caused by a low-protein diet is reflected in an increased severity in dimethylaminoazobenzene carcinogenesis. The liver carcinogen, *N*-dimethylnitrosamine, which must be activated metabolically, is almost without effect in protein-deficient rats whereas strychnine, which is detoxified by the same enzyme system, is more toxic. *See also* NUTRITIONAL EFFECTS ON XENOBIOTIC METABOLISM; NUTRITIONAL TOXICOLOGY.

nutritional effects on xenobiotic metabolism, lipids. Dietary deficiencies in linoleic or unsaturated fats bring about a reduction in cytochrome P450 and related monooxygenase activities. Lipids may also be necessary for the effect of inducers (e.g., phenobarbital) to be expressed fully.

nutritional effects on xenobiotic metabolism, micronutrients. Vitamin deficiencies in general bring about a reduction in monooxygenase activity, although there are exceptions. Riboflavin deficiency, for example, causes an increase in cytochrome P450 and aniline hydroxylation, although at the same time it causes a decrease in benzoapyrene hydroxylation. Decreases in monooxygenase activity are seen in ascorbic acid deficiency as well as in deficiencies of vitamin A and E. Changes in mineral nutrition may also affect monooxygenase activity. In the immature rat, calcium or magnesium deficiency causes a decrease, whereas iron deficiency causes an increase in activity, although not an increase in cytochrome P450. Dietary cobalt, cadmium, manganese and lead all cause an increase in hepatic glutathione levels and a decrease in cytochrome P450 content.

nutritional effects on xenobiotic metabolism, protein. Low-protein diets generally decrease monooxygenase activity, although the effects may vary with sex and the substrate. For example, in the rat, aminopyrine N-demethylation, hexobarbital hydroxylation and aniline hydroxylation activity in the liver are all decreased, but the effect on the first two is greater in males than in females, whereas for aniline hydroxylation the reduction in males and females is similar. These changes appear to be related to the concomitant reductions in the levels of cytochrome P450 and NADPH-cytochrome P450 reductase. The sex and other variations are presumably due to differential effects on cytochrome P450 isozymes. Phase II reactions may also be affected by low dietary protein. For example, chloramphenicol glucuronidation is reduced in protein-deficient guinea pigs, although protein deficiency has no effect on sulfotransferase activity in the rat. *See also* NUTRITIONAL EFFECTS ON TOXICITY.

nutritional effects on xenobiotic metabolism, starvation and dehydration. Starvation generally, but not always, has similar effects to protein deficiency. For example in the male rat, hexobarbital and pentobarbital hydroxylation are decreased, whereas aniline hydroxylation is increased. In the female, all of these activities are stimulated. Water deprivation, at least in some species, causes an increase in cytochrome P450 and hexobarbital metabolism, resulting in a shorter sleeping time. *See also* NUTRITIONAL EFFECTS ON XENOBIOTIC METABOLISM, PROTEIN.

nutritional toxicology. An important aspect of toxicology that deals with the effect of diet on the expression of toxicity and the mechanism of such effects. Areas such as the effects of dietary deficiencies on the activity and induction of xenobiotic-metabolizing enzymes have been studied. Currently there is much interest on the effect of diet on the expression of carcinogenesis and the application of this information to cancer prevention programs. *See also* NUTRITIONAL EFFECTS ON XENOBIOTIC METABOLISM; NUTRITIONAL EFFECTS ON TOXICITY.

Nux vomica alkaloids. *See* STRYCHNINE.

nystatin. *See* ANTIBIOTICS.

O

obligate anaerobe. *See* ANAEROBIC.

obligate nose breathers. Animals that must breathe through the nose rather than through the nose and mouth, such as rats and mice. While human infants are obligate nose breathers, adults can breathe through either nose or mouth. The difference is significant in toxicology, particularly toxicity testing, since the nasopharyngeal region may remove toxicants before they reach the lungs, with such early removal not occurring during mouth breathing.

occupational exposure limit (OEL). Generally the time-weighted average concentrations of an airborne toxicant to which a worker may be exposed during a defined work period.

occupational exposure standard (OES). Occupational exposure standard [usually expressed in air in ppm or mg/m^3, for long-term exposure (8-hour TWA reference period) or short-term exposure (10-minute reference period)] under COSHH Regulations. *See also* conTROL OF SUBSTANCES HAZARDOUS TO HEALTH REGULATIONS.

occupational hazards, poisoning. Many types of poisoning tend to be associated with particular occupations, the following being illustrative examples. Carbon monoxide poisoning may occur among blacksmiths, furnace or foundry workers, brick or cement makers, chimney cleaners, service station attendants, parking attendants, garage workers, miners, refinery workers, plumbers, police officers and sewer workers. Poisoning by chlorinated hydrocarbon solvents is known to occur among rubber cement and plastic cement workers or users, leather workers, dry cleaners, painters, furniture finishers, cloth finishers, paint removers and rubber workers. Lead poisoning may occur among welders, steamfitters, plumbers, painters, ceramic workers, battery makers, miners, pottery makers, electroplaters, printers, service station attendants and junk metal refiners. Methanol poisoning may occur among bookbinders, bronzers, rubber and plastic cement users, dry cleaners, leather workers, printers, painters and woodworkers.

Occupational Safety and Health Act. Administered by the US Occupational Safety and Health Administration (OSHA), this Act regulates health and safety in the workplace. The Act sets standards for worker exposure to specific chemicals, for air concentration values and for monitoring procedures. Construction and environmental controls also come under this act. In addition it provides for research, information, education and training in occupational safety and health. NIOSH (National Institute for Occupational Safety and Health) was established under this act to provide for appropriate studies to ensure that regulatory decisions be based on the best information available.

Occupational Safety and Health Administration (OSHA). In the USA, the government department concerned with health and safety in the workplace. *See also* OCCUPATIONAL SAFETY AND HEALTH ACT.

ochratoxins. A group of toxins produced by *Aspergillus ochraceus* and *Penicillium viridicatum*, the three most important being named ochratoxin A, B and C. Of these, ochratoxin A ((R)-*N*-((5-chloro-3,4-dihydro-8-hydroxy-3-methyl-1-oxo-1H-2-benzopyran-7-yl) carbonyl)-L-phenylalanine), CAS number 303-47-9, is considered the major component. Ochratoxins are frequently found as natural contaminants on peanuts, corn and stored grains. Toxic to humans and livestock but human carcinogenicity is not well proven. There is some limited experimental evidence that ochratoxin A is carcinogenic to animals. *See also* LEWIS, HCDR, NUMBER CHP250.

odorants. Chemicals detected by the sense of smell (olfaction). There are hundreds of distinct odorant receptors in the nasal epithelium, each sensitive to different types of chemicals. This makes the nose a sensitive chemical detector. *See also* ODOROUS COMPOUNDS.

odorous compounds, in water. Odorous compounds contaminating water supplies include chemicals with both industrial or microbiological origins. Industrially derived contaminants include phenol, chlorinated products of phenol, formaldehyde, methylamine, dichloroisopropyl ether, ethylbenzene, 2-methyl-5-ethylpyridine, naphthalene, phenylmethylcarbinol, 1,2,3,4-tetrahydronaphthalene, various chlorinated and non-chlorinated terpenes and sesquiterpenes, alkyl-substituted benzenes and bicyclic aromatics. Biologically derived odorous contaminants include the terpenoid geosmin, 2-methylisoborneol, cadin-4-ene-1-ol, selina-4(14), 7(11)-diene-9-ol, 6-pentyl-α-pyrone, 2-isopropyl-3-methoxypyrazine, *n*-heptanal, mucidone, 1-phenyl-2-propanone, 2-phenylethanol and 5-methyl-3-heptanone. These compounds have created difficulty by reducing the aesthetic quality of drinking and recreational water and by accumulating in aquatic animals (e.g., catfish) thereby reducing the quality of food sources. Few treatments have proven effective in eliminating the odors from water. Although the toxicity of these odorous compounds is not well documented, the toxicity of some similar compounds to higher animals is low.

ODW. *See* OFFICE OF DRINKING WATER.

OECD. *See* ORGANIZATION FOR ECONOMIC COOPERATION AND DEVELOPMENT.

OEL. *See* OCCUPATIONAL EXPOSURE LIMIT.

OES. *See* OCCUPATIONAL EXPOSURE STANDARD.

oestrogen. *See* ESTROGEN.

oestrus. *See* ESTRUS.

Office of Drinking Water (ODW). A division of the US Environmental Protection Agency concerned with the establishment of standards for minimum contamination of drinking water by chemicals and with the regulation of drinking water standards established under federal law.

Office of Pesticide Programs (OPP). A division of the US Environmental Protection Agency (EPA) responsible for the administration of the Federal Insecticide, Fungicide and Rodenticide Act (FIFRA) and for the development of toxicity testing protocols necessary for registration of a pesticide under this act. It operates with the advice and counsel of the FIFRA Scientific Advisory Panel (SAP) comprising a group of non-federal experts. *See also* ENVIRONMENTAL PROTECTION AGENCY; FEDERAL INSECTICIDE, FUNGICIDE AND RODENTICIDE ACT.

Office of Pesticides and Toxic Substances. A division of the US Environmental Protection charged with the administration of federal laws concerning pesticides (e.g., FIFRA) and other chemicals (e.g., TSCA).

Office of Toxic Substances (OTS). A division of the US Environmental Protection Agency.

oil of turpentine. *See* TURPENTINE.

oil spills. The unintentional discharge of crude oil or other petroleum-based liquids into the environment. Oil spills receiving the greatest amount of attention have occurred in the marine environment due to damage to oil tankers or accidents at off-shore drilling rigs and have involved large quantities of oil. The most prominent feature of these massive spills is the damage caused when they reach the shoreline. Although large spills in the marine environment receive worldwide attention, a greater total volume of oil is spilled in the freshwater environment. The immediate effects of oil spills on the ecosystem are usually evident in the form of oil-covered birds, dead fish and the destruction of breeding grounds for marine and estuarine sea life. Environmentalists are particularly concerned about the potential long-term chronic effects, such as disruption of chemotactic responses in certain species, carcinogenic effects of certain constituents in oil, etc. A variety of techniques have been suggested either to contain the oil in a restricted area or to emulsify and disperse the oil to avoid shoreline contamination by the less volatile tars. *See also* ENVIRONMENTAL DISASTERS.

oleander. The common oleander is *Nerium oleander*; the yellow oleander is *Thevetia peruviana* or *T. thevetioides*. All are large evergreen shrubs that are poisonous due to the presence of cardiac glycosides. Common oleander contains at least five cardiac glycosides: oleandrin, digitoxigenin, neriin, folinerin and rosagenin. Although oleander extracts have been used for medicinal purposes, these plants have been recognized as dangerously toxic for centuries.

olfactory. Pertaining to the sense of smell. The olfactory mucosa, located in the nasal turbinates, is important in toxicology for two reasons: (1) it is a rich source of cytochrome P450 and monooxygenase reactions; (2) it is subject to xenobiotic-derived nasal cancer. The latter may be due, in some cases, to the formation of reactive intermediates by isozymes of cytochrome P450.

oligomycin. *See* OXIDATIVE PHOSPHORYLATION INHIBITORS.

oncogenes. Genes that, when activated in cells, can transform the cells from normal to neoplastic. Sometimes oncogenes are carried into normal cells by infecting viruses, particularly RNA viruses or retroviruses. In some cases, however, the oncogene is already present in the normal human cell; it needs only a mutation or other activating event to change it from a harmless, and possibly essential gene, called a proto-oncogene, into a cancer-producing gene. More than 30 oncogenes have been identified in humans. *See also* PROTO-ONCOGENES.

oncology. The study of cancer. *See also* CANCER; CARCINOGEN; CARCINOGENESIS; CARCINOGENICITY.

oncoviruses. *See* RETROVIRUSES.

one-compartment model. A pharmacokinetic model that represents the body as being a single homogeneous unit. This model is most useful for substances that distribute rapidly throughout the body. The blood or plasma is usually used as a reference compartment, and it is assumed that the rate of change of concentration in plasma is a quantitative reflection of the rate of concentration changes in other tissues. Pharmacokinetic parameters that can be calculated from this model include the elimination rate constant, half-life and apparent volume of distribution. The elimination rate constant is typically first-order, but nonlinear kinetics may also be observed, especially after high doses. The pharmacokinetic parameters can be calculated after dosing by various exposure routes including intravenous, oral, intramuscular, dermal or inhalation. *See also* COMPARTMENT; KINETIC EQUATIONS; MULTI-COMPARTMENT MODELS; PHARMACOKINETICS; TOXICOKINETICS; TWO-COMPARTMENT MODEL; VOLUME OF DISTRIBUTION.

one-hit model. *See* LOW-DOSE EXTRAPOLATION.

oocyte. An immature ovum or egg. A stage leading to the formation of a mature ovum or egg.

oogenesis. The process of ovum (egg) formation involving a progression from the stem cell (oogonium) through the primary oocyte and secondary oocyte to the ovum. During this progression, meiosis occurs to produce a haploid gamete. The two meiotic divisions each produce one viable cell with the majority of the cytoplasm and one polar body that has little cytoplasm and degenerates. Therefore, in contrast to spermatogenesis, only one viable gamete is produced for each cell going through oogenesis. The initial stages of the process occur in the ovarian follicle, and the second meiotic division occurs after fertilization.

opiates. *See* NARCOTICS; OPIOIDS.

OPIDN (organophosphate-induced delayed neuropathy). *See* DELAYED NEUROPATHY.

opioids. A group of endogenous peptide chemical messengers (i.e., neurotransmitters/modulators) whose receptors are the target of opiate drugs (e.g., morphine or codeine) and their derivatives. Some classes of opioid peptides include the enkephalins, the endorphins and the dynorphins. Receptors for these peptides occur not only in the CNS, but also in the gastrointestinal tract and other areas of the body. Drugs or toxicants occupying these receptors cause characteristic physiological responses (*See* MORPHINE). The receptors for the endogenous opioids are divided into three major classes: μ; κ; and δ. The μ-receptor is involved in the production of supraspinal anesthesia, respiratory depression, euphoria and physical dependence. Stimulation of κ-receptors results in spinal analgesia, miosis and sedation. The δ-receptors are responsible for dysphoria and hallucinations, as well as respiratory and vasomotor stimulatory effects. *See also* NARCOTICS; OPIUM.

Prototypical drugs for opioid receptors
morphine (R_1 = OH; R_2 = OH)
heroin (R_1 = OCOCH$_3$; R_2 = OCOCH$_3$)

opium (gum opium; crude opium). The air-dried, milky exudation from incised unripe capsules of *Papaver somniferum*. This resin contains two groups of alkaloids: phenanthrenes (including morphine and codeine) and benzylisoquinolines (including papaverine). Morphine is by far the most prevalent alkaloid (10–16%) in opium, and its pharmacological properties account for the licit and illicit use of opium. *See also* CODEINE; HEROIN; MORPHINE; NARCOTICS.

opium alkaloids. Extracted from exudate of unripe capsules of *Papaver somniferum*. *See also* OPIUM.

OPP. *See* OFFICE OF PESTICIDE PROGRAMS.

OPs (organophosphates). *See* ORGANOPHOSPHORUS INSECTICIDES.

optical difference spectra. Absorption spectra in which only the difference in optical density between two samples is recorded. Such spectra are usually used to measure the effect of a ligand on the absorption spectrum of a chromophore under conditions that make difficult the measurement of absolute spectra. Using a split-beam instrument with the chromophore in both cuvettes, a flat baseline is recorded as the two absolute spectra balance each other. On the addition of a reactive ligand to one cuvette, the difference in the absolute spectrum caused by the ligand interaction can be recorded rather than the absolute spectrum of the ligand-chromophore complex. Since particulate enzyme preparations scatter light and light scattering is a function of wavelength, the technique is particularly useful for the characterization of particulate enzymes such as mitochondrial and microsomal cytochromes, where absolute spectra would be seen as variations along a sloping baseline. *See also* CARBON MONOXIDE BINDING, SPECTRAL; CARBOXYHEMOGLOBIN; CYTOCHROME P450, OPTICAL DIFFERENCE SPECTRA.

OPTS. *See* OFFICE OF PESTICIDES AND TOXIC SUBSTANCES.

oral dosing. *See* ADMINISTRATION OF TOXICANTS, ORAL.

organelle evaluation. Cellular organelles (e.g., mitochondria, lysosomes, nuclei, endoplasmic reticulum) may all be affected by toxicants. They may also be involved in toxicant metabolism, and reactive metabolites may mediate the toxic effects. Numerous methods have been used to measure such effects, although none are required by regulatory agencies as part of a toxicity testing protocol. All organelles may be examined for structural changes by electron microscopy, utilizing heavy metal staining, negative staining or freeze-etch techniques. Structural changes can be quantitated by the techniques of ultrastructural morphometry. Biochemical tests either measure marker enzymes characteristic of the organelle in question or measure some function of the particular organelle. The validity of these tests depends on the method of preparation, usually homogenization in an appropriate medium followed by differential centrifugation. Ionic strength, pH and chemical nature of the medium, as well as the temperature and method of homogenization, are all important and must be optimized for each cell type. Tests useful for mitochondrial function include oxygen uptake, oxidative phosphorylation, dehydrogenase enzymes (e.g., malate dehydrogenase), enzymes of heme biosynthesis (e.g., δ-aminolevulinic acid synthetase) and mitochondrial protein synthesis. Marker enzymes for lysosomes include cathespins A, B, C and D, acid phosphatase, aryl sulfatase and acid ribonuclease. Microsomal enzymes utilized in testing include those of the cytochrome P450-dependent monooxygenase system and UDP glucuronosyltransferase. *See also* ENDOPLASMIC RETICULUM; LYSOSOMES; MITOCHONDRIA.

Organization for Economic Cooperation and Development (OECD). An international group of experts from several nations appointed for the production of a set of guidelines for toxicity testing that would be fully acceptable to a number of regulatory bodies within the various countries regardless of where the test is actually carried out. Guidelines for acute oral, dermal and inhalation studies, eye and skin irritation and sensitization, subchronic oral, dermal and inhalation studies, as well as teratogenicity and carcinogenicity studies have all been developed by OECD. OECD Test Guidelines: OECD Expert Group on Good Laboratory Practices (OECD, Paris, 1980). OECD Test Guidelines: Report from the OECD Expert Group on Short Term and Long Term Toxicity (OECD, Paris, 1981). *See also* REGULATORY REQUIREMENTS.

organochlorine insecticides. A large, chemically heterogeneous group of toxic chemicals discussed in more detail under more specific headings. The group contains the cyclodienes (e.g., aldrin), the substituted ethanes (e.g., DDT), cyclohexane derivatives (e.g., lindane) and the complex mixture of chlorinated terpinoids collectively referred to as toxaphene. The only chemical feature in common is the presence of chlorine substituents on an organic parent compound. Despite their earlier importance in agriculture and public health, as a class they are becoming less important

due to problems concerning chronic toxicity, persistence in the environment and, in some cases, *in vivo*, and resistance of pest species to their toxic effects. *See also* CHLORDECONE; CYCLODIENE INSECTICIDES; DDT; LINDANE; MIREX; TOXAPHENE.

organogenesis. The formation of organs and organ systems during development. *See also* ORGANOGENESIS PERIOD.

organogenesis period. The developmental period during which cells migrate, associate and differentiate in such a way as to form the rudiments of the major organs and organ systems. Although all organs are not formed at the same time, they do tend to differentiate at times close to one another during the period of organogenesis, and thus their development is either simultaneous or overlapping. The period of organogenesis is relatively shorter in animals with long gestation periods. For example, in the mouse it is days 6–15 in a 19-day gestation, whereas in humans it is days 21–56 in a 267-day gestation. The period of organogenesis is the most critical for teratogenic effects of chemicals with shorter periods of sensitivity within this time for specific organ systems. *See also* TERATOLOGY TESTING.

organoleptic. Organoleptics are chemicals in the diet that are neither micronutrients nor macronutrients, but rather add flavor, texture, color or aroma to food. If an organoleptic chemical is added to the diet, it is regulated in the USA under the Food, Drug and Cosmetic Act as a food additive. If it is a natural constituent of a foodstuff, it is regulated under the same act but under a different, less stringent, set of standards. *See also* FOOD ADDITIVES.

organometals. Chemical forms of toxic metals in which covalent (or coordinate covalent) bonds exist between the metal and the organic moiety. These forms are often of markedly different toxicity to the inorganic forms of the same metal. Although this may sometimes be due to pharmacokinetic factors (i.e., more of the metal may be concentrated in a sensitive tissue), the intrinsic toxicity of the organometal is often different. *See also* METHYLMERCURY; TRIETHYLLEAD; TRIETHYLTIN; TRIMETHYLTIN; TOXIC METALS.

organophosphate-induced delayed neuropathy (OPIDN). *See* DELAYED NEUROPATHY.

organophosphate poisoning, symptoms and therapy. Organophosphates exert their toxic effects by inhibition of acetylcholinesterase, thus preventing the breakdown of acetylcholine, a situation in which the acetylcholine receptors remain occupied. Since death is the result of respiratory failure, the maintenance of an adequate airway and artificial respiration are of critical importance. Two forms of specific therapy are available. Atropine is used immediately since it competes with acetylcholine for the receptor site, thus preventing the toxic effects of an excess of this neurotransmitter. Subsequently, *N*-methylpyridinium-2-aldoxime (2-PAM) is used in conjunction with atropine, since it reacts with the phosphorylated cholinesterase and removes the phosphorylating group, restoring the enzyme to normal activity. The combination of 2-PAM and atropine is synergistic, being up to 50 times more effective than might be expected from a simple additive effect. *See also* ACETYLCHOLINESTERASE; ATROPINE; *N*-METHYLPYRIDINIUM-2-ALDOXIME.

organophosphorus insecticides (organophosphates; OPs). Phosphates with the generalized structural formulas shown below. They include insecticides such as parathion, malathion and phorate. The first organophosphate used as an insecticide was tetraethylpyrophosphate (TEPP), developed in Germany in 1942. It was highly toxic to mammals, however, as well as being rapidly hydrolyzed. In 1944, parathion and its oxygen analog paraoxon were synthesized in Germany by Schrader. Because of its wide range of insecticidal action and stability in water, it became widely marketed. The mode of action of OPs is the inhibition of acetylcholinesterase (AChE); this inhibition blocks the hydrolysis of the AChE substrate acetylcholine (ACh), a neurotransmitter. The toxic action of OPs is a result of excess stimulation at the neuromuscular junction by an accumulation of acetylcholine, although all synapses using acetylcholine are affected. The active form of the organophosphate is the oxon (P=O), the thion (P=S) being converted *in vivo* to the oxon by the cytochrome P450 monooxygenase system; the oxon then phosphorylates the active site of AChE. The phosphorylated enzyme is only very slowly hydrolyzed to yield free AChE. *See also* ACETYLCHOLINESTERASE; ACETYLCHOLINE; ANTICHOLINESTERASES.

organotins. Dialkyl tins, such as di-*n*-octyltin, are used primarily as heat stabilizers and catalysts while trialkyl tins are used primarily as pesticides. Di-*n*-octyltin is an immunotoxicant, with the primary target appearing to be the T-cells. Tributyltin oxide, CAS number 56-35-9, also causes a reversible atrophy of the thymus and affects the immune system in a number of ways. Like the

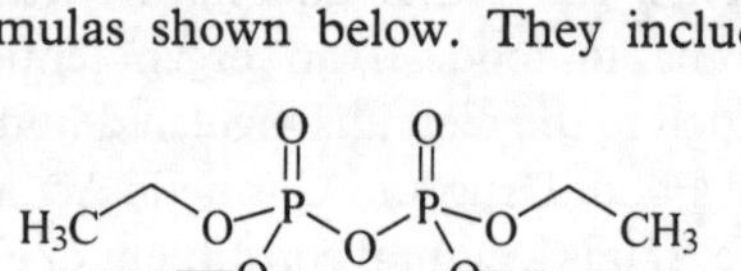

TEPP

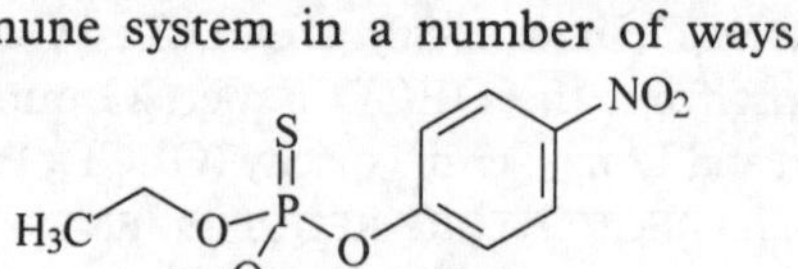

Parathion

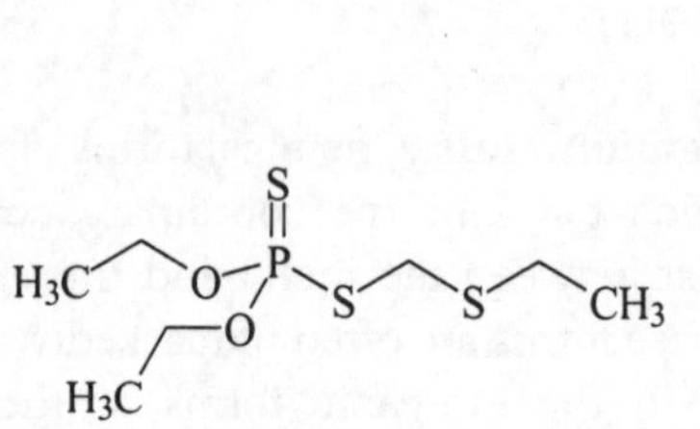

Phorate

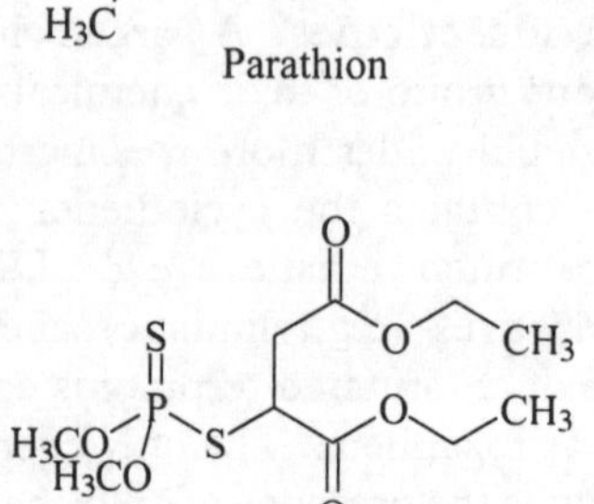

Malathion

Organophosphorus insecticides

dialkyl tins it appears to exert its most significant effects on the T-cells. *See also* DATABASES, TOXICOLOGY; LEWIS, HCDR NUMBER BLL750.

organ toxicity. Any detrimental change in organ physiology, biochemistry or morphology. Toxicants may cause organ toxicity by acting directly on the organ in question or indirectly via disruption of normal physiological mechanisms, including changes in circulation, which can secondarily cause poisoning of a cell. *See also* HEPATOTOXICITY; NEPHROTOXICITY; NEUROTOXICITY; POISON; TOXIC ENDPOINTS.

organ weights, in chronic toxicity testing. *See* TOXIC ENDPOINTS.

organ weights, in subchronic toxicity testing. *See* TOXIC ENDPOINTS.

ornithine carbamyl transferase (ornithine transcarbamoylase). An enzyme that catalyzes the transfer of a carbamyl group from carbamyl phosphate to ornithine to form citrulline; it is a constituent reaction of the urea cycle. This enzyme normally occurs in the mitochondria of liver cells, but only to a minute extent in serum. Since it does not occur to a significant extent in serum, kidney, brain, etc., and only 1 or 2% of the hepatic concentration occurs in small intestine, its presence in serum is a specific indication of damage to liver cells.

ornithine conjugation. An amino acid-conjugating reaction that occurs most commonly in reptiles and birds. It differs from other amino acid conjugations in the nature of the amino acid substrate, which is in this case the non-protein amino acid ornithine ($H_2N(CH_2)_3CH(NH_2)COOH$). *See also* AMINO ACID CONJUGATION; PHASE II REACTIONS.

orosomucoid. *See* α_1-ACID GLYCOPROTEIN.

OSHA. *See* OCCUPATIONAL SAFETY AND HEALTH ADMINISTRATION.

osteolathyrism. *See* LATHYRISM.

osteoporosis. A condition in which bones become weakened, primarily because of the reduction in sex hormones in later years. The sex hormones support bone formation and maintenance. Osteoporosis is particularly prevalent in postmenopausal women and results in numerous stress fractures and broken bones.

OTBE. *See* TRIBUTYLTIN.

OTS. *See* OFFICE OF TOXIC SUBSTANCES.

ouabain   (3-[(6-deoxy-α-l-mannopyranosyl)oxy]-1,5,11α,14,19-pentahydroxycard-20(22)-enolide;   G-strophanthin).   CAS number 630-60-4. One of several cardiac glycosides that have been used clinically as cardiotonic agents and diuretics. Ouabain is obtained from the seeds of *Strophanthus gratus*, *Acokanthera ouabaio* and related species. It was formerly prescribed under the name strophanthuis as the purified seed extract. Ouabain acts as an inhibitor of Na^+/K^+-ATPase, and radioreceptor studies have demonstrated the high affinity binding of ouabain to Na^+/K^+-ATPases. The sensitivity of Na^+/K^+-ATPase to ouabain differs markedly among tissues, with the rat brain enzyme being much more sensitive than the ventricle or kidney enzyme. The i.v. LD50 in rats is 14 mg/kg, with males being more sensitive than females. *See also* CARDIAC GLYCOSIDES; DIGITALIS; NA^+/K^+-ATPASE.

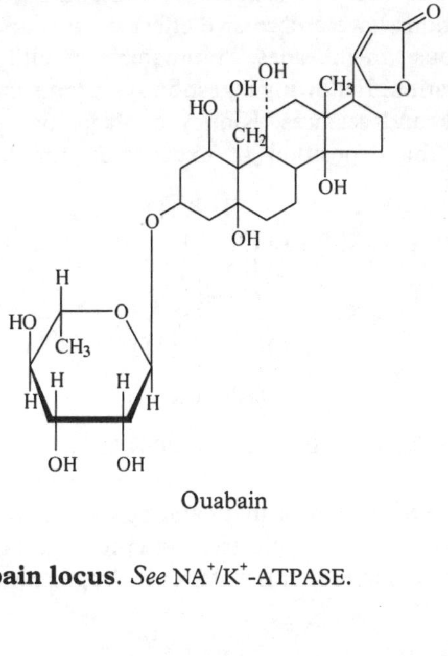

Ouabain

ouabain locus. *See* NA^+/K^+-ATPASE.

ovary. The female gonad responsible for production of the female germ cells (the ova) and of the female sex hormones (the estrogens and progesterone). The active structure within the ovary is the follicle, which develops the ovum and secretes estrogens until ovulation. Following ovulation, the remainder of the follicle involutes and becomes converted into the corpus luteum, which secretes estrogens and progesterone. The above progression occurs for a new follicle or set of follicles with each cycle of the adenohypophyseal gonadotropins; follicle maturation is controlled by follicle-stimulating hormone (FSH) and ovulation and corpus luteum development is controlled by luteinizing hormone (LH).

ovotoxicity. The deleterious effects exhibited in an ovum due to exposure to a toxicant during development, but prior to fertilization.

ovum. The female gamete or egg.

oxalic acid (dicarboxylic acid). CAS number 144-62-7. An acid used in the manufacture of dyes, bleaches, paint removers, dextrin, celluloid, tartaric acid and glycerol. It is also used in a number of industries, including the photographic, engraving and lithographic industries, as well as the metallurgic and pharmaceutical industries. In the workplace the principal route of entry is inhalation of aerosols of oxalic acid solutions, but uptake may also occur by skin absorption and ingestion. Solutions have a corrosive effect on the skin and mucous membranes, ultimately resulting in ulceration. Following ingestion symptoms include shock and seizures. Kidney damage may occur with the deposition of oxalates in the kidney tubules.

$$\underset{HO}{\overset{\displaystyle O}{\underset{\displaystyle \diagup}{\|}}}C - \underset{OH}{\overset{\displaystyle O}{\underset{\displaystyle \diagdown}{\|}}}C$$

Oxalic acid

oxazepam. *See* BENZODIAZEPINES.

oxidases. Enzymes that catalyze oxidation reactions in which the electron acceptor (oxidant) is oxygen, the product is water or hydrogen peroxide (H_2O_2), and the oxygen atoms are not incorporated into the product of the reaction. For example, amino acid oxidases are flavoproteins that catalyze the oxygen-requiring oxidation of amino acids to keto acids with the concomitant formation of hydrogen peroxide. Perhaps the most important example of an oxidase is the cytochrome oxidase which uses electrons from an electron transport chain plus protons from the surrounding medium to reduce oxygen to water. *Compare* OXYGENASES.

oxidation. Formerly oxidation was regarded as a chemical reaction with oxygen; the reverse process, the loss of oxygen, was called reduction. A more general definition, which combines both oxidation and reduction, is that oxidation involves a loss of electrons and reduction a gain of electrons:

$$\text{oxidized state} + ne \underset{\text{oxidation}}{\overset{\text{reduction}}{\rightleftharpoons}} \text{reduced state}$$

Since oxidation and reduction occur simultaneously, two redox systems are always involved.

$$red_1 + ox_2 \rightarrow red_2 + ox_1$$

Every electrode is based on this reaction involving the transfer of electrons, so that when two electrodes are joined in a cell, oxidation occurs at the anode and reduction at the cathode.

***N*-oxidation (nitrogen oxidation)**. Oxidative attack on a nitrogen atom in an organic molecule. Metabolic *N*-oxidation is important in toxicology and can occur in several ways: hydroxylamine (R-NOH) formation, often leading to nitroso (R-NO) and possibly nitro (R-NO₂) products; *N*-oxide formation. The former reaction sequence often is catalyzed by cytochrome P450, the latter by the FAD-containing monooxygenases. Other oxidized nitrogen metabolites include nitroxides (R-NO), oximes (RC=N-O-R) and azoxy compounds (R-N(O)=N-R). Hydroxylamine formation occurs with amines such as aniline and its substituted derivatives. The product of *N*-2-acetylaminofluorene *N*-oxidation is a potent carcinogen and thus, in this case, the reaction is an activation reaction. Oximes can be formed by the *N*-hydroxylation of imines and primary amines.

See also N-2-ACETYLAMINOFLUORENE; CYTO-CHROME P450-DEPENDENT MONOOXYGENASE SYSTEM; FAD-CONTAINING MONOOXYGENASE.

P-oxidation (phosphorus oxidation). Oxidative attack on a phosphorus atom in an organic molecule. The conversion of trisubstituted phosphines to phosphine oxides, such as the oxidation of diphenylmethylphosphine to diphenylmethylphosphine oxide, is not a common metabolic reaction. Formerly thought to be cytochrome P450-dependent monooxygenations phosphines are now known to be oxidized more rapidly by the FAD-containing monooxygenase. *See also* CYTOchrome P450-dependent monooxygenase system; FAD-containing monooxygenase.

S-oxidation (sulfur oxidation). Oxidative attack on a sulfur atom in an organic compound. Metabolic S-oxidation of xenobiotics is an important reaction in the metabolism of drugs and xenobiotics, and is catalyzed by both the FAD-containing monooxygenase and cytochrome P450. Thioethers are oxidized by both of these microsomal monooxygenases to sulfoxides, which may be further oxidized to sulfones. Insecticides of several different chemical classes, including carbamates, organophosphates and chlorinated hydrocarbons are substrates for this reaction. The organophosphates phorate, demeton and others are oxidized to sulfoxides and sulfones, the chlorinated hydrocarbon endosulfan is oxidized to endosulfan sulfate and methiochlor, through a series of sulfoxides and sulfones, to the bissulfone. The carbamate methiocarb is oxidized to the sulfoxide and sulfone, and drugs such as chloropromazine and solvents such as dimethyl sulfoxide, are also subject to S-oxidation. Other sulfur-containing substrates for the FAD-containing monooxygenase include thiols, sulfides and thiocarbamates. The relative role of the two monooxygenases in the oxidation of particular substrate is currently of much interest. *See also* CYTOCHROME P450-DEPENDENT MONOOXYGENASE SYSTEM; FAD-CONTAINING MONOOXYGENASE.

β-oxidation, fatty acids. The principal route for the oxidation of fatty acids. It occurs in the mitochondria and is catalyzed by a series of enzymes that metabolize the fatty acid, in the form of an acyl CoA, to an acetyl CoA and an acyl CoA with a carbon chain two carbon atoms shorter than the original. The initial attack is at the carbon adjacent to the carboxyl group, hence β-oxidation. The process can be repeated until the carbon chain has been broken down into two-carbon units (acetyl CoA). This is an important source of energy since the β-oxidation sequence yields NADH and $FADH_2$, and the acetyl CoA is further oxidized by the tricarboxylic acid cycle. For example, the complete oxidation of one mole of palmitic acid yields 129 moles of ATP. Decreased β-oxidation of fatty acids is a characteristic of fatty liver which results from certain chemical hepatotoxicants (e.g., ethanol). In this case the decreased oxidation is due to the accumulation of acetyl CoA since ethanol affects its oxidation via the tricarboxylic acid cycle. *See also* ω-OXIDATION, FATTY ACIDS; HEPATO-TOXICITY. (*See* equation below.)

ω-oxidation, fatty acids. The oxidation that takes place at the methyl end (i.e., remote from the carboxyl group) of the carbon chain. Both ω- and $ω^{-1}$-oxidations are catalyzed by isozymes of cytochrome P450 in liver and in the kidney. Although it is probable that the liver isozymes involved also oxidize some xenobiotics, oxidation of fatty acids such as laurate appears to be a characteristic as well as somewhat specific reaction for an isozyme of cytochrome P450 found in the kidney. The physiological significance of ω-oxidation of fatty acids is not known. *See also* CYTOCHROME P450, SUBSTRATE SPECIFICITY.

$$n\text{-acyl CoA} + \text{E-FAD} \xrightarrow{\text{acyl CoA dehydrogenase}} trans\text{-}\Delta^2\text{-enoyl CoA} + \text{E-FADH}_2$$

$$trans\text{-}\Delta^2\text{-enoyl Coa} + \text{H}_2\text{O} \xrightarrow{\text{enoyl CoA hydrolase}} \text{L-3-hydroxyacyl CoA}$$

$$\text{L-3-hydroxyacyl CoA} + \text{NAD}^+ \xrightarrow{\text{L-3-hydroxyacyl CoA dehydrogenase}} \text{3-ketoacyl CoA} + \text{NADH} + \text{H}^+$$

$$\text{3-ketoacyl CoA} + \text{CoA} \xrightarrow{\beta\text{-ketothiolase}} \text{acetyl CoA} + (n-2)\text{-acyl CoA}$$

$$R_2CHNH_2 \longrightarrow R_2C(OH)NH_2 \underset{\searrow}{\overset{\nearrow}{}} \begin{array}{l} R_2C{=}O \\[1em] R_2C{-}NH{-}R_2CNOH{-}R_2C{=}O \end{array}$$

Oxidative deamination

oxidation via the tricarboxylic acid cycle. A multi-enzyme pathway formerly known as the citric acid cycle (named for one of the intermediates in the cycle), this is the principal mechanism by which cells oxidize two carbon units, in the form of acetyl co-enzyme A, to yield ATP. The two carbon units are derived from carbohydrates (via glycolysis), from fatty acids (primarily by β-oxidation) and, to a lesser extent, from amino acid degradation.

oxidative deamination. The removal of an amino group from an organic compound, catalyzed by cytochrome P450 and yielding a ketone and ammonia. Deamination of amphetamine, a well-known example, occurs in rabbit liver, but not in dog or rat, both of which hydroxylate the aromatic ring. The reaction is probably not an attack on the nitrogen atom, but rather on the adjacent carbon atom, giving rise to a carbinol amine, which eliminates ammonia, producing a ketone. Another reaction sequence gives rise to an oxime, which is hydrolyzed to yield the ketone. Thus the ketone can be formed by two different metabolic routes. (*See* equation above.)

oxidative desulfuration. *See* DESULFURATION AND OXIDATIVE ESTER CLEAVAGE.

oxidative ester cleavage. *See* DESULFURATION AND OXIDATIVE ESTER CLEAVAGE.

oxidative phosphorylation. The conservation of chemical energy extracted from metabolic oxidations by the phosphorylation of adenosine diphosphate (ADP) by inorganic phosphate to form adenosine triphosphate (ATP) is accomplished at several locations in the energy metabolism pathways. Although a small amount of ATP is formed in glycolysis and the tricarboxylic acid cycle, the majority of ATP is formed by respiratory chain-linked oxidative phosphorylation associated with the electron transport system (respiratory chain,

cytochrome chain) in the mitochondrial inner membrane. In this system, the oxidations are tightly coupled to the phosphorylations through a chemiosmotic mechanism, which uses the energy of the oxidations to pump H^+ across the inner mitochondrial membrane into the intermembrane space, creating an electrochemical proton gradient equivalent to about 160 mV and 1 pH unit. The protons diffuse back to the mitochondrial matrix through an enzyme complex, ATP synthetase (F_oF_1 ATPase), that phosphorylates ADP. Uncouplers of oxidative phosphorylation serve as H^+ ionophores to dissipate the H^+ gradient and thus uncouple the phosphorylations from the oxidations. *See also* ELECTRON TRANSPORT SYSTEM, MITOCHONDRIAL; ELECTRON TRANSPORT SYSTEM INHIBITORS; OXIDATIVE PHOSPHORYLATION INHIBITORS.

oxidative phosphorylation inhibitors. Uncouplers of oxidative phosphorylation uncouple the phosphorylation of ADP to form ATP from the transfer of electrons occurring in the mitochondrial electron transport system, such that the electron transfers continue to occur but ATP production ceases. They serve as H^+ ionophores to dissipate the H^+ gradient which is normally formed during electron transport; without the proton gradient, the energy of fuel oxidations cannot be conserved by ATP synthetase. As a consequence, electron transport and oxygen consumption continue at a higher than normal rate, and the excess energy that cannot be conserved as ATP is given off as heat. A common uncoupler is 2,4-dinitrophenol. Oxidative phosphorylation is also inhibited by the K^+ ionophore valinomycin and the Na^+ and K^+ ionophore gramicidin. These ionophores increase the permeability of the inner mitochondrial membrane to cations and thus perturb the electrochemical gradient required to drive oxidative phosphorylation. Oligomycin inhibits ATP synthetase and therefore also inhibits oxidative phosphorylation. *See also* ELECTRON TRANSPORT

SYSTEM, MITOCHONDRIAL; ELECTRON TRANS-PORT SYSTEM INHIBITORS; OXIDATIVE PHOS-PHORYLATION.

oxidative phosphorylation uncouplers. *See* OXIDATIVE PHOSPHORYLATION INHIBITORS.

oxidative stress. Damage to cells and cellular constituents by reactive oxygen species generated *in situ*. Oxidative stress may be involved in such toxic interactions as DNA damage (including alkylation through peroxidative mechanisms, hydroxylation and single strand breaks), lipid peroxidation, pulmonary and cardiac toxicity. Due to the transitory nature of the most reactive oxygen species, although oxidative stress is often invoked as a mechanism of toxicity, rigorous proof may be lacking. There are a number of protective mechanisms involving glutathione, ascorbic acid, vitamin E, catalase, peroxidase and superoxide dismutase. The expression of toxicity depends on the relative rates of generation of reactive oxygen species and their detoxication. *See also* OXYGEN, REACTIVE SPECIES.

oxidative toxicity. *See* OXIDATIVE STRESS.

N-oxide reduction. *N*-oxides can be reduced either chemically or enzymatically. Both of these types of reactions may be important in the case of the best known xenobiotic substrates, tertiary amine *N*-oxides. Substrates such as imipramine *N*-oxide and *N,N*-dimethylaniline *N*-oxide are reduced by cytochrome P450 and, although FMN and methyl viologen are stimulatory, this stimulation is also cytochrome P450-dependent (being inhibited by carbon monoxide). This activity is highly non-specific as regards cytochrome P450 forms, and it has been suggested that the substrate reacts directly with the heme of the cytochrome. The significance of this reaction in xenobiotic detoxication/intoxication is unclear, since *N*-oxides are common oxidative products of tertiary amines. Possibly the redundant cycling between amine and *N*-oxide is important from a toxicokinetic viewpoint since it would presumably increase the $T_{0.5}$ in the cell. *See also* REDUCTION.

oxidoreductases. *See* ENZYMES.

oximes. Chemicals that contain the -CH=N-OH moiety. Oximes of toxicological interest include products of *N*-oxidation and also the pyridinium-2-aldoximes and pyridinium-4-aldoximes. With phosphorylated cholinesterase, oximes undergo a transphosphorylation reaction which reactivates the catalytic center of the esterase. Although potential cholinesterase inhibitors in themselves, the phosphates of the clinically useful oximes rapidly degrade by internal rearrangement to dialkyl phosphate and the pyridinium nitrile. Although only *N*-methylpyridinium-2-aldoxime (2-PAM) is used in the USA, TMB-4 and obidoxime are used outside the USA. A large number of oximes are of experimental interest. *See also* ACETYLCHOLINESTERASE; ACETYLCHOLINESTERASE, REACTIVATION; ANTICHOLINESTERASES; *N*-OXIDATION; *N*-METHYLPYRIDINIUM-2-ALDOXIME.

oxon. Pentavalent organophosphorus compounds containing the P=O moiety. Oxons are frequently potent inhibitors of cholinesterases and other serine esterases. Organophosphorus compounds containing the P=S moiety that cause poisoning due to the inhibition of cholinesterase must first be activated metabolically by transformation to the corresponding oxon. This activation is catalyzed by cytochrome P450 isozymes and also, in the case of phosphonates, by the flavin-containing monooxygenase.

oxygen (O). Colorless, odorless gas belonging to group VI. It is the most abundant element in the Earth's crust (47.2% by weight) and forms 21% by volume of the atmosphere from which it can be obtained by liquefaction and distillation. Atmospheric oxygen is vital for aerobic respiration. The common form is diatomic (dioxygen, O_2), the liquid and solid forms of which are pale blue in color and are strongly paramagnetic. The gas is sparingly soluble in water and readily soluble in some organic solvents. It is a reactive gas and a strong oxidizing agent, combining with most other elements to form oxides. Its predominant chemistry is in the −2 oxidation state in oxides, alkoxides and ethers.

oxygen radical. *See* OXYGEN, REACTIVE SPECIES.

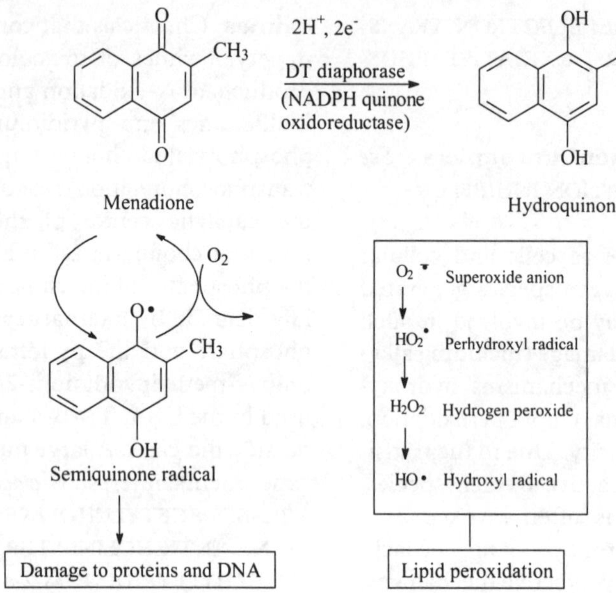

Menadione

Hydroquinone

Semiquinone radical

$O_2^{\bullet-}$	Superoxide anion
$HO_2^{\bullet}$	Perhydroxyl radical
H_2O_2	Hydrogen peroxide
$HO^{\bullet}$	Hydroxyl radical

Damage to proteins and DNA

Lipid peroxidation

oxygen, reactive species. Reactive forms of oxygen formed *in vivo* as a result of several different enzymatic activities. They include superoxide anion, perhydroxyl radical, hydrogen peroxide and hydroxy radical. These reactive species may be formed sequentially as shown in the diagram above. They are formed during such reactions as the autooxidation of semiquinones formed by NADPH-cytochrome P450 reductase and in many cytochrome P450-catalyzed oxidations.

oxygen toxicity. Human adults can tolerate a pure oxygen atmosphere for several hours. After that time, however, there are serious effects on the eye, including constriction of peripheral vision, mydriasis and constriction of the vasculature of the retina. Unlike the situation in premature human infants, however, these symptoms are reversible on return to a normal atmosphere. In the case of premature infants, after being maintained in incubators with oxygen concentrations above ambient, severe ocular problems occur after return to a normal atmosphere. The condition, known as retrolental fibroplasia, is irreversible and is due to the effect of oxygen on the embryonic capillary system, which only becomes fully developed after a full-term pregnancy period. The mechanism of toxicity is not understood, but concomitant inhibition of a number of enzymes involved in energy metabolism has been noted.

oxygenases. Enzymes that catalyze oxidation reactions (usually irreversible) in which oxygen is incorporated from molecular oxygen into the product, often the first oxidative step in the metabolism of stable reduced compounds such as alkanes. Monooxygenases catalyze the incorporation of a single atom of oxygen, the second atom being reduced in the same reaction to water by an electron donor (reductant) which is usually NAD(P)H. Monooxygenase reactions often involve a number of electron transfer components between the electron donor and the substrate, including iron-sulphur proteins, flavoproteins or cytochromes. A typical example is the cytochrome P450-dependent monooxygenase system. Dioxygenases differ from monooxygenases in that both atoms of oxygen from molecular oxygen are incorporated into the product, and a reductant is not involved in the reaction. *Compare* OXIDASES.

oxymorphone. An analgesic narcotic, listed as a controlled substance in the US Code of Federal Regulations.

oxy radical. *See* SUPEROXIDE.

oxy radical scavengers. *See* SUPEROXIDE DIS-MUTASE.

oxytocin. A peptide hormone containing nine amino acids secreted synthesized by the paraventricular and supraoptic nuclei of the hypothalmus and stored and released by the neurohypophysis. It acts in females by inducing uterine contractions during parturition and stimulating milk ejection by the mammary glands. No actions in males are known. Synthetic derivatives of oxytocin are used to induce labor and for therapeutic abortions.

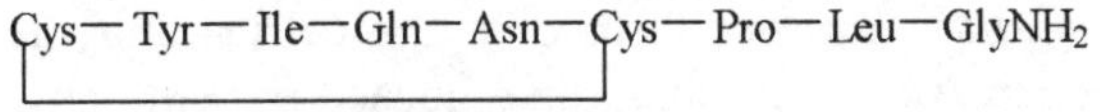

$$Cys—Tyr—Ile—Gln—Asn—Cys—Pro—Leu—GlyNH_2$$

Oxytocin

ozone (O_3). A colorless gas with a pungent odor. Ozone is used as an oxidizing agent in the chemical industry, as a disinfectant for food and water, for bleaching such products as flour, sugar, starch, textiles and paper pulp, for aging liquor and wood, in treating industrial wastes, for drying varnishes and inks, and for deodorizing feathers. Ozone is formed naturally by the action of solar radiation and electrical storms in the atmosphere and forms the protective ozone layer of the atmosphere.

Ozone is also formed around electrical sources such as generators of ultraviolet- or X-rays, mercury vapor lamps, linear accelerators, electric arcs and electrical discharges. Ozone irritates eyes and mucous membranes. Inhalation can lead to choking, coughing, fatigue, bronchial irritation, pulmonary edema and even death from the pulmonary edema. Chronic exposures can result in bronchitis, bronchiolitis and emphysematous and fibrotic changes in the pulmonary parenchyma. Because of its free radical nature, it has produced chromosomal aberrations in experimental situations. The LC50s after a 3-hour exposure are 20 ppm for mice and 50 ppm for guinea pigs. Tolerance to the edematous effects of ozone and other agents such as nitrogen dioxide and phosgene can be induced by brief exposures to ozone. *See also* OZONE LAYER.

ozone layer. A layer of the atmosphere containing ozone (O_3) in addition to O_2, both of which absorb ultraviolet radiation effectively. The wavelengths absorbed are those that are absorbed by DNA and can be mutagenic. Thus the ozone layer is instrumental in preventing excess mutations by ultraviolet radiation and was an important factor allowing the evolution of terrestrial forms of life. Certain pollutants, such as the fluorocarbons used in aerosol products, can damage the ozone layer.

P

^{32}P, post labelling. A technique used to isolate and label nucleotides with ^{32}P, a radioactive isotope of phosphorus. Abnormal nucleotides formed as a result of chemicals that interact with DNA can be separated from the normal nucleotides, providing a measure of DNA adduct formation. It is an important technique in the study of chemical carcinogenesis and mutagenesis.

P$_{53}$. A tumor suppressor gene. It encodes the sequence for a protein that is a transcription factor increasing the rate of transcription of genes that contain the p53 response element while inhibiting transcription of many genes that do not. It arrests cell growth in the G1 phase, when DNA repair occurs and promotes apoptosis. Thus the normal p53 gene protects the cell from neoplastic responses and accumulation of genetic errors. Mutations in the p53 gene are common in many cancers, including those caused by aflatoxin, and it appears that not only are the mutant proteins produced unable to protect the cell but they interfere with the function of the normal p53 protein.

P450. *See* CYTOCHROME P450.

palytoxin. CAS number 77734-91-9. A poisonous material derived from *Palythoa toxica*, a coral that grows in tidal pools near the Hawaiian island of Maui. The toxin ($C_{129}H_{223}N_3O_{54}$) contains 64 disymmetric carbon atoms, and formerly was used by natives to poison their spears.

2-PAM. *See* N-METHYLPYRIDINIUM-2-ALDOXIME.

PAN. *See* PEROXYACETYL NITRATE.

Panadol. *See* ACETAMINOPHEN.

pancreas. A gland located in the loop of the duodenum and connected to it by the pancreatic duct (duct of Wirsung). The pancreas has both exocrine and endocrine functions. The digestive secretion of the pancreas, secreted into the duodenum via the pancreatic duct, contains several digestive enzymes formed in the cells lining the pancreatic acini, including lipase, trypsin, chymotrypsin, carboxypeptidase and pancreatic amylase. The islet cells of the pancreas (islets of Langerhans) secrete two endocrine products—insulin (β-cells) and glucagon (α-cells). When insulin production is deficient, diabetes mellitus results due to inadequate utilization of glucose. The resultant hyperglycemia leads to glycosuria (excess sugar in the urine). Fatty liver may also occur, as well as metabolic acidosis caused by excess ketone bodies (acetone, acetoacetic acid, β-hydroxybutyric acid) formed from the oxidation of fatty acids. Fatty acid oxidation increases whenever glucose oxidation is impaired. *See also* PANCREATIC TOXICITY.

pancreatic toxicity. Although diabetes mellitus is not the result of chemical toxicity, toxicants can cause hyperglycemia, presumably through an effect on the β-cells of the islets of Langerhans. Alloxan, for example, causes diabetes in experimental animals by destruction of the β-cells. Toxicants not specific to the pancreas, such as ethanol and carbon tetrachloride, may stimulate pancreatic exocrine secretions via the pancreatic duct.

papaverine (1-[(3,4-dimethoxyphenyl)methyl]-6,7-dimethoxyisoquinoline; 6,7-dimethoxy-1-veratrylisoquinoline). CAS number 58-74-2. An alkaloid found in crude opium, but chemically and pharmacologically quite different from the opioids. Its major actions are smooth muscle relaxation and coronary and cerebral vasodilation, although demonstrations of clinical efficacy are lacking. The vasodilatory action may be due to the inhibition of cyclic nucleotide phosphodiesterase. Systemic administration of high doses can induce arrhythmias, and the side effects of papaverine include drowsiness, gastrointestinal distress, tachycardia, facial flushing and, potentially, liver toxicity. The LD50 in rats is 750 mg/kg.

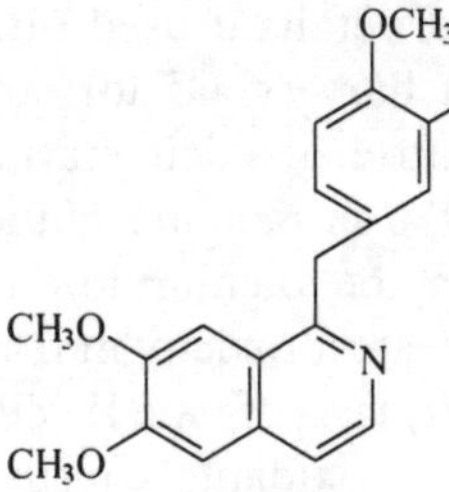

Papaverine

paper chromatography. *See* CHROMATOGRAPHY, PAPER.

papilloma. An exophytic growth pattern of epithelial tumors wherein the tumor cells grow out from a surface much like a cauliflower, with the stalk forming the point of attachment. *See also* ADENOCARCINOMA; ADENOMA.

PAPS (3′-phosphoadenosine-5′-phosphosulfate). A compound involved in the formation of sulfate conjugates of xenobiotics by sulfotransferases. It is formed from ATP in a sequence of reactions involving ATP sulfurylase and adenosine-5-phosphosulfate kinase. *See also* SULFATE CONJUGATION.

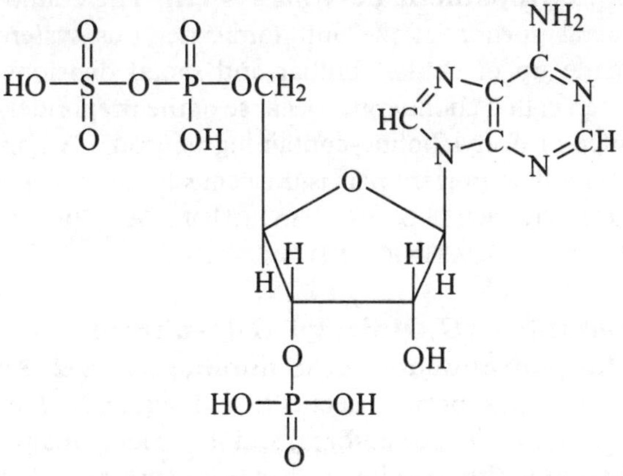

3′-Phosphoadenosine-5′-phosphosulfate

Paracelsus. Philippus Aureolus, also known as Theophrastus Bombastus von Hohenheim, lived from 1493–1541 and is regarded as the father of modern toxicology. His best known work is "On the Miners Sickness and Other Diseases of Miners." His statement that "all substances are poisons; there is none that is not a poison. The right dose differentiates a poison and a remedy" is properly regarded as the basis for the dose response principle on which toxicology and pharmacology both rest.

paracetaldehyde. *See* PARALDEHYDE.

paracetamol. *See* ACETAMINOPHEN.

paraffin. *See* KEROSENE.

paragoric. *See* MORPHINE; OPIOIDS.

paraldehyde (paracetaldehyde). CAS number 123-63-7. A hypnotic; a polymer of acetaldehyde. It is rapid acting, devoid of analgesic properties and has anticonvulsant and antidelirium effects in large doses. High doses produce hypotension and respiratory depression, although hypnotic doses have little effect on these physiological parameters. The use of paraldehyde has largely been restricted to institutionalized patients. Oral administration can irritate the throat and stomach, whereas i.m. injection can cause necrosis and nerve damage. Paraldehyde poisoning has been associated with rapid and labored respiration, acidosis, leukocytosis, hepatitis and nephrosis, pulmonary hemorrhages and edema. Repeated use of the drug can result in tolerance and dependence. The therapeutic uses of paraldehyde have included the treatment of delirium tremens, hyperexcitability and the emergency treatment of convulsions. Paraldehyde can be rapidly oxidized to acetic acid and can react rapidly with plastics. The oral LD50 in rats is 1.65 g/kg. *See also* ACETALDEHYDE; SEDATIVE-HYPNOTICS.

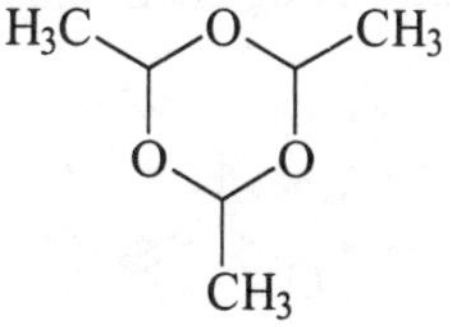

Paraldehyde

paralysis time. A test of the ability of one xenobiotic to affect the metabolism of another. The test is usually carried out by challenging mice with zoxazolamine, which produces a flaccid paralysis of motor function. This paralysis is relatively short-lived and is highly dependent on the blood concentration of the drug which, in turn, is dependent upon the rate of its metabolism by monooxygenases. Thus inhibitors of cytochrome P450 prolong the time of effective paralysis, whereas it is shortened by inducers of this enzyme. *Compare* SLEEPING TIME.

paralytic shellfish poisoning. Poisoning resulting from ingestion of shellfish contaminated with the dinoflagellate *Gonyaulax* that produces saxitoxin. The toxin produces paresthesia, aberrations in sensory perception and proprioception, ataxia, weakness, and respiratory failure. It is also called paresthetic shellfish poisoning. *See also* SAXITONIN.

parametric. If the null hypothesis to be tested includes statements about population parameters such as the mean, then the test is parametric. Parametric statistical tests involve assumptions about the distribution and parameters of the population from which observations are sampled. These assumptions most frequently include normality of distribution and homogeneity of variance. Standard parametric tests used in toxicology include the analysis of variance and the t test. *Compare* NON-PARAMETRIC. *See also* STATISTICS, FUNCTION IN TOXICOLOGY.

paraoxon (*O,O*-diethyl-*O*-(*p*-nitrophenyl) phosphate; E-600). **CAS number 311-45-5**. Although not used as an insecticide, paraoxon is the active metabolite of the widely used insecticide parathion. The parent insecticide is a poor acetylcholinesterase (AChE) inhibitor, but rapidly undergoes desulfuration by microsomal monooxygenases. The resultant paraoxon is a potent anticholinesterase agent. Paraoxon has had limited use in the USA in the management of glaucoma and is

Paraoxon

widely used as a pharmacological research tool as an inhibitor of AChE and other serine esterases. The oral LD50 in rats is 1.8 mg/kg. *See also* ANTICHOLINESTERASES; PARATHION.

paraquat (1,1′-dimethyl-4,4′-bipyridinium). CAS number 4685-14-7. A contact herbicide, crop desiccant and defoliant used on cotton and potato vines, as a harvest aid for soybeans and sometimes for control of illicit marijuana plantings. The oral LD50 in rats and guinea pig is 57 and 22 mg/kg (as the dichloride), respectively. Paraquat causes greatest toxicity in the lung, leading to edema, hyperplasia of type II cells and fibrosis. Paraquat is an oxidant, causing a single-electron oxidation/reduction reaction that depletes cellular NADPH and generates superoxide radicals. Bioaccumulation in the lungs overwhelms detoxification enzymes and results in lipid peroxidation of pulmonary membranes. Irritation and ulceration of mouth and esophagus, abdominal pain and nausea follow oral ingestion. Therapeutic measures include prevention of absorption following oral ingestion by administration of an adsorbent suspension (Fuller's earth) or, if not available, a slurry of activated charcoal. After inhalation, the patient should be removed to fresh air, but supplemental oxygen should not be administered.

Paraquat

parasympathetic nervous system. The craniosacral portion of the autonomic nervous system made up of ocular, bulbar and sacral divisions; often called cholinergic, because of the preponderance of acetylcholine-containing neurons. A particularly important part is the vagus nerve. *See also* ACETYLCHOLINE; ACETYLCHOLINE RECEPTORS, MUSCARINIC AND NICOTINIC.

parathion (*O,O*-diethyl-*O*-(*p*-nitrophenyl)-phosphorothioate). **CAS number 56-38-2**. An organophosphorus insecticide and acaricide. Patents are no longer in force, and it is widely manufactured, although its use has been superseded to some extent by insecticides of lower mammalian toxicity. The oral LD50 in rats is 3.6 mg/kg for males and 13.0 mg/kg for females. It is also readily absorbed through the skin. Parathion is activated to its oxygen analog paraoxon by the microsomal cytochrome P450-dependent monooxygenase system, paraoxon acting as a neurotoxicant by irreversible inhibition of acetylcholinesterase. Symptoms in humans include lachrymation, pupillary constriction, muscular twitching and fibrillation, convulsions, diarrhea, respiratory failure and coma. Therapy in acute poisoning consists of general supportive therapy, respirator, if necessary, atropine and N-methylpyridinium-2-aldoxime (2-PAM). The former interacts with acetylcholine receptors, and the latter reactivates phosphorylated cholinesterase. *See also* ANTICHOLINESTERASES; INSECTICIDES; ORGANOPHOSPHORUS INSECTICIDES; PARAOXON.

Parathion

parathormone. *See* PARATHYROID GLANDS.

parathyroid glands. A set of four glands close to or embedded in the thyroid gland. The parathyroid glands produce the parathyroid hormone (PTH, parathormone). The effect of PTH is to raise blood calcium concentrations by increasing bone resorption, increasing dietary calcium absorption from the digestive tract and decreasing renal excretion of calcium; concurrently it causes increased excretion of phosphorus. A deficiency in PTH can be life-threatening, resulting in tetany because of nervous hyperexcitability. Additional symptoms include cataracts and disturbances of skin, bone, teeth, nails and hair. An excess of PTH causes excessive resorption of bone and therefore bone weakening; the hypercalcemia results in decreased neuromuscular excitability and abnormal calcium deposits, such as kidney stones.

parathyroid hormone (PTH). Single-chain polypeptide of about 75 amino acid residues, secreted by parathyroid gland. Controls blood calcium levels. Low calcium levels stimulate hormone secretion which increases transfer of calcium from bones to blood.

parenteral. *See* ADMINISTRATION OF TOXICANTS, PARENTERAL.

parkinsonism (Parkinson's disease). Movement disorders mediated by changes in the brain basal ganglia in which the major signs are tremor, bradykinesia, rigidity, and disturbance of posture. In Parkinson's disease (an idiopathic disorder with the exception of rare familial genetic occurrences), the primary symptoms result from disruption of dopamine neurotransmission in the extrapyramidal system, specifically in the striatum, due to loss of dopamine neurons. Parkinsonian signs and symptoms (pseudoparkinsonism) also can be caused by toxicants that destroy dopamine neurons, deplete dopamine, or disrupt dopamine neurotransmission. These include the Rauwolfia alkaloid reserpine and dopamine receptor blockers (e.g., the antipsychotic drugs). The toxicant MPTP cause a condition that is strikingly similar to Parkinson's disease, leading to the hypothesis that Parkinson's disease might involve environmental chemicals, although there is little direct evidence in support of this idea. Drugs that increase dopamine function, such as the dopamine precursor L-dopa or the agonist bromocriptine, can provide dramatic improvement and are used clinically to treat this disorder. *See also* L-DOPA; MANGANESE; MPTP; NEUROTOXICOLOGY.

Parkinson's disease. *See* PARKINSONISM.

Parlodel. *See* BROMOCRIPTINE.

particulates. Air pollutants consisting of fine solids or liquid droplets suspended in air, in contrast to gaseous pollutants. The predominant factor affecting deposition of particles in the respiratory system is particle size, and the site of deposition affects the clearance mechanisms available as well as the degree of absorption and the toxic consequences. *See also* AEROSOLS; DUSTS; FUMES; MIST; POLLUTION; SMOG; SMOKE.

partition coefficient. A measure of the relative lipid solubility of a chemical, determined by measuring the partitioning of the compound between a lipid phase and an aqueous phase (e.g., octanol and water). The partition coefficient is important in studies of the uptake of toxicants since compounds with high coefficients (lipophilic compounds) are usually taken up more readily by organisms and tissues. *See also* LIPOPHILIC.

partitioning. The movement of a chemical from one physical location to another. In uptake and transport, it is from one structure or medium to another (e.g., from aqueous solution to cell membrane). In either case, it often involves movement from one physical state to another (i.e., from aqueous solution to lipid, or vice versa). The partition coefficient is a measure of a chemical's relative solubility in aqueous and lipid phases. *See also* COMPARTMENT; ENTRY MECHANISMS; ENTRY MECHANISMS, PASSIVE TRANSPORT; PARTITION COEFFICIENT; TOXICOKINETICS.

passive avoidance. An operant or instrumental learning paradigm to assess learning and/or memory. The procedure typically involves administering punishment (e.g., shock) to an animal contingent upon its moving from one location (e.g., brightly lit chamber) in the test area to another (e.g., dimly lit chamber). To assess learning or memory, the animal is placed back in the test area some time later (e.g., after 24 hours), and the latency to move from one location to the other is measured. A significantly decreased latency relative to control animals is interpreted as evidence of impaired memory. *See also* CONDITIONED AVOIDANCE; NEUROBEHAVIORAL TERATOLOGY; NEUROBEHAVIORAL TOXICOLOGY; POSTNATAL BEHAVIORAL TESTS; TREMORS.

passive transport. *See* ENTRY MECHANISMS, PASSIVE TRANSPORT.

pathology. The study of morphological changes characteristic of abnormal states, including both physiological (endogenous) effects, effects caused by pathogenic organisms and the adverse effects of exogenous physical and chemical agents. It includes changes at the level of gross anatomy, light and electron microscopy. It is particularly important in toxicology for the evaluation of chronic toxicity tests, including carcinogenicity testing. Although still primarily descriptive, more recently quantitative morphometry and histochemical techniques have extended pathology into

valuable studies of the mechanism of toxic action. *See also* CHRONIC TOXICITY TESTING; TOXIC ENDPOINTS.

patulin (4-hydroxy-4H-furo(3,2-c)pyran-2-(6H)one). CAS number 149-29-1. An antimicrobial compound isolated from any of several *Aspergillus* and *Penicillium* species. Patulin is also an animal carcinogen, inhibits K^+-uptake into erythrocytes and inhibits various forms of Na^+/K^+-ATPase.

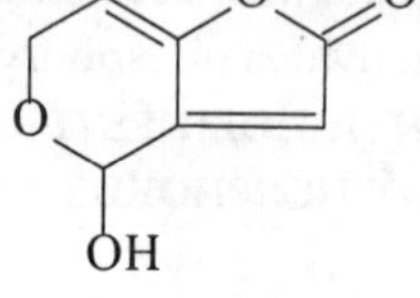

Patulin

Pavlovian conditioning (classical conditioning). A procedure that involves the repeated pairing of a previously neutral stimulus (e.g., tone) with an unconditioned stimulus (e.g., shock) that elicits an unconditioned response (e.g., freezing). Pavlovian conditioning occurs when the previously neutral stimulus, now a conditioned stimulus (CS), reliably elicits a conditioned response (CR) equivalent to the unconditioned response (UCR) previously elicited by the unconditioned stimulus (UCS). The CS is generally presented a short time before presentation of the UCS. *See also* CONDITIONED AVOIDANCE; NEUROBEHAVIORAL TERATOLOGY; NEUROBEHAVIORAL TOXICOLOGY; POSTNATAL BEHAVIORAL TESTS.

PBBs. *See* POLYBROMINATED BIPHENYLS.

PBPK. *See* PHYSIOLOGICALLY-BASED PHARMACOKINETICS.

PCBs. *See* POLYCHLORINATED BIPHENYLS.

PCP. *See* PHENCYCLIDINE.

PD. *See* PROPENSITY TO DUST.

Pearson's product moment correlation. *See* CORRELATION COEFFICIENT.

PEL (Permissible Exposure Level). *See* PERMISSIBLE DOSE.

Penagran. *See* PROMETHAZINE.

penetration, effect of ionization. *See* IONIZATION, AND UPTAKE OF TOXICANTS.

penetration, rate. Assuming that the concentration at the application site is much higher than the absorbed concentration (considered negligible because it is quickly removed), the rate of penetration of non-polar, unionized toxicants in simple systems is believed to follow Fick's law of diffusion. This law, which states that the diffusion constant is equal to the product of the surface area and the concentration divided by the thickness of the membrane, can be expanded to the more experimentally useful equation

$$J = K_m \, C_v \, D_m/d$$

where J = the absorption rate per unit area at steady state (flux), K_m = vehicle partition coefficient, C_v = concentration of penetrant, D_m = diffusion constant of the penetrant in the membrane or tissue and d = the thickness of the membrane. The rate of absorption then depends on two easily controlled, externally determined factors (partition coefficient and concentration of penetrant) and two innate factors (diffusion constant and membrane thickness). Permeability constants for human skin range from 1×10^{-6} to 5×10^{-2} cm/hr. The above equation implies conditions of steady-state penetration not attained until a lag phase has occurred. A plot of the logarithm of the amount unpenetrated versus time should be linear, indicating first-order kinetics. However, this ideal situation is an oversimplification except in simple, usually non-physiological systems, and deviations from first-order kinetics are common due to such factors as differential shunts within the highly lipid membrane, contribution of appendagical shunts, effects of the carrier necessary for application, injury to surface membranes, hydration of the membrane or tissue, binding of the penetrant to the membrane, etc. When first-order kinetics hold, a simple relationship exists between the penetration constant (K) and time necessary for half of the applied dose to penetrate $T_{0.5}$ namely $K = 0.693/T_{0.5}$. When first-order kinetics do not apply,

$T_{0.5}$ may be the only useful number. It should, however, be used only for comparative purposes. *See also* ABSORPTION OF TOXICANTS.

penetration routes, dermal. The skin is a complex, multilayered tissue comprising about 18,000 cm^2 in an average human male. It is relatively impermeable to most ions and aqueous solutions, although it is permeable to a large number of primarily lipophilic toxicants. Three distinct layers— the dermis, the epidermis, the subcutaneous layer—make up this important organ, but the epidermis is the only layer important in the penetration of toxicants. The epidermis is a multilayered tissue varying in thickness from about 0.1 to 0.8 mm. The basal cells of the epidermis proliferate and differentiate as they migrate outward. The columnar cells become rounded and then flattened as they move to form the outer layer (the stratum corneum), the primary barrier to penetration, which consists of layers of flattened dehydrated and highly keratinized cells. The dermis is highly vascular, providing maximal opportunity for transport once molecules enter through the epidermis. The skin may also have a function in the metabolism of topically applied substances before they become available systemically. The skin enzymes are inducible and potentially of toxicological importance both in activation and deactivation of toxicants. Skin metabolic transformations are not presently considered of major significance in cases of rapid penetration, but may have an important first-pass function for compounds that are absorbed slowly. *Compare* PENETRATION ROUTES, GASTROINTESTINAL; PENETRATION ROUTES, PULMONARY.

penetration routes, gastrointestinal. The oral penetration route is important following either accidental or deliberate ingestion of toxicants. Food additives, food toxins and food contaminants and airborne particles excluded from passage to the alveoli and returned to the glottis are all ingested. Ingested toxicants generally enter the body from the stomach or intestine. Some exceptions to this include nicotine, which enters readily through the buccal cavity, and cocaine, which enters through the nasal mucosa. The digestive system is lined by a layer of columnar cells, the distance from the outer membrane to the vasculature being about 40 μm. From this point further transport is easily effected, primarily to the liver, where metabolism is likely to occur. The presence of microvilli, which provide an extremely large surface area, is an important factor in absorption. Although it is generally believed that gastrointestinal absorption is more rapid than dermal absorption, differences in penetration between the dermal and oral routes may be relatively small. Even though the greater surface area of the intestine is a factor in absorption at that location, compounds enter the stomach first and may be rapidly absorbed in that organ. Also, there are appreciable differences in pH within the gastrointestinal tract, a factor that may change permeability characteristics. The stomach tends to be much more acid than the intestine, affecting absorption of ionized compounds such as weak acids. Active transport of toxicants is also known to occur in the gastrointestinal tract in cases where toxicants have structural similarities to endogenous compounds or nutrients normally taken up by active transport mechanisms. A very small number of large molecules, compounds such as bacterial endotoxins, large particles of azo dyes and carrageenens, are apparently absorbed by endocytotic mechanisms in the gastrointestinal tract. *Compare* PENETRATION ROUTES, DERMAL; PENETRATION ROUTES, PULMONARY. *See also* ACTIVE TRANSPORT; ENTEROHEPATIC CIRCULATION; IONIZATION, AND UPTAKE OF TOXICANTS; PHAGOCYTOSIS.

penetration routes, pulmonary. The respiratory system is especially important as a penetration route because of two characteristics. Capillary exchange at the deeper lung recesses causes a toxicant at the lung surface to be separated by only 1–2 μm from the circulation, enabling rapid gas exchange and, in addition, the surface area of the lung is large (50–100 m^2), being about 50 times that of the skin. The classification of toxicant types that are taken up by the respiratory system is complex. Compounds subject to the gas laws include solvents, vapors and gases, and are most easily carried to the alveolar areas. Those in particulate form include aerosols, clouds, particles, fumes, etc. The rate of entry of vapor-phase toxicants is controlled by the alveolar ventilation rate, and the toxicant is presented to the alveoli in an interrupted fashion approximately 20 times per minute. Entry of aerosols and particulates is governed by a number of factors. Particles larger than 5 μm are usually deposited in the nasopharyngeal region. Particles down to 2 μm are deposited in the tracheobronchiolar region, where they are cleared upward by the mucous blanket, which covers the backward-beating cilia. Such particles may move to the glottis and are swallowed, permitting later absorption in the gastrointestinal tract. In addition to upper pathway clearance, lung phagocytosis occurs in both the upper and lower pathways of the respiratory tract. If not phagocytized, particles of 1 μm and smaller may penetrate to the alveolar portion of the lung, and overall removal of alveolar particles is markedly slower than that in the upper respiratory tract. For very small particles and gaseous toxicants, absorption takes place in the alveolar region. Gas in the alveoli equilibrates almost instantaneously with the blood passing through the pulmonary capillary bed, the rate of movement of the gas into or out of the blood being dependent upon solubility in blood. For highly soluble gases, most is transferred to the blood with each breath and little is left in the alveolus. *Compare* PENETRATION ROUTES, DERMAL; PENETRATION ROUTES, GASTROINTESTINAL. *See also* PHAGOCYTOSIS.

penicillamine (3-mercapto-D-valine; Depen). CAS number 52-67-5. A degradation product of penicillins prepared by hydrolysis. It is used as a chelating agent in the treatment of heavy metal poisoning and in copper chelation in Wilson's disease. It has significant side effects, particularly toxic effects on the kidney and aspects of the hemopoietic system. *See also* CHELATING AGENTS.

$$CH_3-\underset{\underset{CH_3}{|}}{\overset{\overset{SH}{|}}{C}}-\overset{\overset{NH_2}{|}}{CH}-\overset{\overset{O}{\parallel}}{C}-OH$$

Penicillamine

penicillins. *See* ANTIBIOTICS.

pentachlorophenol. CAS number 87-86-5. A fungicide and bacteriocide used mainly in the preservation of wood. Entry into the body can occur by inhalation of dust, absorption through the skin or by accidental ingestion. Exposure gives rise to any of a variety of symptoms, including irritation of respiratory mucous membranes, weakness, anorexia, nausea, dizziness and increased body temperature. Pentachlorophenol has been shown to cause fetotoxicity and teratogenesis, and is coming under increasing regulation. IARC has classified pentachlorophenol as possibly carcinogenic to humans. *See also* ATSDR DOCUMENT, MAY 1994; DATABASES, TOXICOLOGY; LEWIS, HCDR, NUMBER PAX250; MERCK INDEX, 12TH EDN, NUMBER 7242.

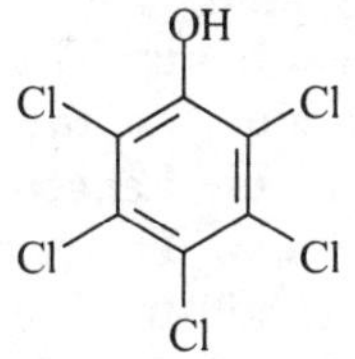

Pentachlorophenol

pentazocine. CAS number 359-83-1. Mixed opioid agonist–antagonist used as an analgesic. This is a narcotic and, in the US, a controlled substance. *See also* MERCK INDEX, 12TH EDN, NUMBER 7261.

Penthrane. *See* METHOXYFLURANE.

pentobarbital (5-ethyl-5-(1-methylbutyl)-2,4,6(1*H*,3*H*,5*H*)-pyrimidinetrione monosodium salt; sodium 5-ethyl-5-(1-methylbutyl) barbiturate; pentobarbital sodium; pentobarbitone sodium; Nembutal). CAS number 76-74-4. A barbiturate that causes CNS depression, apparently due to a facilitation of GABAergic inhibition. It appears that the site of action of pentobarbital may be the macromolecular complex made up of a GABA receptor, chloride channel, benzodiazepine-binding site and picrotoxin-binding site. Barbiturates have been shown to compete for dihydropicrotoxinin-binding sites. In clinical use, barbiturates such as pentobarbital have been largely replaced as sedative-hypnotics by the much safer benzodiazepines. The sedative-hypnotic properties of barbiturates may lead to abuse, as tolerance and dependence are known to occur. In animals, pentobarbital is routinely used for its anesthetic and anticonvulsant properties, as well as for euthanasia. Pentobarbital, like other barbiturates, can induce the metabolism of other

compounds by altering cytochrome P450 activity. The oral LD50 in rats is 118 mg/kg. *See also* BARBITURATES; SEDATIVE-HYPNOTICS.

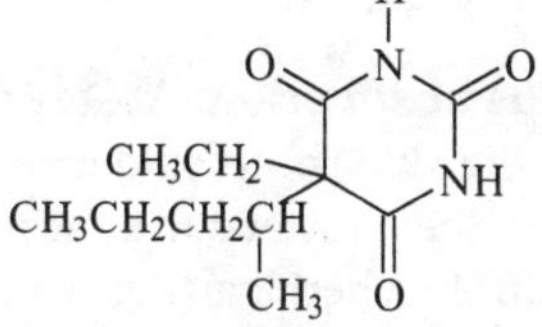

Pentobarbital

Pentothal. *See* THIOPENTAL, SODIUM.

pentylenetetrazole (6,7,8,9-tetrahydro-5*H*-tetrazolo[1,5-*a*]azepine; Metrazol). CAS number 54-95-5. Once believed to be a useful CNS stimulant, as well as an analeptic agent. Because its effective dose is similar to doses that induce seizures, its only present utility is as a diagnostic aid in screening for latent epileptogenic foci, in characterizing the underlying cerebral disorders in individuals with documented cases of epilepsy and in basic research.

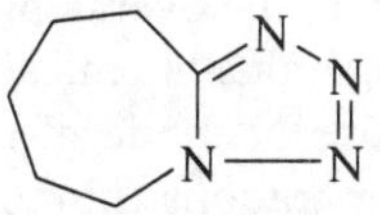

Pentylenetetrazole

pepper. *See* CAPSICUM; CAPSAICIN.

peppermint. *See* ESSENTIAL OILS.

peptide. Compounds that consist of a relatively small number of amino acids linked in peptide bonds (-C(O)NH-). The peptide bond is formed by the elimination of the atoms of water from the amino group of one amino acid and the carboxyl group of another. Although proteins are polypeptides they are usually considered separately because their biological properties are a function of their large size and complex tertiary structure. The term peptide is more commonly used for smaller, more simple molecules with two (dipeptide), three (tripeptide) up to perhaps 20 or 30 amino acids. Such small peptides may have important endogenous functions (e.g., glutathione, a tripeptide), or may be commercial sweetening agents or toxicants. In the latter case they are frequently cyclic and/or contain one or more D-amino acids.

peptides, antibiotics. *See* ANTIBIOTICS.

perchloroethylene. *See* TETRACHLOROETHYL-ENE.

percutaneous absorption. Absorption of chemicals through the skin, both epidermis and dermis. Although this does not occur at appreciable rates for water-soluble chemicals, it is an important route of entry for lipophilic toxicants such as parathion. *See also* PENETRATION ROUTES, DERMAL.

perfusion studies. The perfusion of organs has, in recent years, proven to be a valuable adjunct to toxicological studies. Organ perfusion is the maintenance of the organ either in vascular isolation or removed entirely from the body. This is accomplished by mechanical circulation of an appropriate fluid through the organ's blood system, the many technical problems associated with different organs being solved with an apparatus specially designed for the particular organ. Isolated perfused organs enable the investigator to define the role of that organ in the overall process of interaction with an exogenous chemical, either metabolism, toxicokinetics or mode of action. Unlike *in vitro* cell-free preparations (homogenates, cellular organelles, etc.), cellular integrity and the spatial relationships of cells are maintained. The technique is somewhat limited by the length of time the organ can be maintained in a viable condition and the assessment of changes prior to loss of viability, but it remains a valuable bridge between *in vitro* and *in vivo* experiments. Isolated perfused organs are usually maintained in closed systems since numerous functions must be controlled and monitored continuously. They include the maintenance of perfusion pressure, temperature and humidity, oxygenation of perfusate and continuous sampling of perfusate or other fluids. *See also* PERFUSION STUDIES, BRAIN; PERFUSION STUDIES, HEART; PERFUSION STUDIES, INTESTINES; PERFUSION STUDIES, KIDNEY; PERFUSION STUDIES, LIVER; PERFUSION STUDIES, LUNG; PERFUSION STUDIES, SKIN FLAP.

perfusion studies, brain. Brain perfusion studies have seen little application as yet in toxicology, and the brain does not lend itself to complete isolation. In this case, the brain is partially isolated *in situ* with as many extraneural tissues as possible removed from the artificial circulation. Preparations of varying complexity have been devised, from the perfused rat head to the totally isolated perfused monkey brain, with several intermediate preparations of partially isolated *in situ* brains usually perfused via the carotid artery with an oxygenated fluid such as Krebs–Ringer bicarbonate buffer containing serum albumin or low-molecular-weight dextran. Viability can be determined from spontaneous EEG activity or glucose utilization.

perfusion studies, heart. The first isolated perfused organ technique was the isolated perfused heart preparation of Langendorff, developed almost a century ago. This technique, utilizing aortic perfusion, is still used along with another that utilizes atrial perfusion. In the Langendorff preparation the isolated heart is perfused through the aorta with an oxygenated medium, frequently Krebs–Ringer bicarbonate buffer or one of its variants, although whole blood has been used. Viability is followed by monitoring of heart muscle contraction. Isolated hearts were used initially in studies of cardiac physiology, but have been used extensively in studies of drug metabolism and the action of toxicants on heart muscle.

perfusion studies, intestines. Isolated segments of intestine have been used for many years for studies of absorption, either of nutrients or of exogenous chemicals, or for assessment of the effect of neuroactive compounds on contractility. The use of vascular-perfused isolated intestine has been less common, however. Procedures have been developed in which the intestine is perfused without being isolated via the mesenteric artery and the superior mesentric vein. Not only can blood or perfusion fluid samples be obtained, but also samples of lymph and gut luminal contents. The perfusion fluid is either modified whole blood or Krebs–Ringer buffer. Little use of these preparations has been made in toxicological investigations.

perfusion studies, kidney. The isolated perfused kidney has proven valuable in studies of drug disposition, metabolism and clearance, as well as nephrotoxicity. The rat kidney is commonly used, although dog and rabbit kidney preparations have also been studied. The right renal artery is cannulated via the mesenteric artery, and the ureter is cannulated to collect urinary output. The kidney perfusate may be whole blood; more commonly it is an oxygenated bicarbonate buffer containing insulin, glucose and serum albumin. Glomerular filtration rate, urine flow and sodium and water reabsorption all vary with perfusate composition, and an appropriate compromise must be reached to achieve a viable preparation. Various parameters, including urine flow, glomerular filtration rate and glucose reabsorption, are used to monitor viability.

perfusion studies, liver. The use of the isolated perfused liver has been a valuable and extensively used tool in the study of exogenous compounds, including both their metabolism and effect on liver function. Recent studies using fiber optic light guides have enabled assessment of energy metabolism and monooxygenation through direct non-invasive measurement of pyridine nucleotides. The isolated liver is usually perfused via the portal vein, although simultaneous perfusion of the hepatic artery is also possible. The common bile duct is also cannulated for the collection of bile. Perfusion media vary widely, from heparinized whole blood to modified Krebs–Ringer bicarbonate-buffered solution and including mixtures of the two. Viability criteria used include bile flow, perfusion rate, oxygen consumption and several biochemical parameters, including assessment of glycolysis, the cytochrome P450-dependent monooxygenase system and the biliary excretion of sulfobromophthalein.

perfusion studies, lung. The isolated perfused lung has been valuable in studying non-respiratory functions such as the metabolism of xenobiotics. Isolated perfused lung preparation can, however, be made in such a way that ventilation occurs, and toxicological studies can be carried out in a ventilated lung. The lung is perfused via the pulmonary artery, and the trachea is also cannulated. Ventilation is accomplished by varying the pressure inside the closed chamber within which the lung is suspended, causing air to enter and leave via the tracheal cannula which passes outside of the chamber. Direct ventilation via the tracheal cannula has also been used. Perfusion media vary widely, from

whole blood to that devised by Junod, consisting of a mixture of salts buffered by phosphate and bicarbonate with serum albumin added. Lungs from many species have been successfully perfused, the rabbit probably most commonly. Viability is ascertained by a number of biochemical parameters, including determinations of blood urea nitrogen, pyruvate and lactic dehydrogenase in the perfusate.

perfusion studies, skin flap. The isolated perfused porcine skin flap, as developed by Riviere and co-workers, has proven useful in studies of percutaneous absorption as it permits uptake to be determined in the absence of other organs. This work has been extended into studies of dermal metabolism and the role of these events in toxicodynamics. Skin in the caudolateral epigastric region of the pig is partially isolated and formed into a tubed structure still attached at the base. Following healing of the tubed structure the caudal superficial epigastric artery is cannulated, the structure surgically removed, and the isolated skin flap placed in the perfusion apparatus. The perfusion medium is Krebs–Ringer bicarbonate buffer with added glucose, serum albumin and antibiotics. Viability is assessed from glucose utilization and lactic dehydrogenase release.

perhydroxy radical. *See* SUPEROXIDE.

perinatal period. The developmental period preceding birth; the last third of gestation. *See also* REPRODUCTIVE TOXICITY TESTING.

perinatal/postnatal toxicity tests. *See* REPRODUCTIVE TOXICITY TESTING.

peripheral nervous system. That portion of the nervous system consisting of the nerves and ganglia outside of the spinal cord and brain (central nervous system, CNS).

peripheral neuropathy. A disorder of the peripheral nervous system. Somatic motor, sensory, and autonomic neurons may be equally or preferentially affected. Clinical manifestations reflect the distribution of the pathological changes among somatic motor, sensory and autonomic neurons and include muscle weakness, muscle atrophy, sensory disturbances, and autonomic dysfunction. The disorder may primarily involve neuronal cell body (neuropathy), proximal axon (proximal axonopathy), distal axon (distal axonopathy), Schwann cell or myelin sheath (myelinopathy). Neuropathies may be classified etiologically as toxic, metabolic, hereditary, autoimmune, ischemic, traumatic, neoplastic, infectious or idiopathic. *See also* DEMYELINATION; MYELIN SHEATH.

peritoneal dialysis. *See* DIALYSIS.

permethrin (3-(2,2-dichloroethenyl)-2,2-dimethylcyclopropanecarboxylic acid). CAS number 52645-53-1. A pyrethroid insecticide, one of a group of chemicals whose structures are based on the botanical insecticide, pyrethrin. The mode of action is via an effect on the sodium channels in nerve membranes. Although this mode of action is quite similar to DDT, permethrin is not persistent either *in vivo* or in the environment. Active at low doses and fairly selective in that the acute toxicity is much higher to insects than to mammals although toxicity to fish may cause problems.

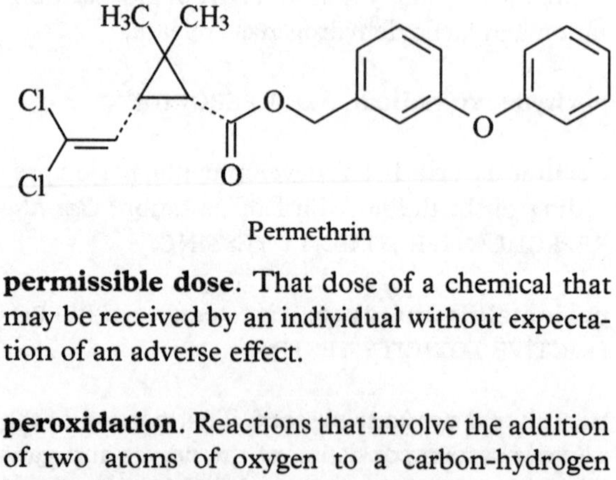

Permethrin

permissible dose. That dose of a chemical that may be received by an individual without expectation of an adverse effect.

peroxidation. Reactions that involve the addition of two atoms of oxygen to a carbon-hydrogen bond. Peroxidations of interest in toxicology include peroxidations of lipids brought about by interaction between lipid free radicals and oxygen, and peroxidation catalyzed by prostaglandin synthase in the formation of prostaglandins from arachidonic acid. Xenobiotic co-substrates can be oxidized, often to active intermediates, during the latter reaction. *See also* CO-OXIDATION, DURING PROSTAGLANDIN SYNTHESIS; LIPID PEROXIDATION.

peroxisome proliferation. A number of chemical agents are known to produce a marked proliferation of peroxisomes in liver cells. They include hypolipidemic agents such as clofibrate and plasticizers such as di(2-ethylhexyl)phthalate. Peroxisome proliferators are often carcinogenic, producing liver tumors, although they are generally negative in short-term tests for genotoxicity, such as the Ames test. It has also been suggested that peroxisome proliferators may function as promoters in carcinogenesis. The mechanism for neither the epigenetic initiation nor the possible promotion is known, but may be due to increased reactive oxygen species formed subsequent to increased H_2O_2 resulting from the proliferation of the peroxisomes. *See also* ACTIVE OXYGEN; PEROXISOMES.

peroxisomes. Cellular organelles that may occur in all cell types, but are particularly prominent in hepatocytes and erythrocytes. Usually 0.5–1.0 μm in diameter, they are bounded by a single membrane and characteristically have high levels of catalase, D-amino acid oxidase and other oxidative enzymes. They appear to have some function associated with lipid metabolism, and are induced by agents such as trichloroethylene and clofibrate. *See also* PEROXISOME PROLIFERATION.

peroxyacetyl nitrate (PAN). A member of a class of compounds, the peroxyacyl nitrates, formed in polluted air as a result of interaction of hydrocarbons and oxides of nitrogen in the presence of oxygen and ultraviolet light. The final step is probably the reaction of nitrogen dioxide with the peroxyacetyl radical. It is a lacrimator and irritant to the mucous membranes and may be involved in the respiratory distress caused by smog.

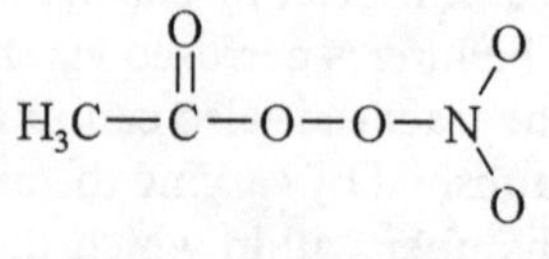

Peroxyacetyl nitrate

peroxy radical. *See* ACTIVE OXYGEN.

pertussigen. *See* PERTUSSIS TOXIN.

pertussis toxin (histamine-sensitizing factor; pertussigen). The gram-negative bacterium *Bordetella pertussis* produces three distinct toxins, one of them being pertussis toxin, a protein of 117,000 daltons, which contains an α-β subunit structure. The LD50 in mice has been reported to be between 0.5 and 4 µg/kg. This toxin is of major importance in the pathogenesis of whooping cough. Pertussis toxin acts on a number of cell types including leukocytes, adipocytes, pancreatic β cells and myocardial cells. The β subunit of the toxin binds to a cell surface, facilitating internalization of the α subunit. Inside the cell, the α subunit catalyzes the transfer of an ADP-ribose moiety from NAD^+ to the guanine nucleotide protein (G_i) responsible for inhibition of adenylate cyclase. Ribosylation uncouples adenylate cyclase from the G_i protein, allowing enhancement of receptor-mediated, GTP-dependent adenylate cyclase activity. The increase in cellular cyclic AMP is hypothesized to mediate many of the adverse effects of the toxin on target cells. Early cold-like symptoms such as a slight fever, sneezing and mild cough progress into a severe paroxysmal cough over a period of one to two weeks. Once the characteristic whooping cough stage has been reached, antipertussis serum is of little use. Antibiotics may prevent secondary infection, but do not stop the cough. *See also* ADENYLATE CYCLASE; CYCLIC AMP; G-PROTEINS.

pesticides. Chemicals specifically developed and produced for use in the control of agricultural and public health pests, to increase production of food and fiber, and to facilitate modern agricultural methods. As commonly used the term does not include chemicals for the control of microorganisms, bacteriocides and antibiotics being considered distinct terms. Although selective toxicity is desirable it is never absolute, and most pesticides are toxic, to a greater or lesser extent, to non-target organisms, including humans. By the very nature of their use they tend to be common contaminants of water, air, food and domestic structures. In most countries there is a body of law governing their development and use. Common classes of pesticides include acaricides, algicides, fungicides, herbicides, insecticides, molluscicides, nemato-cides and rodenticides. *See also* AGRICULTURAL CHEMICALS; FEDERAL INSECTICIDE, FUNGICIDE AND RODENTICIDE ACT.

Pesticide Safety Precautions Scheme. *See* PEST INFESTATION CONTROL LABORATORY.

Pest Infestation Control Laboratory. A part of the Ministry of Agriculture, Fisheries and Food responsible for the Pesticides Safety Precautions Scheme and the Agricultural Chemicals Approval Scheme, which is concerned with safety clearance and efficiency approval of agricultural chemicals intended to be used in the UK.

pethidine. *See* MEPERIDINE.

petrol. *See* GASOLINE.

petroleum. Crude oil, consisting of normal and branched-chain paraffins, cycloparaffins, aromatics and asphaltics (naphthalenes). Petroleum may also contain varying amounts of heavy metals and up to 10% sulfur. It can be distilled into a variety of components, which may be further refined for specific uses. *See also* CRUDE OIL; OIL SPILLS; POLLUTION, FOSSIL FUELS; POLLUTION, PETROLEUM PRODUCTS.

peyote. *Lophophora williamsi*, a small blue green spineless cactus. Small dome-shaped heads are cut off and dried as peyote "buttons". Peyote, which contains many psychoactive β-phenylethylamine and isoquinoline alkaloids, has been used in religious ceremonies for 2–3000 years. The principal hallucinogen is mescaline. *See also* MESCALINE.

PFC assay (plaque-forming assay). *See* JERNE PLAQUE ASSAY.

***Pfiesteria*.** A toxic marine organism that kills fish via infection and produces at least two toxins. Found to date on the US Atlantic coasts of North Carolina and Maryland. Although there are no known human fatalities, intoxication is purported to cause short-term problems such as confusion, fatigue, diarrhea, and breathing difficulties, and may also cause learning and memory problems. The organism can exist as an amoeba on river bottoms. While these amoeba can be inactive and form cysts, they also can secrete zoospores that feed on underwater algae. The zoospores also can transform into toxic dinoflagellates that infect fish.

***p*-glycoprotein**. Membrane transporter also known as multi-drug resistance (MDR) protein which transports intracellular toxicants back into extracellular spaces. It occurs in brain capillary endothelial cells and contributes to the blood–brain barrier. It also extrudes toxicants from oocytes.

phagocytes. Stationary cells within tissue or leukocytes capable of phagocytosis. *See also* PHAGO-CYTOSIS; STEM CELLS.

phagocytosis. A process by which the cell membranes of certain cells flow around particles and engulf them into the interior of the cell. Phagocytosis plays a role in the penetration of toxicants into the body, occurring in the alveoli of the lungs and in the gastrointestinal tract. It is an important feature of the immune system; however, the polymorphonuclear phagocytes (granulocytes) and macrophages both play an important role in resistance to microorganisms. *See also* ENTRY MECHANISMS, ENDOCYTOSIS; IMMUNE SYSTEM; MACRO-PHAGES/MONOCYTES; PENETRATION ROUTES, GASTROINTESTINAL; PENETRATION ROUTES, PULMONARY; STEM CELLS.

Pharmaceutical Manufacturers Association. A US trade association. In 1977 it published guidelines for the testing of drugs and medical devices for safety to humans.

pharmacodynamics. The study of the dynamic changes in a drug or other xenobiotic molecule as it is metabolized, excreted and/or interacts with macromolecules at the site of action. *See also* PROBIT/LOG TRANSFORMS.

pharmacogenetics. The study of the genetic basis for the variation in response to drugs or toxicants. Much of this variation is due to polymorphisms in xenobiotic-metabolizing enzymes. *See also* CYTOCHROME P450, POLYMORPHISMS.

pharmacokinetics. The study of the time course of the absorption, distribution, metabolism and excretion of drugs based upon measurements of concentrations of drugs and metabolites in biological matrices. The term implies the use of mathematical models to obtain parameters that describe the kinetic processes. These parameters may then be used to predict therapeutic or adverse effects using other dosage regimens or routes of administration. *See also* CLEARANCE; COMPART-MENT; FIRST-ORDER KINETICS; FIRST-PASS EFFECT; KINETIC EQUATIONS; MULTI-COM-PONENT MODELS; ONE-COMPARTMENT MODEL; PHYSIOLOGICALLY-BASED PHARMACOKINET-ICS; PROBIT/LOG TRANSFORMS; PROBITS; TOXI-COKINETICS; TWO-COMPARTMENT MODEL; VOLUME OF DISTRIBUTION.

pharmacological antagonism. *See* ANTAGO-NISM, PHARMACOLOGICAL.

pharmacovigilance. Monitoring for suspected adverse reactions to medicines. The observation of all activity tending to provide systematic indications of probable causal links between drugs and adverse reactions in a population but restricted to "harmful reactions to drug doses normally used" (WHO). Overdosage is not considered. The original definition referred to human beings, but veterinary pharmacovigilance is an equally valid concept.

phase I reactions. Reactions that introduce a polar reactive group into lipophilic xenobiotics. In most cases, this group becomes the site for conjugation during phase II reactions. Such reactions include microsomal monooxygenations, cytosolic and mitochondrial oxidations, cooxidations in the prostaglandin synthetase reaction, reductions, hydrolysis and epoxide hydration. The products of phase I reactions may be potent electrophiles that can be conjugated and detoxified in phase II reactions or which may react with nucleophilic groups on cellular constituents, thereby showing greater toxicity than the parent compound. The epoxidation of polycyclic aromatic hydrocarbons is a typical phase I reaction. *See also* CO-OXIDATION, DURING PROSTAGLANDIN SYNTHESIS; EPOX-IDES; HYDROLYSIS; MONOOXYGENATION; NON-MICROSOMAL OXIDATIONS; PHASE II REAC-TIONS; REDUCTION.

phase II reactions. Reactions that involve the conjugation of phase I products and other xenobiotics containing functional groups such as hydroxyl, amino, carboxyl, epoxide or halogen with endogenous metabolites. The endogenous metabolites include sugars, amino acids, glutathione and sulfate. The conjugation products, with rare exceptions, are more polar, less toxic and more readily excreted than their parent compounds. Conjugation reactions usually involve high-energy intermediates and have been classified into two general types: type I (e.g., glycoside and sulfate formation) in which an activated conjugating agent combines with the substrate to yield the conjugated product; type II (e.g., amino acid conjugation) in which the substrate is activated and then combines with an amino acid to yield a conjugated product. The most important conjugation reactions are glycoside formation (particularly glucuronidation), sulfate formation, glutathione conjugation and mercapturic acid formation and acylation (particularly amino acid conjugation). *See also* AMINO ACID CONJUGATION; GLYCOSIDE CONJUGATION; PHASE I REACTIONS; SULFATE CONJUGATION.

phenacemide (N-(aminocarbonyl)benzene-acetamide; (phenylacetyl)urea; Phenurone). CAS number 63-98-9. A straight-chain analog of 5-phenylhydantoin. Its efficacy as an anticonvulsant has not been established, and its toxicity makes it unsuitable for clinical use. Adverse effects include gastrointestinal distress, hepatitis, rash, behavioral changes, aplastic anemia and nephritis. This drug may have some use as an adjunctive treatment in complex partial seizures that are unresponsive to other anticonvulsants. Careful monitoring of patients treated with such a regimen is critical. The oral LD50 in mice and rats is 5.54 and more than 10 mmol/kg, respectively. *See also* ANTICONVULSANTS; PHENYTOIN.

Phenacemide

phenacetin (N-(4-ethoxyphenyl)acetamide; p-acetophenetidide). CAS number 62-44-2. A derivative of p-aminophenol. A large portion of phenacetin is metabolized to acetaminophen, and since acetaminophen has lower toxicity, it is usually preferred. Phenacetin and acetaminophen have the same therapeutic indications as the salicylates (analgesic, antipyretic), except that they lack anti-inflammatory activity. They are much weaker inhibitors *in vitro* of prostaglandin biosynthesis than are the salicylates. Their analgesic and antipyretic action may be due to more potent effects in the CNS. The aniline derivatives sometimes produce relaxation and drowsiness, and some clinicians have suggested that they may produce anti-anxiety effects. Rarely, some patients become habituated to these drugs and use them excessively. Some of their side effects include blood disorders, and abnormal pathways of metabolism may sometimes result in methemoglobin formation and a resulting cyanosis. Beside its effects on the blood, phenacetin has been indicted in the production of kidney damage. In fact in the USA, analgesic mixtures containing phenacetin are required to carry a warning label stating that kidney damage may occur with prolonged use. However, unlike the salicylates, the p-aminophenol derivatives do not cause marked disruption of acid/base balance. The EPA has listed this substance as a carcinogen, as high-dose chronic abuse has resulted in bladder cancer in humans, chronic administration of 2.5% phenacetin in the diet has caused bladder tumors in rats and N-hydroxyphenacetin has caused liver cancer in rats. Finally, phenacetin may perturb male reproductive function. The oral LD50 in rats is 1.65 g/kg. *See also* ACETAMINOPHEN; ANALGESICS; ANTI-INFLAMMATORY AGENTS.

Phenacetin

phenazone. *See* ANTIPYRINE.

phenazopyridine ((3,9-phenylazo)-2,6-pyridinediamine). CAS number 136-40-3. A brick red azo dye used as a urinary tract analgesic. It is now known to be an animal carcinogen. Human acute poisoning is characterized by methemoglobinemia and Heinz body anemia that is more intense in individuals with glucose-6-phosphate dehydrogenase deficiency.

Phenazopyridine

phencyclidine (1-(1-phenylcyclohexyl) piperidine; PCP; "angel dust"). CAS number 77-10-1. An anesthetic first used in the 1950s in animals, and later in humans. The induction of delirium caused its use to be discontinued, but illicit use started in the early 1970s. Phencyclidine and related arylcyclohexylamines are central stimulants, depressants, anesthetics and hallucinogens. Phencyclidine causes a wide range of specific effects, including standard signs of intoxication (e.g., slurred speech, uneven gait), sweating, muscular rigidity, disorganized thought processes, hostility, transient amnesia, analgesia and, at higher doses, tachycardia, convulsions and coma. Tolerance has been demonstrated in both animals and humans. Phencyclidine has been shown to inhibit monoamine re-uptake, and interact with several types of neuroreceptors, including the hypothesized -receptor as well as the glutamate NMDA receptor. The oral LD50 in mice is 76.5 mg/kg. PCP is still manufactured in South Africa (Syclan^R), and used for anesthesia of certain species of wildlife and zoo animals. *See also* KETAMINE.

β-phenethylamine (benzeneethanamine; β-phenylethylamine; 1-amino-2-phenylethane). CAS number 64-04-0. An endogenous primary amine formed by the decarboxylation of phenylalanine. Phenethylamine is related structurally and pharmacologically to amphetamine, an observation that has led to the hypothesis that phenethylamine may be involved in schizophrenia. Increases in phenylacetic acid in the urine of schizophrenics, which is decreased with treatment, were used to support this hypothesis. The increased phenethylamine observed in phenylketonuria has been used to explain the autistic behavior observed in this population. Phenethylamine has also been linked to migraine headaches. Like amphetamine, phenethylamine has anorectic properties and induces hyperactivity in mice and, at high doses, stereotyped behavior in rats. Phenethylamine is a specific substrate for monoamine oxidase type B and so is rapidly metabolized in brain. The behavioral actions of phenethylamine are thought to be mediated by serotonergic as well as catecholaminergic pathways in brain. The LD50 in mice is approximately 470 mg/kg, s.c. *See also* AMPHETAMINE; CATECHOLAMINES.

$CH_2CH_2NH_2$

Phenethylamine

phenobarbital (5-ethyl-5-phenyl-2,4,6(1*H*, 3*H*,5*H*) pyrimidinetrione; 5-ethyl-5-phenyl barbituric acid; phenobarbitone). CAS number 50-06-6. Phenobarbital, like most of the other clinically used sedative-hypnotics has anticonvulsant properties, and it was the first effective antiepileptic agent developed. Phenobarbital both limits the spread of seizures and elevates the seizure threshold, and is especially effective against grand mal (tonic-clonic) epilepsy and cortical focal seizures. The principal side effect of phenobarbital, when used as an antiepileptic, is related to its sedative-hypnotic properties. The incidence of other side effects with phenobarbital is generally low, but withdrawal from barbiturates in an individual dependent on these drugs is marked by convulsions, even in those without a seizure disorder. Phenobarbital is also one of the two major metabolites of primidone, another clinically used antiepileptic drug. In addition to its effects on the nervous system, phenobarbital is also the prototypic inducer of hepatic drug metabolism. It is a predominant inducer of the cytochrome P450 2B subfamily, and can also induce other xenobiotic metabolizing enzymes such as some phase II

Phencyclidine

enzymes. The oral LD50 in rats is 162 mg/kg. *See also* CONVULSIONS; INDUCTION; SEDATIVE-HYPNOTICS.

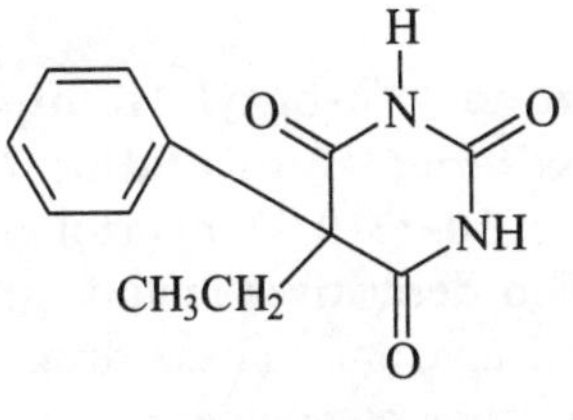

Phenobarbital

phenobarbitone. *See* PHENOBARBITAL.

phenolphthalein (3,3-bis(4-hydroxyphenyl)-1-(3H)-isobenzofuranone). CAS number 77-09-8. A pH indicator that is also active as a cathartic. The glucuronide has been used in studies of hepatobiliary dysfunction caused by toxic chemicals.

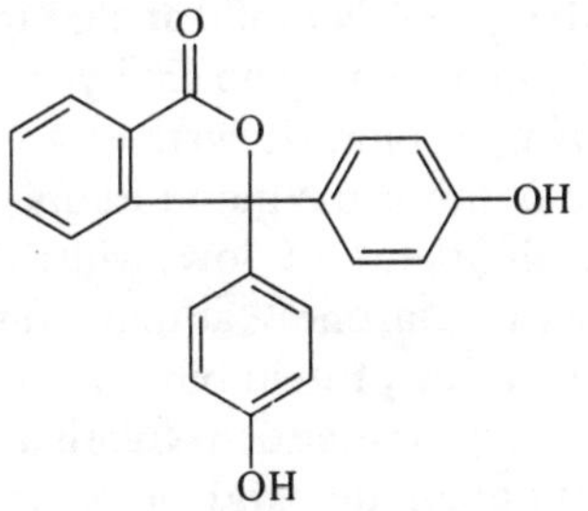

Phenolphthalein

phenols. A class of compounds in which a hydroxyl group is attached directly to a carbon atom of a benzene or other aromatic ring. Considerably more acid than alcohols, they give rise to phenolate ions in solution. The parent compound phenol (carbolic acid) is used as a general disinfectant and is an intermediate in many industrial processes. It is highly corrosive and toxic. Acute poisoning causes nausea, vomiting, circulatory collapse, necrosis of the mouth and gastro-intestinal tract and, in severe cases, death from respiratory failure. The fatal dose for humans is said to be about 15 g, but death has been reported from much lower doses, including doses absorbed through the skin. Chronic poisoning may result in liver and kidney damage, and it has been shown to be a promoter of carcinogenesis in experimental animals.

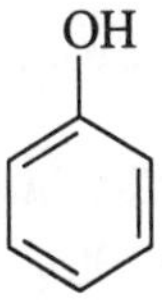

Phenol

phenosulfophthalein. A pH indicator used in the pH 6.8–8.4 range. It is also used clinically to assess kidney function and experimentally to assess tubular activity in investigations of nephrotoxic agents.

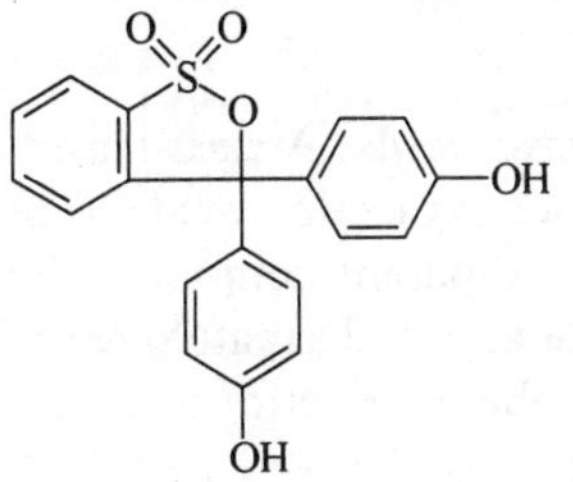

Phenosulfophthalein

phenothiazines. Derivatives of the phenothiazine nucleus; used as antipsychotic and antihistaminic drugs. Derivatives were used as dyestuffs in the late 19th century, and Ehrlich suggested that the resulting aniline dyes might be used to treat psychoses. Promethazine was found during the 1930s to have strong antihistaminic and sedative effects. It and other antihistaminics were used to treat psychoses with little success. However, promethazine did prolong barbiturate sleeping time in rodents, thus suggesting its use as an anesthetic potentiating agent. Chlorpromazine, the prototypic phenothiazine antipsychotic, was synthesized in the search for better anesthetic-potentiating agents and was found to attenuate psychotic symptoms above and beyond simple relief of agitation or anxiety. With all members of this class, there is a secondary nitrogen three carbons removed from the ring which can, in space-filling models, be seen to mimic the elements of dopamine. After the introduction of chlorpromazine in the early 1950s, a search led to other phenothiazine analogs and to the development of the structurally related tricyclic antidepressants. The phenothiazine antipsychotics consist of three classes: (1) the dimethylaminopropyl alkyl side chain (e.g., chlorpromazine); (2) the piperidine side chain (e.g., thioridazine); (3) the piperazine side chain (e.g., trifluoperazine, fluphenazine). This group of antipsychotic drugs works by blocking dopamine receptors. Among its acute toxic side effects are parkinson-like neurological signs; a condition called tardive dyskinesia that is caused by long-term administration. *See also* ANTIHISTAMINES; ANTIPSYCHOTIC DRUGS; CHLORPROMAZINE; DOPAMINE RECEPTORS; PROMETHAZINE; THIORIDAZINE.

phenotype. The visible manifestation of traits determined by an individual's genetic composition (genotype).

phenoxyacetic acids. A class based on substitution of phenoxyacetic acid (CAS number 122-59-8). The parent compound has been used as a fungicide and in dermatology as an exfoliant. Substituted phenoxyacetic acids include herbicides such as alachlor and metolachlor, both of which are under review by the US EPA as suspected carcinogens.

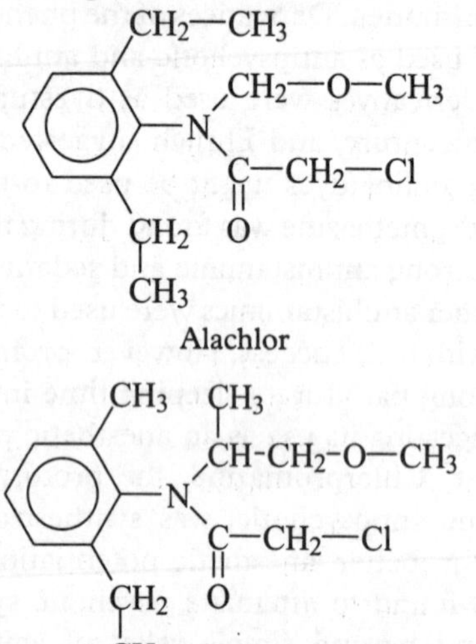

Alachlor

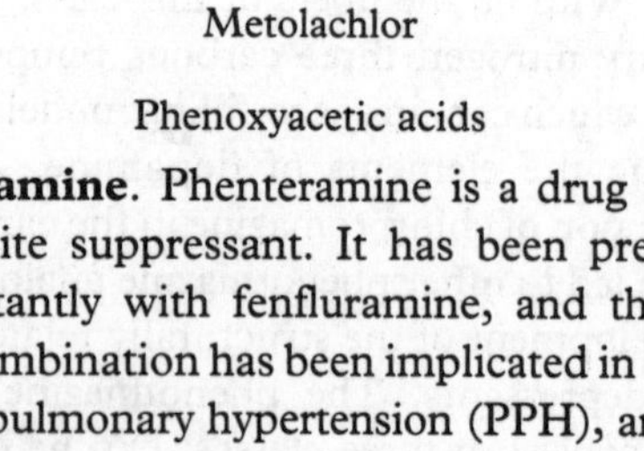

Metolachlor

Phenoxyacetic acids

phenteramine. Phenteramine is a drug used as an appetite suppressant. It has been prescribed concomitantly with fenfluramine, and the "fen-phen" combination has been implicated in causing primary pulmonary hypertension (PPH), an otherwise rare condition in healthy individuals. *See also* FENFLURAMINE.

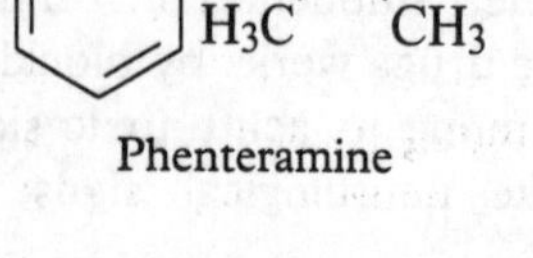

Phenteramine

Phenuron. *See* PHENACEMIDE.

l-phenylalanine mustard. *See* MELPHALAN.

phenylbutazone (4-butyl-1,2-diphenyl-3,5-pyrazolidinedione; Butazolidin; Naprosyn). CAS number 50-33-9. A pyrazolon derivative; other pyrazolon derivatives include aminopyrine, antipyrine and apazone. These drugs tend to be weaker antipyretics or analgesics than the salicylates, but they do have strong anti-inflammatory properties. The main disadvantage of the pyrazolon derivatives is that they may produce serious blood disorders. Agranulocytosis (sudden decrease in white blood cells) may be fatal and can occur in hypersensitive individuals receiving aminopyrine, whereas skin eruptions occasionally occur with antipyrine. These pyrazolon derivatives seem to be more toxic than the other mild analgesics, but they may be useful in patients who are hypersensitive to salicylates. If pyrazolon derivatives are used, it is important to monitor the blood frequently for the possible development of low white blood cell count. Phenylbutazone administration may decrease the plasma protein binding of other drug classes, including oral anticoagulants, oral hypoglycemics, sulfonamides and other anti-inflamatory agents. This may result in potentiated or toxic effects of these other drugs. *See also* ANTI-INFLAMMATORY AGENTS; ANTIPYRINE; APAZONE.

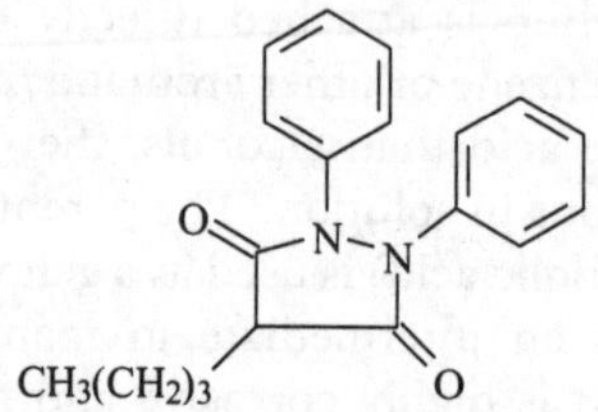

Phenylbutazone

phenylethanolamine *N*-methyltransferase. *See* EPINEPHRINE.

phenylethylene. *See* STYRENE.

phenylisopropylamine. *See* AMPHETAMINES.

phenytoin (diphenylhydantoin; 5,5-diphenyl-2,4-imidazolidinedione; Dilantin). CAS number 57-41-0. A non-sedative anticonvulsant used to treat all classes of seizure disorders except absence seizures. It eliminates generalized tonic-clonic seizures completely, although prodromal signs remain. Phenytoin also eliminates the clonic phase of electroshock-induced seizures, but may prolong or potentiate the tonic phase. Phenytoin appears to act by limiting the spread of seizure activity and reducing the duration of the after-discharge, as opposed to altering the threshold for seizures. This anticonvulsant does not retard the process of kindling as does phenobarbital, carbamazepine, benzodiazepines or sodium valproate. Its mechanism of action is to decrease Na^+ flux, decrease Ca^{2+} influx and delay K^+ efflux. The oral, i.v., and s.c. LD50 in mice are 490, 92 and 110 mg/kg, respectively. Absorption after oral administration is slow and variable, with peak blood levels observed after 3–12 hours. A major metabolite is the p-hydroxyphenyl derivative which is inactive. Side effects include visual disturbances, slurred speech, gastrointestinal distress and drug sensitivity reactions. A major consequence of chronic administration of this drug is gingival hyperplasia. Cardiac arrhythmias, with or without hypotension, and/or CNS depression may occur following i.v. administration at an excessive rate. *See also* ANTICONVULSANTS.

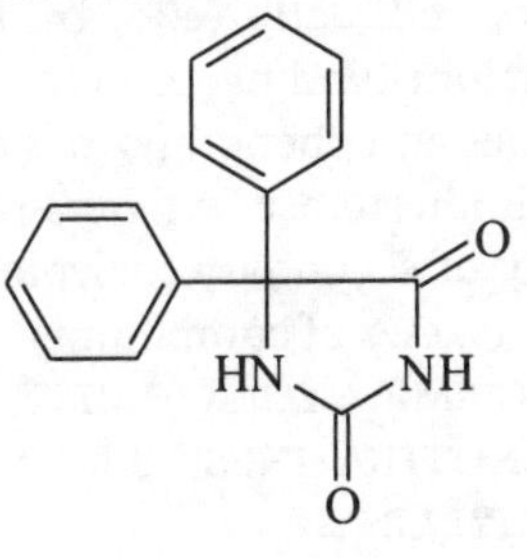

Phenytoin

pheromones. Chemicals, produced by one organisms that affect sexual behavior and/or fertility in members of the opposite gender. They are usually volatile chemicals detected by olfaction.

phorate (*O,O*-diethyl *S*-ethylthiomethyl-phosphorodithioate; thimet; Timet (USSR); Agrimet; Geomet; Granutox; Rampart; Thimenox). CAS number 298-02-2. A soil and systemic insecticide with an oral LD50 in male rats of 2–4 mg/kg and a dermal LD50 in guinea pigs of 20–30 mg/kg. It is a neurotoxicant by virtue of acetylcholinesterase inhibition caused by the cytochrome P450 metabolite phorate oxon. The oxons of the sulfoxide and sulfone are also acetylcholinesterase inhibitors. *See also* ORGANOPHOSPHATE POISONING, SYMPTOMS AND THERAPY; ORGANOPHOSPHORUS INSECTICIDES.

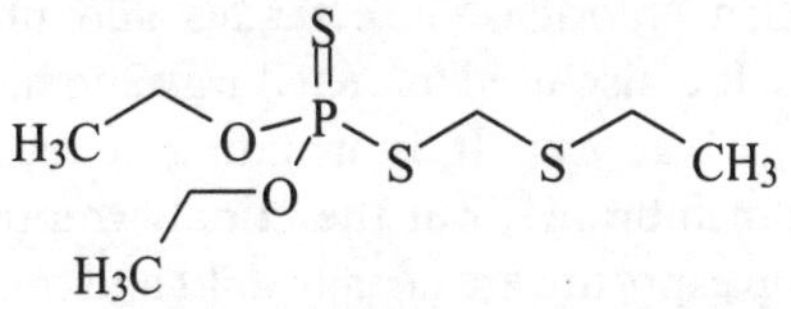

Phorate

phoratoxin. *See* MISTLETOE.

phorbol esters. CAS number 17673-25-5. Diesters of phorbol, particularly 12-*O*-tetradecanoylphorbol 13-acetate, also known as phorbol myristate acetate, have been identified as the potent, highly lipophilic tumor-promoting components in croton oil. They are potent promotors of skin tumors *in vivo* and have been shown to transform cultured fibroblasts and embryonic cells previously exposed to polycyclic aromatic hydrocarbon carcinogens *in vitro*. The structure of phorbol, the parent alcohol is shown below. Phorbol esters also have important effects on leukocytes and on the immune system of the intact animal. There appears to be a specific receptor for phorbol esters on T cells, a finding that may account for the selective toxicity of phorbol esters for T cells. The mechanism of tumor promotion by phorbol esters is still largely unknown, but recent findings suggest an initial cell membrane interaction (often with stimulation of second messenger synthesis and increased protein kinase activity), with subsequent effects on nuclear regulatory events.

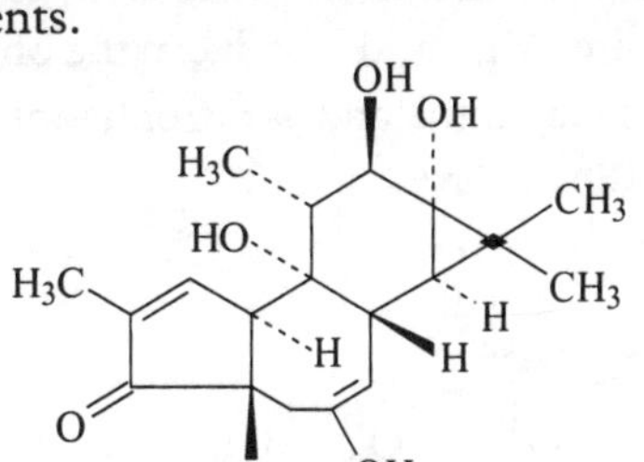

Phorbol

phorbol myristate acetate. *See* PHORBOL ESTERS.

phosgene (COCl₂; carbonic acid dichloride; carbonyl chloride; chloroformyl chloride). CAS number 75-44-5. A colorless, noncombustible gas or volatile liquid. It is used in the synthesis of dyestuffs, isocyanates, carbonic acid esters, acid chlorides, insecticides and pharmaceuticals. It is also used in metallurgy and has been used as a war gas. It is irritating to eyes and mucous membranes, but the initial symptoms of inhalation exposure are usually mild and transient. However, 6–24 hours after exposure, peribronchial edema, pulmonary congestion and alveolar edema occur, leading to death from anoxia. This damage results from the pulmonary hydrolysis of phosgene into HCl and CO_2. Chronic exposures may result in irreversible pulmonary damage such as bronchitis, emphysema and fibrosis. The lethal concentration in air for rats is 50 ppm. Phosgene is the toxic product formed from chloroform by the cytochrome P450-dependent monooxygenase system. Phosgene can be generated from some chlorinated hydrocarbon solvents, such as carbon tetrachloride or methylene chloride, under intense heat, and may be responsible for some solvent-related intoxications and death.

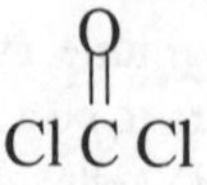

Phosgene

phosphate conjugation. Although phosphorylation of endogenous compounds is a common and essential metabolic reaction, phosphorylation of xenobiotics is uncommon, insects being the only major group of animals in which it is known to occur. The enzyme from cockroach gut utilizes ATP, requires Mg^{2+} and is active in the phosphorylation of α-naphthol and p-nitrophenol. *See also* PHASE II REACTIONS.

phosphates. Inorganic phosphate is a pollutant resulting from excess fertilizer in run-off or from detergents, and it contributes to eutrophication. Soluble fertilizer phosphates, however, are adsorbed strongly to soil particles and move more by soil erosion than by leaching into run-off. An attempt has been made to reduce the use of phosphate-containing detergents.

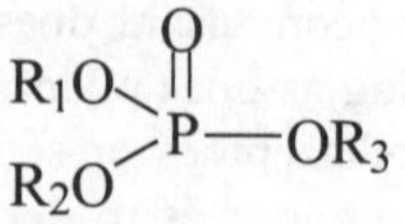

General structure for phosphates

phosphoadenosine-3′-phosphoadenosine-5′-phosphosulfate. *See* PAPS.

phosphodiesterases. Enzymes that hydrolyze the cyclic phosphodiester bond in cyclic nucleotides. The reaction to 5′-monophosphates is generally considered an inactivation reaction, and since this terminates the actions of the cyclic nucleotide, it is an important regulatory step. There are numerous phosphodiesterases, with varying substrate specificities towards different cyclic nucleotides. Toxicants can affect this reaction directly or indirectly (e.g., by affecting the regulatory calcium-binding protein calmodulin). Methylxanthines and phenothiazines are known to inhibit phosphodiesterase activity, although this effect is clearly of secondary toxicological importance for these classes of compounds. *See also* CAFFEINE; CYCLIC AMP; CYCLIC GMP; METHYLXANTHINES; PHENOTHIAZINES; SECOND MESSENGERS; THEOPHYLLINE.

phospholipids. Lipid substances, containing a phosphate group and one or more fatty acid residues, which are essential components of cell membranes. Hydrolysis yields fatty acids, phosphoric acid and a base. They are amphoteric with a polar

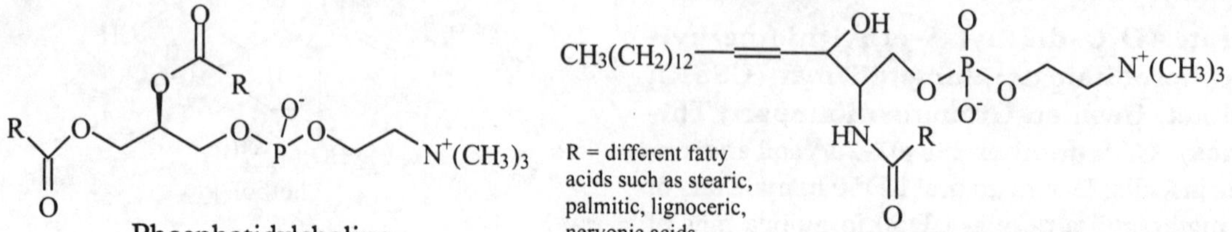

Phosphatidylcholine

R = different fatty acids such as stearic, palmitic, lignoceric, nervonic acids.

Spinghomyelins

Phospholipids

and a non-polar region. Lecithins, cephalins, and related compounds are based on a glycerol backbone, with a phosphate group. In lecithin (phosphatidylcholine), R′ are fatty acid residues, usually one saturated and the other unsaturated. In the cephalins, ethanolamine ($H_2NCH_2CH_2OH$) or serine replace choline. They are used in the food industry as surfactants, emulsifiers and antioxidants. In sphingomyelins R is a fatty acid residue, usually tetracosanoic acid. They occur abundantly in brain tissues in association with cerebrosides, which are similar. On hydrolysis they split into choline, sphingosine, phosphoric acid and a fatty acid.

phosphonates. A class of organophosphorus compounds with at least one phosphorus-carbon bond. It includes insecticides such as EPN, trichlorfon, leptophos and fonofos. These compounds are esters of phosphonic acid with the following general structure. The mode of action of these compounds is cholinesterase inhibition.

$$R_1 \diagdown \overset{\overset{\textstyle O}{\|}}{\underset{R_2O \diagup}{P}} - OR_3$$

General structure for phosphonates

phosphooxythirane ring. A postulated intermediate in the oxidative desulfuration of certain organophosphorus insecticides containing a thionosulfur (P=S); the reaction is mediated by the cytochrome P450-dependent monooxygenase system. *See also* DESULFURATION AND OXIDATIVE ESTER CLEAVAGE.

Phosphooxythirane ring

phosphoproteins. Proteins that may have a phosphate group, usually originating from ATP, covalently added to them by enzymes called protein kinases and possibly removed by protein phosphatases. Protein kinases are an important site for regulation of cellular activities, and the kinase activity itself can be altered by changes in availability of cellular second messengers such as cyclic AMP, diacylglycerol, calcium, etc. The phosphorylation or dephosphorylation of the target protein is often associated with marked changes in physiological/biochemical characteristics (e.g., changes in activity of tyrosine hydroxylase). *See also* SECOND MESSENGERS.

phosphorus (P). CAS number 7723-14-0. A highly reactive element that exists in several physical forms: red, white and yellow. It is a fire and explosion hazard. *See also* ATSDR DOCUMENT, JUNE 1994 FOR WHITE PHOSPHORUS; LEWIS, HCDR, NUMBERS PH0500, PHO740 AND PHO 750.

phosphorylated. The chemical entity resulting from the covalent addition of an inorganic phosphate (such as from ATP) or an organophosphorus moiety (such as from organophosphorus insecticides or nerve agents) to a macromolecule, such as a protein.

phosphotriesterase. *See A*-ESTERASE.

Phosvel. *See* LEPTOPHOS.

photoallergy test. *See* PHOTOTOXICITY TESTS.

photochemical smog. *See* SMOG.

phototoxicity tests. Tests that evaluate the combined dermal effects of light (primarily ultraviolet) and the test chemical. Tests are used for both phototoxicity and photoallergy. The light energy is believed to cause a transient excitation of the toxicant molecule that, on returning to the lower energy state, generates a reactive radical intermediate. In phototoxicity these radicals act directly to cause lesions; in photoallergy they bind to body proteins, which then act as antigens causing the immune system to produce antibodies. These tests are basically modifications of the primary irritation and sensitization tests except that, following application of the test chemical, the treated area is irradiated with ultraviolet light. The differences between the irradiated and non-irradiated animals is a measure of the photo effect. *See also* ACUTE TOXICITY TESTING; DERMAL IRRITATION TESTS; DERMAL SENSITIZATION TESTS.

PHS. *See* PUBLIC HEALTH SERVICE.

phthalic acid esters. Primary plasticizers used in polyvinyl chloride (PVC) products, with di-(2-ethylhexyl) phthalate (DEHP) and di-*n*-butyl phthalate (DBP) being the most prominent. They are widely distributed in materials involved in transportation, construction, clothing, medicine and packaging. The acute toxicities of these compounds are low, i.p. LD50s for DEHP and DBP in mice of 14.2 and 4.0 g/kg, respectively. However, the phthalate esters readily leach out of plastics and are of concern in medical applications such as blood bags, where possible damage to liver or lungs by the leached plasticizer has been suggested. They are known to be peroxisome proliferators and, as such, possible epigenetic carcinogens and/or tumor promotors. Phthalate esters are also widely distributed environmental pollutants, being present in freshwater, marine and terrestrial ecosystems. Phthalate esters may exert detrimental effects on reproduction of some aquatic organisms.

physiological effects on chronic toxicity. *See* CHRONIC TOXICITY TESTING; TESTING VARIABLES, BIOLOGICAL.

physiological effects on xenobiotic metabolism, aging. The effect of senescence on the metabolism of xenobiotics has not been studied extensively. In rats, monooxygenase activity, which reaches a maximum at about 30 days of age, begins to decline some 250 days later, a decrease that may be associated with reduced levels of sex hormones. Glucuronidation also decreases in old animals, whereas monoamine oxidase activity increases.

physiological effects on xenobiotic metabolism, developmental. In mammals, birth initiates an increase in the activity of many hepatic enzymes involved in xenobiotic metabolism. Monooxygenation activity appears to be very low during the last part of pregnancy and to increase after birth, with no obvious differences between immature males and females. This trend is seen in many species although the developmental pattern may vary. The component enzymes of the cytochrome P450-dependent monooxygenase system follow the same general trend, with minor variations. For example, in the rabbit the postnatal increases in cytochrome P450 and its reductase are parallel; in the rat the increase in the reductase is slower than that of the cytochrome. Phase II reactions may also be age-dependent. Glucuronidation of many substrates is low in fetal tissues, but increases with age. The inability of newborn mammals of many species to form glucuronides is associated with deficiencies in both glucuronosyltransferase and its coenzyme uridine diphosphate glucuronic acid (UDPGA). These factors plus slow excretion of the conjugate formed, and the presence of an inhibitor of glucuronidation, pregnanediol, may lead to neonatal jaundice. Glycine conjugations are also low in the newborn. This is due to a lack of glycine, which reaches normal levels at about 30 days of age in the rat and at 8 weeks in the human. Similarly, glutathione conjugation may be impaired, as in fetal and neonatal guinea pigs, due to a deficiency of glutathione. However, in perinatal rats it is the glutathione transferase itself that is barely detectable, adult levels being reached at about 140 days. This pattern of low activity at birth followed by a postnatal increase does not occur in all cases. In the guinea pig, sulfate conjugation and acetylation appear to be fully functional and at adult levels in the fetus, and compounds that are glucuronidated in the adult can be acetylated or conjugated as sulfates in the young.

physiological effects on xenobiotic metabolism, disease. Quantitatively the liver is the most important site for xenobiotic metabolism, and effects on the liver are, therefore, likely to affect the organism's overall capacity for xenobiotic metabolism. Thus, patients with acute hepatitis may have an impaired ability to oxidize drugs, which then show an increase in plasma half-life. Impaired oxidative metabolism has also been shown in patients with chronic hepatitis, cirrhosis or obstructive jaundice. Phase II reactions may also be affected; decreases in acetylation, glucuronidation and a variety of esterase activities have been seen in various liver diseases, whereas hepatic tumors tend to have a lower ability to metabolize foreign compounds than normal liver tissue. Kidney diseases may also affect the overall ability to handle xenobiotics since this organ is one of the main routes for the elimination of xenobiotics and their metabolites. The half-lives of tolbutamide, thiopental, hexobarbital and chloramphenicol are all prolonged in patients with renal impairment.

physiological effects on xenobiotic metabolism, diurnal rhythms. Diurnal rhythms, both in cytochrome P450 levels and in the susceptibility to toxicants, have been described, especially in rodents. Although such changes appear to be related to the light cycle, they may, in fact, be activity-dependent since feeding and other activities in rodents are themselves markedly diurnal.

physiological effects on xenobiotic metabolism, hormones. Hormones other than sex hormones are known to affect the levels of xenobiotic-metabolizing enzymes, but these effects are not well studied or understood. Both increases and decreases in microsomal cytochrome P450-dependent monooxygenation have been reported to occur after treatment with thyroxine. Thyroid hormone can also affect enzymes other than microsomal monooxygenases, but again the effect is complex. For example, liver monoamine oxidase activity is decreased, whereas kidney monoamine oxidase is increased. Adrenalectomy of male rats impairs the hepatic metabolism of aminopyrine and hexobarbital, but the same operation in females has no effect on their metabolism. Cortisone or prednisolone restores activity to normal levels. Similarly, the effect of insulin or alloxan-induced diabetes has variable effects. For example, the *in vitro* metabolism of hexobarbital and aminopyrine is decreased in alloxan-diabetic male rats, whereas it is increased in similarly treated females; no sex differences are seen in the mouse, with both activities showing an increase. Pituitary hormones regulate the function of many other endocrine glands, and hypophysectomy frequently results in a decrease in the activity of xenobiotic-metabolizing enzymes. However, the effects of hypophysectomy or administration of ACTH also gives variable results or results that are sex-dependent. *See also* PHYSIOLOGICAL EFFECTS ON XENOBIOTIC METABOLISM, PREGNANCY.

physiological effects on xenobiotic metabolism, pregnancy. Xenobiotic-metabolizing enzyme activities generally decrease during pregnancy. For example, catechol *O*-methyltransferase and monoamine oxidase decrease, as does glucuronide conjugation, the latter probably being related to increasing levels of progesterone and pregnanediol, both inhibitors of glucuronosyltransferase *in vitro*. A similar effect on sulfate conjugation has been seen in pregnant rats and guinea pigs. Hepatic cytochrome P-450 concentrations may also decrease in pregnancy, with a concomitant decrease in microsomal monooxygenase activity.

physiological effects on xenobiotic metabolism, sex. Metabolism of xenobiotics may vary with the sex of the organism, such variation becoming apparent at puberty and being maintained throughout adult life. Adult male rats carry out many metabolic reactions at higher rates than females, including hexobarbital hydroxylation, aminopyrine *N*-demethylation, glucuronidation of *o*-aminophenol and glutathione conjugation of aryl substrates, although with other substrates such as aniline and zoxazolamine no sex differences are apparent. In humans, sex differences in xenobiotic metabolism are less pronounced. The differences in microsomal monooxygenase activity between males and females are under the control of sex hormones, at least in some species, and sex differences in enzyme activity may vary from tissue to tissue. Differences in toxicity *in vivo* between males and females of various species are known, and such differences may be related to sex-related differences in metabolism. For example, hexobarbital is metabolized faster by males of some species, and females have longer sleeping times. Many of the sex-related differences are related to differences in the distribution of isozymes of the enzymes involved, and sex-specific isozymes of cytochrome P450 have been reported.

physiological tolerance. A form of adaptation that occurs when prior single or repeated exposure to the same concentration of a given agent produces a decreased effect. Alternatively, the term is used when a increased concentration of the agent is necessary to obtain the effects observed with the original concentration. The term refers to compensatory pharmacodynamic changes that take place in the target tissue(s) and include such phenomena as changes in membrane fluidity, receptor affinity or density, allosteric modifications of target tissue, new synthesis or specific biochemical components, etc. Such tolerance may occur rapidly (within minutes or seconds) or may require days, weeks or even months. *See also* ADAPTATION TO TOXICANTS; DEPENDENCE; TOLERANCE.

physiologically-based pharmacokinetics. Differs from classical models in that the compartments are not defined by the data but are real tissues, organs or body regions. The rate constants represent known or inferred physiological processes. Such pharmacokinetic models are more realistic, albeit more complex, than classical models in which both rate constants and compartments are defined by the data, giving rise to the term data-based models as opposed to physiologically-based models.

physostigmine. *See* ESERINE.

picloram. A herbicide. There is some experimental evidence for carcinogenicity, but no evidence for human carcinogenicity. *See also* DATABASES, TOXICOLOGY; LEWIS, HCDR, NUMBER PIB900; MERCK INDEX, 12TH EDN, NUMBER 7552.

picrotoxin (cocculin). A product of the shrub *Anamirta cocculus*, a compound made up of one mole of picrotoxinin plus one mole of picrotin, the latter being inactive. Picrotoxin is highly toxic, particularly in fish, and has an LD50 in mice of 7.2 mg/kg, i.p. Although not used clinically for this purpose, picrotoxin has central and respiratory stimulant properties, and can be used as an antidote to barbiturate poisoning in animals. At larger doses, picrotoxin induces convulsions, salivation, emesis and hypertension. Its action is due to the blockade, centrally, of γ-amino butyric acid (GABA).

picrotoxinin [1aR-(1aα,2aβ,3β,6β,6aβ,8aS*, 8bβ,9R*)]-hexahydro-2a-hydroxy-8b-methyl-9-(1-methyl-ethenyl)-3,6- methano-8H-1,5,7-trioxacyclopenta[*ij*]cycloprop[*a*]azulene-4,8 (3H)-dione. CAS number 17617-45-7. Recent findings support the existence of a picrotoxin-binding site on the ionophore that includes GABA and benzodiazepine recognition sites, as well as a chloride channel. Picrotoxin is absorbed relatively slowly with a short duration of action. It is highly toxic in humans with doses as low as 20 mg

resulting in poisoning. Diazepam can be used effectively as an antidote for picrotoxin poisoning. Picrotoxinin is the toxic component of picrotoxin. The i.p LD50 in mice is approximately 3 mg/kg. *See also* PICROTOXIN.

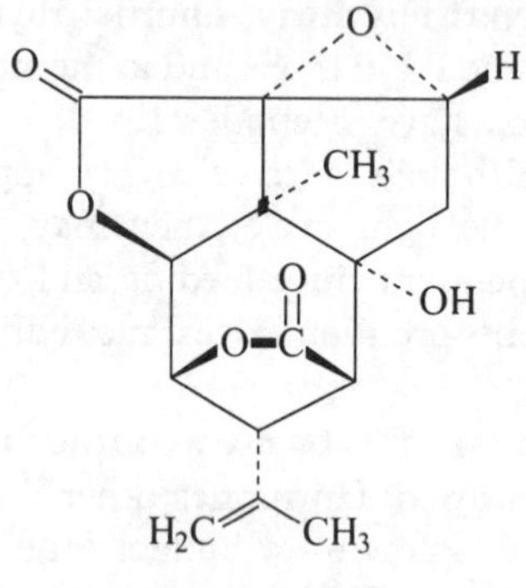

Picrotoxinin

pinocytosis. Engulfment by the cell membrane of a portion of the liquid environment of the cell. It differs from phagocytosis only in that phagocytosis is the engulfment of a solid particle. It is probably not important as a mechanism for toxicant uptake. *Compare* PHAGOCYTOSIS. *See also* ENTRY MECHANISMS, ENDOCYTOSIS.

piperine (1-piperoylpiperidine). CAS number 94-62-2. A methylenedioxyphenyl compound obtained from fruit of various peppers (e.g., *Piper nigrum, P. longum*); mp 130 °C, pK_a 1.98. Acid hydrolysis gives piperidine and piperic acid. It is not toxic to humans, and is responsible for the sharp taste of pepper.

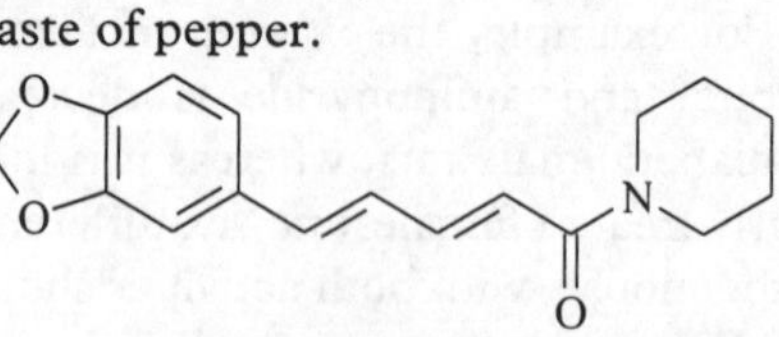

Piperine

piperonyl butoxide (5-[[2-(2-butoxyethoxy) ethoxy]methyl]-6-propyl-1,3-benzodioxole). CAS number 51-03-6. A synergist for the pyrethrins and related insecticides functioning by

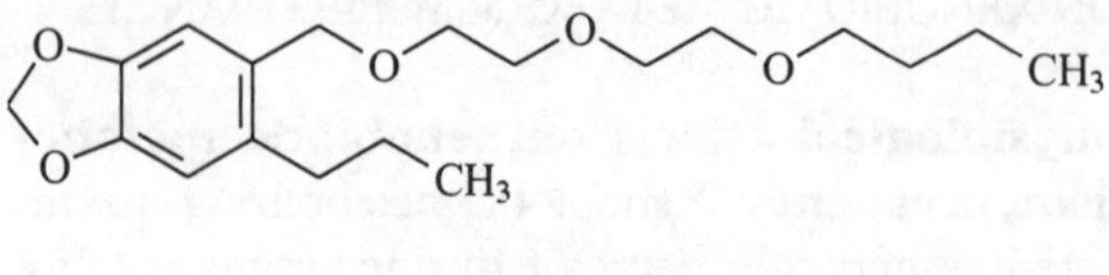

Piperonyl butoxide

acting as an inhibitor of cytochrome P450-mediated detoxication. It is used experimentally as a cytochrome P450 inhibitor both *in vivo* and *in vitro*. The acute oral LD50 in rats and rabbits is about 7500 mg/kg. It is non-carcinogenic, except at very high doses in rats.

pituitary gland (hypophysis). Comprises the anterior pituitary (adenohypophysis), the intermediate lobe and the posterior pituitary (the neurohypophysis), which are under the control of the hypothalamus. It has been called the master gland of the body. *See also* ADENOHYPOPHYSIS; NEUROHYPOPHYSIS; PITUITARY HORMONES.

pituitary gland toxicity. Hypo- or hypersecretion of the pituitary gland can lead to serious endocrine diseases, either directly or via the organs that the tropic hormones stimulate. Examples of directly produced diseases include: gigantism from excess growth hormone in childhood; acromegaly from excess growth hormone in adulthood; dwarfism from inadequate growth hormone in childhood; pituitary cachexia (Simmonds' disease) from inadequate growth hormone in adulthood; diabetes insipidus from inadequate antidiuretic hormone (ADH); edema from excessive ADH that frequently occurs following trauma. Examples of indirectly produced diseases include: Cushing's syndrome from hypersecretion of adrenal glucocorticoids as a result of excessive ACTH; Addison's disease from inadequate ACTH; hyperthyroidism from excessive TSH; hypothyroidism (cretinism in infants, myxedmea in adults) from inadequate TSH; reproductive disorders from inappropriate amounts of the gonadotropins.

pituitary hormones. The anterior pituitary (adeno hypophysis) secretes the following hormones in response to the releasing and inhibitory factors of the hypothalamus: growth hormone (somatotropin); the gonadotropins (follicle-stimulating hormone (FSH) and luteinizing hormone (LH) in the female or interstitial cell-stimulating hormone (ICSH) in the male); adrenocorticotropic hormone (ACTH); thyroid-stimulating hormone (TSH); prolactin. The intermediate lobe secretes melanocyte-stimulating hormone (MSH). The posterior pituitary (neurohypophysis) stores and releases oxytocin and vasopressin (anti-duretic hormone, ADH).

placenta. The structure in the uterus of mammals through which the fetus derives nourishment and eliminates excretory products. It is derived from both fetal and maternal tissue, and a membrane from the placenta encloses the fetus. Blood flow from fetus to and from the placenta is via two umbilical arteries and the umbilical vein, all contained within the umbilical cord. The placenta is important in toxicology as the site of transport of toxicants from the maternal blood to the fetus. *See also* TRANSPLACENTAL.

placental barrier. *See* TRANSPLACENTAL.

placental transfer. *See* TRANSPLACENTAL.

Placidyl. *See* ETHCHLORVYNOL.

plants. *See* POLLUTION, EFFECTS ON PLANTS.

plant toxicants (plant allelochemicals). Chemicals that are believed to have evolved as defense mechanisms against herbivores, particularly insects and mammals. They may be repellent, but not particularly toxic, or they may be acutely toxic to a wide range of organisms. Plant toxicants include many types of chemicals, such as sulfur compounds, lipids, phenols, alkaloids and glycosides. Some of the drugs of abuse such as cocaine, caffeine, nicotine, morphine and the cannabinoids are plant toxicants. Toxic constituents of plants may form part of the human diet. The carcinogen safrole is found in black pepper, and solanine and chaconine, which are cholinesterase inhibitors and possible teratogens, are found in potatoes. Quinones and phenols are widespread in food. Poisoning of domestic animals by plants is still important in veterinary toxicology.

plaque-forming cells (PFC). *See* JERNE PLAQUE ASSAY.

plasma cells. *See* B CELLS.

plasma corticosteroids. *See* ADRENAL GLAND TOXICITY; CORTICOSTEROIDS.

plasma membrane (cell membrane, plasmalemma). Membrane that surrounds prokaryotic and eukaryotic cells and defines the interface between the cell's interior and exterior. Its basic structure is like all biological membranes (often referred to as the fluid mosaic model). Integral proteins are embedded into a lipid bilayer so that the hydrophobic surface of each protein is in the membrane and the polar regions are external. Peripheral proteins are on the surface and bound to a polar region of an integral protein. Integral proteins can drift laterally, but cannot flip-flop. All oligosaccharide residues (of membrane glycolipids and glycoproteins) are found on the noncytoplasmic side of the membrane. Its protein composition and asymmetry reflect its functions at the cell surface (e.g., membrane receptors to bind signalling molecules, such as hormones, in the cells environment; ion pumps to maintain the normal ionic equilibrium with the environment).

plasma protein binding. *See* KINETIC EQUATIONS.

plasma proteins. Approximately 53 characterized proteins that are found in blood plasma subclassed as: globular (e.g., albumin, immunoglobulins); orosomucal (e.g., glycoproteins); lipoproteins (e.g., HDL, LDL); clotting factors. Plasma proteins are synthesized in the liver or reticuloendothelial system. Albumins and lipoproteins nonspecifically bind many drug-like substances in the blood through van der Waals forces and hydrogen bonding. Changes in blood pH or the concentrations of protein constituents, secondary to the physiological alterations of disease, aging, malnutrition, etc. may alter both distribution and clearance of many drugs. A decrease in the albumin concentration results in a decrease in the volume of distribution for many acidic drugs. Increased α-acid glycoprotein (acute-phase reactant protein) plasma concentrations generally increase the extent of protein binding of many basic drugs. Plasma proteins are important in toxicology for several reasons, including transport and storage of toxicants and their metabolites. They also include many antibodies. Transferrin, a β-globulin, is important in iron transport, whereas ceruloplasmin transports copper. The α- and β-lipoproteins transport both endogenous (e.g., steroids) and exogenous chemicals. They are known to be important in the transport of highly lipophilic xenobiotics such as pesticides and polycyclic aromatic hydrocarbons. Depending upon the amount of the protein present, the binding affinity and the number of binding sites, binding to plasma proteins can represent a protective (storage) mechanism or a mechanism permitting rapid transport between tissues. *See also* α$_1$-ACID GLYCOPROTEIN; DISTRIBUTION OF TOXICANTS; TRANSPORT OF TOXICANTS.

plasmid. Plasmids are closed circles of double-stranded DNA, ranging in size from one to 200 kilobases, found in many bacteria and in a few eukaryotic cells. They frequently carry genes conferring antibiotic resistance; infective drug resistance, originally discovered in Shigella, is due to plasmids. Plasmids are widely used as carriers of cloned genes, for example the *E. coli* plasmid pBR322, and numbers of such plasmids may be amplified by treating the donor cells with chloramphenicol, which stops host cell DNA synthesis but not that of the plasmid. Some bacteriophages may exist either as integrated or free copies in the cell, and either case can be termed plasmids. Yeast cells have been found to harbor some plasmids, and the Ti plasmid of *Agrobacterium* can survive in either bacterial or plant cells.

plasmid cloning vector. *See* PLASMID.

plasticizers. Chemicals that are added to plastics to keep them flexible. The most important plasticizers in the polyvinyl chloride (PVC) plastics are the phthalic acid esters, with di-(2-ethylhexyl) phthalate (DEHP) and di-*n*-butyl phthalate (DBP) being the most widely used. Adipic acid esters and citric acid esters are also used as PVC plasticizers. *See also* PHTHALIC ACID ESTERS.

platelets. *See* THROMBOCYTES.

pluripotent stem cells. *See* STEM CELLS.

plutonium (Pu). The toxic effects of inhaled plutonium vary with the dose, high doses in the dog causing death from radiation pneumonitis and pulmonary fibrosis within a relatively short time, those dogs surviving more than 1000 days dying from neoplasias although fibrosis is apparent. If the form inhaled is the relatively insoluble plutonium oxide, much remains in the lung until transported to the lymph nodes. Soluble forms are transported out of the lung and appear in the liver and skeleton. Injected plutonium citrate behaves as the soluble forms mobilized from the lung, causing primarily bone cancers and, less commonly, liver cancers.

PMN. *See* PRE-MANUFACTURE NOTIFICATION.

pneumoconiosis. A respiratory tract disorder resulting from dust inhalation whose main effect is pulmonary fibrosis. The occupations of stone cutting and coal mining lead to this disorder. In the case of coal miners, the disorder is colloquially called black lung disease. Pneumoconiosis is also caused by chronic inhalation of tin dust or fumes.

podophyllotoxin (5,8,8a,9-tetrahydro-9-hydroxy-5-(3,4,5-trimethoxyphenyl)furo [3′,4′,6,7]naphtho[2,3-d]-1,3-dioxol-6(5H)-one). CAS number 518-28-5. An antineoplastic glucoside extracted from the roots and rhizomes of the May apple (*Podophyllum peltatum*). The LD50 in rats is 8.7 mg/kg, i.v., and 15 mg/kg, i.p. Podophyllotoxin causes hematopoietic and lymphoid toxicity by inhibiting nucleoside transport and mitochondrial electron transport. Symptoms of poisoning include nausea, vomiting and alopecia.

Podophyllotoxin

poinsettia. *Euphorbia pulcherrima,* a member of the Euphorbiaceae, the spurge family. It is a popular indoor Christmas plant. Toxic effects have been greatly exaggerated and there are no proven records of fatalities. Poinsettia and other members of the spurge often cause contact dermatitis but without any lasting effects.

point mutation. The smallest alteration in the genetic material is the transformation of a single base-pair. Base-pair transformations are of two types. (1) If the replacement involves the same type of base (e.g., purine to purine, or pyrimidine to pyrimidine) the mutation is called a base-pair transition. (2) If the change is a purine to pyrimidine replacement, it is termed a base-pair transversion. These point mutations can occur by chemical modification, by incorporation of abnormal base analogs into DNA or by alkylation. An example of chemical transformation of bases is that caused by nitrous acid (HNO_2), which results in the transformation of cytosine to uracil or adenine to hypoxanthine; nitrous acid is known to be mutagenic in phage, bacteria and fungi. Most of the chemicals active in the incorporation of abnormal base analogs were developed as drugs for cancer therapy and owe their effectiveness to their ability to produce lethal mutations in rapidly dividing cancer cells. Some examples are 5-bromouracil, 5-fluorodeoxyuridine, 2-aminopurine and 6-mercaptopurine. Alkylating agents (e.g., *N*-dimethylnitrosoamine) are chemicals that can add alkyl groups to DNA. These chemicals yield positively charged carbonium ions which combine with the electron-rich bases in the DNA. Alkylation of DNA results both in mispairing of bases and chromosome breaks. Adenine can be alkylated at three ring nitrogens (N-1, N-3, N-7), whereas guanine can undergo alkylation at either N-3, N-7 or O-6. Cytosine can be alkylated at N-3 and O-2, and thymine at N-3, O-2 and O-4. In addition to alkylation of the purine and pyrimidine bases, the phosphates in the DNA may also undergo alkylation. Although the most frequent site of alkylation is the N-7 of guanine, alkylation at the O-6 position of guanine has most frequently been associated with the mispairing of bases and induction of cancer. *See also* CHROMOSOME ABERRATIONS; FRAMESHIFT MUTATION; MUTATIONS.

poison (toxicant). Any substance that causes a harmful effect when administered to a living organism. Due to the popular connotation that poisons are, by definition, fatal in their effects and that their administration is usually involved with attempted homicide or suicide, most toxicologists prefer the less prejudicial term, toxicant. Poison is a quantitative concept. Almost any substance is harmful at some dose and, at the same time, is harmless at a very low dose. There is a range of possible effects, from subtle long-term chronic toxicity to immediate lethality. For example, aspirin (acetylsalicylic acid) is a relatively safe drug at recommended doses, although chronic use can cause deleterious effects on the gastric mucosa, and it is fatal to humans at a dose of around 0.2–0.5 g/kg. Other toxic chemicals, such as selenium, may be nutritional requirements at lower concentrations. Finally, there is a biological dimension since many compounds are toxic to some species but relatively harmless to others.

Poison Control Centers. A network within the USA to provide expert advice and treatment in cases of poisoning. There are usually several such centers in each state and a state coordinator's office to facilitate communication and organization. Typically centers are associated with medical school hospitals, other hospitals or schools of pharmacy. They are available by telephone for emergency instructions to rescue teams, etc., as well as to practising physicians.

poisoning, emergency treatment. Untrained people should rarely provide first aid to poisoning victims and should never do so if the victim is unconscious or having convulsions. In any case of poisoning or suspected poisoning, professional help should be contacted immediately—the nearest Poison Control Center, hospital Emergency Room or Emergency Rescue Squad. With conscious patients, vomiting will then probably be induced, preferably with syrup of ipecac, although this is never done in the case of acids, bases or petroleum products. In the case of inhaled toxicants the victim is moved to fresh air. With poisoning via dermal contamination, the skin is drenched with water, clothing over the affected area removed and the affected area washed with soap and water. With eye contamination, the eye is washed with a gentle stream of water. If the victims breathing is depressed, artificial respiration is given, preferably by direct inflation or, if available, oxygen is given. Chemical antidotes should not be given. In all cases the patient should be kept warm and either a physician brought to the site or transport arranged to a treatment facility. Since

identification of the poison may be critical, anyone rendering first aid should be sure that the poison, or vomited material, is sent to the treatment facility with the patient (in a sealed container).

poisoning, life support. This involves maintaining an adequate airway, if necessary by catheter, tracheostomy or cricothyroid puncture, and also maintaining adequate pulmonary ventilation. This latter may be by direct, mouth-to-mouth, inflation or by a portable resuscitator. Oxygen is administered, if available. Circulatory failure is usually the result of shock, and emergency therapy appropriate to shock is initiated immediately. The patient is placed in a supine position with lower limbs elevated, body warmth is maintained by blankets, an adequate airway is assured, and adequate circulating blood volume is restored and maintained. If the fall in blood pressure is severe, appropriate drug therapy is initiated along with plasma transfusion. *See also* CATHARSIS; EMESIS; GASTRIC LAVAGE; GASTROTOMY; INTESTINAL LAVAGE.

Poisons Act. UK legislation, passed in 1973, that restricts the sale and use of poisons, as listed in the Poisons List Order 1972. Schedule 1 substances (e.g., apomorphine, atropine, emetine, strychnine) can only be sold by a pharmacist on a medical prescription or on police order. Schedule 2 substances can only be sold by registered pharmacists, and all sales have to be recorded with the purchaser's signature. Schedule 4A drugs (e.g., most barbiturates) and Schedule 4B drugs (e.g., chlorpromazine, tranquilizers) may only be sold on prescription. All substances listed under the Poisons Act must be kept under lock and key, and they should be clearly labeled and their use must be carefully recorded.

pokeweed. *Phytolacca americana*, also known as pokeberry, poke, inkberry, etc. A native weed of the eastern USA, used in folk medicine as a purgative, salve and bronchodilator. Young leaves are eaten in the rural southern USA ("poke salad"). It contains a powerful gastrointestinal irritant, phytolaccine, that can cause effects ranging from a burning sensation of the alimentary tract to severe hemorrhagic gastritis.

pollutant. Any chemical or substance contaminating the environment and contributing to pollution. *See also* POLLUTION.

pollution. Contamination of any aspect of the environment (soil, water, food or the atmosphere) by chemicals, resulting from the discharge or admixture of noxious materials. The chemicals (pollutants) may be naturally occurring or anthropogenic and have the potential for harm to human health, to any aspect of human or natural ecosystems, or to environmental aesthetics or vitality. *See also* AIR POLLUTION; FOOD CONTAMINANTS; POLLUTION, AGRICULTURAL CHEMICALS; POLLUTION, DOMESTIC AND MUNICIPAL WASTES; POLLUTION, EFFECT ON DOMESTIC ANIMALS; POLLUTION, EFFECT ON PLANTS; POLLUTION, EFFECT ON STRUCTURES; POLLUTION, ENERGY SOURCES; POLLUTION, EXHAUST EMISSIONS; POLLUTION, FOSSIL FUELS; POLLUTION, INDUSTRIAL PROCESSES; POLLUTION, INORGANIC CHEMICALS; POLLUTION, LONG-RANGE TRANSPORT; POLLUTION, METALS; POLLUTION, PARTICULATES; POLLUTION, PETROLEUM PRODUCTS; POLLUTION, THERMAL; WATER POLLUTION.

pollution, agricultural chemicals. Pesticides and fertilizers have the potential for contaminating soil, water (surface and ground water) and food sources through direct application, environmental drift, run-off and bioaccumulation. The persistent organochlorine pesticides pose the greatest threat because of their stability and lipophilicity. The more labile organophosphorus, carbamate and pyrethroid insecticides are less serious problems as pollutants. Fertilizer components can lead to enrichment of static and slow-moving surface water, with subsequent algal blooms and eutrophication.

pollution, cadmium. *See* CADMIUM; ITAI-ITAI DISEASE; POLLUTION, METALS.

pollution, domestic and municipal wastes. The water pollution that results from human residential life and urban activities. *See also* DOMESTIC SEWAGE; INDUSTRIAL WASTEWATER.

pollution, effect on domestic animals. Domestic animals can ingest deposited air pollutants in their forage, typically arsenic, lead and molybdenum. Also fluoride released by the fertilizer industry has poisoned domestic animals. *See also* ARSENIC; FLUOROSIS; LEAD; MOLYBDENUM.

pollution, effect on plants. Air pollutants can cause the following effects on vegetation: color changes, including bleaching; necrosis; altered growth; altered reproduction; change in species composition of an ecosystem; increased susceptibility to pests. Serious effects on plants occur in locations close to point sources of pollutants. Some of the effects of pollutants can be attributed to the leaching of nutrients from the soil brought about by acid deposition.

pollution, effect on structures. Air pollution has caused the following effects on structures and various inanimate materials: soiling and darkening; deterioration of marble; corrosion of metal; cracking of rubber; fragility of paper and leather; destruction of fabrics.

pollution, energy sources. The processing and burning of fossil fuels for either heat or power generates smoke, fly ash, sulfur and nitrogen oxides, carbon monoxide, carbon dioxide, metals and organic derivatives. The smoke and carbon monoxide are the result of incomplete combustion. The high sulfur content of some oil and coal leads to sulfur oxides which contribute to acid precipitation. The use of refined petroleum products as an energy source in vehicles leads to exhaust emissions containing smoke, hydrocarbons, lead from tetraethyllead additives, carbon monoxide and nitrogen oxides. Thermal pollution is generated by the cooling mechanisms required at nuclear and electric power plants.

pollution, exhaust emissions. Vehicles burning refined petroleum products for energy produce smoke, carbon monoxide, hydrocarbons and lead particles. Improvement of exhaust emissions has occurred because of the introduction of lead-free gasoline and of catalytic converters which reduce hydrocarbon emissions.

pollution, fossil fuels. The burning of fossil fuels (i.e., primarily coal and oil, including refined petroleum products) produces smoke, hydrocarbons including some carcinogenic polycyclic aromatic hydrocarbons, carbon monoxide, sulfur oxides especially from the higher sulfur oils and coal, carbon dioxide, nitrogen oxides and fly ash from power plants. In addition, spills and continuous leakages pollute the environment with oil, and acid mine drainage from coal mines pollutes water.

pollution, industrial processes. Typical air pollutants arising from industrial processes include: acids (sulfuric, acetic, nitric, phosphoric), solvents, resins, chlorine, ammonia and metals (copper, lead, zinc). Some of these products are discharged routinely into the atmosphere, but they become more serious problems when they are released in transportation accidents. A number of other industrial products pose mainly occupational health hazards; examples include cyanides, chlorides, hydrogen sulfide, hydrogen fluoride, formaldehyde, phosgene and vinyl chloride. Industries also discharge pollutants such as metals and a variety of organic wastes (e.g., PCBs, TCDD, plasticizers, solvents) into water and terrestrial ecosystems, and industrial accidents can result in localized high levels of pollutants. *See also* INDUSTRIAL WASTEWATER.

pollution, inorganic chemicals. In addition to metals and acids, nitrates and phosphates from fertilizers are pollutants and contribute to eutrophication. Phosphates also come from detergents. The intestinal microflora can convert nitrate to nitrite, which can cause methemoglobinemia. *See also* EUTROPHICATION; METHEMOGLOBINEMIA; POLLUTION, AGRICULTURAL CHEMICALS.

pollution, long-range transport. Pollutants can be transported over long distances to points remote from the source. For example, PCBs have been found in the Antarctic and in pristine Arctic lakes. They may be transported as aerosols or particles in the upper atmosphere, as in the case of acid deposition, as residues in migratory animals, as waterborne toxicants in extensive drainage systems or by shipment of finished industrial products.

pollution, mercury. *See* MERCURY; MINAMATA DISEASE; POLLUTION, METALS.

pollution, metals. The primary metal pollutants are lead, mercury, cadmium, zinc, copper, nickel and arsenic. Many of these metals are by-products of industrial processes, or they result from mining or smelting operations. Lead is released in vehicle exhaust emissions. Some metals are present in domestic and municipal waste. Metals can be bioaccumulated by aquatic organisms and therefore occur in high concentrations in upper tropic levels of food chains. Metallothionein is a protective protein in many animals. *See also* ARSENIC; CADMIUM; COPPER; ITAI-ITAI DISEASE; LEAD; MERCURY; METALLOTHIONEIN; MINAMATA DISEASE; NICKEL; ZINC.

pollution, particulates. Particulates suspended in air create visible hazes and smoke that diminish the aesthetic quality of the environment as well as leading to a variety of health effects in humans and animals, primarily respiratory tract problems. Typical particulate pollutants include dusts (e.g., coal or cement dust), fumes (e.g., zinc or lead oxide), mists (e.g., sulfuric acid), smokes (e.g., burning fossil fuels or other materials incompletely), sprays and mineral fibers (e.g., glass, asbestos).

pollution, pesticides. *See* POLLUTION, AGRICULTURAL CHEMICALS.

pollution, petroleum products. Hydrocarbons and sulfur compounds from oil spills, flushing of oil tankers, continuous leakages and improper disposal of petroleum products contribute to water and soil pollution. There can be both acute effects from accidental spills and chronic effects from low-level continuous exposures. *See also* OIL SPILLS.

pollution, thermal. Heated effluents from steel manufacturing or electricity-generating (nuclear and fossil fuels) plants can decrease oxygen content, increase microbial growth and alter species distribution of affected streams and lakes. Although many species can adapt to the increased temperature, some of the economically important species do not adapt well.

polybrominated biphenyls (PBBs). Mixtures of brominated biphenyls with an average bromine content of six atoms per molecule. PBBs have been used as flame retardants, but in view of environmental and health problems such use is being curtailed. Acute toxicity is low; rats given single oral doses of 17 g/kg exhibited no toxic effects. Most poisonings are due to chronic exposure. Chronic doses of 67 mg/kg/day produced anorexia, diarrhea, lachrymation and salivation, dehydration and abortion in pregnant cows. Kidney, gallbladder and thymus changes were noted at necropsy. Extensive subcutaneous edema and hemorrhage occurred in moribund animals. Cattle exposed to contaminated feed in Michigan exhibited the same clinical signs and, in addition, abnormal hoof growth, alopecia, decreased milk production, i.m. hematomas and hepatic changes. Guinea pigs fed 50 ppm PBBs showed effects on the thymus, adrenals and spleen. Exposed humans reported increased incidence of viral and bacterial infections. From this and other evidence, it appears that PBBs have an acute suppressive effect on the immune system. PBBs are potent inducers of renal and hepatic microsomal monooxygenases (cytochrome P450 isozymes). The enzymes are also induced in suckling offspring of female rats fed PBBs. Metabolic transformations and both kidney and biliary excretion of PBBs are low, although milk from exposed cows and persons may contain PBBs. IARC has classified PBBs as possibly carcinogenic to humans; the Department of Health and Human Services has determined that PBBs can reasonably be expected to be carcinogenic. *See also* AROCLORS; ATSDR DOCUMENT, OCTOBER 1993; DATABASES, TOXICOLOGY; POLYCHLORINATED BIPHENYLS.

X = H or Br
Polybrominated biphenyls

polybrominated dibenzo-*p*-dioxins. Similar in structure and toxicity to the polychlorinated dibenzo-*p*-dioxins, although much less well studied. *See also* TCDD.

polychlorinated biphenyls (PCBs). Nonflammable liquids formerly used in heat exchangers, electrical condensers, hydraulic and lubricating fluids, and various inks, adhesives and paints. Most uses have been curtailed due to environmental stability and chronic toxicity of PCBs. Commercial PCBs (e.g., Aroclors) are mixtures of isomers having varying numbers of chlorine atoms per molecule. Acute mammalian toxicity decreases as the level of chlorine increases. In rats, the symptoms of acute intoxication include diarrhea, ataxia and CNS depression. Hemorrhage of lungs, stomach and pancreas, and alterations of liver and kidney also occur. Hepatic monooxogenase activity is elevated by single large doses of PCBs. Monkeys given 300 ppm for 90 days developed alopecia, chloracne, subcutaneous edema, liver hypertrophy, and hypertrophy and hyperplasia of the gastric mucosa. Rabbits given Aroclor 1254 weekly for 14 weeks developed megalohepatocytosis followed by subcapsular midzonal necrosis and fibrotic changes. Repeated dermal applications of several technical-grade PCBs produced hyperplasia and hyperkeratosis of the epidermal and follicular epithelium, liver and kidney changes and atrophy of the thymus. Some of these symptoms may be due to contamination with polychlorodibenzofurans. Moderate repeated doses of PCBs were said to have caused liver tumors in mice, bladder tumors in rats and fetotoxicity in rabbits. In humans, both dermal and oral exposures may lead to chloracne and hepatotoxicity. Acute oral toxicities are generally low. Rat oral LDs range from 4 g/kg (for Aroclor 1221) to 20 g/kg for Aroclor 5460. Symptoms of intoxication following a massive human poisoning episode in Japan included persistent chloracne, skin hyperpigmentation, peripheral neuropathies, blindness, edema, nausea, vomiting and abdominal pain. Newborn infants showed skin discoloration, gingival hyperplasia and skin changes. PCBs are readily absorbed from

X = H or Cl
Polychlorinated biphenyls

the gastrointestinal tract and stored in adipose tissue. The PCBs having a lower percentage of chlorine seem to be excreted more rapidly. Animal studies suggest that enterohepatic circulation of PCBs occurs. The Department of Health and Human Services has determined that PCBs may reasonably be expected to be carcinogens and both IARC and the US EPA have classified them as probable human carcinogens. *See also* ATSDR DOCUMENT, OCTOBER 1993; DATABASES, TOXICOLOGY.

polychlorinated dibenzo-*p*-dioxins. Most information on this class of chemical is derived from studies of TCDD, the most potent of the class. Other polychlorinatated dibenzo-*p*-dioxins also interact with the Ah receptor, are immunotoxic and have similar effects to TCDD, although requiring higher doses. *See also* TCDD.

polychlorocamphene. *See* TOXAPHENE.

polychlorodibenzofurans. Similar in toxicity to polychlorinated dibenzo-*p*-dioxins such as TCDD although less potent. In two poisoning episodes involving contaminated rice oil, one in Taiwan, the other in Japan, not only did the poisoning victims present evidence of compromised immune systems, but the principal tissue residues were polychlorinated dibenzofurans. *See also* POLYCHLORINATED BIPHENYLS; TCDD.

polyclonal antibodies. Produced by B lymphocytes when an antigen is introduced into an immunocompetant host. Although different B lymphocytes each respond to a specific epitope on the antigen molecule and produce an antibody to that epitope only after differentiation, due to the numerous B cells and epitopes a polyclonal antibody as isolated from the serum of the host is a complex mixture of antibodies. Polyclonal antibodies used experimentally for protein identification in such techniques as Western blotting may be made more specific by differential absorption of non-specific components. *See also* MONOCLONAL ANTIBODY.

polycyclic aromatic amines. *See* AROMATIC AMINES.

polycyclic aromatic hydrocarbons. Although some natural products such as coal and crude oil contain polycyclic aromatic hydrocarbons, they are generally associated with incomplete combustion of organic materials and are found in the smoke and residue from the combustion of wood, coal oil, tobacco, etc., as well as tar, creosote and broiled (grilled) foods. Since a number of them are carcinogens (e.g., 3-methylcholanthrene), they have been studied intensively from the point of view of metabolic activation, interaction with DNA and chemical carcinogenesis. Some of these compounds are heterocyclic, containing nitrogen atoms in at

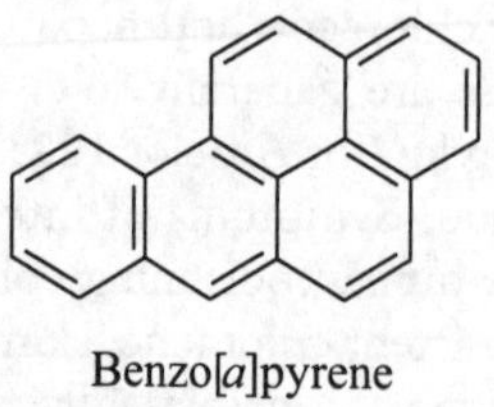

Benzo[*a*]pyrene

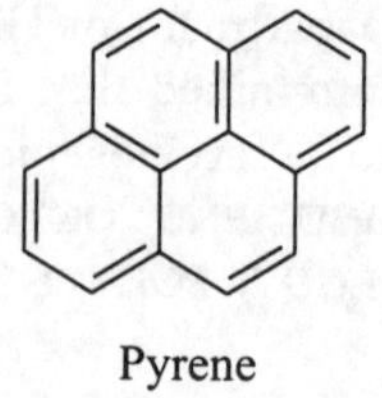

Pyrene

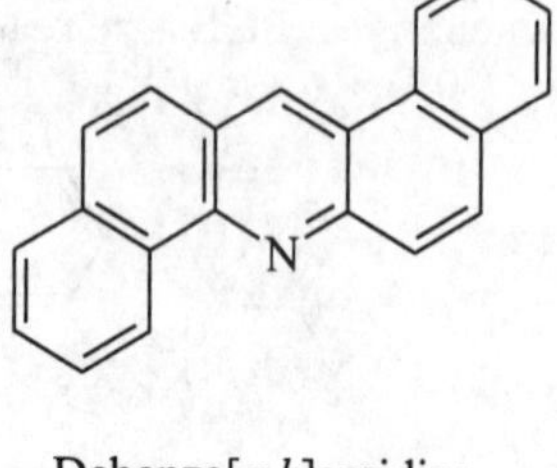

Debenzo[*a,h*]acridine

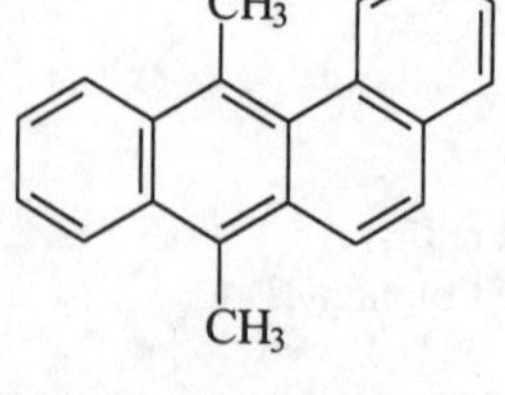

9,10 Dimethyl-1,2-benzanthracene

Polycyclic aromatic hydrocarbons

least one of the rings. Polycyclic aromatic hydrocarbons are often potent inducers of hepatic cytochrome P450, inducing those isozymes associated with aryl hydrocarbon hydroxylase activity through the mechanism that utilizes the Ah receptor. *See also* AH RECEPTORS; ARYL HYDROCARBON HYDROXYLASE; BENZO[*A*] PYRENE; MECHANISMS OF INDUCTION.

polycyclic musk. *See* ACETYLETHYLTETRAMETHYLTETRALIN.

polyene antibiotics. *See* ANTIBIOTICS.

polyhydric alcohols. *See* ALCOHOLS, POLYHYDROXY.

polymerases. Enzymes that catalyze the synthesis of both DNA and RNA. In DNA synthesis the two strands of the double helix unwind and each strand acts as the template for the new complementary strand. Replication involves many proteins including DNA polymerases and a DNA ligase, the activated percursors being the deoxyribonucleoside 5'-triphosphates and synthesis proceeding from 5' to 3' by a nucleophilic attack by the 3'-hydroxyl terminus of the primer strand on the innermost phosphorus atom of the incoming nucleoside triphosphate. DNA polymerases catalyze the elongation of the chain only if the incoming nucleotide is complementary to the base on the strand acting as a template. DNA polymerases also have exonuclease activity that enhances replication fidelity by the removal of mismatched residues. Some of the DNA polymerases also function in DNA repair. RNA is synthesized by a polymerase utilizing a template (DNA) and proceeding from 5' to 3'. Unlike DNA polymerases, it does not require a primer and possesses no nuclease activity. Polymerases are inhibited by many xenobiotics, and their inhibition represents an important mode of toxic action.

polymorphisms. Genetic polymorphisms occur as a result of different alleles at the same gene locus. They arise as a mutational event which leads to an altered gene and often an altered gene product. Genetic polymorphisms have been arbitrarily defined as having a frequency of 1% or more, rarer genetic defects being designated as rare traits. The incidence of polymorphisms differs widely in various racial populations. One of the best known polymorphisms is genetic variation in glucose-6-phosphate dehydrogenase, which can lead to chronic hemolytic anemia. Polymorphisms in drug-metabolizing enzymes are important in toxicology, resulting in interindividual variability in the ability of humans to metabolize drugs, and their relationship to various types of cancer has also been an area of active study. Enzymes which are known to be polymorphic include both *N*-acetyl transferases (NAT 1 and NAT 2). NAT 2 acetylates sulfonamides, isoniazid and a number of arylamine carcinogens. Slow acetylators polymorphic in NAT 2 have been reported to have increased risk of bladder cancer but decreased incidence of colon cancer. There is a homozygous null poymorphism in glutathione *S*-transferase M1 in 50% of Caucasian populations due to a genetic deletion, and the relationship of this polymorphism has been widely studied with respect to many types of cancer. Polymorphisms also occur in other drug-metabolizing enzymes such as paraoxonase, butryl cholinesterase, glutathione *S*-transferase T1 and microsomal epoxide hydrolase. A number of CYP enzymes are polymorphic including CYP2D6 and CYP2C19. *See also* CYTOCHROME P450, POLYMORPHISMS.

polymorphonuclear phagocytes. *See* STEM CELLS.

polyploidy. *See* CHROMOSOME ABERRATIONS.

population at risk. That subgroup of the general population that is more susceptible to the adverse effects of a toxicant or is more likely to be exposed to a toxicant than the general population. *See also* RISK, TOXICOLOGICAL.

population variability. Differences in susceptibility among individuals in a population with respect to their susceptibility to a particular toxicant. While such variability may be expressed through differences in uptake, metabolism, site of action, etc., they are assumed to have a genetic basis.

porphyria. A disorder in which there is increased formation and excretion of porphyrins or their precursors. There are several porphyrias with different causes and effects. Acute intermittent porphyria is characterized by porphyrinuria, acute abdominal pain and neurological disorders. Inherited as an autosomal dominant trait, it is characterized by a deficiency in uroporphyrinogen synthetase and a compensatory increase in δ-aminolevulinic acid synthetase, resulting in an excess of δ-aminolevulinic acid and porphobilinogen. It is episodic in its clinical manifestations and, although not due to xenobiotic toxicity, attacks can be precipitated by barbiturates and other chemicals. Congenital erythropoietic porphyria is inherited as an autosomal recessive trait, resulting in a deficiency in uroporphryrinogen III synthetase. Erythrocytes are prematurely destroyed, and the skin is very light-sensitive. Porphyria erythropoietica is a mild form of porphyria. Porphyria hepatica is caused by disturbances in liver metabolism due to hepatitis or poisoning by heavy metals, benzene hexachloride, etc. *See also* HEME; HEME BIOSYNTHESIS; PORPHYRINS.

porphyrins. A group of pigments found in living cells that act as the prosthetic group for respiratory pigments. They consist of four substituted pyrroles connected in a cyclic arrangement by methylene bridges. A metal (e.g., iron) is central to the molecule and is bound to the nitrogen atoms of the pyrrole rings. Heme is the prosthetic group of hemoglobin and of cytochromes, including cytochrome P450, all of considerable importance in toxicology. *See also* HEME; HEME BIOSYNTHESIS.

porphyrinuria (porphyruria). The excretion of an excessive amounts of porphyrins in the urine. *See also* HEME; HEME BIOSYNTHESIS; PORPHYRIA; PORPHYRINS.

porphyruria. *See* PORPHYRINURIA.

portals of entry. The sites at which xenobiotics enter the body are referred to as portals of entry. They include the skin, the gastrointestinal tract and the respiratory system.

positive control. *See* CONTROLS, IN TESTING.

posterior pituitary. *See* NEUROHYPOPHYSIS.

postnatal behavioral tests. Various tests relying on observational methods and targeting unconditioned or reflexive behaviors have been developed to assess the effects of toxicant exposure *in utero* on the developing nervous system. These tests include the righting reflex, negative geotaxis, open-field behavior, acoustic startle and nursing behavior. These behavioral tests are thought to be estimates of sensorimotor coordination or integration, and have been shown to be sensitive to toxicant exposure. The righting reflex simply involves measuring the latency to assume a quadrapedal position after the animal has been placed on its back. Negative geotaxis involves placing the animal on a screen positioned at an angle (about 30°) with its head oriented downward. The speed with which the animal reorients itself so that its head is up provides the estimate of sensorimotor performance. *See also* AUDITORY STARTLE; CONDITIONED AVOIDANCE; HYPERACTIVITY; LOCOMOTOR BEHAVIOR; NEUROBEHAVIORAL TERATOLOGY; NEUROBEHAVIORAL TOXICOLOGY; PASSIVE AVOIDANCE; PAVLOVIAN CONDITIONING.

postnatal period. The developmental period occurring after birth. Although not specifically excluded from the term, it is generally not used to include adulthood or senescence. In child development, it is used primarily to describe the early (neonatal) post-birth period. In toxicology, it is applied most often in studies of effects initiated *in utero*, but manifested later (e.g., behavioral teratogenesis or the effects on offspring of diethylstilbestrol treatment of the mother).

post-transcriptional. Describing any cellular event that occurs after transcription of RNA from a DNA template. Most frequently the term is applied to nuclear events such as the modification of RNA by tailing and capping which occur prior to translation.

post-translational. Describing any cellular event that occurs in the process of protein synthesis after translation of the messenger RNA into a polypeptide chain. These events are usually cytoplasmic and include protein modifications or differential rates of protein degradation.

potassium cyanide. *See* CYANIDES.

potency. The relationship between the incidence or intensity of an effect and the dose required to produce the effect. Generally used as a standard for comparison of different chemicals. The effect in question may be a deleterious one, as in the case of toxicants, or a therapeutic one, as in the case of drugs.

potentiation. *See* SYNERGISM AND POTENTIATION.

potentiation tests. Since organisms are not exposed to one chemical at a time, potentiation and synergism represent potential sources of hazard. Unfortunately the enormous number of possible combinations of chemicals makes routine screening impossible. Thus it is practical to test for potentiation only when there is some preliminary indication that it is occurring or when either or both of the compounds belong to chemical classes already known to cause potentiation. Such a test can be conducted by comparing the LD50, or other appropriate toxic endpoint, of a mixture of equitoxic doses of the chemicals in question with the same endpoint measured with the two chemicals administered alone. Such methods would be effective in the well-known case of the potentiation of the insecticide malathion by another insecticide EPN, or between malathion and certain contaminants arising during synthesis, such as isomalathion. This example involves inhibition, by EPN or isomalathion, of the carboxylesterase responsible for the detoxication of malathion in mammals. In the case of synergism, in which one of the compounds is relatively non-toxic when given alone, the toxicity of the other compound can be measured when administered alone or after a relatively large dose of the non-toxic compound. *See also* SYNERGISM AND POTENTIATION.

Pozo Rica. *See* ENVIRONMENTAL DISASTERS.

pralidoxime. *See* N-METHYLPYRIDINIUM-2-ALDOXIME.

prechronic studies. Usually used as synonymous with subchronic, it may be used for any study preceding a chronic toxicity study. Its use is often confusing (or confused), and it is best avoided whenever possible.

predisposition, genetic. An inborn (i.e., genetically determined) tendency to react in an unusual, or abnormal, way to a drug or toxicant. Individuals with such genetically determined tendencies may represent a high-risk population for the chemical in question. Such genetic predisposition is often due to the presence of a particular variant of a polymorphic gene coding for a xenobiotic-metabolizing enzyme and can be detected by genotyping procedures. *See also* CYTOCHROME P450, POLYMORPHISMS; POLYMORPHISMS.

Premanufacture Notification (PMN). Most developed countries have PMN systems covering drugs, pesticides and/or industrial chemicals. Under the US Toxic Substances Control Act (TSCA), a manufacturer must notify the EPA 90 days prior to producing a new chemical substance (i.e., a chemical not listed on the EPA inventory). Notification is also required for existing chemicals when new uses might increase production or human and environmental exposure. The PMN includes information on the chemical/toxicological properties of the chemical, the process and level of production and distribution. Assurances must also be provided that processors and consumers have been fully notified of the properties of the chemical. PMN exemptions may be allowed for chemicals that are to be produced in low volumes or used in restricted areas (e.g., at the plant site) or in cases where production, use and disposal does not present unreasonable risk to health or the environment. *See also* TOXIC SUBSTANCES CONTROL ACT.

prenatal period. The developmental period before birth. Prenatal toxicity can result in embryonic or fetal death or teratogenesis. *See also* REPRODUCTIVE TOXICITY TESTING.

preservatives. *See* BACTERIOSTATS.

Preservatives in Food Regulations. Regulations that apply in England and Wales which limit the use of antibiotics as food preservatives in foods for human consumption. Similar regulations exist for Scotland—Preservatives for Foods (Scotland) Regulations.

primaquine. CAS number 90-34-6. Antimalarial.

primary carcinogen. *See* CARCINOGEN, PRIMARY.

primary lung irritants. *See* ASPHYXIANTS; IRRITANTS.

primidone. **CAS number 125-33-7**. Anticonvulsant in human and veterinary medicine.

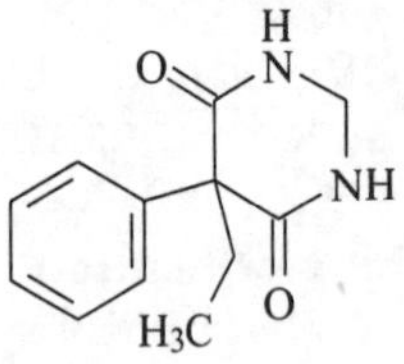

Primidone

Principles and Procedure of Evaluating the Toxicity of Household Substances. Published by the National Academy of Sciences (USA) in 1977, this publication outlines procedures for *in vitro* and *in vivo* tests for acute and chronic toxicity. This is an extensive revision of an earlier report (1964) of the same name. *See also* ACUTE TOXICITY TESTING; CHRONIC TOXICITY TESTING.

Principles for Evaluating Chemicals in the Environment. A report of a National Academy of Sciences (USA) committee called the Committee for the Working Conference on Principles of Protocols for Evaluating Chemicals in the Environment. Published in 1975, it summarized methods to test for toxic effects such as carcinogenicity, mutagenicity and reproductive toxicity. *See also* CHRONIC TOXICITY TESTING.

probability. A quantitative statement about the likelihood of occurrence of a specific outcome. Probability values can range from 0 to 1. *See also* STATISTICS, FUNCTION IN TOXICOLOGY.

probit/log transforms. A plot of the probability unit obtained from the standardized normal distribution versus the logarithm of the concentration or the dose of a substance when a quantal or graded response has been measured. A linear plot provides evidence that the distribution is log normal. Estimates of the ED50 and LD50, as well as the standard deviation for the distribution, can then be made. *See also* PHARMACODYNAMICS; PROBITS; TOXICODYNAMICS.

probits. A method of analysis of dose–response data. A probability unit is obtained by modification of the standard variate of the standardized normal distribution by addition of a constant value of 5 (to avoid negative numbers). Conversion of cumulative percent response to probits followed by plots against concentration or dose can give useful information about the distribution of the response and estimates of ED50 or LD50 values. *See also* PHARMACODYNAMICS; PROBIT/LOG TRANSFORMS; TOXICODYNAMICS.

procainamide. **CAS number 614-39-1**. Antiarrhythmic.

procarbazine (*N*-4-isopropylcarbamoyl benzyl-*N*-methylhydrazine). **CAS number 366-70-1**. A substituted hydrazine developed as an antineoplastic agent. It has been found to be carcinogenic in several species, the mechanism being, presumably and by analogy with 1,2-dimethyl hydrazine, the release of the methyl carbonium ion. This compound is also known to be immunosuppressive and to have adverse effects on the reproductive system.

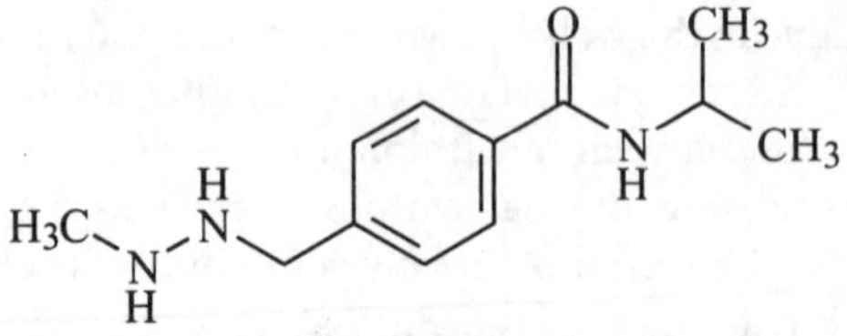

Procarbazine

procarcinogen. *See* CARCINOGEN, PROXIMATE.

procaryote. *See* PROKARYOTE.

Procytox. *See* CYCLOPHOSPHAMIDE.

product licence. British term (from UK Medicines Act, 1968) for Marketing Authorization. *See also* MARKETING AUTHORIZATION.

proestrus. *See* ESTROUS CYCLE.

progesterone (**pregn-4-ene-3,20-dione; D-pregnen-3,20-dione; progestin; progestagen**). **CAS number 57-83-0**. A steroid hormone functioning in the maintenance of pregnancy, the prevention of ovulation and the preparation of the mammary glands for lactation. The endogenous sources are the corpus luteum, the placenta of pregnancy and the adrenal gland; the hormone is also produced synthetically. In humans, progesterone, or similar compounds, alone or in combination with estrogens, is used in oral contraceptives and in treatment of abnormal uterine bleeding, dysmenorrhea, premenstrual tension, endometriosis, threatened or habitual abortion, suppression of postpartum lactation, endometrial carcinoma and suppression of testicular function in males. Side effects include depression or elation of mood and easy fatigue.

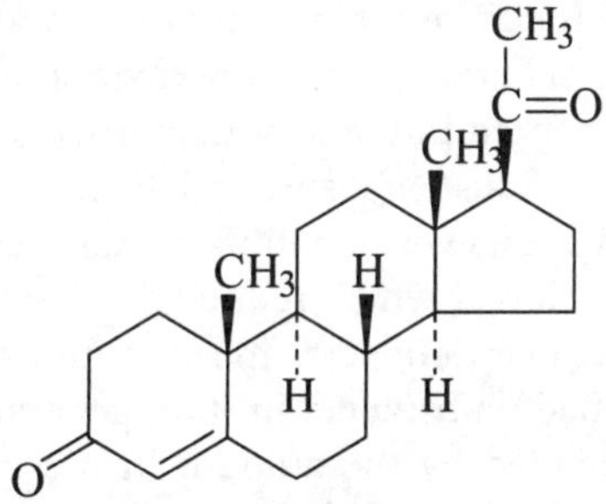

Progesterone

progression. The acquisition of a phenotypic alteration in a neoplasm leading to a less-differentiated state or more aggressive, malignant behavior. *See also* CARCINOGEN; INITIATION; NEOPLASM; PROMOTION.

prokaryote mutagenicity tests. *In vitro* test systems that detect either forward or reverse mutations in a variety of bacterial strains are being used to assess the mutagenicity of chemicals. Strains of *Salmonella typhimurium*, *Escherichia coli* and *Bacillus subtilis* are commonly used. Mutations occurring include alterations in histidine, tryptophan or galactose metabolism, or the ability to repair damaged DNA. Mutagens can be detected by these short-term tests and, because of their effects on DNA, the potential carcinogenicity of these compounds is implied. Direct-acting mutagens, as well as those requiring metabolic activation, by addition of the rat liver S-9 fraction, can be determined. *See also* AMES TEST; BACTERIAL MUTAGENESIS; DNA REPAIR; MUTATION; S-9 FRACTION.

prokaryotes. Simple unicellular organisms, primarily the bacteria and cyanobacteria, that do not have nuclei to house their genetic material. They have very few subcellular structures. Because of their rapid reproductive rate, they are used in a variety of tests for mutagenicity. *See also* PROKARYOTE MUTAGENICITY TESTS.

prolactin. The hormone from the adenohypophysis, consisting of single chain of 198 amino acid residues with three disulphide linkages that stimulates lactation by the mammary glands, in conjunction with the effects of estrogen, progesterone and oxytocin. Prolactin secretion is normally suppressed by the hypothalamic prolactin inhibitory factor until after parturition. In birds stimulates secretion of crop milk by the crop glands.

proliferative dust. *See* DUST, PROLIFERATIVE.

promethazine (*N,N*,α-trimethyl-10*H*-phenothiazine-10-ethanamine; 10-(2-dimethylaminopropyl)phenothiazine; **Phenagran**). **CAS number 60-87-7**. A phenothiazine that acts by blocking H$_1$ histamine receptors. This action causes inhibition of the effects of histamine on smooth muscle, including the gastrointestinal tract and respiratory smooth muscle. Promethazine, like many other H$_1$ antagonists, does not inhibit histamine-induced gastric acid secretion. Whereas CNS depression is the typical response to therapeutic doses of H$_1$ antagonists, these drugs may cause central stimulant effects in higher doses. Promethazine, like several other H$_1$ antagonists, is also effective in treating motion sickness, probably owing to its antimuscarinic effects. Side effects include sedation, dizziness, fatigue, blurred vision, euphoria, insomnia and tremors. Loss of appetite, nausea, vomiting and constipation or diarrhea may also be associated with use of this drug. H$_1$ antagonists may cause hallucinations, excitement, incoordination and convulsions if inadvertently taken

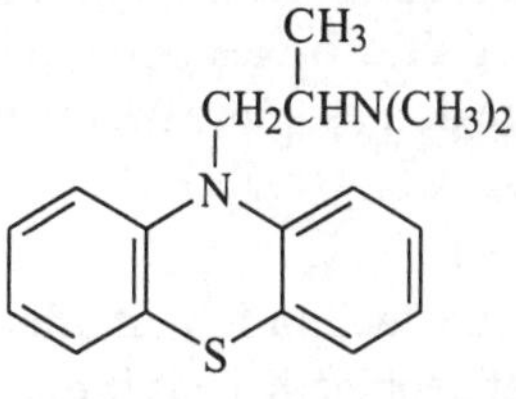

Promethazine

by children. The LD50 in rats is 400 mg/kg, s.c., and in mice is 55 mg/kg, i.v. *See also* ANTIHISTAMINES; PHENOTHIAZINES.

prometon. *See* TRIAZINE HERBICIDES.

prometryon. *See* TRIAZINE HERBICIDES.

promoter. (1) A chemical that can increase the incidence of response to a carcinogen previously administered to the test species, or shorten the latency period for the carcinogenic response. It stimulates the carcinogenic response induced or initiated by another chemical. A promoter is capable of altering the expression of genetic information of the cell. Examples of such agents include hormones, drugs, plant products, phorbol esters and ethanol, which in themselves do not directly react with the genetic material, but rather affect its expression by a variety of mechanisms, including their interaction with cell surface receptors or the cytoplasmic and nuclear protein receptors, or by an alteration of other cellular components and functions. Many, but not all, promoting agents stimulate an increase in DNA synthesis and/or cell replication in the target cells.

(2) Region on a DNA molecule upstream from the coding sequence to which the RNA polymerase initially binds prior to the initiation of transcription. The nucleotide sequence of the promoter determines the nature of the polymerase that associates with it. This is significant since a range of different RNA polymerases occurs in eukaryotic cells. Some genes have internal promoter sequences, for example the small ribosomal RNA gene coding for 5S RNA. Certain consensus sequences within the promoter region seem to be particularly important in the binding of RNA polymerase, and these are known as CAT and TATA boxes. The promoter region extends from some 40 nucleotides to about five nucleotides upstream from the start of the gene-coding region, the CAT and TATA boxes being located within the promoter region as short six or seven nucleotide sequences.

promotion. The facilitation of the growth and development of neoplastic cells into a tumor. This process is manifested by enhancement of carcinogenesis when the agent is given after a carcinogen. *See also* CARCINOGENESIS; INITIATION; NEOPLASM; TUMOR.

propazine. *See* TRIAZINE HERBICIDES.

2-propenal. *See* ACROLEIN.

propenamide. *See* ACRYLAMIDE.

propenenitrile. *See* ACRYLONITRILE.

propensity to dust (PD). Compound substances, even if finely divided powders, produce dusts which can vary markedly in composition to the parent material. If the more toxic substances is over-represented in the dust then obviously safety assessment of dust exposure will differ from that of the parent. Likewise manufacturing techniques can be developed which reduce the propensity to dust. The PD is defined as the amount (% w/w) of the specified substance in the generated dust sample, divided by the amount in the initial test substance. A test technique such as the Stauber–Heubach test is used to produce the dust sample. *See also* STAUBER–HEUBACH TEST.

propetamphos. Organophosphorus compound used for the control of ectoparasites as well as a wide range of household pests. Cholinesterase inhibitor. In the USA is a restricted use pesticide (i.e., licensed applicator only). *See also* DATABASES, TOXICOLOGY; MERCK INDEX, 12TH EDN, NUMBER 8000; ORGANOPHOSPHORUS INSECTICIDES; ORGANOPHOSPHOROUS POISONING, SYMPTOMS AND THERAPY.

propham. *See* CARBAMATE AND THIOCARBAMATE HERBICIDES.

prophase. *See* MITOSIS.

Proposition 65, California. A ballot initiative voted into law in 1986 by the voters of the state of California. Popularly known as Proposition 65, a name derived from its position on the ballot, correctly known the Safe Drinking Water and Toxic Enforcement Act of 1986. The primary purpose of the act is to prohibit contamination of drinking water with carcinogens or reproductive toxicants. Among other provisions the law requires the governor to publish lists of known carcinogens and reproductive toxicants and prohibits the release of such chemicals into the environment.

propoxyphene (α-[2-(dimethylamino)-1-methylethyl]-α-phenylbenzeneethanol propanoate; Darvon). CAS number 469-62-5. An opioid analgesic similar in structure to methadone. It is a much less potent analgesic than morphine and is devoid of antipyretic or anti-inflammatory effects. Its side effects are qualitatively similar to codeine. The clinical indications for propoxyphene are much the same as for aspirin. It is used when the degree of analgesia required is less than that produced by morphine. Recent clinical trials suggest that propoxyphene is no more effective in controlling mild pain than is aspirin. Because they act by different mechanisms, aspirin and propoxyphene have often been given in combination. Recently, there has been a trend away from use of propoxyphene because its weak analgesic properties do not compensate for other problems with its use. Interestingly, the analgesic activity of propoxyphene resides largely in the dextrorotatory isomer, whereas the antitussive effect is produced primarily by the levorotatory isomer. The oral LD50 in rats is 84 mg/kg.

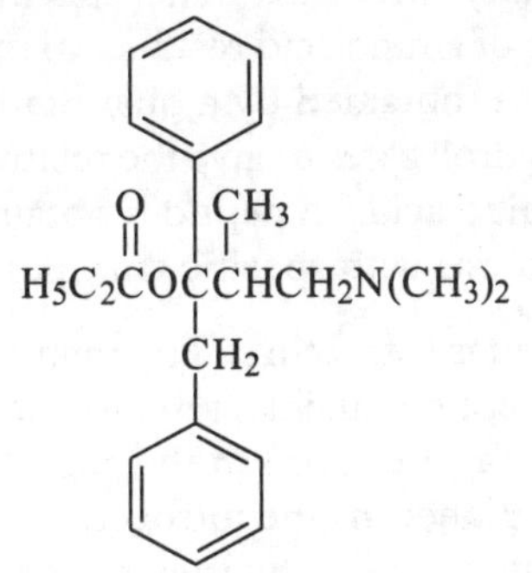

$$H_5C_2COCCHCH_2N(CH_3)_2$$

Propoxyphene

propylene dichoride. *See* DICHLOROPROPANE.

propylene glycol. CAS number 57-55-6. Similar in almost all respects to ethylene glycol, although perhaps less acutely toxic. *See also* ETHYLENE GLYCOL.

propylthiouracil (2,3-dihydro-6-propyl-2-thioxo-4(1H)-pyrdinone). CAS number 51-52-5. An antithyroid agent that may cause cholestasis in the liver. This compound is a substrate for thiol S-methyltransferase, and this enzyme may be important in its deactivation *in vivo*.

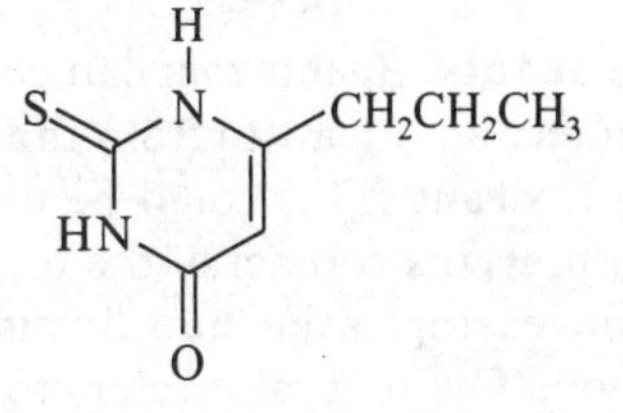

Propylthiouracil

prospective epidemiological study. *See* EPIDEMIOLOGICAL STUDIES, PROSPECTIVE.

prostaglandins. A group of chemically related hormone-like substances that are formed from essential fatty acids and occur in most mammalian tissues and body fluids. They are all unsaturated derivatives of prostanoic acid. The two main types differ in their oxygen function at C-9: in series E (PGE) it is carboxyl, whereas in series F (PGF) it is hydroxyl. They exhibit a wide range of pharmacological activities, but are best known for their potent effect on smooth muscle, particularly in stimulating contraction and relaxation of the human uterus.

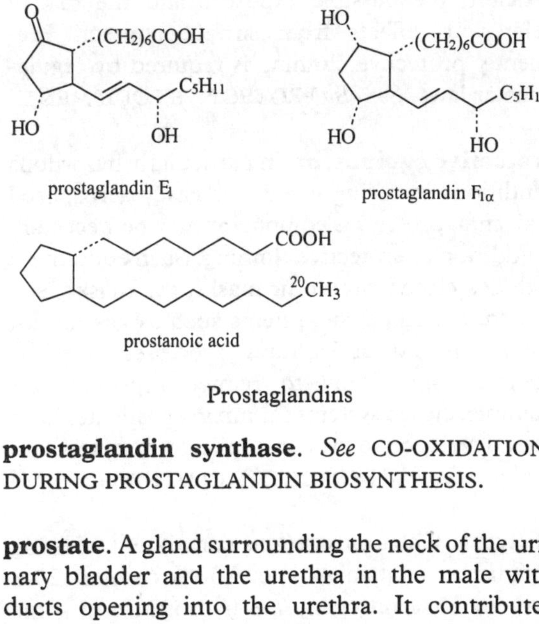

prostaglandin E₁   prostaglandin F₁α

prostanoic acid

Prostaglandins

prostaglandin synthase. *See* CO-OXIDATION, DURING PROSTAGLANDIN BIOSYNTHESIS.

prostate. A gland surrounding the neck of the urinary bladder and the urethra in the male with ducts opening into the urethra. It contributes about one-third of the seminal fluid in human males. Prostatic secretion contains acid phosphatase, and its concentration in seminal fluid is taken as an indicator of prostatic function.

Prostigmine. *See* NEOSTIGMINE.

protective agents. Agents that can completely or partially protect an organism from the deleterious effects of a toxicant. This could be a mechanical barrier that prevents contact of the organism with the toxicant; examples include dusting powders and collodion. The term also refers to a chemical that can be used prophylactically to prevent the toxic effects of another chemical. As an example, a carbamate anticholinesterase can be used to protect against the toxicity of organophosphate anticholinesterases, such as the nerve gases, by transiently occupying the active site of acetylcholinesterase until the circulating levels of organophosphate can be reduced.

protective clothing. The prevention of toxic effects from chemicals, particularly in the workplace, in changing situations such as industrial fires and in certain cases in agriculture may require protective clothing. This may consist of rubberized or plastic coveralls, gloves and goggles. The nature and degree of protection should be dictated by the physical and chemical characteristics of the toxicant, the possible exposure and the risk of deleterious effects from surface contact. Frequently protective clothing is required by regulations or laws. *See also* PROTECTIVE EQUIPMENT.

protective equipment. In particularly hazardous conditions involving volatile or easily aerosolized toxicants, protective equipment may be necessary in addition to protective clothing. Such equipment includes closed-circuit air masks, gas masks, etc. In addition to personal items such as gas masks, industrial and agricultural processes may be designed specifically to reduce exposure; for example, closed systems for mixing pesticides have been developed to protect applicators, mixers and loaders. *See also* PROTECTIVE CLOTHING.

proteins. Chief nitrogenous constituent of living organisms, containing about 50% carbon, 25% oxygen, 15% nitrogen, 7% hydrogen and some sulphur. Protein molecules consist of one or several long-chains (polypeptides) of amino acids linked in a characteristic sequence. In spite of their high relative molecular mass (up to many millions), many proteins have been crystallized or purified until they behave as a homogeneous substance. They are precipitated from solution by ethanol, propanone and concentrated salt solutions, and undergo denaturation (i.e., alteration of the tertiary structure of the molecule) by changes in pH, by UV radiation, by heat and by some organic solvents. Proteins are dipolar ions which migrate in an electric field and have characteristic isoelectric points. Proteins may be broadly classed as: (1) globular proteins which are compact rounded, water-soluble molecules (e.g., enzymes, antibodies, carrier proteins—hemoglobin—and storage proteins—casein); (2) fibrous or structural proteins which are insoluble in water (e.g., keratins, collagens). In classifying of proteins, a single protein may fall into more than one class (*see* Table 5).

Structure of proteins. The grosser structure of proteins has been determined by X-ray diffraction patterns, and their shapes and sizes by sedimentation velocity, diffusion and light-scattering techniques. The three-dimensional arrangement of proteins is important in determining the properties of the protein (e.g., the specific enzyme activity).

(1) Primary structure. The specific covalent sequence of amino acid residues in the polypeptide chains, obtained by a quantitative analysis of acid hydrolyzates to give the relative amounts of the amino acids in peptides obtained by partial hydrolysis with specific enzymes.

(2) Secondary structure. The manner in which the polypeptide chains are coiled according to the rules: (a) the atoms in the peptide link lie in the same plane; (b) the nitrogen, hydrogen and oxygen atoms of a hydrogen bond are in a straight line; (c) every NH and every CO group is engaged in bonding. There are two possible conformations. (i) The α-helix, in which hydrogen bonds form between a carbonyl oxygen and the NH of the fourth residue along the same chain. This produces a stable structure with 3.5 residues per turn, each with a pitch of 0.544 nm. The majority of polypeptides have a right-

Table 5 Classification of proteinss

Type	Occurrence, examples	Properties
Simple proteins		
Albumins	Present in all living tissues; oval-bumin (egg), lactalbumin (milk)	Soluble in water, dilute salt solutions
Globulins	Myosin (muscle), fibrinogen (blood), edestin (hemp seed)	Weakly acidic; insoluble in water, soluble in dilute salt solutions
Protamines	Present in fish sperm (e.g., salamine) associated with nucleic acids	Simplest proteins; strongly basic, soluble in water, not coagulated on heating. Low M_r (~3000), contain high levels of arginine, no S-containing amino acids
Histones	Associated with nucleic acids in thymus and pancreas (not found in plants)	Similar to protamines, but wider range of amino acids, basic, soluble in water, coagulates on heating
Prolamines (gliadins)	Present in seeds of cereals, gliadin (wheat), zein (corn)	Insoluble in water, soluble in 70% aq. EtOH, dilute acids and alkalis. Hydrolysis gives much Pro, Gln, but no Lys or Trp
Glutelins	Present in cereals; glutenin (wheat)	Insoluble in water, soluble in dilute acids and alkalis
Scleroproteins	Present in skeletal and connective tissues of animals; (1) collagen (skin, tendons, cartilage, ligaments); (2) keratins (horn, wool); (3) elastin (elastic tissue, ligaments, arterial walls)	Insoluble in water, resistance to proteolytic enzymes. (1) Most abundant protein in body, mainly Pro, Gly, Hyp. (2) Unattacked by pepsin or trypsin. (3) Struc-turally related to collagen, but contains about 30% Gly, 30% Leu, 15% Pro
Conjugated proteins (containing a prosthetic group)		
Phosphoproteins	Casein (milk), phosphovitin (egg yolk)	Contain phosphates, not coagulated by heat
Nucleoproteins	Nuclei of all cells, chromosomes; plant viruses and bacteriophages are pure nucleoprotein	Nucleic acid linked via salt bridges to protamines or histones; soluble in bases, insoluble in acids
Lipoproteins	Present in blood and lymph, functioning in the transport of lipids from small intestine to the liver	Prosthetic group is lipid moiety of variable compomposition. α-lipoprotein of serum contains glyceride, phosphatide and cholesterol (35% total complex); β-lipoprotein contains some glyceride, phosphatide and cholesterol (75% of total complex)
Glycoproteins (mucoproteins)	Present in mucus (saliva, gastric juice), and as hormones, antigens, certain enzymes	Carbohydrate prosthetic group (about 45% of complex) may contain D-galactose, D-mannose, N-acetyl-D-glucosamine and sialic acid. Aqueous solutions are very viscous

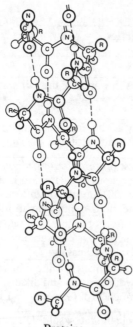

Proteins
α-Helix (right-handed) of a protein chain

Proteins
β-pleated sheet

handed helix on account of the preponderance of the L-configuration of naturally occurring amino acids. (ii) The β-pleated sheet in which the hydrogen bonds link different polypeptide chains, as in fibroin, a constituent of silk.

(3) Tertiary structure. The three-dimensional structure established by the folding of the helical polypeptide chains due to bonding which is strong enough to overcome the hydrogen bonding responsible for the secondary structure. Such bonding includes the disulphide linkages, ionic interactions (pH-dependent) and stronger hydrogen bonds. Folding is characteristic for each protein and occurs in such a way as to expose the maximum number of hydrophilic (polar) groups and enclose a maximum number of hydrophobic (non-polar) groups within its interior.

(4) Quaternary structure. This describes the way in which multiple subunits (not always the same) can aggregate to form a large complex.

The polypeptide chains are held together by dispersion and electrostatic forces (e.g., in hemoglobin and tobacco mosaic virus). In viruses, the protein complex usually forms a protective sheath around the core nucleic acid.

protein binding. Covalent binding to proteins is important in the mode of toxic action of many toxicants. Non-covalent binding is important in transport and distribution of toxicants and their metabolic products. A number of factors define the physiological and biological significance of protein binding. The number of ligand molecules bound per protein molecule (v) and the maximum number of binding sites (n) define the definitive capacity of the protein. The binding affinity ($K_{binding}$ or $1/K_{diss}$) is also important. If the protein has only one binding site for the toxicant, a single affinity constant describes the strength of the interaction. Usually, more than one binding site is present with each site having its intrinsic binding constant, k_1, k_2,..., k_n. This is especially true where hydrophobic binding and van der Waals forces contribute to non-specific, low-affinity binding. The chemical nature of the binding site is of critical importance in determining binding characteristics. The three-dimensional molecular structure of the binding site, the environment of the protein, the general location in the overall protein molecule and allosteric effects are doubtless all factors that influence binding, although studies with toxicants have not yet provided adequate elucidation of these factors. *See also* BINDING;

DISTRIBUTION OF TOXICANTS; EQUILIBRIUM DIALYSIS; K_D; RADIORECEPTOR ASSAYS; SCATCHARD PLOT.

protein synthesis. Cellular mechanisms leading to the production of proteins. The levels of protein structure above that of primary structure are acquired as a result of self-assembly, the amino acid sequence adopting the helical or sheet form and hydrogen bonds forming cross-links between amino acids. Protein primary structure is determined by the coding sequence of a specific gene. Production of the protein is a two-stage process, involving transcription and translation. In transcription, a messenger RNA (mRNA) is synthesized from the gene coding sequence by an RNA polymerase. Following processing and migration from the nucleus, the mRNA associates with ribosomes in the cytoplasm where translation begins. (In bacteria, where there is no subdivision into nucleus and cytoplasm, translation and transcription occur almost simultaneously, the mRNA being translated into protein before its transcription from the gene is completed.) Translation involves the assembly of aminoacyl tRNA molecules along the nucleotide coding triplets of the mRNA. Peptide bonds are then formed between adjacent amino acids, and the polypeptide chain gradually elongates.

proteinuria. The appearance of protein in the urine. Since the protein is commonly albumin, proteinuria is often referred to as albuminuria. Proteinuria may be a symptom of poisoning by compounds that affect renal function, such as arsenic or mercurials. *See also* DIAGNOSTIC FEATURES, URINARY TRACT.

proto-oncogenes. The normal cellular gene that can become an oncogene. These genes are apparently easily modified to form cancer-inducing genetic sequences. They may be distinguished from oncogenes in text by the presence of a "c" prefix before the oncogene designation.

Prozac. *See* SELECTIVE SEROTONIN RE-UPTAKE INHIBITORS.

Prunus species. Members of the genus *Prunus* contain amygdalin, a cyanogenic diglucoside, D-mandelonitrile-beta-D-gentiobioside, usually in the kernels of the pits. Prunasin is the hydrolysis product D-mandelonitrile-beta-D-glucoside. They include *P. armenica*, apricot; *P. dulcis*, bitter almond; *P. persica*, peach; *P. serotina*, black or wild cherry; *P. virginiana* v. melanocarpa, choke cherry. Amygdalin becomes dangerous when hydrolyzed by emulsin in the crushed seed or by some human gut microorganisms to yield cyanide. Laetrile, a purported cancer cure, is largely amygdalin. Controlled clinical trials have failed to support its efficacy, and some deaths have resulted from its use. *See also* AMYGDALIN.

pseudoephedrine. *See* EPHEDRINE.

Pseudonitizshia. A diatom that contaminated mussels in Canada in 1987 leading to four deaths and many cases of "amnesic shellfish poisoning." *See also* DOMOIC ACID.

pseudoparkinsonism. *See* PARKINSONISM.

psilocin. *See* PSILOCYBIN.

psilocybin (3[2-(dimethylamino)ethyl]indol-4-ol dihydrogen phosphate ester; *O*-phosphoryl-4-hydroxy-*N,N*-dimethyltryptamine). **CAS number 520-52-5.** A hallucinogenic (psychedelic) agent that occurs naturally in certain fungi of the genera *Psilocybe*, *Stropharia* and *Conocybe*. These so-called "magic mushrooms" were

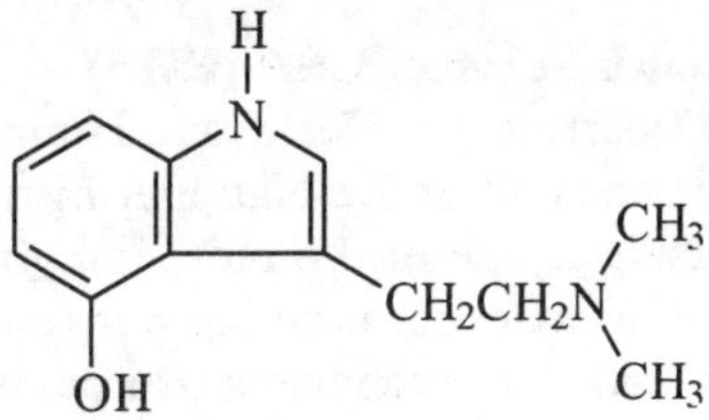

Psilocin

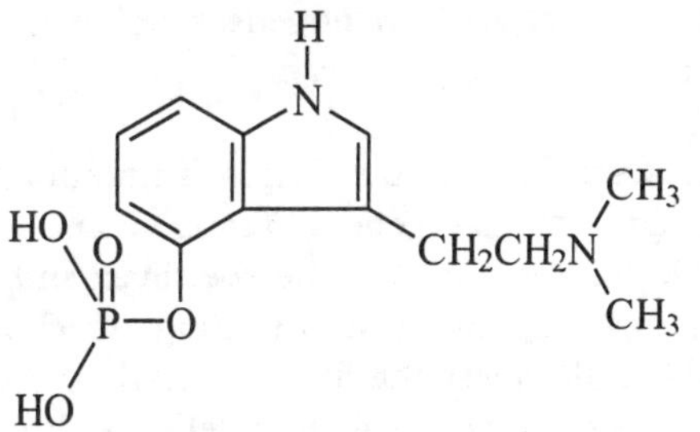

Psilocybin

known as Teonanacatl and were used in ancient Aztec religious rites. Psilocybin may catalyze the onset of severe emotional problems or psychosis in predisposed individuals. The mechanism of action is not known, although an interaction with central serotonin receptors would be consistent with speculations concerning other classes of hallucinogens. Intoxication causes perceptual alterations and illusions, including changes in touch, taste and odor. Vividly colored closed-eye imagery is pronounced with psilocybin, and the thinking process is substantially altered. At high doses, it causes hallucinations and loss of contact with reality. Acute panic reactions can be treated in a quiet, supportive environment, whereas diazepam has been used for management of severe anxiety. Psilocin is a minor hallucinogenic constituent of the same species of mushroom. See also HALLUCINOGENS.

psychedelic agents. See HALLUCINOGENS.

psychological effects. Effects on higher nervous functions in humans, i.e., changes in mental states, perceptions and moods. Many drugs and toxicants affect higher mental states and, for this reason, may be used in religious ceremonies or may be abused.

psychotomimetic agents. See HALLUCINOGENS.

Public Health Service, USA (PHS). A division of the US Department of Health and Human Services. Administers all of the National Institutes of Health making it one of the most important US government agencies for carrying out research in toxicology and for supporting, through extramural programs, toxicological research. Among its mandated responsibilities is the publication of an Annual Report on Carcinogens, prepared by the National Toxicology Program.

puffer fish. Fish of the family Tetraodontidae, particularly of the genera *Tetradon* and *Fugu*. Tetrodotoxin is found in the roe, liver and skin. Eating this fish may cause poisoning, which is frequently fatal, unless the fish is expertly prepared. Nevertheless, it is considered a delicacy (Fugu) in Japan. Clinical signs include motor inco-

ordination, numbness of the skin, salivation and diarrhea, followed by generalized paralysis and death in many cases. See also TETRODOTOXIN.

pulmonary compliance. See COMPLIANCE, PULMONARY.

pulmonary edema. The presence of excess fluid in the lungs. Although it may occur in a number of diseases, if due to poisoning it is usually caused by irritants that injure the pulmonary epithelium. Cholinesterase inhibitors may increase bronchial secretion and cause pulmonary edema. Pulmonary edema interferes with oxygen uptake and can be fatal. See also EDEMA; MAINTENANCE THERAPY, RESPIRATION.

pulmonary excretion. See EXCRETION, PULMONARY.

pulmonary penetration. See PENETRATION ROUTES, PULMONARY.

pulmonary resistance. Respiratory resistance is of two types, one due to the elastic recoil of the thorax and lungs, and the other being the frictional resistance to the flow of air through the airways. In both cases the work of the respiratory musculature is necessary to overcome the resistance. Factors affecting either the diameter or elasticity of the airways or the efficacy of the muscles will affect the efficiency of respiration.

pulmonary toxicity. The effects of compounds that exert their toxic effects on the respiratory system, primarily the lungs. Because the lung has such a large surface area and because such a large volume of air is passed over its surface (10,000–20,000 liters per day for the average adult human), the lung is the major interface between organisms and their environment. Pulmonary diseases caused by agents associated with occupations, such as stone quarrying, coal mining and textiles, have been known for centuries. The problem is more complex today because new volatile agents, such as gasoline additives and exhaust particles, pesticides, plastics, solvents, deodorant and cosmetic sprays, and construction materials, are constantly being added to our environment. In addition, the entire blood volume passes through the lung one to five times a minute, exposing the lung to circulating toxins and drugs. Although many different agents may damage the lung, the patterns of cellular injury and repair are relatively constant. One of the most obvious is irritation caused by volatile compounds such as ammonia or chlorine gas that, if severe or persistent, may lead to constriction of airways and edema of the lung. Intense damage to cells lining the airways, such as that which follows exposure to agents such as ozone, nitrogen oxides and phosgene, often results in increased permeability of membranes, edema and even necrosis. Fibrosis, or formation of collagenous tissue, was one of the earliest recognized forms of occupational diseases. Silicosis results from inhalation of various forms of silica. Asbestosis, resulting from inhalation of asbestos fibers, is of considerable concern since it is now known to be associated with increased risk of lung cancer. Numerous agents, including microorganisms, spores, dust and chemicals, are known to elicit allergic responses. Examples are farmer's lung resulting from spores of a mold that grows on damp hay, mushroom picker's lung, maple bark stripper's disease from spores of a fungus growing on maple trees and cheese washer's lung from Pencillium spores. Perhaps the most severe response of the lung to injury is cancer, the primary causative agent being inhaled cigarette smoke. *See also* ASBESTOSIS; PULMONARY TOXICITY, BIOTRANSFORMATION AND REACTIVE METABOLITES; SILICOSIS.

pulmonary toxicity, biotransformation and reactive metabolites. The activation of pulmonary toxicants varies according to the site of formation of the active intermediate or the nature of the reactive intermediate. The parent compound may be activated in the liver, and the reactive metabolite transported to the lung. Such metabolites, although reactive, have sufficient stability that a part of that formed in the liver reaches the lung. These activated compounds lead to covalent binding and damage to both liver and lung tissues. The best known example of lung toxicity by this mechanism is the damage to pulmonary endothelial cells by certain pyrrolizidine alkaloids (e.g., monocrotaline). Xenobiotics entering the lung, either from inhaled air or the circulatory system, may be metabolized to the toxic intermediate within the lung itself. Although the concentration of activating enzymes of the cytochrome P450 monooxygenase system in the lung is less than that in the liver, the concentration varies between different cell types with the highest concentration in the non-ciliated bronchiolar epithelial (Clara) cells of the terminal bronchioles. The complement of cytochrome P450 isozymes in the lung is different from that of the liver; in the rabbit, for example, two of the cytochrome P450 isozymes that comprise more than 70% of pulmonary cytochrome P450 are minor components of the hepatic cytochrome P450 monooxygenase system. The best known example of a toxic compound activated in the lung is 4-ipomeanol, a naturally occurring furan derivative from moldy sweet potatoes that causes severe lung injury in cattle. Pulmonary injury by 4-ipomeanol is caused by a highly reactive alkylating metabolite, probably an epoxide produced by cytochrome P450 isozymes. Since the two major lung cytochrome P450 isozymes both readily metabolize 4-ipomeanol, activation by the lung is much greater than that of the liver, which contains significantly lower levels of these two isozymes. The Clara cells in which these two isozymes are concentrated are most affected by 4-ipomeanol toxicity. Other toxic lung furans, such as the atmospheric contaminants 2-methylfuran and 3-methylfuran, may also exert their toxicity through the formation of reactive metabolites, probably reactive aldehydes. The presence of the cytochrome P450 system in Clara cells is of toxicological significance since many cytotoxic and carcinogenic chemicals require activation by this enzyme system. Thus the Clara cells may be a major site for the formation of the ultimate toxicant or carcinogen, as well as a primary target for the effects of activated chemicals. Another means of metabolic activation is the cyclic reduction/oxidation of the parent compound, resulting in high rates of consumption of NADPH and production of superoxide anion. Either the depletion of NADPH and/or the formation of reactive oxygen radicals can lead to cellular injury. For example, systemic administration of paraquat initiates a progression of degenerative and potentially lethal lesions in the lung. The redox cycling of paraquat causes two damaging cellular events: (1) the generation of active oxygen species (superoxide anion, hydrogen peroxide, and hydroxy radical) which are highly reactive toward tissue macromolecules; (2) the depletion of cellular reducing equivalents (NADPH, reduced glutathione) which are essential for normal function. Other lung toxicants such as oxygen, bleomycin and nitrofurantoin may have similar mechanisms. *See also* CLARA CELLS; IPOMEANOL; PARAQUAT; PULMONARY TOXICITY; PYRROLIZIDINE ALKALOIDS.

pulmonary toxicity, induction. *See* PULMONARY TOXICITY, BIOTRANSFORMATION AND REACTIVE METABOLITES.

purines. A group of organic bases with fused five- and six-membered rings best known as components of DNA and RNA (e.g. adenine, guanine) although such purines as caffeine, theobromine and theophylline are important in toxicology. Purines may occur in the free state but are usually combined with ribose as nucleosides, with ribose and phosphoric acid as nucleotides or in DNA and RNA.

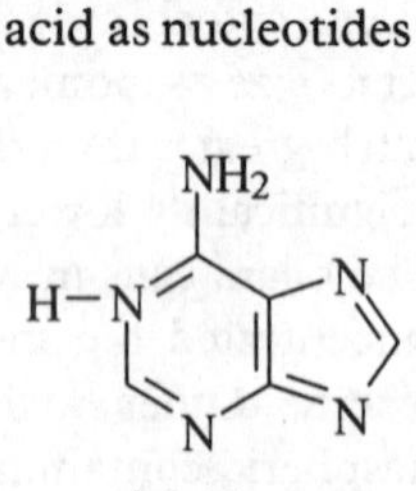

Adenine

Purinethol. *See* 6-MERCAPTOPURINE.

pydrin. *See* FENVALERATE.

pyrazolon derivatives. *See* ANTIPYRINE; PHENYLBUTAZONE.

pyrene. *See* POLYCYCLIC AROMATIC HYDROCARBONS.

pyrethrins. The six insecticidal constituents of the extract of the pyrethrum flowers *Pyrethrum* (Chrysanthemum) *cinerariae* (folium). Pyrethrins I and II are most prominent, existing in the ratio 71:21:7 for pyrethrin (I and II), cinerin (I and II), jasmolin (I and II). Pyrethrins are potent, non-systemic, contact insecticides, causing rapid paralysis or knockdown and death at a later stage in a variety of insects. They exhibit low vertebrate toxicity with an acute oral LD50 in rats of 1.2 g/kg.

The mechanism of action involves modification of nerve membrane Na^+ channels. Opening and closing of the Na^+ channel is slowed, resulting in increased Na^+ permeability and depolarization leading to hyperexcitability. Symptoms in humans include gastrointestinal irritation, nausea, vomiting, diarrhea, numbness of tongue and lips, syncope, hyperexcitability, incoordination, convulsions, muscular paralysis, collapse and death due to respiratory paralysis. Treatment involves gastric lavage, emetics, cathartics, demulcents, artificial respiration if necessary and short-acting barbiturates for convulsions.

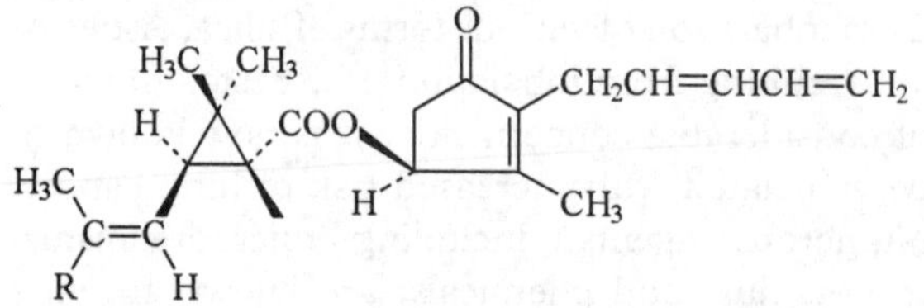

Pyrethrin I

pyrethroid insecticides. A relatively new class of synthetic insecticides based on the pyrethrins, insecticides of botanical origin. They are characterized by a high selectivity index and a failure to accumulate either *in vivo* or in the environment. Their mode of action appears to be similar to that of the pyrethrins, namely interaction at the Na^+ channel, having the effect of causing repetitive discharges and hyperexcitability. This class includes compounds such as fenvalerate, resmethrin, bioresmethrin and permethrin. *See also* FENVALERATE; PYRETHRINS.

pyrethrum. The insecticidal extract of the pyrethrum flower *Pyrethrum* (Chrysanthemum) *cinerariae* (folium). *See also* PYRETHRINS.

pyridine. CAS number 110-86-1. A solvent and synthetic intermediate. Appears to have very low toxicity to humans. Acute inhalation may cause neurological effects, long-term inhalation may cause liver damage. No known carcinogenic effects. *See also* ATSDR DOCUMENT, SEPTEMBER 1992; DATABASES, TOXICOLOGY; LEWIS, HCDR, NUMBER POP250.

pyridostigmine (3-[[(dimethylamino)carbonyl]oxy]-1-methylpyridinium). A synthetic eserine analog; more effective in the treatment of myasthenia gravis and with fewer undesirable side effects than eserine. Since pyridostigmine is a dimethylcarbamate, recovery of the inhibited acetylcholinesterase is slower than with eserine. Because of its quaternary ammonium nature, its actions are limited primarily to the peripheral nervous system. Pyridostigmine is occasionally used in treatment of glaucoma. *See also* ANTICHOLINESTERASES; ESERINE.

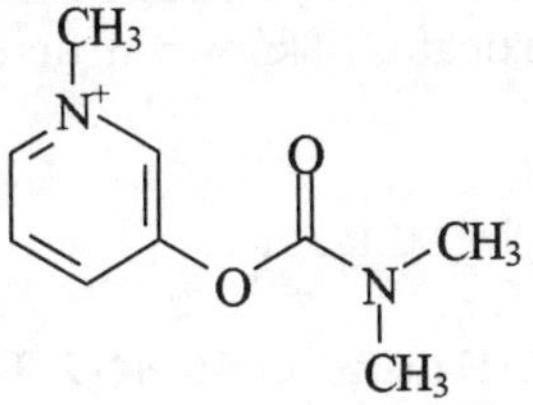

Pyridostigmine

pyrimidines. Six-membered heterocyclic compounds containing two nitrogens. Best known as constituents of DNA and RNA.

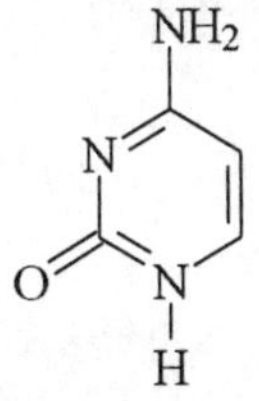

pyrocatechol. *See* CATECHOL.

Cytosine

pyrrolizidine alkaloids. Highly toxic alkaloids produced by plants of the genera *Crotolaria*, *Senecio* and *Heliotropium*. Monocrotaline is a typical pyrrolizidine alkaloid. Pyrrolizidine alkaloids are potent hepatotoxicants and carcinogens. These compounds may contribute to human liver cancer incidence in some parts of the world, in others they are the cause of acute poisoning episodes in food animals. Pyrrolizidine alkaloids are activated to electrophilic intermediates by cytochrome P450.

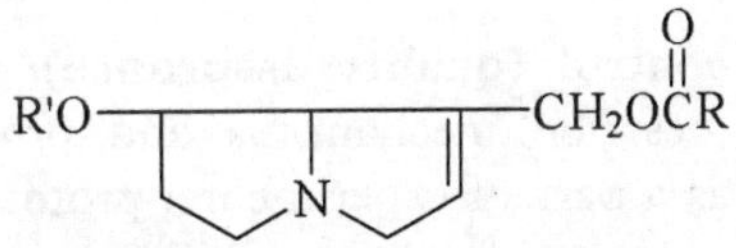

Pyrrolizidine alkaloids, general formula

Q

Q★. *See* CANCER POTENCY FACTOR.

q1★. The symbol used to denote the 95% upper bound estimate of the linearized slope of the dose response curve in the low dose region.

QSAR. *See* QUANTITATIVE STRUCTURE–ACTIVITY RELATIONSHIPS.

quality assurance. *See* QUALITY CONTROL.

quality control (quality assurance). A term used to describe mechanisms and procedures planned as a part of experimental protocols that are designed to reduce the possibility of error, particularly human error. Integral parts of quality control include the design of procedures in such a way as to minimize the possibility of human error, the collection of data not only on the results of the experiments, but also on the daily activities, personnel involved, etc., and the proper training of all laboratory and animal room personnel. Activity and results forms must be designed in such a way that omissions are immediately apparent. Quality control is critical in long-term testing procedures such as carcinogenesis and other chronic toxicity tests, since these studies may take years to complete and involve many animals. Although essential at all stages of such experiments, quality control is particularly important in the area of facility design and maintenance, quarantine and pretest screening of animals, the dosing of animals and the proper identification and tracking of pathology samples. *See also* CARCINOGENICITY TESTING; CHRONIC TOXICITY TESTING.

quantitative structure–activity relationships (QSAR). The relationship between the physical and/or chemical properties of chemicals and their ability to cause a particular effect, enter into particular reactions, etc. The goal of QSAR studies in toxicology is to develop procedures whereby the toxicity of a compound can be predicted from its chemical structure by analogy with the properties of other toxicants of known structure and toxic properties.

quicksilver. *See* MERCURY.

quinidine. CAS number 56-54-2. Isomeric with quinine; mp (anhyd.) 174–175 °C. Chemical properties are similar to quinine; salts are more soluble than those of quinine. Antimalarial and antiarrhythmic.

quinine. CAS number 130-95-0. Antimalarial, still used primarily for treatment of plasmodium resistant to synthetic antimalarials. Also used as antipyretic for colds, influenza, and cramp; quinine has toxic effects on the eye, apparently due to an immune reaction, and on male reproductive capacity.

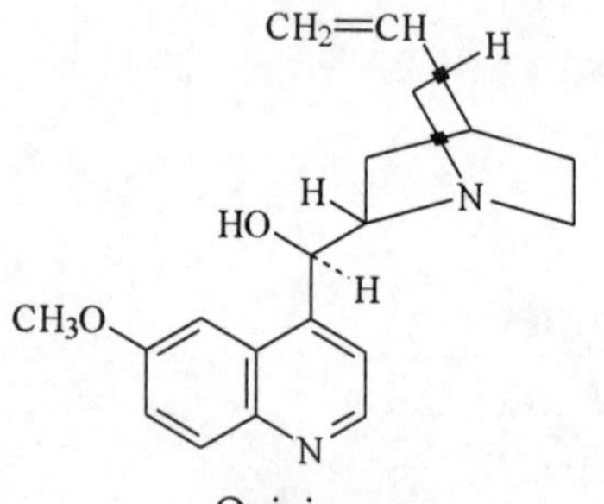

Quinine

quinoline. CAS number 91-22-5. Antimalarial.

quinolinic acid (2,3-pyridinedicarboxylic acid). CAS number 89-00-9. Focal injection of quinolinic acid into specific areas of the brain produces neuronal damage although sparing axons of passage. Similarities between the biochemical and morphological profiles of these lesions and human neuropathy seen in neurodegenerative diseases have led to the proposal that endogenous excitotoxins may play a role in such neurodegenerative disease states. Quinolinic acid is an intermediate in the kynurenine pathway of tryptophan metabolism and has been detected in the brains of several mammals including man. The neuroexcitatory action is thought to be mediated via interaction with the N-methyl-D-aspartate (NMDA) receptor of the glutamate family. No mechanism for quinolinic acid removal, nor for synaptic inactivation, has been found, and consequently accumulation of concentrations capable of inducing neuronal degeneration and death may occur. *See also* EXCITOTOXINS.

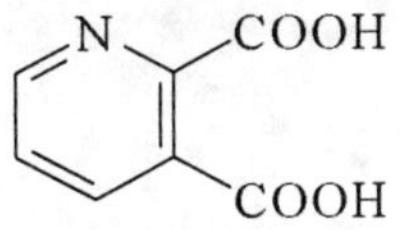

Quinolinic acid

R

radial immunodiffusion (RID). *See* IMMUNO-ASSAY.

radiation. Energy in the form of electromagnetic waves, radiant energy or energy emitted from a radioactive source or nuclear reactor in the form of particles which possess mass and which may or may not be electrically charged (e.g., α- or β-particles and neutrons). Radiation is used in medicine in the form of X-rays, and in industry as a sterilizing agent, and polymerizaton initiator. Radiation forms the basis of all types of spectroscopic analysis. The detection of radiation forms the basis for the use of radioactive atoms as tracers in biochemical toxicology.

radiation carcinogenesis. One of the major stochastic effects and probably the most important late somatic effect of ionizing radiation. A clear relationship has been established between radiation dose and excess risk of cancer in irradiated human populations and in animal experiments. The cytopathological changes in irradiated cells are numerous, varied and complex, yet quite similar to those seen following other types of cellular injury.

radiation dose equivalent (dose equivalent). A measure of the effect of ionizing radiation on the substance or tissue that absorbs it. Since the effect of radiation in one kind of biological tissue or organ is different from the effect in another issue or organ, and some types of radiation are more harmful than others, the absorbed dose, which can be measured, is multiplied by weighing factors stipulated by the International Commission on Equivalence, for which the SI unit is the sievert. The value in sieverts represents the risk to health from that amount of radiation had it been absorbed uniformly throughout the body.

radioactive isotope (radioisotope). Isotope of an element that is intrinsically unstable and is likely to emit ionizing radiation as a result of radioactive decay to a more stable form. Such isotopes are used as radioactive tracers (e.g., ^{14}C, ^{32}P) while others are used in therapy (e.g., ^{125}I). Decay characteristics of some commonly used radioactive isotopes are as shown in Table 6.

radioactive labeling (radiolabeling). A means of identifying molecules and their biological or chemical products by the presence of a radioactive isotope (e.g., ^{14}C, ^{3}H, ^{35}S and ^{32}P). The substitution of a radioactive atom for its non-radioactive isomer changes the chemical properties of the molecule only slightly. Moreover, enzymes or receptors seldom can distinguish between labeled and unlabeled molecules. Using such methods as autoradiography and scintillation counting it is possible to trace the fate of the labeled molecule in metabolic pathway(s). A large number of compounds of biochemical interest including drugs, hormones, metabolite analogues, antimetabolites and their metabolites are available labeled with ^{14}C, ^{3}H, ^{32}P or ^{125}I.

radioactivity. Manifestation of spontaneous nuclear transformation in which energy is emitted. Radioactivity can be natural, caused by the decay of naturally occurring radioactive isotopes, or induced by bombardment with high-energy particles, frequently neutrons. In toxicology, radioactivity is of interest because of its potential health effects and for the use of radioactive isotopes as tracers in metabolic and mechanism of action studies.

radioallergosorbent test (RAST). *See* IMMUNOASSAY.

Table 6 Some radioactive isotopes used in toxicology and medicine

Isotope	Half life	Type of decay[a]
Cadmium-109	462 days	EM
Calcium-45	164 days	β
Carbon-14	5730 years	β
Chlorine-36	3×10^5 years	β + EM
Chromium-51	27 days	EM
Cobalt-60	5.27 years	β
Iodine-125	60 days	EM
Iodine-131	8 days	β
Iron-55	2.69 years	EM
Iron-59	44 days	β
Manganese-54	312 days	EM
Phosphorous-32	14.3 days	β
Radium-226	1600 years	α
Sodium-22	2.60 years	β + EM
Strontium-85	64 days	EM
Strontium-89	50 days	β
Strontium-90	28.6 years	β
Sulphur-35	87.4 days	β
Tritium (hydrogen-3)	12.43 years	β
Zinc-65	243 days	β + EM

[a]β, beta particles; α, alpha particles; EM, electromagnetic radiation.

radioimmunoassay (RIA). A competitive binding assay based on a test ligand, a radiolabeled ligand and an antibody. Typically, a test ligand is added to a known amount of antibody and radiolabeled ligand. After separation of the antibody-ligand complex from free ligand and free antibody, the amount of bound ligand can be determined directly by radioactive counting. The number of counts of labeled ligand bound is inversely proportional to the concentration of unlabeled ligand added. The discovery of the RIA in the early 1960s revolutionized biological research because of the ease of use and high sensitivities of these types of assays. *See also* ELISA; IMMUNOASSAY; RADIORECEPTOR ASSAYS.

radioligand binding methods. *See* RADIORECEPTOR ASSAYS.

radioreceptor assays. Assays used to characterize the interaction of ligands with specific high-affinity recognition sites. Frequently, these recognition sites have intrinsic biological roles (e.g., neurotransmitter receptors or enzymes). Radioreceptor assays are based on the law of mass action and are used in toxicology for three distinct purposes: (1) To characterize the interaction of a toxicant with a physiological recognition site (e.g., ouabain with the Na^+/K^+-ATPase or α-bungarotoxin with the cholinergic receptor). Two common techniques are used for this purpose: (a) radiolabeling the toxicant of interest; or (b) determining how the toxicant competes for a well-characterized radioligand. In either case, the equilibrium and kinetic analyses use methods essentially identical to those used in enzyme kinetics. (2) To characterize how intoxication perturbs a site of physiological importance, such as a neurotransmitter receptor. (3) As analytical tools for indirectly quantifying analytes in test samples. The radioimmunoassay is the most common application of analytical radioreceptor assays, but endogenous binding proteins (e.g., neurotransmitter receptors) have also been used. *See also* EADIE-HOFSTEE PLOT; ENZYME KINETICS; K_D; K_M; LINEWEAVER–BURK PLOT; METABOLITE INHIBITORY COMPLEXES; MICHAELIS–MENTEN EQUATION; RADIORECEPTOR ASSAYS; WOOLF PLOT; XENOBIOTIC METABOLISM, INHIBITION.

radon (Rn). Radioactive gas belonging to Group 8A; the product of radioactive decay of the heavy elements. Of the 20 isotopes known, the important ones, ^{222}Rn (thoron, Th) from thorium (half-life: 54.5 s) and ^{219}Rn (actinon, An) from actinium (half-life: 3.92 s), are α-emitters. Radon is used as a radiation source and as a gaseous tracer. It creates a hazard in uranium mines and is believed to be hazardous in homes with a high background level. While the data derived from uranium miners show clearly that there is an increased risk for lung cancer, that from exposure in the home is less clear. It appears that smokers are at increased risk for lung cancer due to radon, implying an interaction between radon and tobacco smoke in cancer causation, but a statistically significant increased risk for lung cancer due to radon among non-smokers has yet to be determined, although the results are often suggestive of such an increase.

rainbow trout (*Oncorhyncus gairdneri*). A standard fish species for aquatic toxicology tests. *See also* AQUATIC BIOASSAY.

Rampart. *See* PHORATE.

randomization. A procedure for assigning subjects to experimental conditions such that the probability of being assigned to an experimental condition is equally likely for all subjects. The purpose of randomization is to decrease the probability that the effects of the independent variable are confounded by other variables such as age, gender, etc. Such confounding variables may be plausible rival hypotheses to the hypothesis being tested. Randomization is perhaps the most important mechanism for eliminating threats to both the internal and external validity of the experiment. *See also* STATISTICS, FUNCTION IN TOXICOLOGY.

ranitidine. Histamine H_2-receptor antagonist that inhibits gastric acid secretion. Gastric alcohol dehydrogenase inhibitor.

rapid acetylators. *See* FAST AND SLOW ACETYLATORS.

RAST (radioallergosorbent test). *See* IMMUNOASSAY.

rate-doubling concentration. As defined in the Committee 17 Report, the concentration of chemical that would be required to produce the same amount of mutational activity in a given unit of time as would have been expected to occur spontaneously in the particular test system under consideration. *See also* MOLECULAR DOSIMETRY; SPECIES EXTRAPOLATION.

rattlesnake venom. The product of the venom glands of snakes belonging to the family Crotalidae; it is injected into the victim via two mobile, needle-sharp teeth. The venom contains many noxious agents, rather than one specific toxin. The lung appears to be the major target organ, where increased vascular permeability causes pulmonary congestion and hemorrhage, in addition to hemolysis. Symptoms include local bleeding, severe pain, superficial edema of rapid onset, hemorrhagic blister formation and fang marks. Common field emergency treatments such as incision and suction, tourniquets and ice packs are more damaging than useful. The spread of venom is limited by avoidance of unnecessary motion. Antivenins should be started as soon as possible. *See also* SNAKE VENOMS.

Rauwolfia alkaloids. *See* RESERPINE.

RC Path. *See* ROYAL COLLEGE OF PATHOLOGISTS.

RCRA. *See* RESOURCE CONSERVATION AND RECOVERY ACT.

reabsorption. *See* ABSORPTION OF TOXICANTS; ADMINISTRATION OF TOXICANTS, RECTAL.

reactivation, acetylcholinesterase. *See* ACETYLCHOLINESTERASE, REACTIVATION.

reactive intermediates (reactive metabolites). Chemical compounds, produced during the metabolism of xenobiotics, that are more chemically reactive than the parent compound. Although they are susceptible to detoxication by conjugation reactions as a consequence of their increased reactivity, they have a greater potential for adverse effects than the parent compound. A well-known example is the metabolism of benzo[*a*]pyrene to its carcinogenic dihydrodiol epoxide derivative by cytochrome P450 and epoxide hydrolase. Reactive intermediates involved in toxic effects include epoxides, quinones, free radicals, reactive oxygen species and a small number of unstable conjugation products. *See also* ACTIVATION; PHASE I REACTIONS; XENOBIOTIC METABOLISM.

reactive oxygen species. *See* OXYGEN, REACTIVE SPECIES.

rebaudioside. Naturally sweet diterpenoid glucoside extracted from a South American plant, *Stevia rebaudiana*. Rebaudioside is non-calorific and is not fermentable. Sold commercially in Asia. *See* STEVIOSIDE; SWEETENING AGENTS.

Rebelate. *See* DIMETHOATE.

recalcitrant molecules, in environment. Molecules that persist in the environment and are resistant to degradation by physical (e.g., ultraviolet light), chemical (e.g., hydrolysis, oxidation/reduction) or biological (e.g., metabolism) factors.

receptor. A high-affinity binding site for a particular ligand. Receptors almost always have specificity for ligands with selected structural features. Although the term may be used generally for any high-affinity binding site, the most important class of receptors are those whose purpose is to interact with biologically endogenous ligands, thereby facilitating cell–cell or intracellular communication. One very important class comprises the cell surface receptors, such as those that bind neurotransmitters and neuromodulators (e.g., muscarinic or nicotinic cholinergic receptors, α- and β-adrenergic receptors, dopamine receptors, GABA receptors, glutamate receptors and opioid peptide receptors) and those that interact with hormones (e.g., insulin, TRH, somatostatin). Other receptors are cytoplasmic, for example, for ligands such as steroid hormones, calcium (calmodulin and troponin C) or carcinogenic polycyclic aromatic hydrocarbons (Ah receptor). Interaction with receptors (as either an agonist or antagonists) is an important mechanism by which many toxicants or drugs produce toxic sequelae. In addition, many toxicants that do not act directly on receptors may cause physiological effects by causing compensatory changes or damage to receptor systems. The understanding of the action of toxicants on receptors often requires an awareness of the biochemical events that are associated with these receptors, including second messenger biosynthesis (e.g., cyclic AMP or phosphoinositols) and ion conductance. *See also* ACETYLCHOLINE RECEPTORS, MUSCARINIC AND NICOTINIC; B_{MAX}; CHLORIDE CHANNEL; GABA; K_D; RADIORECEPTOR ASSAYS; SECOND MESSENGERS; SODIUM CHANNEL.

recombinant DNA. The manipulation of segments of DNA from one organism into the DNA of another ("gene splicing"). Such DNA is then replicated and expressed in the host organism. Recombinant DNA techniques are valuable research tools in toxicology, enabling proteins of interest to be isolated, sequenced and expressed separately from closely related proteins.

recombination. *See* MITOTIC RECOMBINATION.

rectal administration. *See* ADMINISTRATION OF TOXICANTS, RECTAL.

red blood cells. *See* ERYTHROCYTES.

reduction. A chemical process, opposite to that of oxidation, in which there is a gain of electrons by the reducing agent and a decrease in the oxidation state. In organic chemistry, the most obvious effect of reduction is the increase in the proportion of hydrogen and the decrease in the number of multiple bonds in the molecule. Specific reducing agents include hydrogen and lithium tetrahydridoaluminate. Functional groups in organic molecules such as nitro, diazo, carbonyl, disulfide, sulfoxide and alkene are susceptible to enzymatic or, in some cases, non-enzymatic, reduction. In certain cases, such as the reduction of the double bond in cinnamic acid ($C_6H_5CH=CHCOOH$), the reaction has been attributed to the intestinal microflora. *See also* ALDEHYDE AND KETONE REDUCTION; AZO REDUCTION; DISULFIDE REDUCTION; NITRO REDUCTION; OXIDATION; OXIDATION STATE; SULFOXIDE REDUCTION.

redux. *See* FENFLURAMINE.

re-entry intervals. The time periods following application of pesticides to fields during which workers may not re-enter the area. They are established on a case-by-case basis, but generally speaking for insecticides, particularly cholinesterase inhibitors such as the organophosphates, they are established in the USA by the Office of Pesticide Programs of the EPA under the authority established by the Federal Insecticide, Fungicide and Rodenticide Act (FIFRA). *See also* FEDERAL INSECTICIDE, FUNGICIDE AND RODENTICIDE ACT.

reference dose (RfD). An estimate, with approximately an order of magnitude uncertainty, of the daily exposure of a toxicant to the human population that is likely to be without adverse

effects after lifetime exposure at that level. The units for the RfD are mg toxicant/kg body weight/day for oral exposure or mg toxicant/m^3 of air breathed for inhalation exposures.

Reglone. *See* DIQUAT.

regulator gene. Gene whose function is to control the transcriptional activity of other genes, either adjacent or distant in the genome. In bacteria, the same regulatory gene may affect a series of non-adjacent operons. The presence of regulator genes in eukaryotes is in many situations hypothetical, although the products of genes with a common sequence known as a homeo boxes seem likely to have regulatory functions in regard to other genes.

regulatory requirements. In toxicology, the data from toxicity testing that must be submitted to any government agency empowered to regulate the manufacture, sale, distribution or disposal of chemicals. *See also* ACUTE TOXICITY TESTING; CANADIAN HEALTH PROTECTION BRANCH; CHRONIC TOXICITY TESTING; CONSUMER PRODUCTS SAFETY COMMISSION; ENVIRONMENTAL PROTECTION AGENCY; FEDERAL INSECTICIDE, FUNGICIDE AND RODENTICIDE ACT; FOOD AND DRUG ADMINISTRATION; GOOD LABORATORY PRACTICES; INTERAGENCY REGULATORY LIAISON GROUP; PHARMACEUTICAL MANUFACTURERS ASSOCATION; REPRODUCTIVE TOXICITY TESTING; SUBCHRONIC TOXICITY TESTING; TOXIC SUBSTANCES CONTROL ACT.

regulatory toxicology. The branch of applied toxicology that is concerned with the formulation and administration of regulations governing the manufacture, sale and use of toxicants and potential toxicants, as well as their release into the environment. In most countries this is done by regulatory agencies operating within a framework of laws passed by the legislative bodies of the country in question. Much of regulatory toxicology is concerned with evaluation of risk based on data gathered from toxicity tests prescribed in the regulations. Actions taken may vary from requirements for warning labels, to use restrictions or, in some cases, to a ban that makes illegal any manufacture or use of the toxicant in question.

relative teratogenicity index. *See* TERATO-GENIC HAZARD POTENTIAL.

renal clearance. *See* KINETIC EQUATIONS, RENAL CLEARANCE.

renal damage. *See* NEPHROTOXICITY.

renal excretion. *See* EXCRETION, RENAL; MAINTENANCE THERAPY, BLOOD; MAINTENANCE THERAPY, URINARY TRACT; MAINTENANCE THERAPY, WATER AND ELECTROLYTE BALANCE; RENAL FAILURE.

renal failure (Bright's disease; renal dropsy). The loss of the ability of the kidney to maintain salt and water balance, acid and potassium excretion, bicarbonate reabsorption, phosphate excretion and nitrogenous waste (urea) excretion. Renal failure results in a progressive systemic acidosis, volume overload, congestive heart failure, high blood pressure, osteomalacia, secondary hyperparathyroidism and death. There are two types of renal failure: (1) oliguric, the most common form with all of the above manifestations accompanied by marked reduction in urine flow; (2) nonoliguric, the relatively uncommon form with either increased or normal urine flow. Causes of renal failure include uncontrolled hypertension, toxins, heavy metal poisoning, drugs, vascular insults and inflammatory diseases of the kidney. *See also* DIAGNOSTIC FEATURES, URINARY TRACT; NEPHROTOXICITY.

renal toxicity. *See* NEPHROTOXICITY.

reportable quantity. The quantity of a hazardous substance that is considered reportable under CERCLA. Reportable quantities are either one pound (347 g)/24 hours or, in the case of certain compounds, an amount established by regulation under CERCLA or the Clean Water Act per 24 hours. *See also* CERCLA; CLEAN WATER ACT.

Report on the Review of Flavourings in Food. A report of the Food Additives and Contaminants Committee (UK) that recommended that flavorings should be controlled by a permitted list, with no flavorings being authorized unless on this list.

reproductive failure, in birds. The decline in bird populations in recent years is related, in part, to diminished reproductive success which may be due to eggshell thinning, possibly caused by organochlorine insecticide contamination. Also methylmercury and PCBs exert adverse effects on reproduction by reducing egg production and causing mortality in young birds. *See also* EGGSHELL THINNING; METHYLMERCURY; POLYCHLORINATED BIPHENYLS.

reproductive system. Organ systems in male and female organisms with the function of producing male and female, usually haploid, gametes. In viviparous species such as mammals the female reproductive system is also the site for the fertilization of the ova and the prenatal development of the young. Toxic effects on the reproductive systems and on the developing young are very important endpoints in toxicology. *See also* OVARY, REPRODUCTIVE TOXICITY, SERTOLI CELLS, SPERM; SPERMATOCYTE, SPERMATOGENESIS, SPERMATOGONIA; SPERMATOZOA; TERATOGENESIS, TERATOGENIC; TERATOLOGY; UTERUS.

reproductive toxicity, male. Adverse effects on the male reproductive system, including the associated endocrine tissues, caused by exposure to toxicants. May be apparent as visible microscopic abnormalities and/or expressed at the functional level through deficits in sexual behavior, fertility, pregnancy outcomes, etc. *See also* REPRODUCTIVE TOXICITY TESTING.

reproductive toxicity testing. Many complex protocols exist in reproductive toxicity testing with few objective criteria to facilitate a preference. Furthermore, the terminology used in teratology is extensive, highly specialized and varies between research groups. The following embodies the general features of the most common protocols. The subject is divided into four areas: (1) fertility and general reproductive performance—single-generation studies; (2) fertility and general reproductive performance—multi-generation studies; (3) teratology; (4) the effect of chemicals in late pregnancy and lactation (perinatal/postnatal). As with all forms of *in vivo* tests utilizing experimental animals, the principles of animal husbandry as they apply to facilities, cages, environmental controls, diet, etc. should be closely adhered to. *See also* ACUTE TOXICITY TESTING; CHRONIC TOXICITY TESTING; REPRODUCTIVE TOXICITY TESTING, MULTI-GENERATION; REPRODUCTIVE TOXICITY TESTING, PERINATAL/POSTNATAL; REPRODUCTIVE TOXICITY TESTING, SINGLE-GENERATION; SUBCHRONIC TOXICITY TESTING.

reproductive toxicity testing, multi-generation. Tests that are carried out using rodents, usually rats, with the test compound being administered to both males and females, from weaning of the F_0 generation to the end of the test, usually three generations in length. The test compound is administered in the food or drinking water, usually at three levels. The high level is approximately one-tenth of the LD50, the low dose is one that subchronic studies indicate does not cause toxicity in dams or fetuses of the F_1 generation. The intermediate dose(s) are equally spaced on a logarithmic scale between low and high doses. Enough females from the F_0 group and enough survivors of the F_1 and F_2 group are provided so that each generation of each treatment group and the controls have 20 pregnant females per dose level. After males and females of the initial group have been treated for 60 days they are mated to produce the first F_1 litter. After birth the pups are weighed, sexed and examined for external abnormalities, and the litters are then culled to a constant number of pups (usually 10). Pup weight and survival are measured until weaning, when the pups are sacrificed and autopsied to detect internal abnormalities, obtain organ weights, etc. The parents are again mated after the first litter is weaned. The pups of the second litter are treated in the same way as the first, except that enough are permitted to survive to produce the 20 or more males and females for the next generation. Again each pair is allowed to produce two litters, which are treated in the same way as those of the first generation, again setting aside enough animals to produce the two litters of the third generation. Since this is the final generation, in addition to examining weanlings as described above, a selected number are subjected to a complete histological examination. The following endpoints are evaluated: (1) fertility index, the number of pregnancies relative to the number of matings; (2) the number of live births, relative to the total number of births; (3) gender and initial weight of pups; (4) growth rate of pups; (5) survival of pups relative to number born (or relative to number to which litters are culled); (6) gross deformities at birth; (7) internal abnormalities at weaning; (8) histological changes at weaning (third generation only). As with the single-generation test, males or females of any generation can be mated to untreated individuals of the opposite sex to determine the sex specificity of any effect observed. *See also* CHRONIC TOXICITY TESTING; FERTILITY INDEX; GROWTH INDEX; REPRODUCTIVE TOXICITY TESTING, PERINATAL/POSTNATAL; REPRODUCTIVE TOXICITY TESTING, SINGLE-GENERATION; SEX RATIO; VIABILITY INDEX; WEANING INDEX.

reproductive toxicity testing, perinatal/postnatal. Tests that are usually carried out on rats. Typically 20 pregnant females per dosage group are treated during the final third of gestation and through lactation to weaning (day 15 of pregnancy through day 21 post partum). The duration of gestation and delivery problems, as well as the number and size of pups in the naturally delivered litter, are observed as is the growth performance of the offspring. Groups may be treated only to parturition or only postpartum in order to separate pre- and postnatal effects. Cross-fostering of pups to untreated dams may also be used to the same end. Behavioral testing of the pups has also been suggested, as well as other physiological tests and histological examination. *See also* CHRONIC TOXICITY TESTING; FERTILITY INDEX; GROWTH INDEX; SEX RATIO; VIABILITY INDEX; WEANING INDEX.

reproductive toxicity testing, single-generation. Tests that are usually carried out on rats. Typically 20 males are treated with the test compound for 60 days prior to mating and 20 females for 14 days prior to mating; treatment times are selected to coincide with the time for spermatogenesis and ovulation. After mating, the females are treated through pregnancy and until the pups are weaned. The test compound is administered either in the feed, in the drinking water or by gavage. The high dose is either that which causes some, but not excessive, maternal toxicity or that which just fails to cause maternal toxicity. The low dose is either that to which humans are expected to be exposed or a dose that gives measurable tissue levels, but no measurable toxicity. The intermediate dose(s) are evenly spaced, on a logarithmic scale, between the low and high doses. The rats are placed in cohabitation, with one male and one female caged together. Mating is confirmed by the appearance of spermatozoa in the daily vaginal smear or by the appearance of a copulatory plug. Half the females are killed at mid-gestation and examined for pre- and postimplantation lethality; the other half are permitted to bear and nurse their pups, the litters being culled to a constant number, usually 10, after three to four days. At weaning, the pups are sacrificed and autopsied for gross and internal abnormalities. Because both males and females are treated, it is not possible to distinguish between maternal and paternal effects. This can be determined, however, by treating additional animals to the stage of mating and then outcrossing them to untreated members of the opposite sex. The endpoints observed are as follows: (1) preimplantation death, the number of corpora lutea in the ovaries relative to the number of implantation sites; (2) postimplantation deaths, the number of resorption sites in the uterus relative to the number of implantation sites; (3) gross effects on the male or female reproductive system; (4) duration of gestation; (5) litter size and condition, number of dead and live pups, weight of pups, gender of pups, gross morphological variation in pups; (6) subsequent survival and performance of dam and pups, weight gain, mortality, etc.; (7) gross and visceral abnormalities in weanlings. Although detailed examination of the pups is possible, this is generally carried out under the protocol described for teratology testing. It has been suggested that a number of weanlings be left to develop and be tested later for behavioral and/or physiological deficits. *See also* CHRONIC TOXICITY TESTING; FERTILITY INDEX; GROWTH INDEX; REPRODUCTIVE TOXICITY TESTING, MULTI-GENERATION; SEX RATIO; VIABILITY INDEX; WEANING INDEX.

RER (rough endoplasmic reticulum). *See* ENDOPLASMIC RETICULUM.

reserpine (11,17α-dimethoxy-18β-[(3,4,5-trimethoxybenzoyl)oxy]yohimban-16-carboxylic acid methyl ester). **CAS number 50-55-5**. One of the Rauwolfia alkaloids (from *Rauwolfia serpentina*). Reserpine causes depletion of monoamines from presynaptic nerve terminals, both in the central and peripheral nervous systems, presumably by interfering with amine storage mechanisms. For this reason, reserpine has sedative, hypotensive, antipsychotic and antimanic properties and has been commonly used for all of these purposes. However, both the side effects and lack of specificity are significant disadvantages, and with the development of more selective drugs in each of these classes, reserpine is of little clinical use at present. Adverse effects may include nightmares, severe depression, abdominal cramps, diarrhea and hypotension. Reserpine has been listed by the EPA as a carcinogen, and some evidence exists that rates of breast cancer are increased in reserpine-treated women. *See also* CATECHOLAMINES.

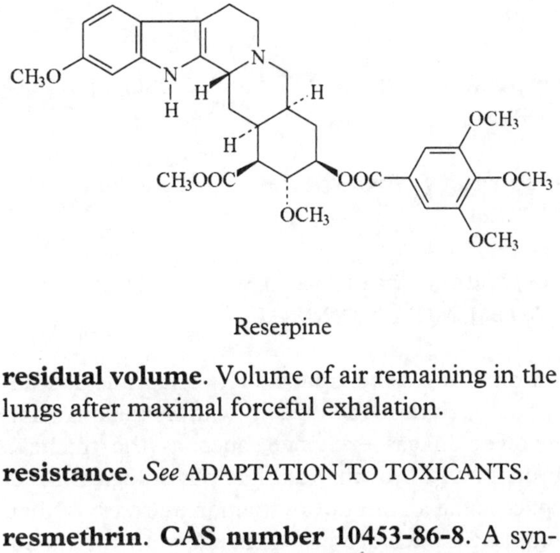

Reserpine

residual volume. Volume of air remaining in the lungs after maximal forceful exhalation.

resistance. *See* ADAPTATION TO TOXICANTS.

resmethrin. **CAS number 10453-86-8**. A synthetic pyrethroid effective against a wide range of insects. Resmethrin has low mammalian toxicity, with an acute dermal LD50 in rats of about 2000 mg/kg. A dose of 3000 mg/kg/ day for 90 days had

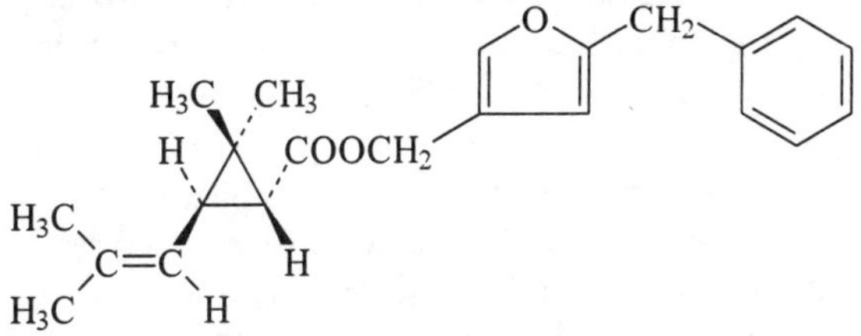

Resmethrin

no effect. The mode of action is via an effect on the sodium channels, leading to hyperexcitability. *See also* PYRETHROID INSECTICIDES.

Resource Conservation and Recovery Act (RCRA). Administered by the EPA, this Act is the most important one governing the disposal of hazardous wastes in the USA. It promulgates standards for the identification of hazardous wastes, their transportation and their disposal. Included in the disploral are the siting and construction criteria for landfills and other disposal facilities, as well as the regulation of owners and operators of such facilities.

respirable dust. Defined as dust whose size is less than 10 μm in size. *See also* DUST, RESPIRABLE.

respiratory acidosis. *See* ACIDOSIS, RESPIRATORY.

respiratory alkalosis. *See* ALKALOSIS, RESPIRATORY.

respiratory bronchioles. *See* RESPIRATORY SYSTEM.

respiratory chain. *See* ELECTRON TRANSPORT SYSTEM, MITOCHONDRIAL.

respiratory dead space. The anatomical dead space includes the space within regions not involved in gas exchange, such as the trachea, bronchi and bronchioles. The physiological dead space is the amount of ventilation in excess of that required to achieve gas exchange with the blood flow at a particular time (i.e., wasted ventilation).

respiratory depression. The reduced respiration rate that can occur in many conditions as a result of disease, following injury, etc. In toxicology, it is important as a complication in poisoning due particularly to CNS depressants such as opioids and barbiturates, which presumably act on the respiratory center in the brain. Since maintenance of respiration is critical in treatment, artificial respiration, respirators, etc. are used immediately in such cases. *See also* MAINTENANCE THERAPY, RESPIRATION.

respiratory rate. The number of inspiration/expiration cycles per unit time.

respiratory resistance. *See* PULMONARY RESISTANCE.

respiratory sensitization. Type I or anaphylactic reactions involving the respiratory system. Such sensitization can be a response to chemicals, as in chemically induced respiratory allergies or asthma.

respiratory system (respiratory tract). The respiratory system consists of three regions. (1) The nasopharyngeal region, which consists of the nasal region and the pharynx, is involved in filtering large particles. The nasal epithelium is also an important site for monooxygenation of xenobiotics. (2) The tracheobronchial region consists of airways connecting the nasopharynx to the alveoli, these airways being the trachea, bronchi and bronchioles. They all have ciliated epithelium covered by a thin layer of mucus. (3) The pulmonary region of the lung, which consists of alveolar ducts and sacs, is the region in which gas exchange takes place. The respiratory system has over 40 specialized cell types concerned with its many specialized functions including gas exchange, phagocytosis, detoxication, ciliary action, mucous secretion and surfactant secretion. *See also* ALVEOLUS.

respiratory tract. *See* RESPIRATORY SYSTEM.

restriction endonucleases. Some commonly used restriction endonucleases, with the organism from which they are recovered and the sequence that they recognize and cleave are shown in Table 7 (N = any base).

restriction mapping. Technique of ordering type II restriction endonuclease cleavage sites on a DNA fragment. Restriction maps are usually constructed by complete digestion of a target molecule with a number of different restriction endonucleases. Sequential complete digests allow the relative position of different restriction sites to be determined. Restriction fragments produced in such analyses are then sized by electrophoresis using agarose gel. In this system the mobility of DNA fragments within defined size ranges is

Table 7   Restriction endonucleases used in molecular biology

Microorganism	Name of enzyme	Sequence
Arthrobacter luteus	Alu I	AG↓CT
Bacillus amyloliquefaciens	Bam HI	G↓GATCC
B. centrosporus	Bcn I	CC↓GGG
B. subtilis	Bsu RI	GG↓CC
Caryophanon latum	Cla I	AT↓CGAT
Desulphovibrio desulphuricans	Dde I	C↓TNAG
Diplococcus pneumoniae	Dpn I	GA↓TC
Enterobacter cloacae	Eca I	G↓GTNACC
Escherichia coli	Eco RV	GATAT↓C
E. coli	Eco RI	G↓AATTC
E. coli	Eco RII	↓CC(A/T)GG
Fasubacterium nucleatum	Fnu Di	GG↓CC
Haemophilus haemolyticus	Hha I	GCG↓C
H. influenzae	Hin d III	A↓AGCTT
H. influenzae	Hinf I	G↓ANTC
H. parainfluenzae	Hpa I	GTT↓AAC
H. parainfluenzae	Hpa II	C↓CGG
Klebsiella pneumoniae	Kpn I	GGTAC↓C
Moraxella bovis	Mbo I	↓GATC
Nocardia aerocolonigenes	Nae I	GCC↓GGC
N. rubra	Nru I	TCG↓CGA
Proteus vulgaris	Pvu I	CGAT↓CG
Providencia stuartii	Pst I	CTGCA↓G
Serratia marcescens	Sma I	CCC↓GGG
Staphylococcus aureus	Sau 3A	↓GATC
Streptomyces achromogenes	Sac I	GAGCT↓C
Strept. albus	Sal I	G↓TCGAC
Strept. aureofaciens	Sau I	CC↓TNAGG
Strept. lavendulae	Sla I	C↓TCGAG
Strept. tubercidicus	Stu I	AGG↓CCT
Thermus aquaticus	Taq I	T↓CGA
Xanthomonas badrii	Xba I	T↓CTAGA
X. holcicola	Xho I	C↓CTGAG
X. malvacearum	Xma III	C↓GGCCG

proportioned to the $\log_{10} M_r$. The use of DNA standards of known molecular weight allows the construction of calibration curves from which the size of unknown restriction fragments can be determined. The diagram shows how a simple restriction map may be constructed. *See also* RESTRICTION ENDONUCLEASES.

restrictive lung disease. Lung disease in which the expansion of the lung is restricted because of changes in the supportive structures of the lung, disease of the pleura or of the chest wall, or of the neuromuscular system associated with the breathing cycle.

retardation. *See* MENTAL RETARDATION.

retention. *See* DEPOSITION.

reticulocytes. Immature erythrocytes that still possess an endoplasmic reticulum. The maturation of an erythrocyte is as follows: bone marrow erythroblast (derived from the pluripotent stem cell) to marrow reticulocyte to circulating reticulocyte to circulating erythrocyte. *See also* STEM CELLS.

retinopathy. Any non-inflammatory disease of or damage to the retina. Retinopathies can be produced by a number of compounds that are retinotoxic, including the anti-inflammatory drugs, chloroquine and indomethacin, as well as certain phenothiazines. High concentrations of oxygen (hyperoxia) can also be retinotoxic as evidenced by the development of retrolental fibroplasia in preterm infants in hyperoxic incubators. Retinopathies are also a common secondary complication of diabetes mellitus. Experimental retinopathies have been induced in animals using iodoacetate, diabetogenic agents and diaminodiphenoxyalkanes. *See also* CHLOROQUINE; DIABETES MELLITUS.

retiolental fibroplasia. *See* OXYGEN TOXICITY.

retrospective epidemiological studies. *See* EPIDEMIOLOGICAL STUDIES, RETROSPECTIVE.

retroviruses (leucoviruses). Group of single-stranded RNA viruses that are characterized by their possessing reverse transcriptase, which transcribes the RNA genome into DNA during the replicative cycle. The transcribed viral DNA is then integrated into the host cell DNA and is replicated with it. The genomes of most retroviruses consist of a set of four genes: *gag*, which codes for the capsid protein of the virus; *pol*, which codes for the reverse transcriptase; *env*, which codes for a protein forming spikes on the outer envelope; *onc*, which is an oncogene. Many retroviruses are oncogenic, owing this property to the possession of oncogenes. Closely related sequences that are present in cellular genomes and code for normal proteins are termed proto-oncogenes. The termini of the retroviral genome consists of repeat sequences, which facilitate the integration of the retroviral DNA into the genome of the host cell. Retroviruses include Rous' sarcoma virus, mouse leukemia viruses such as malony leukemia virus, mouse mammary tumor viruses such as Bittner mouse milk factor virus, feline leukemia viruses, and the human HTLV viruses including the AIDS virus. Retroviruses have, in the past, been known as leucoviruses or oncornaviruses.

reversed phase chromatography. *See* CHROMATOGRAPHY, REVERSED-PHASE.

reversed phase liquid chromatography. *See* CHROMATOGRAPHY, REVERSED-PHASE HIGH-PERFORMANCE LIQUID.

reverse mutation. A mutation that changes a mutant gene, causing it to revert to the original wild-type gene. *See also* AMES TEST; MUTATION.

reverse transcriptase (RNA-dependent DNA polymerase). Enzyme possessed by retroviruses that allows transcription of DNA from an RNA template. Such an enzyme has never been isolated from other sources, but speculation about its possible occurrence continues. Such an enzyme is widely used experimentally in genetic engineering to allow the formation of complementary DNA (cDNA) from purified RNA. The discovery of this enzyme faulted the widely held central dogma, which stated that the information flow in nature was always from DNA to RNA.

reversible effect. An effect which is not permanent. In toxicology it is usually used for adverse effects that diminish once exposure to a toxicant is ended. *See also* IRREVERSIBLE EFFECT.

reversible inhibition. *See* XENOBIOTIC METABOLISM, REVERSIBLE INHIBITION.

RfC. *See* INHALATION REFERENCE CONCENTRATION.

RfD. *See* REFERENCE DOSE.

rhinitis. Inflammation or irrition of the nasal mucosa resulting in nasal dysfunction: stuffy nose, excess nasal discharge, nasal pain, and nasal itching. May be caused by sensory irritants, allergic responses or infectious disease.

rhododendron. An ornamental plant belonging to the family Ericaceae and to the same genus (*Rhododendron*) as azalea, a genus containing several hundred species. The toxins are a complex mixture, mainly of diterpenic polyalcohols, that has not been fully characterized, but includes grayanotoxins and andromedotoxin (potent hypotensive agents).

rhodotoxin. *See* GRAYANOTOXIN.

Rhothane. *See* DDD.

rhubarb (*Rheum rhabarbarum*). A vegetable, the stems of which are used for pies, jams, etc. The leaf is toxic, containing a high level of soluble oxalates.

RIA. *See* RADIOIMMUNOASSAY.

ribonucleic acid. *See* RNA.

ricin. A toxic lectin and hemagglutinin from the castor plant, *Ricinus communis*; now known to be a mixture of several different proteins of which two agglutinins and two toxins have been isolated. Ricin is extremely toxic, the i.p. LD50 in mice is approximately 1.0 μg ricin N/kg body weight. At lower doses it has antitumor activity. Although the seeds (castor beans) of *Ricinus communis* are toxic,

the toxicity is not due entirely to ricin. Other toxic products are present, and ricin, in any case, would be expected to be hydrolyzed by proteolytic enzymes. *See also* CASTOR BEAN; LECTINS; RICININE; RICINOLEIC ACID.

ricinine (**1,2-dihydro-4-methoxy-1-methyl-2-oxo-3-pyridinecarbonitrile**). **CAS number 524-40-3**. A toxic compound produced by the castor plant *Ricinus communis*. It causes nausea, vomiting, gastroenteritis, liver and kidney damage and, in severe cases, convulsions, coma, hypotension, respiratory depression and death. No specific therapy is available.

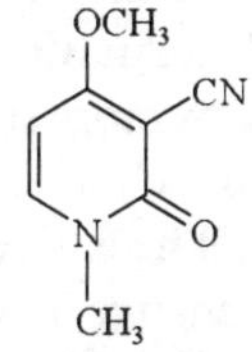

Ricinine

ricinoleic acid (**[R-(Z)]-12-hydroxy-9-octadecanoic acid**). **CAS number 141-22-0**. A fatty acid that comprises most of the fatty acid components of the triglyceride fraction of castor oil, the cathartic oil obtained from the seeds of the castor plant *Ricinus communis*.

$$CH_3(CH_2)_5\overset{\overset{\displaystyle OH}{|}}{C}HCH_2CH=CH(CH_2)_7\overset{\overset{\displaystyle O}{\|}}{C}OH$$

Ricinoleic acid

RID (radial immunodiffusion). *See* IMMUNOASSAY.

risk. The probability of harm.

risk, toxicological. The probability that some adverse effect (e.g., cancer) will result from a given exposure to a chemical; it is the estimated frequency of occurrence of an event in a population. Risk may be expressed in absolute terms (e.g., one in one million or 10^{-6}) or in terms of relative risk (the ratio of the risk in an exposed population to that in an equivalent unexposed population). *See also* RISK ASSESSMENT.

risk analysis. *See* RISK ASSESSMENT.

risk assessment (risk analysis). The process by which the potential adverse health effects (usually carcinogenicity) of human exposure to chemicals are characterized; it includes the development of both qualitative and quantitative expressions of risk. The process of risk assessment may be divided into four major components: (1) hazard identification; (2) dose–response assessment (high-dose to low-dose extrapolation); (3) exposure assessment; (4) risk characterization. *See also* DOSE–RESPONSE ASSESSMENT; EXPOSURE ASSESSMENT; HAZARD IDENTIFICATION; RISK CHARACTERIZATION.

risk assessment, environmental (ecological). The process that evaluates the probability that adverse ecological effects may occur (or are occurring) as a result of one or more stressors. The stressors may be one or more chemicals and/or physical or biological changes. The endpoints are also multiple and include any change in a valued characteristic of the ecosystem in question. Although the current methodology is derived from human health risk assessment, the multiple, interacting stressors and complex endpoints make precision a problem. A great deal of effort is currently being expended to develop risk assessment analysis methods that are more specific for effects on ecosystems.

risk characterization. The final step in the risk assessment process; it utilizes the exposure and dose–response assessments to estimate the probable incidence of adverse health effects under various conditions of human exposure. *See also* RISK ASSESSMENT.

risk factor. Any characteristic such as race, gender, age, body type (e.g., obesity or malnourishment) or life style (e.g., smoking, use of drugs of abuse or occupational exposure) that is associated with increased risk of adverse effect.

risk management. The process of evaluating alternative regulatory options and selecting between them. Risk management is not a scientific process, but involves consideration of the social, economic and political implications of a series of possible regulatory options. Risk assessment is one of the bases of risk management. *See also* RISK ASSESSMENT.

risk specific dose. The dose corresponding to a specific level of risk.

RNA (ribonucleic acid). Group of polynucleotides consisting of the sugar ribose associated with purine and pyrimidine bases (uracil rather than thymine, as found in DNA). Most RNA molecules are single-stranded, although they may form double-stranded, hydrogen-bonded duplexes. They can also hybridize with complementary strands of DNA. RNA exists in cells in a number of discrete categories, such as hnRNA (heterogeneous nuclear RNA), snRNA (small nuclear RNA), rRNA (ribosomal RNA), tRNA (transfer RNA) and mRNA (messenger RNA). RNA also constitutes the sole genetic material of many groups of viruses (e.g., retroviruses).

RNA polymerase (DNA-dependent RNA polymerases, transcriptases). Group of enzymes for catalyzing the synthesis of RNA from a DNA template (sense strand). Bacteria possess only a single type of RNA polymerases, but eukaryotic cells possess at least four. They are designated: type I (pol I), which is responsible for synthesis of ribosomal RNA (except 5S RNA); type II (pol II), which is responsible for synthesis of messenger RNA (and its precursor, heterogenous nuclear RNA); type III (pol III), which is responsible for synthesis of transfer RNA and the small ribosomal 5 SRNA; type IV, which is the RNA polymerase of the mitochondria. RNA polymerases are sensitive to various antibiotics: for example, pol II is sensitive to α-amanitin and pol I to actinomycin D. Since a single species of RNA polymerase is responsible for synthesis of all messenger RNA, the specificity of gene expression is clearly not determined by the polymerase enzyme, but since the promoter sequence (see promoter) upstream of the initiation site of the coding sequence is recognized by the enzyme, differences in the sequence of the promoter between different genes will affect transcription rates. RNA polymerases are complex proteins. The bacterial enzyme consists of a core enzyme comprising *a-*, *b-* and *b'-*subunits, and a sigma factor, which recognizes the pribnow box. *See also* DNA POLYMERASE; REVERSE TRANSCRIPTASE.

RNA-RNA viruses. *See* VIRUSES.

rodenticides. Chemicals used for the control of rodents, particularly rats and mice. They include anticoagulants such as warfarin, alkaloids such as strychnine sulfate, glycosides such as Scillaren A and B, fluorides such as sodium fluoroacetate, inorganics such as thallium sulfate and thioureas such as α-naphthylthiourea (ANTU). The main toxicological problems associated with rodenticides are due to accidental or suicidal ingestion of the compounds. Fluoroacetate (compound 1081) and fluoroacetamide (compound 1080) are highly toxic, affecting the tricarboxylic acid cycle. Warfarin is an anticoagulant and red squill a cardiac poison, whereas ANTU causes massive pulmonary edema and strychnine is a neurotoxicant. *See also* FLUORACETATE, FLUOROACETAMIDE.

rosary pea. *See* ABRIN.

rotenone. CAS number 83-79-4. The most active of several rotenoids produced by certain legumes, especially *Derris* and *Lonchocarpus* species. Although once widely used as an insecticide, rotenone is now used primarily as a fish poison. The mode of action of rotenone is inhibition of the mitochondrial electron transport system, specifically at the NADH-coenzyme Q oxidoreductase complex. The oral LD50 in rats is 132 mg/kg.

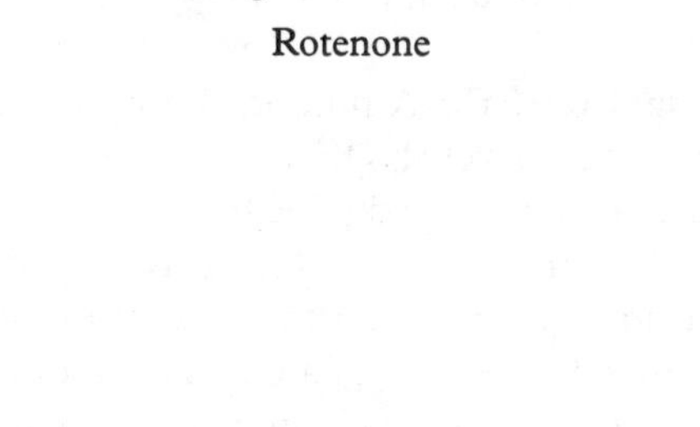

Rotenone

rough endoplasmic reticulum. *See* ENDOPLASMIC RETICULUM.

route of exposure. *See* EXPOSURE; PORTALS OF ENTRY.

Royal College of Pathologists (RC Path). A UK professional body, which awards a Diploma in Toxicology (Dip. Tox.).

RPE. Abbreviation for respiratory protective equipment.

Rubomycin. *See* DAUNORUBICIN.

run-off, environmental. Run-off from rains dissolves or suspends some pollutants and carries these pollutants from the plants or soil into adjacent water. This is particularly significant in the case of agrochemicals which are carried from the crops and their fields into nearby drainage ditches, streams, rivers, ponds or lakes. Run-off of fertilizers can result in eutrophication. Run-off of pesticides can result in entry of toxicants into the food chain with subsequent bioaccumulation into higher trophic levels. Urban run-off can contain dissolved air pollutants, as well as other pollutants derived from industrial, transportation and residential sources, and thus may contain inorganic nutrients (which can result in eutrophication), heavy metals, carcinogens and other organic compounds. Acid mine drainage from coal mining decreases pH and may leach heavy metals from the land. Run-off may also contain dissolved dust or suspended sediments which greatly affect the clarity of the water.

ryanodine. (3-(1H-pyrrole-2-carboxylate)). **CAS number 15662-33-6**. Insecticidal compound isolated from *Ryania speciosa*. Calcium channel blocker.

S

S-9 fraction. A subcellular enzyme preparation used in *in vitro* toxicity testing for the purpose of determining whether the test chemical requires metabolic activation to exert its mutagenic effect. First developed for the Ames test, it is usually the supernatant fraction prepared by centrifugation of a rat liver homogenate at about 9000 g for 10–20 minutes. It consists primarily of the cytosolic fraction, containing the cytosolic enzymes, and the microsomal fraction, containing the enzymes of the cytochrome P450-dependent monooxygenase system, epoxide hydrolase, etc. For routine testing, the rats are usually treated with Aroclor 1254, a mixture of polychlorinated biphenyls, in order to induce cytochrome P450 isozymes. In experimental studies, S-9 fractions from both induced and uninduced rats have been used, as well as S-9 fractions from other organs and species. *See also* AMES TEST; CYTOCHROME P450; *IN VITRO* TOXICITY TESTS; MICROSOMES.

saccharin (1,2-benzisothiazol-3(2H)-one-1,1-dioxide). CAS number 81-07-2. Discovered in 1879, this compound has been used by diabetics for many years and, in more recent years, as a non-nutritive sweetener in a variety of soft drinks and diet foods. It is listed by the EPA as a carcinogen, although the studies involved have been controversial, as have attempts to regulate its use. Early studies were complicated by contaminants in the saccharin. Later a two-generation study using 5% dietary saccharin showed a small increase in bladder tumors in mice. Interpretation of these results is complicated by the fact that saccharin has been shown to be a promoter for other bladder carcinogens, such as *N*-methylnitrosourea. Thus it is not clear whether saccharin is a carcinogen and a promoter, or whether it acts indirectly via an effect on indole metabolism. Regulation of saccharin is equally controversial. Unregulated in some coun-

tries (e.g., the UK), it is banned in others, such as Canada. It was first banned in the USA by the FDA, and then a moratorium was placed on the ban by legislative action. *See also* SWEETENING AGENTS.

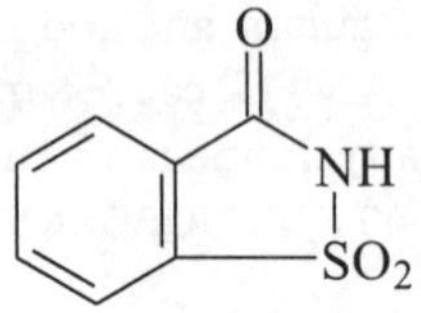

Saccharin

Saccharomyces cerevisiae. A species of yeast most frequently used in *in vitro* tests to detect the mutagenic potential of chemicals. *See also* EUKARYOTE MUTAGENICITY TESTS; YEAST MUTATION TEST.

SADR. *See* SUSPECTED ADVERSE DRUG REACTION.

Safe Drinking Water Act. A US act setting standards for drinking water to protect the public health. It authorizes research relating to causes, diagnosis, treatment, control and prevention of human diseases and other impairments resulting, directly or indirectly, from contaminants in drinking water.

safety. Freedom from risk.

safety factor (SF). A number by which the no observed effect level (NOEL) is divided to obtain the acceptable daily intake (ADI) of a chemical for regulatory purposes. The factor is intended to account for the uncertainties inherent in estimating the potential effects of a chemical on humans from results obtained with surrogate test species. The safety factor allows for possible differences in sensitivity between the test animal species and humans, as well as for variations in the sensitivity of individuals within the human population. The size of the safety factor (e.g., 10–1000) varies depending on the confidence in the database and the nature of the adverse effect. Small safety factors indicate a high degree of confidence in the data, an extensive database and/or the availability of human data. Large safety factors are indicative of an inadequate, uncertain database and/or the severity of the unexpected toxic effect. The use of safety factors tends to be restricted to chemicals causing only non-carcinogenic effects. If a NOEL cannot be established then the ADI concept (and hence a SF) is not applicable. It is assumed that man is ten times more sensitive than the most sensitive test animal, and that within the human population there is a tenfold range in individual sensitivity. Thus a factor of SF = 100 is applied if there is adequate data, i.e., a 90-day feeding trial. If the compound has been extensively studied in man in well-controlled studies and a NOEL in man (particularly for pharmacological effects) can be established, then it may be appropriate to set SF = 10. Epidemiological data from man alone is not sufficient to set a reduced SF. If animal studies indicate teratogenic effects at doses which do not cause maternal toxicity, then SF = 1000 will usually be appropriate. If the compound is a non-genotoxic carcinogen with a threshold then a SF of up to 1000 should be set, depending on the carcinogenic mechanism involved. The "usual" values for SFs are 100, 200, 500 or 1000. *See also* ACCEPTABLE DAILY INTAKE; NO OBSERVED EFFECT LEVEL.

safrole (5-(2-propenyl-1,3-benzodioxole)). CAS number 94-59-7. A naturally occurring methylenedioxyphenyl compound found in black peppers and in oil of sassafras; safrole has been used as a flavoring and in perfumery. It has been shown to be a carcinogen in animal studies, causing liver tumors in rats at a concentration of 0.5% in the diet. The active metabolite appears to be the sulfate ester of the 1'-hydroxy derivative. As a methylenedioxyphenyl compound, it forms a type

Safrole

III spectrum with reduced cytochrome P450 and inhibits cytochrome P450-dependent monooxygenations.

Salem sarcoid. Common name for lung pathology caused by beryllium used in the defense and aerospace industries. *See also* BERYLLIOSIS.

salicylates. Useful analgesic agents (e.g., aspirin). Salicylic acid is too irritating internally to be useful, but drugs with similar effects are used. Salicylate poisoning is initially characterized by respiratory stimulation (unlike narcotic analgesics, which produce respiratory depression in large overdosage). The resulting hyperventilation produces a respiratory alkalosis through increased respiratory excretion of carbon dioxide. After this initial respiratory stimulation, exceedingly high doses of salicylates may produce a respiratory paralysis resulting in respiratory acidosis. It is difficult for the body to compensate for the respiratory acidosis that occurs in the later stages of poisoning since neutralizing bicarbonate ions were excreted in urine as the body compensated for respiratory alkalosis during the initial stages of overdosage. In the later stages of early poisoning, a metabolic acidosis is also observed. The metabolic acidosis results from a number of factors, including the formation of acid derivatives from salicylic acid and deranged carbohydrate metabolism. These changes in acid/base balance are exceedingly serious. Children can succumb in a matter of hours to the dehydration that results from changes in acid/base balance, although death usually results from respiratory failure. Treatment of salicylate poisoning is symptomatic. *See also* ANTIINFLAMMATORY AGENTS; FOOD COLORS.

salmonella poisoning. Caused by bacteria of the genus *Salmonella*. Since the bacterium is heat labile and susceptible to the acid pH of the stomach, large numbers of organisms are required to produce poisoning, although drug resistant strains are a cause for concern. Animal products such as eggs, meat and poultry are the principal sources and the principal effect is an inflammatory diarrhea caused when the organism invades the intestinal mucosa. More serious effects may occur when bacteremia occurs, especially in the immune impaired individual. Chloramphenicol is the drug of choice but should not be given in mild cases.

Salmonella typhimurium. Several strains of this bacterium with mutations in the histidine biosynthesis pathway are used in the Ames test and other prokaryote mutagenicity tests to detect chemicals with mutagenic potential. *See also* AMES TEST; BACTERIAL MUTAGENESIS; MUTATION; PROKARYOTE MUTAGENICITY TESTS.

salsolinol. *See* TETRAHYDROISOQUINOLINES.

sampling. In addition to having accurate and sensitive analytical techniques, toxicological data are dependent upon appropriate sampling to ensure that data are properly representative. This is particularly the case with environmental samples which are often observations of active events rather than the results of controlled experiments. Thus, care must be taken to assure that the sample is representative of the object of study, and special attention must be paid to sampling procedures. Sampling accomplishes a number of objectives, depending on the type of area being studied. In large environmental areas, such as wilderness regions, lakes or rivers, it can provide data on both the concentration of pollutants and the extent of pollution. In urban areas, continous sampling can provide information on the types of pollutants humans are exposed to, either by inhalation or by ingestion, as well as changes in these parameters with time. In industrial areas, hazardous conditions can be detected and sources of pollution identified. As pollution controls are implemented, sampling can provide a chronicle of the changes that occur. Sampling in industrial areas in the USA can document compliance with existing OSHA and EPA regulations. The many methods available for sampling the environment can be divided into air, soil, water and tissue sampling. Tissue sampling is also of particular interest in experimental laboratory and forensic studies. *See also* SAMPLING, AIR; SAMPLING, SOIL; SAMPLING, TISSUES; SAMPLING, WATER.

sampling, air. Most pollutants entering the atmosphere come from fuel combustion, industrial processes and solid waste disposal. Additional sources, such as atomic explosions, forest fires, solid dusts, volcanoes, natural gaseous emissions, and agricultural burning, contribute less to the level of atmospheric pollution, although locally they may be of primary importance. To affect terrestrial animals and plants, particulate pollutants must be in a size range that allows them to enter the organism. Such liquid suspensions include fogs (small particles) and mists (large particles) produced from atomization, condensation or entrainment of liquids by gases, and solids—including dusts, fumes and smokes produced by crushing, metal vaporization and combustion of organic materials, respectively. Air samplers are designed to collect the particulate matter in the size range most detrimental to humans (0.5–5 µm). An air sampler generally consists of an inlet to direct air into a collector, a filter to screen out larger particles that might interfere with an analysis, a collector where the sample is deposited, a flowmeter and valve to calibrate the air flow and a pump to pull air through the system. In recent years, samplers have been miniaturized so that they can be connected to individuals while they are working, walking or riding, allowing estimation of individual exposure. Many air samplers use various types of filters to collect solid particulate matter, such as asbestos, which is collected on glass fiber filters with pores 20 µm in diameter or less. Membrane filters with pores 0.01–10 µm in diameter are used to collect dusts and silica. Liquid-containing collectors called impingers are used to trap mineral dusts and pesticides. Mineral dusts are collected in large impingers that have flow rates of 10–50 liters of air per minute passing through them; insecticides are collected in smaller "midget" impingers that handle flows of 2–4.5 liters of air per minute. Depending upon the pollutant being sought, the entrapping liquid is distilled water, alcohol, ethylene glycol, hexylene glycol or some other solvent. Small glass tubes approximately 7 cm × 0.5 cm containing activated charcoal are used to entrap organic vapors in air. Absorbents have been developed to collect specific organic compounds, including industrial organics, pesticides and formaldehyde. Another type of sampler requires no pump; the compound to be monitored diffuses through a porous membrane and is collected on an adsorbent. Polyurethane foam (PUF) has become a popular trapping medium for pesticides because of the ease of handling and the rapid desorption of compounds from it.

sampling, forensic. *See* SAMPLING, TISSUES.

sampling, pharmacokinetics. *See* SAMPLING, TISSUES.

sampling, soil. The behavior of environmental pollutants deposited on land is complicated by interactions with organic and inorganic components, liquid-gas phases in the environment, as well as the living and non-living components of the soil. Depending upon its chemical and physical structure, the pollutant can remain in one location for long or short periods, be absorbed into plant tissue or move into the soil by diffusion. Movement is also affected by external forces, such as being dissolved or suspended in water or adsorbed onto inorganic and organic soil components. Thus, sampling for pollutants in soils can be difficult. To obtain representative samples, the chemical and physical characteristics of the sampling site(s) must be considered, as well as possible reactions of the pollutant with soil components and the degree of variability in the sampling area. Site(s) can then be divided into homogeneous areas and samples collected. The number of samples depends upon the functions of variance and the degree of accuracy required. Many types of soil samplers are available, but coring devices are preferred because they allow determination of vertical distribution of the pollutant. They can be either steel tubes, which vary from 2.5 to 7.6 cm in diameter and from 60 to 100 cm in length (for hand use) or are large mechanically operated boring tubes that have dimensions of 10 cm × 200 cm. Another type of coring equipment is a wheel to which small tubes are attached so that large numbers of small subsamples can be taken, thus allowing more uniform sampling over a site. Specialty samplers with large diameters (about 25 cm) may incorporate a blade to slice a core of soil from a particular depth.

sampling, tissues. Environmental surveys of plants and animals for pollutants are conducted in contaminated areas. Many of the surveys are conducted during hunting and fishing seasons, when tissues are removed for analysis for suspected contaminants by federal and state laboratories. Such sampling can help determine the concentration, extent of contamination within a given species and the area of contamination. Many environmental pollutants are known to concentrate in specific tissues. These organs are removed from recently killed animals for analysis; samples are either pooled with others from the same species or are assayed separately as single subsamples. When plant material is gathered for analysis, it is either divided into roots, stems, leaves, flowers and/or fruit, or the whole plant is analyzed as a single entity. Experimental studies, particularly those involving the metabolism or mode of action of toxic compounds in animals (or, less often, plants) may be conducted either *in vivo* or *in vitro*. Since individual organisms or enzyme preparations are treated with known compounds, the question of random sampling techniques does not arise as it does with environmental samples. Enough replication is needed for statistical verification of significance. In metabolic studies, the question of reactive (therefore unstable) products and intermediates is of critical concern, and the reaction must be stopped and the sample processed using techniques that minimize degradation. The initial sampling step is therefore to stop the reaction, usually by a protein precipitant. Although traditional compounds such as trichloroacetic acid are effective protein precipitants, they are usually undesirable. Water-miscible organic solvents such as ethanol or acetone are milder, whereas a mixture of a miscible and an immiscible solvent (e.g., chloroform/methanol) not only denatures the protein but also effects a preliminary separation into water- and organo-soluble products. Rapid freezing is a mild method of stopping reactions, but low temperature during the subsequent handling is necessary. In toxicokinetic (pharmacokinetic) studies involving sequential sacrifice and tissue examination, it is critical to obtain uncontaminated organ samples. Apart from contamination by blood, this can be avoided by careful dissection and rinsing of the organs in ice cold buffer, saline or other appropriate solution. Blood samples are obtained by cardiac puncture, and blood contamination of organ samples is minimized by careful bleeding of the animal at sacrifice or, if necessary, by perfusion of the organ in question. Since forensic toxicology deals primarily with sudden or unexplained death, the range of potential toxicants is extremely large. However, the analyst does not usually begin examination of the samples until all preliminary studies (autopsy, pathology) are complete, thereby reducing the number of possible toxicants. Since further sampling would involve exhumation or be impossible, in the case of cremation, adequate sampling and sample preservation are essential. Body fluids must be collected in a proper way: blood by cardiac puncture, never from the body cavity; urine from the urinary bladder; bile collected intact as part of the ligated gallbladder; etc. Adequate sample size is important. Blood can be analyzed for carbon monoxide, ethanol and other alcohols, barbiturates, tranquilizers and other drugs; at least 100 ml should be collected. Urine is useful for analysis of both endogenous and exogenous chemicals, and the entire content of the bladder is retained. The liver frequently contains high levels of toxicants and/or their metabolites, and it and the kidney are the most important solid tissues for forensic analysis; 100–200 g of liver and the equivalent of one kidney are usually retained. An unusual requirement with important legal ramifications is that of possession. An unbroken chain of identifiable possession must be maintained. All transfers are marked on the samples as to time and date, and all transfers must be signed by both parties. The security of samples during time of possession must be verifiable as a matter of law.

sampling, water. The most important factors to be considered in obtaining representative samples of water are the nature of the pollutant and the point at which it enters the aquatic environment. Such pollutants may be contributed by agricultural, industrial, municipal or other sources, such as spills from wrecks or train derailments. The simplest method of collecting water is the "grab" technique, in which a container is lowered into the water, rinsed, filled and capped. A Van Dorn type sampler is frequently used to obtain water at greater depths. In the USA, continuous monitoring is required to obtain data for management decisions necessary to comply with the Clean Water Act. Continuous monitoring devices consist of a pump (floating, peristaltic, submersible or tank-mounted) to draw water into collecting

devices (generally glass or plastic bottles), metering devices to determine flow rates and a timer to implement periodic sampling. To reduce the large number and volume of samples, collectors containing membranes with small pores (about 4.5 μm) to entrap metal-containing pollutants, or ion exchange resins, resin-loaded filter paper or long-chain hydrocarbons (e.g., C18) bonded to silica to bind organic pollutants, are often used as this allows several liters of water to pass through, leaving only the entrapped pollutants. Once samples are collected, ideally they should be frozen in solid carbon dioxide (dry ice). If they are not analyzed soon after collection, they should be stored frozen at temperatures of –20 °C or lower.

Sangara. *See* ENVIRONMENTAL DISASTERS.

Santox. *See* EPN.

saprobic classification (saprobien classification). A classification of river organisms according to their tolerance of organic pollution. (a) The polysaprobic group, including sewage fungus, bloodworms and the rat-tailed maggot (*Eristalis tenax*), can live in grossly polluted water in which decomposition is primarily anaerobic. (b) The alpha-mesosaprobic group, including the waterlouse (*Asellus*), can tolerate polluted water where decomposition is partly aerobic and partly anaerobic. (c) The beta-mesosaprobic group, including Canadian pondweed (*Elodea canadensis*), some caddis-fly larvae (trichoptera), the eel (*Anguilla anguilla*) and the three-spined stickleback (*Gasterosteus aculeatus*), can tolerate mildly polluted water. (d) The oligosaprobic group, including stone-fly nymphs (*Plecoptera*) and the river trout (*Salmo trutta fario*) are restricted to non-polluted water, which may contain the mineralized products of self-purification from organic pollution. *See also* BIOTIC INDEX.

SAR. *See* QUANTITATIVE STRUCTURE-ACTIVITY RELATIONSHIP.

SARA. *See* COMPREHENSIVE ENVIRONMENTAL RESPONSE, COMPENSATION AND LIABILITY ACT.

L-sarcolysine. *See* MELPHALAN.

sarcoma. A tumor, often highly malignant, that is made up of cells similar to embryonic connective tissue. Sarcomas may be composed of closely packed cells in a fibrillar or homogeneous matrix.

sarcoplasmic reticulum. The modified endoplasmic reticulum in muscle fibers that functions to actively sequester calcium ions using a calcium ATPase. The extensive membrane system of the sarcoplasmic reticulum overlies the sarcomeres and lies in close proximity to the transverse (T) tubules system; an action potential in the T tubules increases the permeability of the sarcoplasmic reticulum to calcium. Calcium diffuses into the sarcomeres and triggers excitation-contraction (e-c) coupling by binding to its receptor troponin C. At the end of the action potential, calcium is removed from the sarcoplasm by the calcium ATPase of the sarcoplasmic reticulum to reverse e-c coupling. Ryanodine, one of the components of the natural insecticide Ryania, interferes with e-c coupling.

sarin (GB; isopropyl methylphosphono-fluoride). CAS number 107-44-8. One of a family of volatile, liquid, anticholinesterase nerve agents that reacts irreversibly with the enzyme cholinesterase, thereby permitting a deleterious accumulation of acetylcholine at nerve endings, which can lead to rapid death. Sarin is a neurotoxicant and causes running nose, maximal miosis, eye pain, twitching eyelids, difficulty in accomodation, chest tightness, salivation, coughing and sneezing, nausea, heartburn, fatigue, muscle fasciculation, insomnia, diarrhea, frequent urination, dyspnea, ataxia, slow reaction, convulsions and, ultimately, coma, respiratory paralysis and death. The LD50s are as follows: man, 14 µg/kg, i.v.; monkey, 20 µg/kg, i.v.; rat, 45 µg/kg, i.v. and 112 µg/kg, i.m.; rabbit, 14 µg/kg, i.v. and 60 µg/kg, i.m. It acts as an irreversible inhibitor of acetylcholinesterase. Therapy includes general supportive measures, and a

Sarin

respirator if necessary, along with atropine and N-methylpyridinium-2-aldoxime. The former interacts with acetylcholine muscarinic receptors, and the latter reactivates phosphorylated cholinesterase. Diazepam may be used to alleviate convulsions. *See also* ANTICHOLINESTERASE; G GAS; INHIBITION; ORGANOPHOSPHORUS INSECTICIDES.

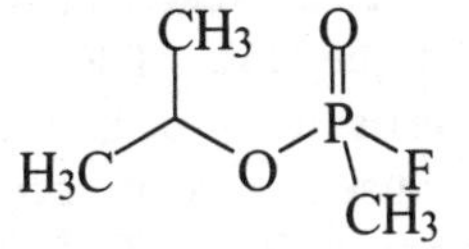

saxitoxin (STX; paralytic shellfish poison). CAS number 35554-08-6. A small, water-soluble molecule synthesized by the marine dinoflagellates *Gonyaulax catenalla* and *G. excavata*. During seasons when dinoflagellates "bloom", filter-feeding shellfish become contaminated with accumulated toxin and are toxic when eaten. STX blocks nerve membrane sodium channels in nanomolar concentrations when applied externally. STX competes with tetrodotoxin (TTX) for binding to sodium channels. The mechanism of action on nerves is the same as that of TTX, although recovery from STX block occurs slightly faster than that after TTX block. The i.p. LD50 in mice is 10 µg/kg. Symptoms in humans within 30 minutes of ingestion include tingling and burning in face, lips, tongue and eventually the whole body, parathesia followed by numbness, ataxia, general motor incoordination, confusion and headache. Death due to respiratory paralysis occurs within 12 hours. Treatment is restricted to symptoms. There is no antidote, and emesis is advisable. Artificial respiration is given if necessary. Prostigmine methylsulfate (1 ml of 1:2000 solution, i.v.) is helpful.

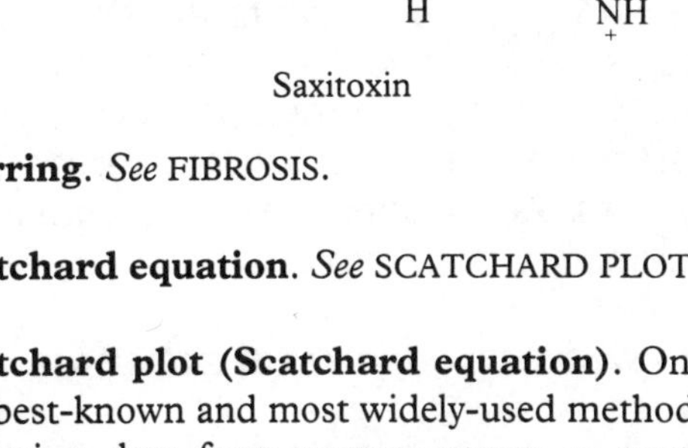

Saxitoxin

scarring. *See* FIBROSIS.

Scatchard equation. *See* SCATCHARD PLOT.

Scatchard plot (Scatchard equation). One of the best-known and most widely-used methods of analyzing data from enzyme assays or protein-ligand binding (radioreceptor) studies. The Scatchard equation is derived from Michaelis–Menten kinetics. For radioreceptor assays, the equation is of the form

$$\frac{B}{[F]} = \frac{1}{K_D} \times B + \frac{B_{max}}{K_D}$$

In this equation, B is the moles of ligand bound, [F] is the concentration of the free ligand, K_D is the dissociation constant of the toxicant and B_{max} is the number of sites exhibiting such affinity. When $B/[F]$ is plotted against B, a straight line is consistent with one population of binding sites with similar affinities. After graphical analysis (Scatchard plots), the slope is $-1/K_D$, and the intercept on the abscissa is an estimate of B_{max} (the theoretical number of binding sites). When more than one class of binding sites with different affinities exists (a situation that is probably the commonest one for toxicants), the Scatchard plot yields a curvilinear plot, from which estimates of the affinities and densities may be obtained by suitable methods (e.g., nonlinear regression), but not by direct estimations from tangents. Despite the widespread use of the Scatchard plot, its application is often flawed by improper experimental design. An alternate form of this equation, sometimes called the Woolf plot, has been demonstrated to be less subject to experimental variance. In enzyme assays, the Scatchard equation is of the form

$$\frac{v}{[S]} = \frac{1}{K_m} \times v + \frac{V_{max}}{K_m}$$

where v is the amount of product formed, [S] is the concentration of the substrate, K_m is the Michaelis constant and V_{max} is the maximal theoretical velocity of the reaction. Interpretation of Scatchard plots from enzyme data requires similar constraints. *See also* B_{MAX}; EADIE–HOFSTEE PLOT; ENZYME KINETICS; K_D; K_M; LINEWEAVER–BURK PLOT; METABOLITE INHIBITORY COMPLEXES; MICHAELIS–MENTEN EQUATION; RADIORECEPTOR ASSAYS; WOOLF PLOT; XENOBIOTIC METABOLISM, INHIBITION.

SCE. *See* SISTER CHROMATID EXCHANGE.

SCF. *See* SCIENTIFIC COMMITTEE FOR FOOD.

Scheffe's test. A procedure for conducting multiple post hoc comparison tests following a significant main effect. All possible comparisons among individual means can be evaluated while holding the experiment-wise error rate or the probability of making a type I error at alpha. Because the test is based on the F distribution, the F ratio for each comparison is tested against a critical F that is equal to the critical F for the main effect of treatment multiplied by the number of treatments minus one. A less-frequent reference to Scheffe's test may be to Scheffe's test for homogeneity of variance, a test that is fairly insensitive to violations of the assumption of normality. *See also* DUNCAN'S MULTIPLE RANGE TEST; STATISTICS, FUNCTION IN TOXICOLOGY.

Scientific Committee for Food. An EC committee. Food additives assessed as safe by the committee are given E numbers.

scombroid poisoning. A seafood poisoning named for the fish family Scombroidae, which contains some of the fish species frequently causing the toxicosis. The poisoning results most frequently from fish such as tuna, skipjacks, bonitos and mahi-mahi. The poisoning occurs about 2 to 16 hours following ingestion of fish which have typically not been kept sufficiently chilled before cooking, and is the result of the presence of histamine and other toxic factors. It is usually not fatal.

scopolamine ([7(*S*)-(1α,2β,4β,5α,7β)]-α-(hydroxymethyl)benzeneacetic acid-9-methyl-3-oxa-9-azatricyclo[3.3.1.0^{2,4}]non-7-yl ester; 6β,7β-epoxy-3β-tropanyl *S*-(−)-tropate; 6,7-epoxytropine tropate; scopine tropate; hyoscine). **CAS number 51-34-3**. A belladonna plant alkaloid that exerts its pharmacodynamic effects by blocking muscarinic acetylcholine receptor sites. The s.c. LD50 of scopolamine hydrobromide in mice is 3.8 g/kg. Scopolamine crosses the blood–brain barrier, and its antimuscarinic effects include, in therapeutic doses, drowsiness, euphoria, amnesia, fatigue, loss of REM sleep and, at higher doses, restlessness or even delirium. Scopolamine can be used to treat motion sickness and parkinsonian tremor. The effects of scopolamine may be greater in the CNS than atropine, and it may be a better antidote for organophosphate intoxication. *See also* ACETYLCHOLINE; ACETYLCHOLINE RECEPTORS, MUSCARINIC AND NICOTINIC; ATROPINE.

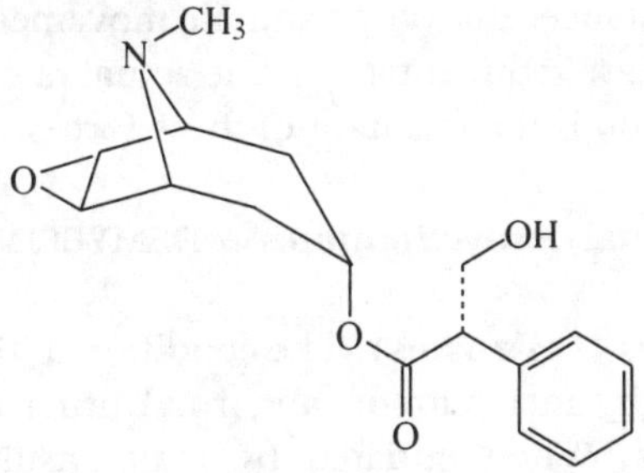

Scopolamine

scorpamine. *See* SCORPION VENOM.

scorpion. A sub-group of the Arachnida containing over 600 known species, all of which cause painful stings in humans. Fortunately, only a small number of species are dangerous. The latter includes *Centruroides sculpturatus*, found throughout the desert south-west of the USA and in northern Mexico. In adults the results of envenomation are similar in severity to a bee or wasp sting and usually resolve in about 10 hours without long-term effects. In children the effects are more extensive and may be serious, even fatal. *See also* SCORPION VENOM.

scorpion venom (scorpamine). The most toxic venoms are produced by scorpions of the family Buthidae. The neurotoxin is a small basic protein (Mr = 7000) containing hyaluronidase components. Toxicity depends on the presence of disulfide bonds and lysine residues. It potentiates the release of acetylcholine by motor neurons and postganglionic autonomic neurons. Axonal Na^+ permeability is increased. Symptoms include local inflammation and pain, restlessness, malaise, sympathetic discharge, cardiac arrhythmia and respiratory compromise. All cases of severe poisoning must be treated with antiscorpion serum as soon as possible. Small children are particularly vulnerable to scorpion stings. *See also* NEUROTRANSMITTERS.

Scottish Home and Health Department. *See* MINISTRY OF AGRICULTURE, FISHERIES AND FOOD.

scrotum. Structure in the male containing the testicles and part of the spermatic cord. Although not a common site of toxic action, it is of note in this regard since the original observations of Sir Percival Pott who, in 1775, observed the association between occupation as a chimney sweep and the occurrence of scrotal cancer.

SDS-polyacrylamide gel electrophoresis. Modification of polyacrylamide gel electrophoresis in which the solution of proteins to be analyzed is dialyzed against a solution of the detergent sodium dodecyl sulphate (SDS). The proteins bind to the SDS and all become negatively charged, having similar weight-to-charge ratios. In an electric field, electrophoretic separation will occur dependent on the proteins' size and shape. Use of differing concentrations of polyacrylamide gel permits different molecular weight ranges to be analyzed. It is usual to reduce the disulphide bonds in the protein by treatment with 2-mercaptoethanol; this results in the reduced proteins having similar shapes, so separation will be by size alone. It should be noted, however, that SDS binds less to heavily glycosylated proteins than to unglycosylated proteins of similar molecular weight. *See also* ELECTROPHORESIS.

SDWA. *See* SAFE DRINKING WATER ACT.

secobarbital (5-(1-methylbutyl)-5-(2-propenyl)-2,4,6(1*H*,3*H*,5*H*)-pyrimidinetrione monosodium salt; sodium 5-allyl-5-(1-methylbutyl)barbiturate; Seconal). CAS number 84-43-3. A barbiturate sedative-hypnotic with a long half-life, the abuse of which can lead to tolerance and dependence. The oral LD50 in rats is 125 mg/kg. *See also* BARBITURATES; PENTOBARBITAL; SEDATIVE-HYPNOTICS.

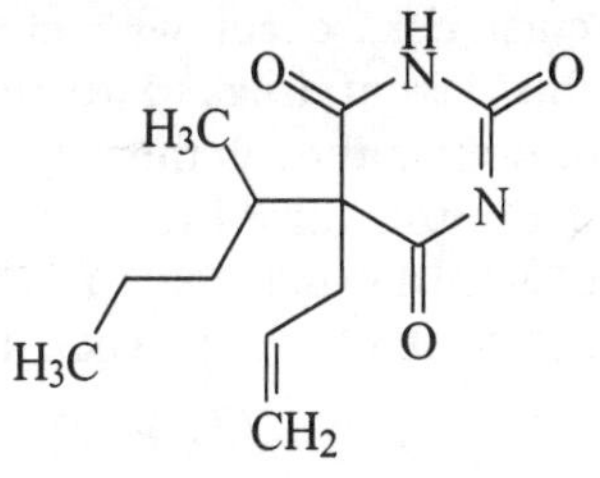

Secobarbital

secondhand smoke. Tobacco smoke, either main-stream or side-stream, produced by smokers and inhaled by non-smokers. It is becoming clear that secondhand smoke can have deleterious health effects even though they are considerably less than the effects of tobacco smoke on smokers. *See also* MAIN-STREAM SMOKE; SIDE-STREAM SMOKE.

second messengers. Compounds whose synthesis can be stimulated or inhibited by the binding of a hormone or neurotransmitter ("first messenger") to a receptor. The most well-known of the second messengers are cyclic AMP and cyclic GMP, but breakdown products of phospholipids (diacylglycerol, phosphoinositols, etc.) also fit in this category. These second messengers may affect one or many other sites, causing important cellular changes that may lead to a variety of functional alterations. Frequently, toxicants may have primary actions by directly or indirectly altering second messenger concentrations (e.g., forskolin or cholera or pertussis toxin). *See also* CYCLIC AMP; CYCLIC GMP.

Sedatine. *See* ANTIPYRINE.

sedative-hypnotics (sleeping pills). A class of drugs used to produce drowsiness and promote sleep. The classical sedative-hypnotic agents are the barbiturates; however, their use has been largely superseded by the benzodiazepines, mainly for reasons of safety. The benzodiazepines have a much higher therapeutic index because they cause little respiratory or cardiovascular depression. Several other classes of drugs with actions similar to the barbiturates are still occasionally used, including the chloral derivatives, tertiary alcohols (e.g., ethchlorvynol) and glutethimide. Sedative-hypnotics are likely to be abused by some individuals, and their prescription should be carefully monitored. Particular risks occur with chronic high-dose use of this class of drugs (particularly during abrupt withdrawal), although the benzodiazepines are much safer in this regard too. *See also* BARBITURATES; BENZODIAZEPINES; CHLORAL DERIVATIVES; GLUTETHIMIDE; MINOR TRANQUILIZERS.

sedatives. *See* SEDATIVE-HYPNOTICS.

sedimentation. Deposition of particles from the atmosphere onto solid or liquid media, deposition of particles in the small airways of the lung. In both cases gravity acts to increase sedimentation while air resistance, buoyancy and air movements tend to decrease sedimentation. The actual rate of sedimentation is the resultant of these forces.

segmental demyelination. *See* DEMYELINATION.

seizures (epilepsies). The condition in the brain caused by intermittent, abnormal firing of CNS neurons. When initiated by toxic insult, these sudden and transitory seizures are called secondary or symptomatic epilepsies. They may be generalized seizures that are bilateral in nature, the most common type of which is the grand mal. This is characterized by sudden onset (sometimes preceded by an aura) and loss of consciousness, followed by tonic-clonic contractions. At the conclusion of a grand mal seizure, the patient is usually lethargic and disoriented, and has postictal depression in which he or she may sleep for approximately 30 minutes. Petit mal (absence seizure) or partial seizures are also seen. The electroencephalograph (EEG) is a valuable diagnostic tool in epilepsy, and diagnosis can sometimes be made on the basis of EEG records during periods when symptomatic episodes are not occurring. Many agents may induce seizures. This may be through direct action on the nervous system as with picrotoxin or pentylenetetrazole or indirectly through physiological disturbances. *See also* CLONIC; TONIC.

selective serotonin re-uptake inhibitors (SSRIs). Drugs that bind to the serotonin neurotransporter and inhibit its function. The transporter normally is responsible for the active scavenging of serotonin from the synapse, and the blockade of this function increases synaptic availability of serotonin. This, in turn, initiates neuro-compensatory events that give these drugs their antidepressant properties. SSRIs have a much higher therapeutic index and are better tolerated during initial therapy than tricyclic antidepressants because they lack anticholinergic properties, and do not significantly affect catecholamine uptake as do tricyclic antidepressants. Examples include drugs such as fluoxetine (Prozac), sertaline (Zoloft) and paroxetine(Paxil). *See also* TRICYCLIC ANTIDEPRESSANTS.

selective toxicity. *See* SELECTIVITY.

selectivity (selective toxicity). A characteristic of the relationship between toxic chemicals and living organisms, whereby a particular chemical may be highly toxic to one species, but relatively innocuous to another. The search for selective toxicants is an important aspect of comparative toxicology since chemicals toxic to target species (e.g., insecticides to pest species of insects, antibiotics to disease organisms), but innocuous to non-target species (e.g., humans) are extremely valuable in agriculture and medicine. The mechanisms involved vary from differential penetration rates through different metabolic pathways to differences in receptor molecules at the site of toxic action.

selenium (Se). An element that is an essential trace metal (e.g., as a natural component of glutathione peroxidase). The requirement for selenium is of the order of 50–70 μg/day, and the LD50 ranges between 1.5–6 mg/kg, depending on compound and species. Most selenium compounds are water-soluble, and many can be biotransformed in glutathione-dependent reactions. In acute intoxication, a garlic-like odor of the breath is sometimes detected. An endemic human intoxication occurred in China during the 1960s. Loss of hair, teeth and nails were the most common signs, with lesions of the skin, mottled teeth and nervous symptoms seen less frequently. Toxicity can result from high intakes of selenium from natural sources, dietary supplements or industrial exposure. In animals, consumption of accumulator plants may cause an relatively acute condition called "blind staggers," selenium toxicity with a syndrome including impaired vision, depressed appetite and a tendency to wander in circles, followed by paralysis and death from respiratory failure. There is no conclusive evidence linking selenium to mutagenic or carcinogenic events in man. An extremely interesting observation is the fact that selenium may spare or alleviate the toxic effects of other metals, including mercury, lead, cadmium and arsenic, and that some of these other metals may also protect against selenium toxicity. *See also* ATSDR DOCUMENT, APRIL 1994.

semen. Fluid containing spermatozoa discharged through the male urethra. Semen contains the mixed products of several glands, including the prostate and bulbourethral, as well as the spermatozoa produced by the testes.

semen analysis. Although used widely for determination of infertility in men, semen analysis is not widely used in toxicity studies using experimental animals. It is clear that reproductive effects on males should often be detectable in semen and that such tests could be valuable.

seminal vesicles. A pair of sac-like structures, located behind the bladder and connected to the vasa deferentia. Although not present in all species (e.g., dog, cat), in man it produces about 60% of the seminal fluid. Its secretion is an alkaline fluid which neutralizes the acidity of the female reproductive tract to maintain the viability of the sperm.

semustine. *See* 1-(2-CHLOROETHYL)-3-CYCLOHEXYL-1-NITROSOUREA.

sensitive population. A population which might have enhanced sensitivity to the toxic effects of a chemical compared with the general population. Examples could include infants and children, or the aged, or those with respiratory system impairment. Sensitive populations may result from the occurence of polymorphisms in the genes encoding the enzymes responsible for the metabolism of xenobiotics creating subgroups of poor metabolizers and normal or high metabolizers. Such subgroups will vary in their responses to the toxic or therapeutic effects of xenobiotics metabolized by the enzyme in question. *See also* CYTOCHROME P450, POLYMORPHISMS; POLYMORPHISMS.

sensitization. An allergic reaction to a material that occurs after a previous contact. The sensitization reaction is more severe than after the initial contact, may be elicited by a lower dose and is not necessarily on the same site. *See also* DERMAL SENSITIZATION TESTS; PHOTOTOXICITY TESTS.

sensory irritants. An irritant is any non-corrosive substance that on immediate, prolonged or repeated contact with normal living tissue produces a local inflammatory reaction. Sensory irritants are a subset of irritants that affect primarily the sense organs, particularly the eyes, nose and mucus membranes. Typically they stimulate the trigeminal nerve endings.

sentinel species. A species that is extremely sensitive to the effects of a given pollutant or class of pollutants. The species can be observed as a monitor for the presence of the pollutant. When the sentinel species shows adverse effects (physiological, biochemical, behavioral, etc.), then it can be assumed that the pollutant is at a level that poses a threat to the ecosystem.

separation and identification. *See* CHROMATOGRAPHY; EXTRACTION; SOLVENT PARTITIONING; SPECTROMETRY; SPECTROSCOPY.

SER (smooth endoplasmic reticulum). *See* ENDOPLASMIC RETICULUM.

serine esterases. Esterases that include a serine residue in the active site. They are important in toxicology because the serine residue can be phosphorylated, and thereby inhibited, by organophosphorus compounds. Although the best studied example is acetylcholinesterase, other serine esterases (carboxylesterases, etc.) are known to be targets for these compounds. *See also* ACETYLCHOLINESTERASE; NERVE GASES; ORGANOPHOSPHORUS INSECTICIDES.

serine proteases. Enzymes capable of hydrolyzing proteins (having a serine residue at the active site). This serine makes them susceptible to inhibition by the same organophosphorus compounds (insecticides and nerve agents) that phosphorylate the serine at the active site of acetylcholinesterase. *See also* NERVE GASES; ORGANOPHOSPHORUS INSECTICIDES.

serotonin (5-hydroxytryptamine; 5-HT; 5-hydroxy-(2-aminoethyl)indole). **CAS number 50-67-9**. A neurotransmitter in the CNS and a regulator of smooth muscle contraction in the periphery (e.g., intestinal tract). Serotonin is biosynthesized by the hydroxylation of dietary tryptophan to form 5-hydroxytryptophan, which is subsequently decarboxylated to form serotonin. Anatomically, neurons in the brain that utilize serotonin for neurotransmission are restricted to clusters of cells in the brainstem (e.g., raphe nuclei) that send diffuse projections to the forebrain and spinal cord. The cellular action of serotonin on brain cells exhibiting electrical activity is thought to be predominantly inhibitory. Serotonin has been implicated in diverse brain functions, such as sleep–wake cycles, eating, thermoregulation and reproductive behavior, as well as in the mechanism of action of psychoactive drugs such as hallucinogens and antidepressants. *See also* 5-HYDROXYINDOLEACETIC ACID; NEUROTRANSMITTERS.

Serotonin

serotonin receptors. There are currently at least 15 different receptors for the neurotransmitter serotonin. Most of these receptors are in the G-protein coupled receptor superfamily (5-HT$_1$, 5-HT$_2$, ..., 5-HT$_7$), but one (5-HT$_3$) is an ionotropic receptor. Serotonin receptors are thought to play a major role in mediating the toxic effects of hallucinogenic drugs like LSD and mescaline. *See also* SEROTONIN; NEUROTRANSMITTERS.

Sertoli cells. Accessory (non-germinal) cells within the seminiferous tubules of the testes which envelop the developing germ cells as they undergo spermiogenesis. Since the Sertoli cells are connected by tight junctions, they are responsible for the blood–testis barrier which retards passage of chemicals from the blood into the germ cells. Sertoli cells are responsible for removing most of the spermatid cytoplasm by phagocytosis during spermiogenesis. In addition, because Sertoli cells exclusively contain FSH receptors, they mediate the effects of FSH within the seminiferous tubules. *See also* GERM CELLS.

serum alkaline phosphatase. *See* LIVER ENZYMES, IN BLOOD.

serum enzymes. *See* LIVER ENZYMES, IN BLOOD.

SETAC. *See* SOCIETY OF ENVIRONMENTAL TOXICOLOGY AND CHEMISTRY.

Seveso. A village near Milan, Italy, contaminated by an accidental discharge of dioxin (TCDD) following an explosion in 1976 at the Icmesa factory which was manufacturing the herbicide 2,4,5-T. The population of Seveso (700 people) was evacuated, more than 600 domestic animals were destroyed, and contaminated vegetation burned within an 8-kilometer radius. People heavily exposed to the dioxin suffered from chloracne, but there were no deaths and no evidence of lasting damage to health. *See also* ENVIRONMENTAL DISASTERS; SEVESO DIRECTIVE.

Seveso Directive. Following the Seveso TCDD incident, an EEC directive, agreed to by environment ministers of the member states in December 1981, was issued. It obliges industries to notify the authorities, their own workers and local residents of stocks they hold of dangerous chemicals and restricts the quantities of specified substances that may be stored within 500 meters of one another. *See also* SEVESO.

Sevin. *See* CARBARYL.

sewage treatment. In most communities the domestic sewage from individual residences is carried to a central treatment facility via a sewage system. At the sewage treatment facility, the sewage undergoes primary treatment, secondary treatment and, in a few cases, tertiary treatment. In primary treatment, the sewage passes through a bar screen (to remove large objects which may damage pumps), grit chamber (to remove heavy objects, e.g., rocks, glass), flotation basin (where oil, grease and floating objects are removed) and a primary sedimentation basin (where suspended solids settle out). In secondary treatment, the dissolved organic matter and remaining suspended solids are removed (by a trickling filter system or an activated sludge system), and potential pathogenic microorganisms are killed by chlorination. Tertiary treatment is designed to remove inorganic phosphorus and nitrogen in order to prevent eutrophication in a receiving water system. In some rural communities, sewage treatment may be accomplished in an oxidation pond. In areas where no sewage collection system is present, a septic tank coupled with a filter bed is used to treat the sewage.

sex-linked recessive mutation test. A test for mutagenicity that utilizes *Drosophila melanogaster* (the fruit fly) males with a marker (yellow body) on the X chromosome. The males are treated with the test compound and are mated with females at selected times after treatment (so that effects on spermatozoa, spermatids or spermatocytes can be distinguished). The F1 progeny are mated in brother–sister matings, and the F2 males are observed for the presence of the marker; if no yellow bodies are present, then a lethal mutation on the X chromosome from the original treated male is indicated. *See also* EUKARYOTE MUTAGENICITY TESTS.

sex ratio. The ratio of one sex to another in any group of animals; usually used with regard to progeny of a particular mating. In reproductive toxicity testing, it is determined at several preselected intervals post partum (e.g., 0, 4, 7, 14 and 21 days postpartum) to determine whether or not any mortality observed as a result of treatment with the test chemical is sex-specific. *See also* FERTILITY INDEX; GROWTH INDEX; REPRODUCTIVE TOXICITY TESTING; VIABILITY INDEX; WEANING INDEX.

SGOT (serum glutamic-oxaloacetic transaminase). *See* LIVER ENZYMES, IN BLOOD.

SGPT (serum glutamic-pyruvic transaminase). *See* LIVER ENZYMES, IN BLOOD.

sheepshead minnow (*Cyprindon variegatus*). A standard fish species for toxicology tests. *See also* AQUATIC BIOASSAY.

shellfish poisoning. *See* CIGUATARA; DOMOIC ACID; PFIESTERIA.

shock. Primary shock is fainting or collapse with low blood pressure, usually resulting from cerebral anoxia due to injury, as a response to pain (physical or psychological) or to certain toxicants. Primary shock usually responds readily to treatment. Secondary shock results when the peripheral blood flow remains inadequate to return sufficient blood to the heart for normal oxygen transport to the tissues. It may progress to coma and may be fatal. Shock may be a symptom of poisoning due to a wide variety of toxicants. *See also* DIAGNOSTIC FEATURES; MAINTENANCE THERAPY.

short-term exposure limit (STEL). *See* THRESHOLD LIMIT VALUE, SHORT-TERM EXPOSURE LIMIT.

sick building syndrome. *See* INDOOR AIR POLLUTION.

side-stream smoke. Tobacco smoke produced by cigarettes other than that smoked by the user, e.g., from the burning tip of the cigarette. Side-stream smoke is a contributor to secondhand smoke. *See* MAIN-STREAM SMOKE; SECOND-HAND SMOKE.

Silent Spring. Published by biologist Rachel Carson in 1962, this book was one of the first works to raise environmental awareness. Its main theme was the effects heavy pesticide usage may have had on natural animal populations. The book was a major influence in initiating the American environmental movement.

silica (silicon dioxide, SiO₂). CAS number 14808-60-7. Common in nature as sand, quartz, agate, etc. It is highly insoluble in water and organic solvents, and is used in the manufacture of glass, ceramics and abrasives. Inhalation of the dust for extended periods can give rise to a fibrous condition of the lungs known as silicosis, and is an occupational hazard in some mining activities, including stone cutting. Silica also causes perturbations in the immune system which may lead to schleroderma, an autoimmune disease, and is a suspected human carcinogen, causing cancer of the bronchus.

silicon dioxide. *See* SILICA.

silicosis. A condition that results from the inhalation of silica. It involves first the uptake of the particles by macrophages and lysosomal incorporation, followed by rupture of the lysosomal membrane and release of lysosomal enzymes into the cytoplasm of the macrophages. Thus the macrophage is digested by its own enzymes, and after lysis the free silica is released to be ingested by fresh macrophages, and the cycle continues. It is also thought that the damaged macrophages release a chemical that initiates collagen formation in the lung tissue. *See also* SILICA.

simazine. *See* TRIAZINE HERBICIDES.

simulated ecosystem. *See* ECOLOGICAL EFFECTS, SIMULATED ECOSYSTEM.

simulated field tests. *See* ECOLOGICAL EFFECTS, SIMULATED FIELD TESTS.

single dose toxicity. A UK term synonymous with the EC's acute toxicity. *See also* ACUTE TOXICITY.

singlet oxygen. *See* ACTIVE OXYGEN.

sintomycetin. *See* CHLORAMPHENICOL.

sister chromatid exchange (SCE). An exchange of chromatin between two sister chromatids at the same locus, occurring because of a break in both of the DNA strands. This can be induced by clastogenic agents. *See also* CLASTOGEN; SISTER CHROMATID EXCHANGE TEST.

sister chromatid exchange test (SCE test). A test for chromosome aberrations that assesses the amount of sister chromatid exchange (SCE) induced by a test chemical. Cells from an animal treated *in vivo* or cultured cells, usually Chinese hamster ovary cells exposed *in vitro*, are cultured in the presence of 5-bromo-2'-deoxyuridine during two cycles of DNA replication. Following staining with a fluorescent dye, observation under ultraviolet light will reveal the extent of the SCEs. The *in vitro* test should be run with and without the S-9 fraction from rat liver and should be conducted with positive and negative controls. The SCE test is useful for detecting DNA-alkylating agents. *See also* CHROMOSOME ABERRATION TESTS; CHINESE HAMSTER OVARY CELLS; S-9 FRACTION; SISTER CHROMATID EXCHANGE.

sitosterol (24-ethylcholesterol, $C_{29}H_{50}O$). One of at least six sterols present in wheat germ oil. CAS number for α-sitosterol 474-40-8. β-sitosterol (CAS number 83-46-5) has been used as an anti-cholesteremic and for treatment of prostatic adenoma.

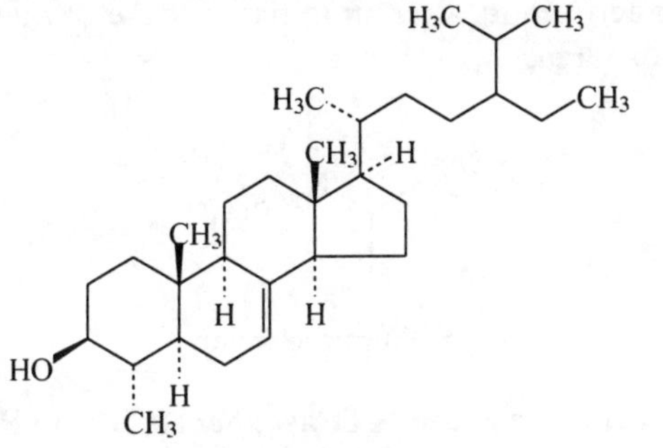

α-Sitosterol

skeletal examination. Examination for morphological skeletal abnormalities conducted to evaluate the effect of chemicals in teratogenesis tests. *See also* TERATOGENIC EFFECTS, SKELETAL ABNORMALITIES; TOXIC ENDPOINTS, TERATOLOGY.

SKF-525A. A potent inhibitor of cytochrome P450-dependent monooxygenation either *in vitro* or *in vivo*; it has been widely used in studies of the effect of monooxygenation in detoxication, activation and interactions between xenobiotics. Its effectiveness as an inhibitor is related to its ability to form a stable metabolite inhibitory complex with the reduced cytochrome. *See also* CYTOCHROME P450-DEPENDENT MONOOXYGENASE SYSTEM.

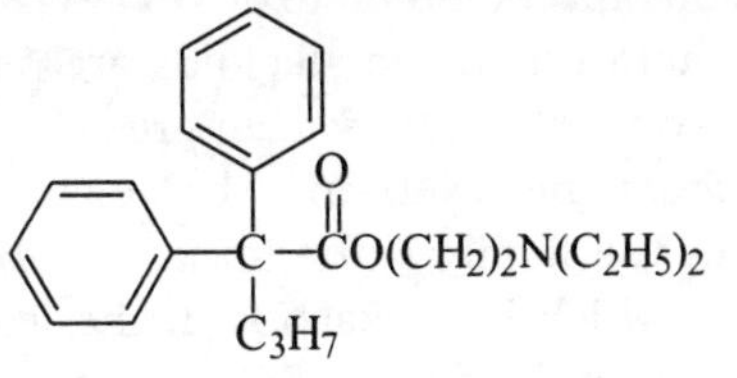

SKF-525A

skin. *See* DIAGNOSTIC FEATURES, SKIN; PENETRATION ROUTES, DERMAL.

skin painting. *See* ADMINISTRATION OF TOXICANTS, DERMAL.

skin sensitization test. *See* DERMAL SENSITIZATION TEST.

skin testing. *See* DERMAL TOXICITY TESTS.

skin toxicity tests. *See* DERMAL TOXICITY TESTS.

sleeping pills. *See* SEDATIVE-HYPNOTICS.

sleeping time. A test of the ability of one xenobiotic to affect the metabolism of another. It is usually carried out using mice and the drug hexobarbital. Hexobarbital-induced sleep is highly dependent upon the blood concentration of hexobarbital, which in turn is dependent upon the rate of metabolism by monooxygenase enzymes. Thus, inhibitors of cytochrome P450 prolong hexobarbital-induced sleep, whereas it is shortened by inducers of this enzyme. *Compare* PARALYSIS TIME.

slow acetylators. *See* FAST AND SLOW ACETYLATORS.

small intestine. *See* INTESTINE.

smog. Originally coined to refer to the mixture of smoke and fog that was formerly characteristic of severe air pollution episodes in cities such as London. The term is now used more commonly to refer to irritating photochemical (oxidizing) air pollution caused by the effects of bright sunlight on automobile exhaust gases which periodically affects cities such as Los Angeles and Denver. *See also* AIR POLLUTION.

smoke. Small particulate matter contributing to air pollution, with particle diameter in the range of 0.05–1.0 μm. The particles result from the incomplete combustion of fossil fuels or other organic material.

smooth endoplasmic reticulum. *See* ENDOPLASMIC RETICULUM.

snake venoms. Many types of snakes, as well as other reptiles, have highly developed secretory glands which can produce poisons (venoms) that may be delivered to a victim during biting.

Generally, this mechanism is important in the ability of the snake to procure food. Venoms often contain several active components that may work syner- gistically to intoxicate the target animal. A detailed study of the individual components therefore may not provide full understanding of the actions of the intact venom. Snake venoms are often classified according to the primary toxic effect (e.g., neurotoxin, cardiotoxin, hemotoxin, myotoxin), but the toxic effects of the venom may involve multiple tissues. *See also* α-BUNGAR-OTOXIN; β-BUNGAROTOXIN; COBRA VENOM; MOMBA TOXINS, RATTLESNAKE VENOM.

snorting. Colloquial term for insufflation. Particularly applied to the abuse of cocaine.

Society for Environmental Toxicology and Chemistry (SETAC). A scientific society promoting investigations in toxicology and analytical chemistry as they relate to the environment. The Executive Office is in Pensacola, Florida.

Society of Toxicology (SOT). Principal US professional society for the advancement of all aspects of the science of toxicology. Holds annual meetings and publishes important toxicology journals, including *Toxicology and Applied Toxicology* and *Fundamental and Applied Toxicology*. SOT also has regional and specialty sections. Headquarters are located in Reston, Virginia.

SOD. *See* SUPEROXIDE DISMUTASE.

sodium channel (Na⁺ channel). A small pore in excitable membranes that opens and closes in response to membrane potential changes. The sodium channel is selectively permeable to sodium ions thereby allowing the ions to enter the cell to generate an action potential. The sodium channels are widely distributed in nerves and muscles with a density ranging from 25 to 500 channels per μm^2 of membrane. The sodium channel is a protein consisting of 1820 amino acid residues and exhibits four repeated homology units. It is an important site of action of various therapeutic and toxic agents, including local anesthetics, antiepileptic drugs, antiarrhythmic drugs and the pyrethroid insecticides and DDT. Tetrodotoxin and saxitoxin are highly specific and potent blockers of the

sodium channel. Hille, B. Ionic Channels of Excitable Membranes (Sinauer, Sunderland, 1984). *See also* SAXITOXIN; TETRODOTOXIN.

sodium cyanide. *See* CYANIDES.

sodium cyclamate. Non-nutritive sweetener. Evidence that cyclamate is a carcinogenic initiator is equivocal but is less so for its activity as a carcinogenic promotor. Cyclamate is a promotor for rat bladder tumors after an initiation dose of methylnitrosourea.

Sodium cyclamate

sodium/potassium ATPase. *See* NA⁺/K⁺ ATPASE.

sodium sacharride. *See* SACCHARIN.

soft-tissue examination. Examination for non-skeletal morphological abnormalities conducted to evaluate the effect of chemicals in teratogenesis tests. *See also* TERATOGENIC EFFECTS, VISCERAL ANOMALIES; TOXIC ENDPOINTS, TERATOLOGY.

soil sampling. *See* SAMPLING, SOIL.

solanum family. The plant family Solanaceae contains a number of poisonous species due to the presence in them of alkaloids such as solanine. The Irish, or common, potato (*Solanum tuberosum*) is among the solanaceous plants known to contain solanine or other toxic alkaloids. In the normal potato tuber, the alkaloids are present in non-toxic amounts; however, in green or stressed potato tubers the levels may be toxic. Another member of the family is the tomato, *Lycopersicon esculentum*, which has alkaloids in the leaves and vines but not in the fruit. Other well-known toxic plants in this family include *S. dulcamara*, the deadly nightshade, as well as a variety of other nightshade species. Sweet potato, *Ipomoea batatas*, is not a member of this family and, although it may contain a toxic furanoterpenoid, ipomearone, it is seldom associated with episodes of acute poisoning. *Nicotiana tabacum*, tobacco, as well as other *Nicotiana* species, are also members of the solanaceae. Smoking *N. tabacum* has been established as a cause of lung and other cancers and is also associated, possibly due to high content of nicotine, with cardiovascular and other health deficits. *See also* NICTONINE, TOBACCO.

solvent abuse. The inhalation of various solvents to obtain a "high" or "rush." The mechanisms responsible for this are unclear, but probably involve a combination of solvent-induced hypoxia plus neural mechanisms similar to those evoked by inhalational anesthetics. There is a high degree of toxicity (both to the nervous system and peripheral organs) from such abuse. Agents that are used include gasoline and many commercial solvents.

solvent partitioning. A technique that distributes a solute between two immiscible liquids (e.g., octanol/water). The solute will distribute between the two layers of liquids according to a partition coefficient defined for that given pair of immiscible solvents. For example if solute X had a partitioning coefficient of 1 for solvent A and solvent B then it would be equally distributed between both solvents. If X had a partitioning coefficient of 3 for the same solvents, there would be three times more X in one solvent than the other. The higher the partition coefficient the greater the fraction of solute moved per transfer. A mixture containing solutes X, Y and Z, each with a different partition coefficient, can be separated by repetitive partitions of the mixture between two immiscible solvents.

solvents. In toxicology, this term usually refers to industrial solvents. Solvents belong to many different chemical classes, and a number of these are known to cause problems of toxicity to humans. They include: aliphatic hydrocarbons (e.g., hexane); halogenated aliphatic hydrogens (e.g., methylene chloride); aliphatic alcohols (e.g., methanol); glycols and glycol ethers (e.g., propylene and propylene glycol); aromatic hydrocarbons (e.g., toluene).

soman (GD; pinacolyl methylphosphonofluoridate; 1,2,2-trimethyl propyl methylphosphonofluoridate). CAS number 96-64-0. One of a family of volatile, liquid anticholinesterase nerve agents. Soman reacts irreversibly with the enzyme cholinesterase (ChE), thereby permitting a deleterious accumulation of acetylcholine at nerve endings, which can lead to rapid death. Soman causes miosis, salivation, lachrymation, muscular twitching and fasciculations, diarrhea, frequent urination, convulsions, coma, respiratory failure and death. These autonomic, central and somatic neuromuscular systems are responsible for the lethal actions of GD. The half-time for aging of the soman-ChE complex is 2 to 5 minutes. There is little spontaneous or oxime-induced reactivation of enzyme activity after severe soman poisoning, thus the oximes are relatively ineffective against GD nerve gas. LD50 values are: rhesus monkey, 7 µg/kg, s.c.; rabbit, 16 µg/kg, s.c. and 9 µg/ kg, i.v.; rat, 110 µg/kg, s.c. and 50 µg/kg, i.v.; dog 50 µg/kg, i.v. Therapy includes general supportive measures, a respirator if necessary and atropine, oxime (HI-6) and the anticonvulsant diazepam. The atropine blocks excessive stimulation of acetylcholine muscarinic receptors, the oxime reactivates phosphorylated cholinesterase, and diazepam is used for its anticonvulsant activity. *See also* ANTICHOLINESTERASES; G GAS; ORGANOPHOSPHORUS INSECTICIDES.

Soman

somatic mutation. A mutation in a cell other than one in the germ line (i.e., in any cell other than those that give rise to cells that carry the genetic information to the next generation). Mutations in somatic cells are important in toxicology since there is considerable evidence that somatic mutation is the first step in the cell transformation leading to cancer. The correlation between mutagenic and carcinogenic potential arises from this mechanism. *See also* CARCINOGENESIS; MUTATION.

somatotropin. *See* GROWTH HORMONE.

sorbitol. *See* SWEETENING AGENTS.

sorbitol dehydrogenase. *See* LIVER ENZYMES, IN BLOOD.

SOT. *See* SOCIETY OF TOXICOLOGY.

Southern blotting. A transfer technique (named after the inventor E. Southern) that allows DNA fragments that have been separated on the basis of size by agarose gel electrophoresis to be immobilized by transfer to a solid support. DNA fragments within the gel are denatured at room temperature in alkali. The gel is then neutralized, and transfer of the DNA to the solid support is achieved by capillary action in sodium chloride-sodium citrate buffer. The DNA is normally fixed to the supporting matrix by baking at 80 °C. The relative positions of DNA in the gel remain unchanged by the transfer process. The presence of specific DNA bands transferred to the solid support can be detected using complementary radioactive probes. *Compare* NORTHERN BLOTTING; WESTERN BLOTTING.

special transport. *See* ENTRY MECHANISMS, SPECIAL TRANSPORT.

species differences. Differences between species are of critical importance in toxicology, particularly in toxicity testing in which experimental animals of various species are used as models for humans. Species vary from one another in their uptake, metabolism and susceptibility to toxicants. With few exceptions, the differences do not vary predictably along systematic lines, and even closely related species may vary in one aspect, but not another. As a result of this variation, no one species is an appropriate model for human toxic responses, and the best model for the particular phenomenon under study must be found by investigation. *See also* COMPARATIVE TOXICOLOGY; COMPARATIVE VARIATION IN XENOBIOTIC METABOLISM, *IN VITRO* METABOLISM; COMPARATIVE VARIATION IN XENOBIOTIC METABOLISM, *IN VIVO* METABOLISM; COMPARATIVE VARIATION IN XENOBIOTIC METABOLISM, *IN VIVO* TOXICITY; SPECIES EXTRAPOLATION.

species extrapolation. One of the major problems in risk assessment is extrapolation from one species, the experimental animal, to another, usually humans. This arises, in part, from not knowing how a particular biological function may vary with size. Many physiological functions appear to be related to some exponent of body weight, the exponent varying with the function in question. In toxicity studies, the manner in which the dose is expressed is critical, and studies have compared such expressions as mg/kg body weight/day, mg/m^2 body surface/day and mg/kg body weight/lifetime as the basis for extrapolation. Since the ultimate test of extrapolations to humans is comparison with epidemiological data, this remains a difficult question since little data are available. However, it has been claimed that mg/kg/day and mg/m^2/day provide for more accurate extrapolation between species than mg/kg/lifetime. *See also* EXTRAPOLATION; EXTRAPOLATION, TO HUMANS; LOW-DOSE EXTRAPOLATION; RISK ASSESSMENT.

specific locus test. An *in vivo* gene mutation test in mice that uses wild-type males treated with the test chemical. These males are mated to females with recessive genes for visible phenotypes. Any F1 progeny not demonstrating the wild-type phenotypic characteristics would indicate a mutated gene in a specific genetic marker. *See also* EUKARYOTE MUTAGENICITY TESTS.

spectra, optical difference. *See* OPTICAL DIFFERENCE SPECTRA.

spectral binding constant. *See* K_s.

spectrometry. The generic term referring to identification and/or quantification of compounds or elements based of how they absorb or emit energy, usually electromagnetic radiation. The energy that is measured by a spectrometer may be directly emitted by the material of interest (e.g., gamma spectrometry), may result from signals induced by irradiation (e.g., nuclear magnetic resonance spectrometry) or may simply be a measure of the absorption of irradiation (e.g., ultraviolet spectrometry). These methods can provide both structural and quantitative data about an unknown material. The methods most commonly used in toxicology include atomic absorption spectrometry, electron spin resonance, flame photometry, liquid scintillation spectrometry, mass spectrometry, nuclear magnetic resonance spectrometry and ultraviolet/visible and infrared spectrometry. *See also* SPECTROSCOPY.

spectrometry, atomic absorption (AAS). Atoms of the element being determined are irradiated with a light source emitting the spectral lines of that element. The amount of light absorbed at one of these wavelengths is proportional to the concentrations of the element in the solution used to generate the atoms. The atoms are generated from a solution of salts of the element by atomizing the solution in a flame or by heating a small quantity of the solution rapidly to high temperature. The beam of light from the source, typically a hollow cathode lamp, is directed through the flux of atoms into a monochromator and, finally, to a photomultiplier tube which measures the decrease in light intensity due to absorption by the atoms. This technique produces sensitive analyses of individual elements. Sensitivity depends upon the element employed. A major problem is non-specific absorption, but this interference is often circumvented by subtracting background using a second light source. *Compare* FLAME PHOTOMETRY.

spectrometry, electron spin resonance (ESR; electron paramagnetic resonance spectroscopy). A technique similar to nuclear magnetic resonance (NMR) except that observation is of unpaired electrons rather than nuclei. Unpaired electrons are relatively rare, but are a feature of radical species, triplet electronic states and of a few unusual molecules. The electron has a spin of $\frac{1}{2}$, and in a magnetic field has two energy levels. Transitions between these levels may be induced (e.g., radiofrequency radiation). The unpaired electron may couple with nuclei in the molecule to produce the hyperfine coupling similar to the nuclear spin-spin splitting observed in NMR. Structural information about the radical can then be deduced from these data. Compounds that do not contain an unpaired electron can be studied by a method called spin-labeling in which a stable free radical is bonded to the molecule. Detailed information about the molecular environment in the vicinity of the label can then be deduced.

spectrometry, gamma (gamma counting). The technique used to measure the decay of radioactive isotopes that emit gamma rays. In the most common equipment, the sample is placed in a counting well, which is formed from a crystal of an inorganic salt, usually sodium iodide doped with thallium. Gamma rays from nuclear disintegration produce scintillations in the crystal, and the excited electrons in the scintillation crystal can decay to a number of optical states. The resulting photons are detected by a photomultiplier tube in concordance with a pulse height analyzer. The efficiency of any such instrument (the number of counts relative to the number of decays) depends upon the geometry of the crystal, the placement of photomultiplier windows, peak spread of the resultant photons, etc. Although not as widely used in toxicology as liquid scintillation spectrometry, gamma spectrometry allows the counting of appropriate isotopes without the need for chemical treatment of the sample. *See also* SPECTROMETRY, LIQUID SCINTILLATION.

spectrometry, infrared (IR; infrared spectrophotometry). The infrared spectrum of a molecule is the result of the absorption of electromagnetic radiation of appropriate energy giving rise to stretching and bending within the molecule. In order for the molecule to absorb energy, a change in the dipole moment of that molecule must occur. Infrared spectrometers are of several types. Early instruments used prisms for dispersion of the radiation; more modern instruments have employed gratings and, most recently, interferometers for this purpose. The interferometer-based instruments scan very rapidly allowing the instrument to be coupled to a gas or liquid chromatograph with the direct observation of spectra of individual components of mixtures as they are separated by these techniques. The range of wavelengths most commonly observed are from 400 to 4000 cm^{-1} (i.e., mid-infrared). Resolution is dependent upon the phase (gas, liquid or solid) employed, but is usually about 1–4 cm^{-1}. Detection limits when signal averaging is employed are as low as a few nanograms. IR spectroscopy is most useful for the identification of compounds because the spectra are unique even for structurally similar compounds. Functional groups in organic molecules have characteristic absorption that allows their presence in the molecule to be deduced regardless of any other structural features of the compound.

spectrometry, laser. In fluorescence and Raman spectroscopy, the use of laser light, because of its greater power and coherence, can increase the resolution and sensitivity.

spectrometry, liquid scintillation (liquid scintillation counting). The most versatile and sensitive technique for the detection and measurement of radioactivity. It can be used for alpha-, beta- and gamma-emitters and electron-capturing radionuclides, and is commonly employed in toxicology for toxicokinetic studies, radioreceptor assays, radioimmunoassays, etc. Essentially, a liquid scintillator acts as an energy transducer, converting the nuclear energy into light. The resulting photons of light are detected by photomultipliers, whose output is coincidence-gated and discriminated and, after appropriate logic analysis, converted to counts. The solution used for liquid scintillation spectrometry consists of a solvent containing one or more solutes called fluors or scintillators. The process involves absorption of energy by the solvent molecules, formation of solvent excited states, energy transfer from the solvent to fluors, followed by fluorescent emission by the fluors. Despite its wide applicability and ease of use, many factors can affect this procedure, ranging from inefficiencies of energy transfer from solvent to fluors, lack of quantitative emission, spontaneous emission of light from chemical reactions, etc.; proper use of the method requires consideration of these factors.

spectrometry, mass (MS; GC/MS). A technique in which a molecule is ionized. These ions and various fragment ions of the molecule are separated according to their mass, and the abundance of each ion is determined by an ion detector. The ions are usually generated by bombarding the sample with a beam of energetic electrons in a high vacuum. Either positive or negative ions so produced are then directed into a mass separator— either a magnetic field or a set of charged rods (quadrapole). The ions of each mass-to-charge (m/e) ratio are detected and amplified by the ion detector. The scan of m/e with time is accomplished by varying the accelerating voltage or the voltage on the quadrapole rods. A few picograms of compound may be sufficient to produce a spectrum. If the molecule simply loses an electron, the resulting radical cation has m/e equal to the molecular weight of the compound. If a high-resolution spectrometer is employed, the molecular formula may be deduced. Many elements exist with more than one isotope in reasonable natural abundance. The presence of and number of atoms of these elements may be deduced from the ion clusters that are produced.

spectrometry, nuclear magnetic resonance (NMR). A technique based upon transitions of spinning nuclei in an applied magnetic field. The nuclei of each isotope with non-zero spin angular momentum are characterized by a nuclear magnetic moment $f(\mu)$. Commonly observed nuclei ^1H, ^{13}C, ^{31}P, ^{19}F and ^{15}N all have spin ½. In a magnetic field, the spins orient themselves with or against the applied field, and the incidence of radiofrequency energy causes transitions between these states. A given isotope (e.g., ^1H) has a single condition for resonance, but local electric fields in the molecule shield the nucleus from the applied field. These local electrical fields vary from one ^1H to another in the molecule, thus each different type of hydrogen atom has a unique condition for resonance. This gives rise to a spectrum of resonances for different types of hydrogens in various electronic environments (chemical shifts). Other nuclei behave similarly, but each has resonance conditions that are different from one another by many orders of magnitude more than the differences caused by local electronic fields for a given isotope. Thus, one may observe only one isotope at a time. In addition to the information about types of atoms present obtained from chemical shifts data, high-resolution spectra show fine structure due to interaction of one nucleus with other nuclei with nuclear spin in the molecule (spin-spin splitting). These data provide insights into the ways in which atoms are connected to one another in the molecule. NMR is a relatively insensitive technique; detection limits even with signal averaging are in the milligram region, ^1H being much more sensitive than most other nuclei. Fourier transform techniques with short scan times and extensive signal averaging are necessary if spectra are to be obtained on small quantities. These limitations have made it very difficult to successfully couple this instrumentation to modern chromatographic separation technologies.

spectrometry, ultraviolet/visible (UV). A technique based upon the absorption by a molecule of electromagnetic energy in the ultraviolet and visible region of the spectrum (180–800 nm). These absorptions occur by virtue of transitions of electrons from one molecular energy level to higher ones. The transitions may be from bonding or non-bonding electrons. The bands are typically broad because multiple but unresolved transitions may occur from and to a multiplicity of closely spaced vibrational energy levels. The instrumentation is usually double beam so that solvent or matrix may be spectrally substracted from sample. Some functional groups have characteristic absorptions. Conjugated systems of double bands produce shifts to longer wavelengths. Detection limits may be as low as a few micrograms. This technique is used extensively for quantitative analysis because it is sensitive and precise. A common application is for detection in high-performance liquid chromatography systems. Spectra are almost always determined in solution, and choice of solvent may be important because significant solvent shifts can be observed. Interactions between solute components in mixtures can also produce shifts in the spectra of one or both components.

spectrophotometer (spectrometer). Device for recording the frequency and intensity of absorption or emission of electromagnetic radiation. The exact nature of the instrument depends on the range of wavelengths and the form of the material to be studied (*see* Table 8). The output of a spectrophotometer is usually in the form of a graph of intensity against wavelength or frequency.

spectroscopy. A general term referring to the identification of elements on the basis of the inherent physical characteristics, such as absorption or emission of energy. *See also* SPECTROMETRY.

speed. *See* METHAMPHETAMINE.

sperm. *See* SPERMATOGENESIS.

spermatocyte. One of the intermediate cells in spermatogenesis. Spermatogonia—the stem cells—give rise to primary spermatocytes which are diploid. Primary spermatocytes undergo the first meiotic division to yield secondary spermatocytes, which undergo the second meiotic division to yield spermatids.

spermatogenesis. The process of male gametogenesis in which spermatozoa are formed from the stem cells, the spermatogonia. During this progression, meiosis occurs, giving rise to haploid germ cells. The sequence of cells is spermatogonia, mitosis to primary spermatocyte, first meiotic division to secondary spermatocyte, second meiotic division to spermatid, transformation to spermatozoa (sperm). For each primary spermatocyte undergoing division, four spermatids and therefore four spermatozoa arise. The process of spermatids becoming transformed into functional spermatozoa is called spermiogenesis and involves removal of most of the cytoplasm and acquisition of a flagellum. *See also* GERM CELLS; SPERMATOCYTE.

spermatozoa. *See* SPERMATOGENSIS.

spermatozoan (sperm). Male gamete. *See also* REPRODUCTIVE TOXICITY, MALE; SPERMATOGENESIS.

spermiogenesis. *See* SERTOLI CELLS; SPERMATOGENESIS.

spider. A large sub-group of the Arachnida with some 20,000 species in the USA alone. Only two of these are non-venomous but only some 50 species have mouthparts capable of penetrating human skin. The venomous spiders likely to represent serious problems to humans all belong to two genera, *Latrodectus* (the widow spiders) and *Loxosceles* (the brown recluse spiders).

spider, black widow. *Latrodectus mactans*, a member of a genus collectively known as the widow spiders. The venom is extremely toxic and is primarily neurotoxic, producing little local tissue reaction. Although the complex venom contains many components, including hyaluronidase, phosphodiesterase, GABA and 5-hydroxytrypamine,

Table 8   Spectrophotometer

Technique spectroscopy	Radiation	Source	Intensity control	Frequency control	Sample holder	Detector
Mössbauer	Gamma	Radioactive nuclei	Amount of source	Change source	Supported solid	Geiger counter, scintillation counter
X-ray	X	e-bombarded metal	Flux of electrons	Target metal + crystal grating	:	:
Atomic	Vacuum UV	Discharge lamp	Energy into source + slits, diaphragm	Filters + grating monochromator	Quartz cuvette	Photomultiplier, photographic plate, photocell
Fluorescence	UV	D_2-discharge lamp Tungsten lamp	:	:	:	:
Electronic	Visible	:	:	:	Glass cuvette	:
Raman		Laser	:	:	:	:
Vibration	IR	Nernst glower, glow bar	:	:	KBr disk, mull	Thermocouple, bolometer
Vibration-rotation	Far-IR	IR laser, mercury discharge	Energy into source	:	:	:
Rotation	Microwave	Klystron magnetron	:	:	Low P gas	:
Electron spin resonance	Radio	Backward wave oscillator	:	Sweep magnetic or electric field	Quartz tube	Silicon-tungsten crystal
Nuclear magnetic resonance	Radio	Radio transmitter	:	:	:	Radio receiver

the high molecular weight neurotoxin (c. 130,000 daltons) appears to be responsible for the high toxicity to mammals. *See also* BLACK WIDOW SPIDER VENOM.

spider, brown recluse. Although technically the term brown recluse applies to *Loxosceles reclusa,* this genus contains many species (13 are native to the USA). Probably the most dangerous species is *L. laeta,* a native of South America. The most serious effect of brown recluse venom is the production of necrotic lesions in the skin, lesions that may become extensive and take many months to heal. The venom is primarily cytotoxic and is very complex, including such enzymes as hyaluronidase, collagenase, esterases, proteases, phospholipase, deoxyribonuclease and ribonuclease, but the factor(s) responsible for the skin lesions is not known with certainty.

spin trapping. Method of detecting and identifying free radicals by reaction with a molecule to produce a more stable radical that may be studied by electron spin resonance spectroscopy. Nitroxides and nitrones are often used as traps. The ESR spectrum of a radical formed from a nitroxide is split into three by the nitrogen-14 nucleus and then further by protons of the trapped radical.

$$t\text{-RCNO} + (\text{R}') \rightarrow t\text{-RC(R}')\text{CNO}'$$

Nitrones trap the radical one atom further removed from the site of the unpaired electron (oxygen atom) which makes the interpretation of the resulting spectrum more difficult

$$\text{R}_2\text{C}^+\text{=N}^-+\text{N(R)O} + (\text{R}) \rightarrow \text{R}_2\text{R}'\text{CN(R)O}$$

spindle poisons. Antimitotic agents; agents, usually chemical, that disrupt the structure and/or function of the mitotic or meiotic spindle. The term was first applied to the plant alkaloid colchicine, which promotes disassembly of microtubules by binding to tubulin dimers. Many other agents (e.g., vinblastine, vincristine, non-physiological temperature, elevated pressure, nitrous oxide, taxol, nocodozole, deuterium oxide and chloral hydrate) affect the structure and/or function of the spindle.

spirits of turpentine. *See* TURPENTINE.

spironolactone. CAS number 52-01-7. Diuretic and cytochrome P450 inducer; affects thyroid function by modifying the circulating levels of thyroid hormones.

spleen. An abdominal organ largely composed of lymphoid tissue. It has two primary functions. It contains B and T lymphocytes, and therefore plays an important role in the immune response. It also removes and breaks down old, damaged or defective erythrocytes from circulation. In addition, the spleen may serve as a reservoir for erythrocytes which can be expelled into the blood stream following blood loss. *See also* B CELLS; LYMPHATIC SYSTEM; T CELLS.

spray. *See* AEROSOL.

spring water. *See* GROUND WATER.

squamous cell carcinoma. A malignant neoplasm derived from squamous epithelium.

SSRIs. *See* SELECTIVE SEROTONIN RE-UPTAKE INHIBITORS.

stachybotryotoxicosis. *See* TRICOTHECENES.

stagnant hypoxia. *See* HYPOXIA.

standardized mortality ratio. Number of deaths expressed as a percentage of the number of deaths expected in a group, drawn from the general population, with the same age and gender characteristics. Used in epidemiology as a standard to allow comparisons among groups.

Staphylococcus aureus. Probably the most important cause of bacterial food-borne illness. Vomiting, nausea, diarrhea and abdominal pain are caused by heat-stable enterotoxins, although vomiting and nausea are most common and most severe. Rarely, the condition may progress to toxic shock.

starvation. *See* NUTRITIONAL EFFECTS ON METABOLISM, STARVATION AND DEHYDRATION.

statistics. Numerical indices that are computed from a sample of observations. Such indices provide descriptive information regarding the distribution of the observations in the sample or inferences about the population from which the sample of observations was taken. Descriptive statistics include mean, median, mode, standard deviation, range, coefficient of variation and other measures of the sample distribution. Inferential statistics are used for hypothesis testing and include both parametric and non-parametric statistics such as ANOVA and Mann–Whitney *U* test. Statistics is of wide general importance in all areas of toxicology, but is particularly critical in chronic testing, epidemiology and risk assessment. *See also* BIOMATHEMATICS; STATISTICS, FUNCTION IN TOXICOLOGY.

statistics, function in toxicology. The function of statistics is primarily in parameter estimation and hypothesis testing. Parameter estimation involves obtaining a statistic (quantitative measure of some property of a sample) that is a good estimate of the population parameter. Hypothesis testing or significance testing involves determining if differences in sample statistics (e.g., means) are of sufficient magnitude to reject the null hypothesis of no difference between population parameters. This decision is based upon a comparison of the obtained value of the statistic with its critical value at the alpha level that was selected *a priori*. *See also* PROBABILITY; STUDENT'S *T* TEST.

Stauber–Heubach Test. A method of measuring the amount of dust produced from a substance under well-defined experimental conditions. An amount representative of respirable dust is collected on a filter in a Heubach dustmeter; this may be simply weighed, or if the parent substance is a compound mixture subjected to chemical analysis. A propensity to dust for materials can thus be established.

Steering Group on Food Surveillance. A UK group that has made requests to the Committee on Toxicity of Chemicals in Food, Consumer Products and the Environment to consider the levels of metals in foods and the health implications. The group has also considered the levels of polychlorinated biphenyls.

STEL. *See* THRESHOLD LIMIT VALUE, SHORT-TERM EXPOSURE LIMIT.

stem cells. Precursors of all the cells in the blood and lymphoid systems. They reside in the bone marrow in postnatal life and are self-regenerating. The stem cell differentiates, under stimuli that are not entirely understood, into percursor cells of the erythroid (red blood cells) and leukocyte (white blood cells) lineages. These precursors may then migrate to other locations (e.g., pre-T cells to the thymus) or remain in the bone marrow (e.g., bone marrow reticulocytes) to mature fully. Among the cell types that arise from the stem cell are erythrocytes, platelets, granulocytes (neutrophils—also called polymorphonuclear granulocytes, basophils and eosinophils), lymphocytes (B cells and T cells), plasma cells (B cell progeny), monocytes and macrophages (monocyte progeny). Many drugs and chemicals can damage the bone marrow stem cells and either reduce overall cellularity or affect one or more cell lineages preferentially, thus skewing production of circulating cells. Since bone marrow cells are actively dividing, the chemotherapeutic agents that affect cell division (e.g., cyclophosphamide) cause significant bone marrow hypoplasia. Benzene is also a potent bone marrow toxicant and can lead to anemia, lymphocytopenia, leukopenia, etc. Histological examination of bone marrow is a common toxicological screening procedure since effects on the stem cells and early progenitor cells are likely to have profound consequences for the immune system. If bone marrow cellularity is depressed, progenitor cell assays are often used to determine if a particular cell lineage is being preferentially affected. *See also* IMMUNOSUPPRESSION.

stepholidine. The most important of the tetrahydroprotoberberine alkaloids isolated from extracts of the Chinese herb *Stephania*. Stepholidine can affect the nervous system via actions at dopamine receptors.

Stepholidine

stercobilinogen. *See* UROBILINOGEN.

steroids. Lipids containing a perhydrocyclopentanophenanthrene ring. Two important classes of hormones are steroids: (1) the sex hormones from the gonads and the adrenal cortex; (2) the glucocorticoids and mineralocorticoids from the adrenal cortex. Other important endogenous steroids include the bile acids and vitamin D. Some exogenous steroids are carcinogenic and others have therapeutic applications. The sterols, bile acids, cardiac aglycones (*see* DIGITALIS), sex hormones, corticosteroids, toad poisons and steroid sapogenins belong to this large group of compounds. Many synthetic steroids are known; some are valuable medicinals. *See also* ADRENAL GLAND; ANDROGENS; BILE ACIDS.

sterols. Alcohols containing the C-19 ring structure, exemplified by cholesterol, that vary considerably in their peripheral structural features, stereochemistry and degree of ring saturation. They are present in all animal and plant cells (also in some bacteria), often partially esterified with higher fatty acids. *See also* CHOLESTEROL; ERGOSTEROL; LANOSTEROL; SITOSTEROL; STIGMASTEROL.

stevioside. *See* SWEETENING AGENTS.

stigmasterol (3β-hydroxy-24-ethyl-Δ^{5,22}-cholestadiene). **CAS number 83-48-7**. Plant sterol (mp 170 °C); isolated from soya bean oil.

Stigmasterol

stilbestrol. *See* DIETHYLSTILBESTROL.

stimulants. Classes of drugs with different pharmacological and toxicological properties that share the general property of increasing the state of activity of the nervous system. Each of these classes of compounds gives rise to specific toxicological concerns. Stimulants include drugs like amphetamine, cocaine or methylphenidate, which facilitate catecholamine neurotransmission, and methylxanthines (e.g., caffeine, theophylline), which work by interacting with purine receptors. Although compounds like picrotoxin or strychnine have sometimes been called stimulants or analeptics, they do not share the true stimulant properties of amphetamine or cocaine. *See also* AMPHETAMINES; ANALEPTICS; CAFFEINE; COCAINE.

stimulus-oriented behavior. *See* BEHAVIOR.

Stilphostrol. *See* DIETHYLSTILBESTROL.

Stoddard solvent. A colorless solvent mixture related to the naphthas. It is used in dry cleaning, in degreasing and as a paint thinner. It, or its components, can enter the body by inhalation, ingestion or through the skin. Local symptoms include irritation of the mucous membranes and dermatitis; systemic effects include dizziness. Although Stoddard's solvent is not considered highly toxic some of its constituents are known to be toxic. *See also* ATSDR DOCUMENT, MAY 1993; NAPHTHA.

stonefish. Scorpaenids or scorpionfish are members of the family *Scorpaenidae*, a large family of venomous fish consisting of about 30 genera and ca. 350 species, at least 80 of which have caused venomous injuries in humans. The most dangerous is a scorpionfish belonging to the genus *Synanceia* (Synanceja) and commonly called the stonefish. While scorpionfish are widely distributed, the greatest number of species, including the two stonefish species *S. horrida* (*trachnis*) and *S. verrucosa*, are indigenous to the Indian and Pacific oceans and the Red Sea. Stonefish contain a venom apparatus consisting of 13 dorsal spines and pairs of venom glands located in the spines. Local manifestations of poisoning include radiating pain, local paralysis, numbness of the skin and an area of ischemia surrounded by erythema and ecchymosis about the wound, extensive swelling, induration and edema of the limb, regional lymphadenopathy, and tissue necrosis and sloughing of the wound site. Systemic manifestations include respiratory distress, cardiac arrythmias, hypotension, generalized muscular weakness, convulsions, paralysis and death. Complications may include infection of the wound site, cutaneous granulomas and indolent ulcers and neuropathies. The stonefish venom causes a conduction block due to slow depolarization of the muscle membrane. In addition, it may contain cytolytic toxins that play a role in toxicity.

STP. *See* DOM.

strain differences. *See* COMPARATIVE VARIATION IN XENOBIOTIC METABOLISM; TESTING VARIABLES, BIOLOGICAL.

streptococcus. Food poisoning in the form of an influenza-like syndrome may be caused by *Streptococcus* species, usually from contamination of high-protein food by food handlers and/or improper refrigeration.

streptomycins. *See* ANTIBIOTICS.

streptozocin (streptozotocin; 2-deoxy-2-[[(methylnitrosoamino)carbonyl]amino]-*d*-glucopyranose). CAS number 18883-66-4. A substituted *N*-methylnitrosamine; an antibiotic that has been used as an antineoplastic and in the treatment of malignant pancreatic insulinoma. Adverse effects include nausea and vomiting, and renal (proximal tubular) and hepatic damage. Anemia, leukopenia or thrombocytopenia also occur in about 20% of patients. Streptozotocin has become the preferred diabetogenic agent, selectively destroying pancreatic beta-cells and causing chemically induced diabetes when administered to animals at approximately 50 mg/kg, i.v. Streptozotocin acts by inhibiting synthesis of DNA in mammalian cells and in microorganisms by alkylating the bases in DNA. The i.v. LD50 in rats is 138 mg/

Streptozotocin

kg, whereas in dogs it is 25–50 mg/kg. *See also* DIABETES MELLITUS; NITROSAMINES; ANTIBIOTICS.

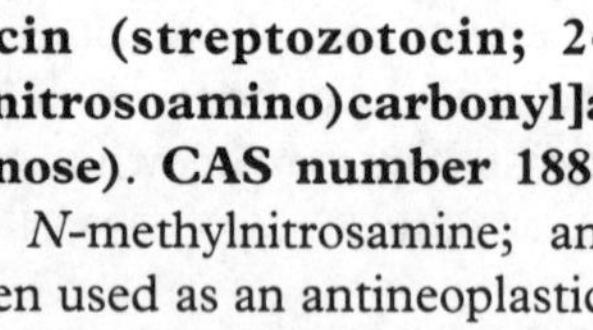

stress effects. *See* ENVIRONMENTAL EFFECTS ON XENOBIOTIC METABOLISM, ALTITUDE; ENVIRONMENTAL EFFECTS ON XENOBIOTIC METABOLISM, IONIZING RADIATION; ENVIRONMENTAL EFFECTS ON XENOBIOTIC METABOLISM, LIGHT; ENVIRONMENTAL EFFECTS ON XENOBIOTIC METABOLISM, MOISTURE; ENVIRONMENTAL EFFECTS ON XENOBIOTIC METABOLISM, NOISE; ENVIRONMENTAL EFFECTS ON XENOBIOTIC METABOLISM, TEMPERATURE.

strontium (Sr). Interest in strontium is related to concern over the presence of ^{90}Sr in fission products and the possibility of its occurrence as fall-out or in nuclear waste. Strontium is readily absorbed by calcium uptake mechanisms and is deposited largely in bone. Relatively low doses, regardless of route of uptake, cause bone cancer, although there is considerable species differences with regard to rate of occurrence. For example, occurrence of bone cancer is high in dogs and low in swine.

strophanthius. *See* OUABAIN.

structure–activity relationships. *See* QUANTITATIVE STRUCTURE–ACTIVITY RELATIONSHIPS.

structures. *See* POLLUTION, EFFECTS ON STRUCTURES.

strychnine (strychnidin-10-one). CAS number 57-24-9. The extremely poisonous principal alkaloid from the seeds of *Strychnos nux vomica*. A muscle relaxant used to kill vermin and in homeopathic medicine, which interferes with spinal cord glycine function. Strychnine poisoning results in

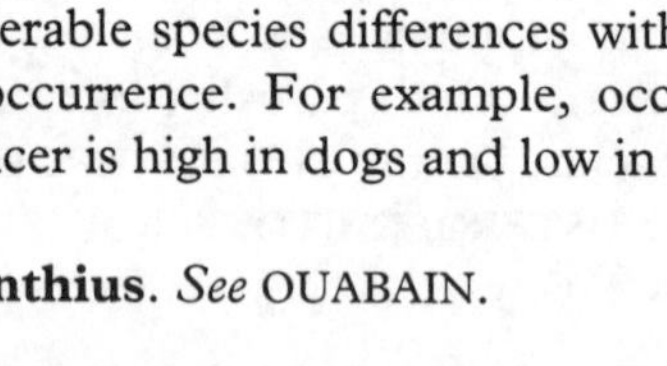

Strychnine

hypersensitivity to sensory stimuli and convulsions that impair respiration and result in respiratory and metabolic acidosis. Death may occur after as few as two to five such convulsions. Treatment of strychnine poisoning includes i.v. administration of diazepam or a short-acting barbiturate. Strychnine, although having a role in research, has no therapeutic utility as an analeptic agent or stimulant. Its primary use is as a rodenticide. Its actions occur primarily, but not exclusively, in the spinal cord. Strychnine blocks inhibition in the CNS as opposed to enhancing excitation. Its potent convulsant properties are due to the antagonism of the inhibitory effects of glycine. *See also* ANALEPTICS; STIMULANTS.

Student's *t* test. A procedure for testing hypotheses about means when the population variance is unknown. Tests of significance are based on the Student's *t* distribution. The most frequently employed *t* statistic is computed by taking the ratio of the difference between the sample means minus the difference between the hypothesized population means to the standard error of the sample mean difference. The most frequent use of the *t* test is to test hypotheses concerning the difference between two means. In the case of two sets of observations from the same set of subjects, a correlated or paired *t* test is appropriate. *See also* STATISTICS, FUNCTION IN TOXICOLOGY.

STX. *See* SAXITOXIN.

styral. *See* STYRENE.

styrene (cinnamene; cinnamol; ethenylbenzene; phenylethylene; styral; vinylbenzene). CAS number 100-42-5. An aromatic organic compound used in the manufacture of plastics, including crystalline polystyrene, rubber-modified impact polystyrene, acrylonitrile-butadiene-styrene terpolymer (ABS), styrene-acrylonitrile copolymer (SAN), styrene-butadiene rubber (SBR), resins, insulators and dyes. The TLV-TWA is 50 ppm, STEL is 100 ppm) and the LD50 in rats is 5 g/kg. Styrene causes irritation to eyes and respiratory passages. It is a CNS depressant and causes pulmonary edema, cardiac arrhythmia and renal and hepatic damage. The effect on the CNS is due to amino acid depletion by disruption

of transport (glutamic, serine, threonine) through the blood–brain barrier. In addition, styrene lowers the concentration of DNA and RNA in leukocytes and causes dysproteinemia, lipoprotein shift and GSH depletion in the liver. In humans, symptoms include cutaneous irritation, headache, fatigue, weakness, depression and peripheral neuropathy. In case of acute poisoning, the patient should be moved to fresh air and artifical respiration carried out. The eyes or skin should be flushed with water. IARC has designated styrene as a possible human carcinogen. *See also* ATSDR DOCUMENT, SEPTEMBER 1992.

Styrene

subacute exposure. *See* EXPOSURE, SUBACUTE.

subacute toxicity testing. *See* SUBCHRONIC TOXICITY TESTING.

subchronic exposure. *See* EXPOSURE, SUBCHRONIC.

subchronic toxicity. Toxicity due to exposure to quantities of a toxicant that do not cause any evident acute toxicity for a time period that is extended, but is not so long as to constitute a significant part of the lifespan of the species in question. In subchronic toxicity tests using mammals, a 30–90-day period is considered appropriate. *See also* SUBCHRONIC TOXICITY TESTING.

subchronic toxicity testing. Subchronic tests measure toxicity caused by repeated dosing over an extended period, but not one that constitutes a significant portion of the expected lifespan of the test species. A 90-day oral study in the rat or dog would be typical, as would a 30-day dermal study or a 30–90-day inhalation study. Such tests are also called subacute, a term that is inaccurate and should be avoided. Subchronic tests provide information on essentially all types of chronic toxicity other than carcinogenicity and are used to establish the dose regimens for chronic studies. They are frequently used for the determination of the no observable effect level (NOEL), a value often used in risk assessment calculations. Subchronic tests also provide information on target organs and on the potential of the test chemical to accumulate in the organism. *See also* NO OBSERVABLE EFFECT LEVEL; SUBCHRONIC TOXICITY TESTING, DERMAL; SUBCHRONIC TOXICITY TESTING, FEEDING; SUBCHRONIC TOXICITY TESTING, INHALATION; SUBCHRONIC TOXICITY TESTING, ENDPOINTS; TESTING VARIABLES, BIOLOGICAL; TESTING VARIABLES, NON-BIOLOGICAL; TOXICITY TESTING.

subchronic toxicity testing, dermal. Dermal tests are important when the expected route of human exposure is by skin contact, as with many industrial chemicals, pesticides, etc. Test compounds, either undiluted or in a suitable solvent, are usually applied weekly to shaved or clipped areas on the back of the animal. Solvent selection is difficult since many affect the skin, causing either drying or irritation, whereas others may affect the rate of penetration of the test chemical. Corn oil, ethanol or carboxymethylcellulose are preferred to dimethyl sulfoxide or acetone. Restraining collars may be used to prevent ingestion of the test chemical as a result of grooming by the animal. The criteria for environment, dose selection, species selection, etc. are not greatly different to those used for subchronic feeding tests nor are the endpoints to be evaluated. In addition, the skin at the point of application is examined since local effects may be as important as systemic ones. *See also* SUBCHRONIC TOXICITY TESTING, FEEDING; TESTING VARIABLES, BIOLOGICAL; TESTING VARIABLES, NON-BIOLOGICAL; TOXIC ENDPOINTS.

subchronic toxicity testing, endpoints. The endpoints examined in both chronic and subchronic tests are similar, covering a wide variety of physiological, clinical, biochemical and pathological parameters. *See also* TOXIC ENDPOINTS.

subchronic toxicity testing, feeding. These tests usually take the form of 90-day feeding tests in which chemicals are administered in the diet, less commonly in the drinking water, and only when necessary by gavage, since the last involves handling and stress. Numerous biological and experimental variables must be controlled; the number of possible endpoints is also large, and record-keeping and data analysis present problems. Dose selection, preparation and administration are all also important variables. Subchronic studies are usually conducted using three, less often four, dose levels. The highest level is one which produces obvious toxicity, but not high mortality, the lowest slight or no mortality, whereas the intermediate dose(s) cause effects clearly intermediate between the high and low dose. Estimation of dose from acute tests can be difficult, particularly with chemicals that accumulate in the body, and a 14-day range-finding study may be necessary. Ideally the route of administration should mimic the expected route of exposure in humans, but in practice the chemical is usually administered ad libitum in the diet. Measurement of food consumption and pair feeding with controls is recommended, except in cases in which accurate measurement of food consumption is important, in which case the animals may be fed by gavage or via capsules containing the toxicant. Subchronic studies are usually conducted with 10–20 of each sex of a rodent species at each dose level or on four to eight of each sex of a larger species (e.g., dog) at each dose level. Animals should be drawn from a larger group and randomly assigned to control or treatment groups, but the mean weights and ages of the subgroups should not vary significantly from each other at the beginning of the experiment. *See also* TESTING VARIABLES, BIOLOGICAL; TESTING VARIABLES, NON-BIOLOGICAL; TOXIC ENDPOINTS.

subchronic toxicity testing, inhalation. Inhalation studies are necessary when the expected route of exposure to humans is expected to be via the lungs. Animals are commonly exposed for 6 to 8 hours per day, 5 days per week, in chambers of the type described in elsewhere (*see* ADMINISTRATION OF TOXICANTS, INHALATION). Even though food is removed during exposure, exposure tends to be in part dermal and, due to grooming of the fur, in part oral. Environmental and biological parameters are the same as for other subchronic tests, as are the routine endpoints to be measured. Particular attention is paid to effects on the tissues of the nasal cavity and the lungs since these are the areas of maximum exposure. *See also*   SUBCHRONIC   TOXICITY   TESTING,

FEEDING; TESTING VARIABLES, BIOLOGICAL; TESTING VARIABLES, NON-BIOLOGICAL; TOXIC ENDPOINTS.

subcutaneous administration. *See* ADMINISTRATION OF TOXICANTS, INJECTION.

succinylcholine (suxamethonium). CAS numbers of bromide, chloride and iodide forms are 55-94-7, 71-27-2 and 541-19-5 respectively. A synthetic muscle relaxant with a curare-like action. Although the selectivity and superficial nature of the paralysis produced by succinylcholine mirrors that of tubocurarine, the specific action is quite different. Succinylcholine is classified as a depolarizing blocking agent, and it blocks acetylcholine receptors by persistent depolarization rather than by the competitive antagonism seen with true curarimimetics. In addition, succinylcholine is inactivated by cholinesterases, limiting the duration of its action. The i.v. LD50 in mice is 0.45 mg/kg.

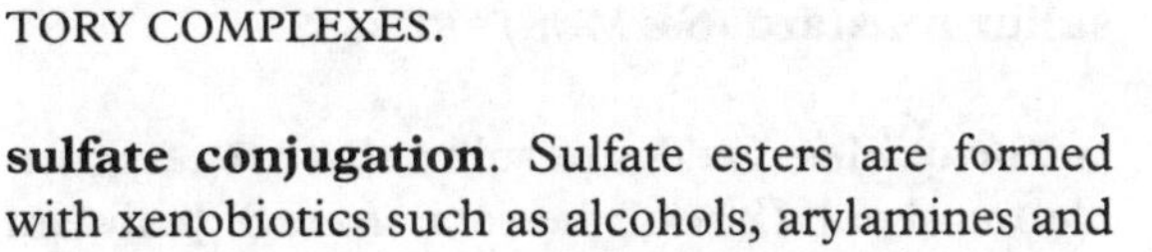

Succinylcholine bromide

suicide substrates. *See* METABOLITE INHIBITORY COMPLEXES.

sulfate conjugation. Sulfate esters are formed with xenobiotics such as alcohols, arylamines and phenols in a process requiring the prior activation of sulfate ions to 3'-phosphoadenosine-5'-phosphosulfate (PAPS). Although sulfate esters are water-soluble and easily eliminated, their formation requires the consumption of ATP. The formation of PAPS requires the sequential action of ATP sulfurylase and adenosine 5'-phosphosulfate kinase. ATP sulfurylase from rat liver is a large molecule of some 500,000 daltons. It can utilize several group VI anions other than sulfate. However, the resultant anhydrides are unstable, and thus these other anions can deplete the cell of ATP. The kinase is not well characterized from mammalian tissues, but that from yeast shows a high affinity for APS, and the reaction is essentially

irreversible. The final step is catalyzed by a group of sulfotransferases, which includes aryl sulfotransferase, hydroxysteroid sulfotransferase, estrone sulfotransferase and bile salt sulfotransferase. Four distinct aryl sulfotransferases have been separated from rat liver, each of which catalyzes the sulfation of a variety of phenols and catecholamines. They differ in pH optimum, relative substrate specificity and immunological properties, although all have molecular weights of 61,000–64,000 daltons. Hydroxysteroid sulfotransferase also exists in several forms, and it is important not only as a detoxication enzyme, but also in the synthesis and possibly transport of steroids. Estrone sulfotransferase, which has been purified from bovine adrenal gland, conjugates hydroxyl groups on the A ring of sterols. Bile salt sulfotransferase detoxifies bile salts and has been purified from both liver and kidney, the two forms appearing to be distinct entities. *See also* PAPS.

sulfhemoglobin. An ill-defined term first used to describe derivatives of hemoglobin generated by *in vitro* exposure to hydrogen sulfide. These derivatives have, however, not been characterized and appear to play no role in hydrogen sulfide poisoning. It is now used in an even less appropriate way to describe pigments generated *in vivo* in the absence of hydrogen sulfide. They appear to be of little toxicological significance, although they may be associated with the formation of Heinz bodies. *See also* HEINZ BODIES; HYPOXIA.

sulfobromophthalein, in hepatotoxicity. CAS number 71-67-0. A blue dye used in the assessment of hepatobiliary dysfunction. The concentration in plasma is monitored since dye removal from the blood is delayed in hepatic dysfunction.

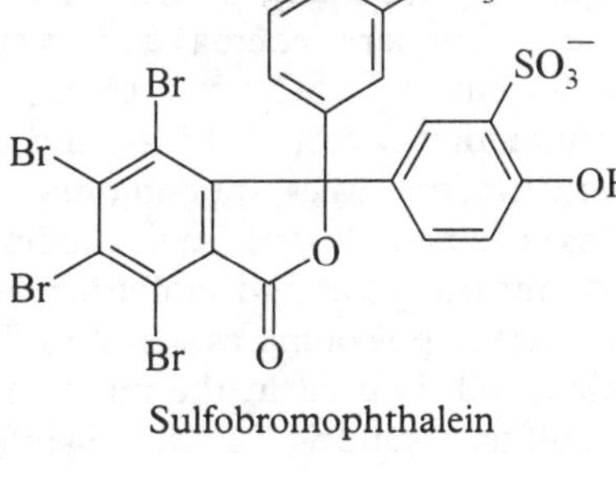

Sulfobromophthalein

Experimentally the appearance of sulfobromphthalein in the bile can also be measured. *See also* HEPATOTOXICITY.

sulfonamides. Organic compounds containing the -SO$_2$NR$_2$ group. Includes the so-called "sulfa drugs" such as sulfanilamide, sulfadiazine and sulfathiazole, which have been used as bacteriocidal agents since the 1930s. Mode of action is the inhibition of bacterial folic acid synthesis by inhibiting uptake of the folic acid precursor, *p*-aminobenzoic acid, into the bacterial cell.

sulfotransferases. *See* SULFATE CONJUGATION.

sulfoxidation. The addition of an oxygen atom to a sulfur atom in an organic molecule (e.g., a sulfide or thioether sulfur) to form a sulfoxide. Although this reaction can proceed non-enzymatically, the most important sulfoxidations are catalyzed by the cytochrome P450-dependent monooxygenase system or the FAD-containing monooxygenase. *See also* MONOOXYGENASES; *S*-OXIDATION.

$$R'C-S-CR'' \longrightarrow R'C-\overset{\overset{\displaystyle O}{\uparrow}}{S}-CR''$$

Sulfoxidation

sulfoxide reduction. A reduction that has been reported to occur in mammalian tissues. In some cases, soluble hepatic thioredoxin-dependent enzymes are responsible. Oxidation in the endoplasmic reticulum followed by reduction in the cytoplasm may initiate recyling which could extend the half-life *in vivo* of some xenobiotics. *See also* REDUCTION.

sulfur dioxide (SO$_2$; sulfur oxide). A nonflammable gas; an eye, skin and mucous membrane irritant and a respiratory poison. It reacts with water to form sulfurous acid. SO$_2$ affects the upper respiratory tract and bronchi mainly, but may cause pulmonary edema and respiratory paralysis. Specifically, SO$_2$ can cause rhinitis, cough, conjunctivitis, corneal burns and opacity, bronchoconstriction, rales, pneumonia, fatigue, altered sense of smell, dyspnea, a thickening of the respiratory mucous layer and inhibition of ciliary movement. Acute poisoning can lead to death by asphyxiation. SO$_2$ is used in the manufacture of sodium sulfite, sulfuric acid, disinfectants, fumigants, glass, wine, ice and industrial and edible protein. It is also used as a bleach, in leather tanning, in brewing, in preserving and in refrigeration. It is released as a by-product of ore smelting, coal and fuel oil combustion, paper manufacturing and petroleum refining and, as such, contributes heavily to air pollution. It is one of the most important contributors to acid precipitation. SO$_2$ has also been shown to enhance the carcinogenicity of polycyclic aromatic hydrocarbons.

sulfuric acid (H$_2$SO$_4$). CAS number 7664-93-9. A designated hazardous substance (EPA). It is an oily liquid usually sold as 95% sulfuric acid. It is used in the synthesis of a variety of chemicals, including various sulfates, acetic acid, citric acid and phenol, and also in the manufacture of fertilizers, nitrate explosives, dyes, drugs and detergents. Sulfuric acid is also used as a dehydrating agent and as an electrolyte in batteries. Its toxic effects are due to skin contact or to inhalation of sulfuric acid aerosols generated during industrial processes. Because of its affinity for water and the exothermic nature of the reaction, concentrated sulfuric acid burns the skin, mucous membranes and eyes. Ingestion is often fatal due to perforation of the esophagus or stomach. Dilute sulfuric acid does not have this effect, but is an irritant to mucous membranes. Chronic exposure to sulfuric acid aerosols etches tooth enamel.

sulfur mustard. *See* MUSTARD GAS.

sulfur oxides. Oxides of sulfur that are responsible for about 18% of the total average pollutant content of air. The major oxide of concern is sulfur dioxide (SO$_2$), which is generated primarily by the burning of sulfur-containing fossil fuels. Although not highly toxic from an acute standpoint, SO$_2$ increases respiratory tract mucous secretion and causes mild bronchoconstriction. Asthmatics are particularly sensitive. Some of the atmospheric SO$_2$ can be converted to sulfuric acid, ammonium sulfate and other sulfates, as well as stable sulfite complexes. Sulfuric acid increases airway resistance and is a major contributor to acid precipitation.

sumicidin. *See* FENVALERATE.

sunset yellow. *See* FOOD COLORS.

Superfund. *See* COMPREHENSIVE ENVIRON-MENTAL RESPONSE, COMPENSATION AND LIABILITY ACT.

Superfund Amendments and Reauthorization Act (SARA). *See* COMPREHENSIVE ENVIRONMENTAL RESPONSE, COMPENSATION AND LIABILITY ACT.

superoxide (O_2^-). A product of the univalent reduction of O_2 or the univalent oxidation of H_2O_2. The superoxide radical (O_2^-) or its corresponding acid (perhydroxyl radical, $HO_2^\bullet$; $pK_a = 4.8$) is generated both enzymatically and non-enzymatically in biological systems. Superoxide can also be produced by cathodic reduction of O_2 in an aprotic solvent, as well as by ultrasonication, pulse radiolysis or photolysis of water. By virtue of a relatively negative dioxygen/superoxide couple ($E° = -0.31$ V) superoxide is a stronger reductant than it is an oxidant (i.e., it readily reduces oxidized cytochrome c). Detection methods include optical spectroscopy, electron spin resonance, mass spectrometry and detection of its presence based on its ability to reduce readily measurable oxidants such as cytochrome c or tetrazolium salts. Due to its reductive ability as well as the spontaneous disproportionation that proceeds with a rate constant of about $10^5 M^{-1}sec^{-1}$ ($O_2^- + O_2^- + 2H^+ \rightarrow H_2O_2 + O_2$), the steady-state concentrations of the oxy radicals are usually low at physiological conditions. *See also* ACTIVE OXYGEN.

superoxide dismutase (SOD). A group of metalloenzymes that catalyze a disproportionation reaction in which superoxide is reduced to hydrogen peroxide according to the following equation

$$O_2^- + O_2^- + 2H^+ \rightarrow H_2O_2 + O_2$$

Three forms of the protein have been described, a copper- and zinc-containing protein, a manganese-containing protein and an iron-containing protein. The copper-zinc protein is found predominantly in eukaryotes, has a molecular weight of about 30,000, consists of two subunits and is inhibited by CN^- and H_2O_2. The iron enzyme is found predominantly in prokaryotes, has a molecular weight of about 40,000, consists of two subunits and is resistant to CN^-, but is inhibited by H_2O_2. The manganese enzyme is found in both

prokaryotes and eukaryotes, has a molecular weight of about 40,000–80,000 (depending upon source) and is resistant to CN^- and H_2O_2. *See also* ACTIVE OXYGEN; SUPEROXIDE.

suppressor T cells. *See* T CELLS.

suprarenal gland. *See* ADRENAL GLAND.

surface–activity relationship. *See* QUANTITATIVE STRUCTURE–ACTIVITY RELATIONSHIP.

surface area scaling factor. An intra- and interspecies scaling factor used in cancer risk assessment to convert animal doses to an equivalent human dose. Expressed in mg/m^2/day. Body surface is approximately proportional to the basal metabolic rate and the ratio of surface area to metabolic rate tends to be constant from one species to another. Since surface area is approximately proportional to body weight to the 2/3 power, the scaling factor can be reduced to mg per body weight 2/3. This scaling factor is used in cancer risk assessment by the US EPA.

surface water. Water in the hydrological cycle that is held or moves on the surface of the ground in lakes, rivers, streams, oceans, and swamps, and is subject to pollution from direct contamination or surface run-off.

Surital. *See* THIAMYLAL.

suspected adverse drug reaction (SADR). For medicines, any product report indicating that there has been or may have been an adverse reaction to a product (including suspected lack of efficacy), including reports that have not been fully investigated and reports which subsequent investigations have shown to be unrelated to the use of a particular product. *See also* ADVERSE DRUG REACTION.

suspension, under FIFRA. Under the Federal Insecticide, Fungicide and Rodenticide Act (FIFRA), a suspension order is used to effect an immediate ban on the production and sale of a pesticide considered to pose an imminent hazard to humans or the environment. Despite its misleading name, a suspension order is more expeditious than a cancellation order for removing a pesticide from commerce. Suspension orders are of two types: ordinary and emergency. In the former case, the registrant is given notice of the order and an opportunity for a hearing prior to the suspension taking effect; in the latter, no prior notice need be provided. *See also* CANCELLATION, UNDER FIFRA; FEDERAL INSECTICIDE, FUNGICIDE AND RODENTICIDE ACT.

suxamethonium. *See* SUCCINYLCHOLINE.

sweetening agents. Nutritive sweetening agents (sucrose, lactose, maltose and fructose) are usually extracted from plants or other natural sources such as honey. Non-nutritive agents include compounds that have no calorific value in the human diet and are believed to be non-toxic to humans. Non-nutritive sweetening agents are used in weight-reduction regimens and by diabetics. *See also* ACESULPHAME K; DL-AMINOAMALONYL-D-ALANINE ISOPROPYL ESTER; ASPARTAME; REBAUDIOSIDE; SODIUM SACCHARIDE; 1′,4,6′-TRICHLOROGALACTOSUCROSE; XYLITOL.

sweet glycosides. *See* SWEETENING AGENTS.

sweet potato. *See* SOLANUM FAMILY.

sympathetic nervous system. The thoracolumbar portion of the autonomic nervous system that contains both pre- and postganglionic fibers. Much of the sympathetic nervous system is adrenergic in nature. *See also* NOREPINEPHRINE.

synapse. The specialized structure at which a neuron communicates directly with a target cell, usually another neuron or muscle cell. There are several structures in the synapse that may be affected by toxicants. These include receptors and the enzymatic systems used to terminate the actions of the neurotransmitters (uptake or degrading enzymes). In addition, some neurotoxicants cause direct damage to the synapse and related elements of the nerve terminal, thereby affecting synaptic function. *See also* NEUROTOXICOLOGY; NEUROTRANSMITTERS; RECEPTOR.

synergism, of pesticides. Apart from synergism as a phenomenon of concern during multiple chemical exposure, synergists have been developed for practical application in the case of pesticides. The best known are the methylenedioxyphenyl insecticide synergists such as piperonyl butoxide or dicarboximides such as MGK 264. These compounds increase the toxicity of certain insecticides by their ability to inhibit cytochrome P450-dependent monooxygenations. *See also* METHYLENEDIOXY RING CLEAVAGE; PIPERONYL BUTOXIDE; SYNERGISM AND POTENTIATION.

synergism and potentiation. A toxicity that is greater when two compounds are given simultaneously or sequentially than would be expected from a consideration of the toxicities of the compounds given alone. In an attempt to make uniform the use of these terms, it has been suggested that insofar as toxic effects are concerned, they be used as follows: both involve toxicity greater than would be expected from the toxicities of the compounds administered separately, but in the case of synergism one compound has little or no intrinsic toxicity when administered alone, whereas in the case of potentiation both compounds have appreciable toxicity when administered alone. They are, however, frequently (particularly with reference to clinical drugs) used in the opposite manner or indeed without clear definition. No consensus on the correct definition of these terms has yet been reached.

synthomycin. *See* CHLORAMPHENICOL.

syrup of ipecac. *See* IPECAC, SYRUP OF.

systemic. A systemic toxicant affects the body as a whole or, at the very least, acts in a region of the body other than the portal of entry.

systemic insecticide. Insecticides that are taken in and then translocated throughout a plant or animal, rendering the host lethal to insect pests. In the case of plant systemics these insecticides may be less harmful to wildlife than contact poisons because insects not actually feeding on the treated plants may escape their effects.

T

2,4,5-T (2,4,5-trichlorophenoxyacetic acid). **CAS number 93-76-5**. A post-emergence herbicide used for the control of shrubs and trees. The acute oral LD50 is 300 mg/kg in rats and 100 mg/kg in dogs. There is no evidence of carcinogenicity in long-term chronic studies in rats. Most of the problems associated with 2,4,5-T appear to be due to TCDD, a contaminant. *See also* TCDD.

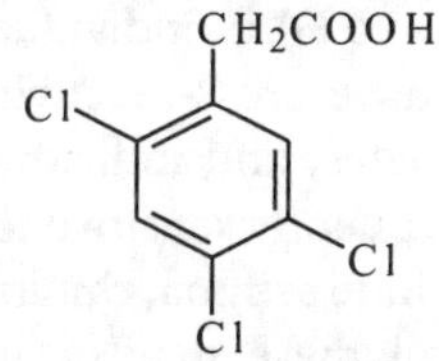

2,4,5-Trichlorophenoxyacetic acid (2,4,5-T)

$T_{0.5}$. Conventional abbreviation for half-life. *See also* HALF-LIFE.

T-2 toxin. *See* TRICOTHECENES.

T3 (triiodothyronine). *See* THYROID.

T4 (thyroxine). *See* THYROID.

tabun (GA; ethyl phosphorodimethylamido-cyanidate). **CAS number 77-81-6**. One of a family of volatile, liquid anticholinesterase nerve agents that reacts irreversibly with the enzyme cholinesterase, thereby permitting a deleterious accumulation of acetylcholine at nerve endings, which can lead to rapid death. Tabun is a neurotoxic agent with an i.v. LD50 in monkeys of 50 μg/kg and in rabbits of 63 μg/kg; the s.c. LD50 in rabbits is 300 μg/kg. This neurotoxicant causes runny nose, tightness of chest, dimness of vision and pinpointing of the eye pupils, difficulty in breathing, drooling and excessive sweating, nausea, vomiting, cramps, involuntary defecation and urination, twitching, jerking and staggering, headache, drowsiness, coma and convulsions, followed by cessation of breathing and death. Therapy includes general supportive measures and respirator, if necessary, along with atropine and 2-PAM. The former interacts with acetylcholine muscarinic receptors, and the latter reactivates phosphorylated cholinesterase. Diazepam may be used to alleviate convulsions. *See also* ANTICHOLINESTERASES; G GAS; ORGANOPHOSPHORUS INSECTICIDES.

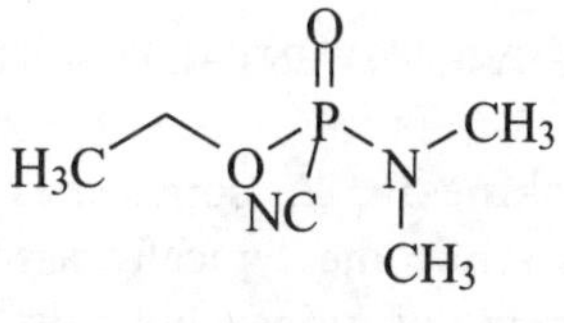

Tabun

tachycardia. Rapid heartbeat, above 100 beats per minute. Tachycardia is often a symptom of acute poisoning.

Tagamet. *See* CIMETIDINE.

talc (talcum; $Mg_6(SiO_2)OH_4$). A finely powdered hydrous magnesium silicate. It is used in a variety of industrial processes and products, including rubber, paints, lubricants, insulating materials, cosmetics and toiletries, such as baby and dusting powders. Acute inhalation of large quantities of talc, such as infants aspirating a massive amount of powder, has caused death within hours because of drying of the mucous membranes, clogging of the smaller airways, pulmonary edema and pneumonia. Chronic inhalation of talc, such as occurs in talc miners, leads to talcosis (a pneumoconiosis) involving pulmonary fibrosis and pleural sclerosis. Lymph nodes can also be affected. There are recent unproven suggestions that talc can result in cervical or ovarian cancer. Some talc is contaminated with asbestos. *See also* FIBROSIS; PNEUMOCONIOSIS.

talcosis. *See* TALC.

talcum. *See* TALC.

tamoxifen. **CAS number 10540-29-1**. A non-steroidal estrogen antagonist. Used in the palliative treatment of breast cancer, and its use in breast cancer prevention has been suggested. It is, however, an hepatocarcinogen in the rat, and its use often causes unwanted side effects.

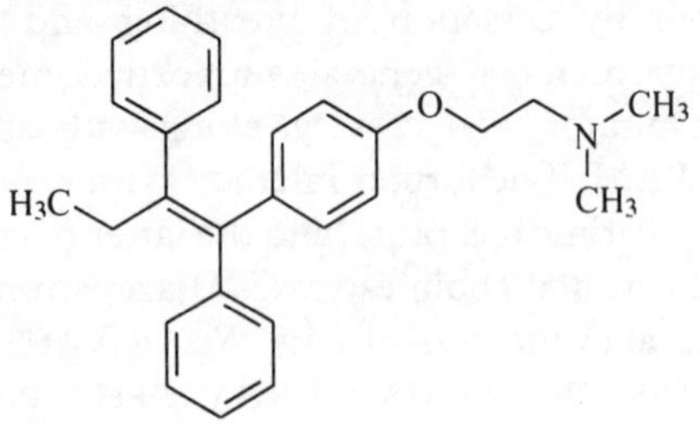

Tamoxifen

Tanio. *See* ENVIRONMENTAL DISASTERS.

tardive dyskinesia. A sometimes irreversible neurological syndrome typically associated with the long-term use of antipsychotic drugs. This disorder is seen in approximately 10–20% of patients treated with classical (now called "typical") antipsychotic drugs, and manifests itself by pronounced buccal-lingual-masticatory movements, as well as choreoathetotic movements. The iatrogenic nature of this syndrome is somewhat controversial; descriptions of similar conditions occurred in the literature prior to the use of the first antipsychotic drug, chlorpromazine. Sex and age have been shown to correlate positively with the disorder, with postmenopausal women being at greatest risk. Although there is no effective treatment for this disorder, increased doses of antipsychotic drugs will suppress tardive-related movements. *See also* ANTIPSYCHOTIC DRUGS; CHLORPROMAZINE; DOPAMINE RECEPTORS.

target dose. The amount or concentration of a chemical that gets to the site of action, causing a measurable effect.

target organ/system. That organ, or organ system, in which the principal adverse effect of a toxicant is manifested.

tarone test. A statistical test used in carcinogenicity studies to evaluate the significance of the time of observation of tumor rather than death as an endpoint. This test is only appropriate under certain defined conditions such as when the number of animals dying early with a lethal tumor is large and control survival has been large.

tartrazine (trisodium salt of 5-hydroxyl-1-(p-sulfophenyl)-4-(p-sulfophenylazo)pyrazole-3-carboxylic acid; FD&C Yellow No. 5; E102). **CAS number 1934-21-0**. A food color that is often used in dairy products, juices, jams and marmalades, catsup, pickles, etc., as well as in pharmaceuticals. The major metabolite is sulfanilic acid, with lesser amounts of p-acetoamido-benzenesulfonic acid. A small, but significant number (about 1–5%) of individuals with aspirin sensitivity also have cross-reactivity to tartrazine and other benzoates, and individuals sensitive to tartrazine are frequently sensitive to aspirin. Allergic reactions include asthma, rhinitis, urticaria and angioedema, and these may be life-threatening. Pharmaceuticals containing this color are therefore labeled. *See also* FOOD COLORS.

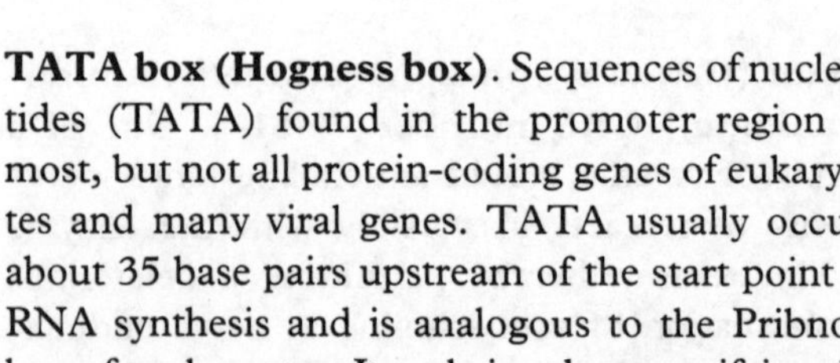

Tartrazine

TATA box (Hogness box). Sequences of nucleotides (TATA) found in the promoter region of most, but not all protein-coding genes of eukaryotes and many viral genes. TATA usually occurs about 35 base pairs upstream of the start point of RNA synthesis and is analogous to the Pribnow box of prokaryotes. Its role involves specifying the precise initiation site for RNA polymerase II.

taurine conjugation. An unusual form of amino acid conjugation involving the non-protein amino acid taurine (CAS number 107-35-7). Although a common, albeit minor, route of conjugation for bile acid, phenylacetic and indolylacetic acids in most species, it is extensive in a small number of vertebrate species, including the pigeon and the ferret. *See also* AMINO ACID CONJUGATION; PHASE II REACTIONS.

$$H_2NCH_2CH_2SO_3H$$

Taurine

taxol (Paclitaxel). CAS number 33069-62-4. An antineoplastic agent from the yew *Taxus cuspidata* and *T. brevifolia*, with the highest concentrations occurring in the needles and bark. Taxol prevents the dissociation of microtubules into tubulin. *See also* YEW.

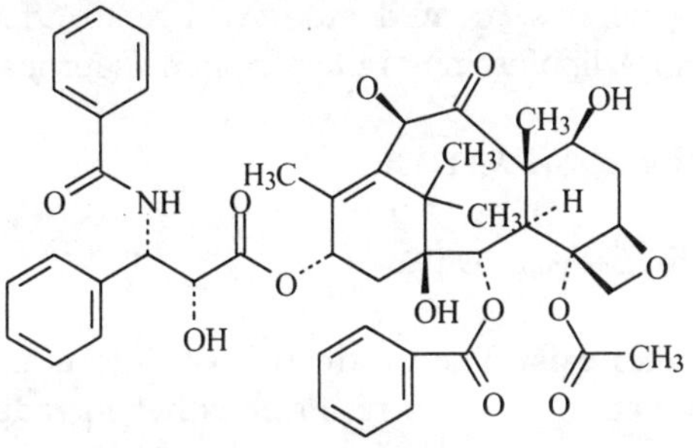

Taxol

TBTO (tributyltin oxide). *See* TRIBUTYLTIN.

TCA. *See* TRICHLOROACETIC ACID.

TCDD (Dioxin; 2,3,7,8-tetrachlorodibenzo-*p*-dioxin). CAS number 1746-01-6. A contaminant of 2,4,5-trichlorophenol and 2,4,5-trichlorophenoxyacetic acid (the herbicide 2,4,5-T) formed at high temperatures during synthesis of organochlorine compounds. It is frequently referred to, inaccurately, as dioxin, its unsubstituted parent compound. It has an oral LD50 of 0.022 mg/kg in male and 0.045 mg/kg in female rats. The oral LD50 in guinea pigs of either sex is 0.001 mg/kg. EPA lists TCDD as a carcinogen, although DNA adducts have not been detected. It is possibly a promoter. The mode of action is unknown, although enzyme induction and toxicity are both correlated with TCDD binding to the Ah receptor. The symptoms in humans include chloracne, porphyrinuria and porhyria cutanea

TCDD

tarda, and therapy is symptomatic only. *See also* AH LOCUS; AH RECEPTOR; MECHANISM OF INDUCTION.

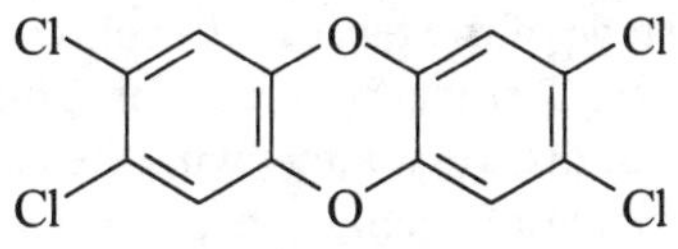

TCDD-binding protein. *See* AH RECEPTOR.

T cells (T lymphocytes; thymus-dependent lymphocytes; thymus-derived lymphocytes). The descendants of pluripotent bone marrow stem cell that have migrated to, and matured in, the thymus and bear characteristic cell-surface markers. These immunocompetent T cells then populate the lymph nodes, spleen and other secondary lymphoid organs where they interact with B cells and accessory cells to induce antibody production. They also interact with other T cells and accessory cells to generate cell-mediated responses, such as delayed-type hypersensitivity, graft rejection and resistance to tumors and viral infections. Many of these cell interactions are restricted by glycoproteins encoded in the major histocompatability complex (MHC), some of which are expressed in nearly all tissues (class I) and some of which are expressed primarily on lymphoid cells (class II). There are several broad classes of T cells—helper T cells, cytotoxic T cells, suppressor T cells—as well as numerous putative subpopulations of T cells, each bearing distinguishing cell-surface markers or combinations of markers. The function of most markers is unknown, and the correspondence between a given marker and a functional cell type is rarely absolute.

helper T cells. Cells that assist antigen-specific B cells to proliferate and differentiate into mature antibody-producing plasma cells. They also assist in the maturation of cytotoxic T cells and are probably regulated by suppressor T cells. They are restricted to interactions with cells bearing the appropriate class II MHC molecules.

cytotoxic T cells (cytolytic T cells, killer T cells). Antigen-specific T cells that can kill other cells via mechanisms that do not involve antibody. They are the primary effector cells of the cell-mediated immune response. Cytotoxic T cells recognize antigen in conjunction with class I MHC molecules.

suppressor T cells. Cells that down-regulate normal humoral (antibody) and cell-mediated immune responses, as well as being crucial to some forms of tolerance to self and to foreign proteins. Most immune responses generate both helper and suppressor populations, and the ratio between these populations is often more important than the absolute cell count. The route of administration, size of dose, type of antigen and timing of antigen presentation will favor the development of one population over the other.

The AIDS virus affects the ratio by destroying helper T cells (the normal helper: suppressor ratio of 2:1 is reversed) as does Cyclosporin A, an immunosuppressive drug used in transplant patients. Diethylstilbestrol (DES) affects the helper:suppressor ratio, but it is unclear whether it inhibits the helper cell population and/or induces the suppressor cell population. Alcohol abuse has been reported to affect T-cell function. Phorbol diesters also adversely affect T cells. *In vitro*, T-cell populations are typically quantified by their associated markers and the functional integrity of the purified populations assessed by lymphoproliferative assays. *In vivo*, T-cell function is assessed by testing delayed-type hypersensitivity reactions, skin graft rejection, resistance to tumors or other model systems not involving antibody production. *See also* B CELLS; MACROPHAGES/MONOCYTES.

TCP (tri-*o*-cresyl phosphate). *See* TOCP.

TDI. *See* TOLUENE DIISOCYANATE.

TD$_{Lo}$. Toxic low dose.

tear gas. *See* C AGENTS.

Tegretal. *See* CARBAMAZEPINE.

Tellurium (Te). A member element of group IVa in the Periodic Table with both metallic and non-metallic properties. Tellurium compounds of biological interest include the elemental form, as well as compounds with valences of +2 (telluride), +4 (tellurite) and +6 (tellurate). Commercial applications of tellurium include its use as a coloring agent and as an alloy with other metals. Industrial hazards generally involve the volatile forms including tellurium dioxide and hydrogen telluride rather than the less toxic elemental form. Exposure to potassium tellurite may also occur; this compound is known to cause hemolysis of erythrocytes, probably via its reduction product, telluride. Other non-nervous system effects of exposure to tellurium compounds include weight loss, blue/black discoloration of skin and a characteristic garlic breath odor. Animal models have clearly implicated tellurium in induction of specific neuropathological findings. These include its action as a teratogen in the induction of communicating hydrocephalus (treated rats give rise to affected offspring), lipofuscinosis and peripheral neuropathy.

telophase. *See* MITOSIS.

Temik. *See* ALDICARB.

teratogenesis. The production of defects in the reproduction process, resulting either in reduced productivity due to fetal or embryonic mortality or in the birth of offspring with physical, mental, behavioral or developmental defects. Compounds causing such defects are known as teratogens. *See also* TERATOGENESIS, CRITICAL PERIODS; TERATOGENESIS, DOSE-RESPONSE; TERATOGENESIS, GENETIC FACTORS.

teratogenesis, critical periods. The process of embryogenesis involves cell proliferation, differentiation, migration and finally organogenesis; all of which occur in a precisely timed sequence. The first two weeks in human embryonic development is a time of rapid cell proliferation. After fertilization, the cells divide rapidly forming the blastocyst, with little morphological differentiation. Very few specific teratogenic effects occur at this time, with death of the embryo due to substantial damage to undifferentiated cells being the major effect. The time of greatest susceptibility to teratogens, at least in the induction of gross anatomical defects, occurs during the next period, that of germ layer formation and organogenesis. The type of teratogenic response is determined by the developmental stage of the fetus at the time of exposure (i.e., there are "critical periods" for different malformations of organ systems, with the early events in organ formation being most sensitive). Histogenesis and functional development generally begin before organogenesis is completed, and continue into the subsequent growth phases. Adverse influences at this time do not usually result in gross malformations, but can result in functional abnormalities that may be manifested only by growth retardation or, more seriously, may result in fetal death due to interference with some critical biological function.

teratogenesis, dose-response. Most teratogens appear to have a threshold or "no-effect" level below which there are no observable malformations. Abnormal development frequently appears to depend upon destruction of a critical number of cells above the level that can be restored quickly; destruction of less than this critical mass produces no persistent effect, whereas destruction of an excessive number results in fetal death or malformation.

teratogenesis, genetic factors. Susceptibility to teratogens depends on the genotype of the organism, including species as well as strain differences. This variation in response may be due in part to differences in maternal metabolism, distribution or transplacental passage of the compound, resulting in differential exposure to the ultimate teratogenic agent. For example, rabbits and mice are very susceptible to cleft palate induction by cortisone, whereas rats are not. Thalidomide is very species-specific; humans and other higher primates are extremely sensitive to its effects, whereas most other mammals are resistant, with only some rabbit and mouse strains reacting to large doses.

teratogenic effects. Although many teratogenic effects are possible (morphological, physiological, behavioral), it is the morphological effects that have been studied most intensively. They include external malformations, visceral anomalies and skeletal abnormalities. *See also* TERATOGENIC EFFECTS, EXTERNAL MALFORMATIONS; TERATOGENIC EFFECTS, SKELETAL ABNORMALITIES; TERATOGENIC EFFECTS, VISCERAL ANOMALIES; TERATOLOGY TESTING; TOXIC ENDPOINTS, TERATOLOGY.

teratogenic effects, external malformations. The anomalies described below have been observed in rats; many similar lesions have been

recorded in humans. Malformations of the brain, cranium or spinal cord include: encephalocele, a protrusion of the brain through an opening of the skull, where the cerebrum is well-formed and covered by transparent connective tissue; exencephaly, a lack of skull with disorganized outward growth of the brain; microcephaly, a small head on a normal-sized body; hydrocephaly, a marked enlargement of the ventricles of the cerebrum; craniorachischisis, an exposed brain and spinal cord; spina bifida, non-fusion of spinal processes in which the covering ectoderm usually is missing and the spinal cord is visible. In the nose, enlarged nares or single naris may occur. Teratogenic lesions of the eye include: microphthalmia, small eye; anophthalmia, lack of eye; and open eye with no apparent eyelid. Anotia, the absence of the external ear, or microtia, small ear, may also occur. Various malformations of the jaw include: micrognathia, small lower jaw; agnathia, the absence of lower jaw; aglossia, the lack of a tongue. Astomia, lack of mouth opening, bifid (or forked) tongue and cleft lip, which may be either a unilateral or bilateral cleft of the upper lip, may also occur. Cleft palate, a cleft or separation of the median portion of the palate, is also seen. Common limb malformations include: clubfoot, a foot that has grown in a twisted manner, resulting in an abnormal shape or position; micromelia, abnormal shortness of the limb; hemimelia, the absence of any of the long bones, resulting in a shortened limb; phocomelia, the absence of all the long bones of a limb, the feet being attached directly to the body.

teratogenic effects, skeletal abnormalities. The descriptions below are derived from rats; however, many similar lesions have been recorded from humans. Polydactyly is the presence of extra digits. Since five is the normal number in the mouse, a polydactylous fetus would have six or more. Syndactyly is the fusion of two or more digits. Oligodactyly is the absence of one or more digits. Brachydactyly is smallness of one or more digits. The ribs may be any aberrant shape (wavy ribs) or there may be extra ribs on either side. Ribs may be missing on either side or ribs may be fused anywhere along the length of the rib. Finally, in branched ribs, the ribs may have a single base and then be branched. The tail may be short usually because of a lack of vertebrae or the tail may be missing or corkscrew-shaped.

teratogenic effects, visceral anomalies. These effects are noted in rats, but many similar anomalies have been reported in humans. In the intestines, an umbilical hernia, a protrusion of the intestines into the umbilical cord, or ecotopic intestines, an extrusion of the intestines outside the body wall, may be present. In enlarged heart either the atrium or ventricle may be enlarged, whereas in dextrocardia there is a rotation of the heart axis to the right. Enlarged lungs with all lobes enlarged may be seen, or conversely there may be small lung in which all lobes are usually small and the lobes may have an immature appearance. Undescended testes, in which the testes are located anterior to the bladder instead of lateral may occur, and this may be bilateral or unilateral. In agenesis of testes one or both testes is missing, whereas in agenesis of uterus one or both horns of the uterus is missing. Hydronephrosis is a fluid-filled kidney that is often grossly enlarged, a condition which can be accompanied by hydroureter, or enlarged, fluid-filled ureter. The kidneys can be fused, appearing as one misshapen kidney with two ureters, or one or both kidneys may be missing. Misshapen kidney may be small, enlarged, spherical or odd-shaped.

teratogenic factors. *See* TERATOGENIC MECHANISMS (10 ENTRIES); TOXIC ENDPOINTS, TERATOLOGY.

teratogenic hazard potential. Attempts have been made to develop indices that distinguish between teratogenic compounds with little or no adult toxicity and compounds that are both toxic to adults and teratogenic. Such an index should also express the relationship between the two. As yet no final solution has been found to this problem, but the two best known attempts are those of Johnson, whose measure of teratogenic hazard potential is equal to log (lowest adult lethal dose/lowest teratogenic dose), and that of Fabro *et al.* The latter developed the relative teratogenicity index, which is equal to LD01 adult/TD05, where TD05 is the dose necessary to cause 5% more malformations than in controls. Both of these suffer

from a variety of statistical and experimental problems, not least of which is the fact that the slopes of the dose-response curves for teratogenicity and adult mortality may be quite different.

teratogenicity index. *See* TERATOGENIC HAZARD POTENTIAL.

teratogenicity testing. *See* TERATOLOGY TESTING.

teratogenic mechanisms. Many different types of compounds may cause similar abnormalities if they are administered during the same critical period. This has led to the proposal that there are certain common mechanisms by which teratogenic agents are able to initiate abnormal development, the teratogenic agent initiating one or more of these mechanisms resulting in abnormal embryogenesis. These toxic events lead to too few cells or cell products for normal morphogenesis or functional development; cell death or tissue necrosis is one of the most frequent signs of chemical or physical damage to the developing embryo. Although cell death above normal physiological levels does not inevitably lead to malformation, there may be too few cells or cell products to effect localized morphogenesis or functional development. Since the initiating events of abnormal development usually occur at the subcellular or molecular level, the damage is not readily detected until cell death, morphological damage or functional disability is observed. *See also* TERATOGENIC MECHANISMS, CHROMOSOMAL ABNORMALITIES; TERATOGENIC MECHANISMS, ENERGY SUPPLY; TERATOGENIC MECHANISMS, ENZYME INHIBITION; TERATOGENIC MECHANISMS, MEMBRANE STRUCTURE; TERATOGENIC MECHANISMS, MITOTIC INTERFERENCE; TERATOGENIC MECHANISMS, MUTATION; TERATOGENIC MECHANISMS, NUCLEIC ACID FUNCTION; TERATOGENIC MECHANISMS, NUTRITIONAL DEFICIENCIES; TERATOGENIC MECHANISMS, OSMOLARITY.

teratogenic mechanisms, chromosomal abnormalities. Chromosomal abnormalities (e.g., excess of chromosomes, deficiencies and rearrangements resulting from non-disjunction or breaks in the chromosomes) probably account for less than 3% of human developmental errors, because an excess or deficiency of chromosomal material, apart from that of the sex chromosomes, is usually lethal. Advanced maternal age is a factor in non-disjunction in germ cells, as is aging of germ cells in the genital tract prior to fertilization. Other causes of chromosomal abnormalities include viral infection, irradiation and chemical agents. *See also* CHROMOSOME ABERRATIONS.

teratogenic mechanisms, energy supply. The growth of the embryo requires high-energy utilization, and factors that interfere with energy supply are associated with teratogenesis. They include inadequate glucose supply (dietary deficiency, induced hypoglycemia), interference with glycolysis (iodoacetate, 6-aminonicotinamide), inhibition of citric acid cycle (riboflavin deficiency, 6-aminonicotinamide) and blockage of the terminal electron transport system (hypoxia, cyanide, 2,4-dinitrophenol). *See also* ELECTRON TRANSPORT INHIBITORS.

teratogenic mechanisms, enzyme inhibition. Chemicals that inhibit enzymes, especially those involved in intermediary metabolism, can alter fetal growth and development. Other chemicals are known to be both mutagenic and teratogenic by inhibiting DNA repair enzymes or by inhibiting polymerases necessary for formation of the mitotic spindle.

teratogenic mechanisms, membrane structure. Altered membrane permeability can lead to osmolar imbalance and result in changes in osmolarity as a teratogenic mechanism. The solvent DMSO and excess vitamin A may act in this way to cause teratogenic effects. *See also* TERATOGENIC MECHANISMS, OSMOLARITY.

teratogenic mechanisms, mitotic interference. Certain "cytotoxic" chemicals, such as hydroxyurea or irradiation slow or arrest DNA synthesis, thereby inhibiting mitosis. Chemicals, such as colchicine or vincristine, interfere with spindle formation and prevent the chromosomes from separating at anaphase. The resulting tetraploid cells usually lead to fetotoxicity. Irradiation or radiomimetic chemicals may also lead to "stickiness" or "bridges" between chromatids

preventing proper separation of chromosomes. Any or all of these events are believed to be possible mechanisms of teratogenicity. *See also* SPINDLE POISONS.

teratogenic mechanisms, mutation. It has been estimated that some 20–30% of human developmental errors are due to mutations in the germ cells; such changes are hereditary. If the mutations occur in somatic cells, then the alteration will be transmitted to all descendants of that cell, but it will not be inherited. However, somatic mutations in the early embryo may affect enough cells to produce a structural or functional defect. Mutagens include such agents as ionizing radiation, chemicals such as nitrous acid, alkylating agents, most carcinogens and agents that interfere with DNA repair mechanisms. *See also* MUTAGENESIS; MUTATION.

teratogenic mechanisms, nucleic acid function. Many antibiotics and antineoplastic drugs are teratogenic by interfering with nucleic acid replication, transcription or RNA translation, including cytotoxic chemicals such as cytosine arabinoside, which inhibits DNA polymerase, and 6-mercaptopurine, which blocks incorporation of adenine and guanine into DNA. Agents that block protein synthesis are generally embryolethal above the no effect dose. Growth retardation occurs at lower doses, but at higher doses inhibition of protein synthesis leads to embryo death rather than malformation.

teratogenic mechanisms, nutritional deficiencies. Lack of metabolic precursors or substrates is a well-established mechanism of teratogenesis. Specific dietary deficiencies, especially of vitamins and minerals, are growth-inhibiting, teratogenic or embryolethal. Embryos frequently show teratogenic symptoms before the mother shows signs of deficiencies, contrary to the widespread belief that the embryo will receive nutrients at the mother's expense. Swayback, a disease of lambs due to copper deficiency in pregnant sheep, is characterized by paralysis of the hind limbs, lack of coordination and, in some cases, blindness. It can be prevented by copper supplementation of the diet of pregnant ewes. Endemic cretinism, characterized by mental and physical retardation, potbelly, large tongue and faces similar to Down's syndrome, occurs where the iodine content of the soil is extremely low, and can be eliminated by the addition of iodized salt to the diet. Failure of materials to be absorbed from the maternal digestive system, as with excess zinc or sulfate preventing adequate copper absorption, or failure of placental transport of essential metabolites may also be the cause of teratogenic effects. *See also* TERATOGENIC MECHANISMS, ENERGY SUPPLY.

teratogenic mechanisms, osmolarity. Abnormal fluid accumulations may cause tissue distortions sufficient to lead to malformations. For example, hypoxia in chick embryos leads to edema, hematomas and blisters, which subsequently give rise to abnormal embryogenesis in eye, brain and limbs. Trypan blue, hypertonic solutions and adrenal hormones are also known to give rise to this "edema syndrome" and resulting malformations, although it is frequently difficult to separate cause from simultaneous effect.

teratogens. *See* TERATOGENESIS.

teratology. Study of birth defects. The study of abnormal development between conception and birth. In toxicology, abnormal development due to chemicals is of primary importance.

teratology testing. Although in teratology tests the test chemical may be administered from implantation to parturition, it is usually administered only during the period of major organogenesis, and observations, which may be extended throughout life, are usually made immediately prior to birth. The endpoints observed are mainly morphological (i.e., structural changes and malformations), although embryofetal mortality is also measured. Teratology studies are almost always carried out in a rodent species, usually the rat, occasionally also the rabbit, but only rarely in non-human primates or dogs. Enough females are used so that, given normal fertility for the strain, there are 20 pregnant females in each dosage group of rodents or 10 pregnant females per dosage group of non-rodents. The test chemical is administered in the diet, in the drinking water or by gavage. The high-dose level is one that causes some maternal toxicity, but less than 10%

maternal mortality. The low dose is one at which no maternal toxicity is apparent, and intermediate dose(s) are spaced evenly, on a logarithmic scale, between the low and high doses. Compound administration is generally such that the dam is exposed during the period of major organogenesis (i.e., days 6–15 of gestation in the case of the rat or mouse, and days 6–18 in the case of the rabbit). Tests are terminated by dissection of the dams on the day before normal delivery is expected. The uterus is examined for implantation and resorption sites and for live and dead fetuses and the ovaries for corpora lutea. In rodent studies, one-third of the fetuses are examined for soft tissue malformations and two-thirds for skeletal malformations. In non-rodents, all fetuses are examined for both soft tissue and skeletal malformations. Endpoints that may be examined include maternal toxicity, embryofetal toxicity, external malformations and soft tissue and skeletal malformations. *See also* CHRONIC TOXICITY TESTING; EMBRYOFETAL TOXICITY; MATERNAL TOXICITY; TOXIC ENDPOINTS, TERATOLOGY.

terbutaline. CAS number 23031-25-6. Bronchodilator.

terfenadine (α-[4-(1,1-dimethylethyl)phenyl]-4-(hydroxydiphenylmethyl)-1-piperidinebutanol). CAS number 50679-08-8. A selective H_1 histamine receptor blocker used for treatment of histamine-mediated allergic responses. Terfenadine is non-sedating because it does not cross the blood–brain barrier, and also has very low anticholinergic effects. It can cause rare, but potentially life threatening, cardiac arrhythmias by lengthening of the QT interval. Other cardiac problems also can occur if high plasma levels of unaltered terfenadine accumulate. *See also* ANTIHISTAMINES.

Terfenadine

terrestrial–aquatic ecosystem. A model ecosystem involving both terrestrial and aquatic environments and appropriate organisms in each environment. *See also* AQUATIC ECOSYSTEM; MODEL ECOSYSTEMS; SIMULATED ECOSYSTEMS; TERRESTRIAL ECOSYSTEM.

terrestrial ecosystem. An ecosystem involving strictly substrate and above-ground, but not aquatic elements. Model terrestrial ecosystems have also been developed to study the fate of chemicals in the environment. *See also* MODEL ECOSYSTEMS.

test evaluation, acute. *See* TOXIC ENDPOINTS.

test evaluation, chronic. *See* TOXIC ENDPOINTS.

test evaluation, subchronic. *See* TOXIC ENDPOINTS.

testing. *See* TOXICITY TESTING.

testing sequences. Considering all of the tests for acute and chronic toxicity, either *in vivo* or *in vitro*, it is impractical to test completely all of the chemicals of commerce and their derivatives and degradation products. The challenge of toxicity testing therefore is to delimit the most effective set or sequence of tests necessary to describe the toxicity and potential hazard of a particular chemical or mixture of chemicals. The recent emphasis on *in vitro* or short-term test development has been based on the need to find substitutes for lifetime feeding studies in experimental animals or to enable priorities to be established for chronic testing of chemicals. However, regulatory agencies worldwide have failed to agree either on test sequences or on when short-term tests may be substituted for chronic tests. As a result, short-term tests are usually required in addition to the other tests that were required before their development. However, sequences of tests from the following categories have been suggested: gene mutations; structural chromosome aberrations; other genotoxicity tests, such as DNA damage and repair; numerical chromosome aberrations, as appropriate. Following review of such test sequences a decision is reached on whether or not to start long-term chronic studies.

testing variables, biological. Probably the most important single biological variable is the species of test organism. Although the species with the greatest pharmacokinetic and metabolic similarity to humans for the compound in question should be used, this information is seldom available. In practice, the most common rodents used are rats, and the most common non-rodents are dogs. The particular genetic strain may also be important. Inbred rodent strains are used to reduce variability, although different strains may show different responses. Ideally, age should be matched to the expected exposure period in terms of the stage of human development that is most likely to be exposed. This is not often done, however, and either young adult or adolescent animals that are still growing are used in almost all cases. Since sex may also be an important variable, both sexes are routinely used. Good animal care is critical since toxicity may vary with diet, disease and environmental factors. Animals should be quarantined before being admitted to the test area, their diet should be optimum for the species, and the facility should be kept clean. Regular inspection by a veterinarian is essential since animals showing unusual symptoms not related to the treatment must be removed from the test and autopsied. *See also* TOXICITY TESTING.

testing variables, non-biological. Environmental variables may affect toxicity evaluations, either directly or through effects on animal health. Deviations from optimum temperature and humidity for the test species may cause stress. Stress can also arise from housing more than one test species in the same room. Many toxic or metabolic effects show diurnal variations related to photoperiod. Cage design and the nature of the bedding have also been shown to affect the toxic response. Cleanliness is related closely to animal health and the transmission of disease. Dose selection, preparation and administration are also important non-biological variables. Optimum housing conditions for *in vivo* toxicity tests are clean rooms, each containing a single species, with the temperature, humidity and photoperiod being optimal for the test species. Cages should be the optimum design for the species, bedding should be inert relative to enzyme induction or other toxic effects, and individual cages should be used whenever possible. To avoid effects from non-specific variations in the diet, if possible, enough feed from the same batch should be obtained for the entire study, part being set aside for the controls while the remainder is mixed with the test chemical at the various dose levels. Food storage conditions should ensure that the chemical remains stable and the nutritional value is maintained with periodic analysis to ensure the identity and concentration of the test chemical remains unchanged. *See also* TOXICITY TESTING.

testis. The male gonad whose primary structures are the seminiferous tubules in which spermatogenesis occurs and the interstitial cells (Leydig cells) which secrete androgens.

testosterone (17β-hydroxyandrost-4-en-3-one). CAS number 58-22-0. The primary circulating androgen, but must be metabolized to dihydrotestosterone (DHT) for activity. It controls development and maintenance of male sex organs and secondary sex characteristics. Used, together with synthetic analogues, in treatment of disorders due to impaired secretion of natural hormone. It is produced primarily by the testicular Leydig cells, under the influence of the pituitary gonadotropin interstitial cell-stimulating hormone (ICSH). Testosterone can cause virilization of female fetuses. Excess testosterone in the adult female, such as from the adrenogenital syndrome, causes masculinization. The i.p. LD100 in female rats is 325 mg/kg. A number of testosterone derivatives, mostly esters, are used therapeutically as androgens. *See also* ANABOLIC STEROIDS; ANDROGENS.

Testosterone

tetanospasmin. *See* TETANUS TOXIN.

tetanus. An acute disease caused by the toxicity of the toxin produced by *Clostridium tetani*, growing anaerobically at the site of an injury. Frequently fatal, it is characterized by persistent tonic spasm of certain voluntary muscles. The term also refers to a normal, sustained contraction, and is used to describe experimentally induced sustained muscle contractions or toxicant-induced sustained muscle contractions by, for example, strychnine. *See also* TETANUS TOXIN.

tetanus toxin (tetanospasmin). A 150,000-dalton neurotoxic protein composed of one heavy and one light peptide chain linked by a disulfide bond. It is heat-labile and easily oxidized. The excitotoxin is produced by the gram-positive obligate anaerobe *Clostridium tetani*. *C. tetani* spores are found in soil throughout the world. The toxin blocks the release of amino acid neurotransmitters from inhibitory interneurons in the ventral horn of the spinal cord. The toxin binds to presynaptic endings of motor neurons and is internalized, thereby gaining entry to the CNS. It is transported by retrograde intra-axonal transport to the cell bodies in the spinal cord. Transsynaptic transport of the toxin accounts for the presence and primary action of the toxin on interneurons of the spinal cord. *C. tetani* infection occurs in deep wounds under anaerobic conditions. The toxin is absorbed by the nervous system, and symptoms of the disease include muscle stiffness progressing to rigidity and convulsive spasms. Profuse sweating and tachycardia are common. Congestive heart failure may arise from hypoxia or by a direct action of the toxin on autonomic neurons and myocardial cells. The fatality rate is 50–60%. Intensive life support measures must be undertaken to ensure adequate hydration and ventilation. Antiserum will bind free toxin and should be used early in treatment. Antibiotics may increase toxin release to the detriment of the patient. It is believed to be retrogradely transported in neurons. *See also* NEUROTRANSMITTERS; TETANUS.

tetraalkyl lead. Compounds such as tetraethyl lead (CAS number 78-00-2) and tetramethyl lead (CAS number 75-74-1) are listed as extremely hazardous by the US EPA. Particularly toxic to the central nervous system. *See also* LEWIS, HCDR, NUMBERS TCF250 AND TDR500.

2,5,7,8-tetrachlorodibenzo-*p*-dioxin. *See* TCDD.

tetrachloroethane. **CAS number 79-34-5**. Not widely produced in the USA at present, but formerly used as a degreasing agent. *See also* ATSDR DOCUMENT, AUGUST 1994.

tetrachloroethylene (perchloroethylene). **CAS number 127-18-4**. Dry cleaning solvent and metal degreasing agent. Inhalation can cause dizziness, headaches, confusion and nausea. High dose animal studies showed tetrachloroethylene to cause liver and kidney damage and tumors. Although no direct evidence exists the Department of Health and Human Services has determined that tetrachloroethylene may be anticipated to be a human carcinogen. *See also* ATSDR DOCUMENT, APRIL 1993; LEWIS, HCDR, NUMBER PCF275; DRY-CLEANING SOLVENTS.

Tetrachloroethylene

tetracyclines. A family of antibiotics effective against gram-positive bacteria. The acute oral LD50 in rats is greater than 400 mg/kg. Effects of continued use in humans include fatty liver and renal disease. Photosensitivity may also result. Tetracyclines tend to be deposited at sites of active calcification in teeth and bones. Effects seen after birth on teeth exposed to tetracyclines *in utero* may be severe. *See also* ANTIBIOTICS.

Tetracycline

tetraethyl lead. *See* TETRAALKYL LEAD.

tetraethyltin. *See* TRIETHYLTIN.

Δ⁹-*trans*-tetrahydrocannabinol (THC). **CAS number 1972-08-3**. The cannabinoid that is the major psychoactive compound present in *Cannabis sativa*. It was first isolated by Gaoni and Mechoulam in 1964, and these authors reported the first successful synthesis in 1965. When THC has been administered to man in controlled experiments, it produces pharmacological effects identical to those produced by marijuana. The pharmacological effects of this compound are complex and difficult to classify because it affects structures of the CNS responsible for different functions. For example, THC produces limbic cortical effects characterized by euphoric, contemplative and non-aggressive states; thalamo-cortical effects characterized by increases in extero- and proprioception; temporal lobe effects characterized by changes in the perception of time and short-term memory; hypothalamic-pituitary effects characterized by suppression of luteotropic hormone pulses; bulbar effects characterized by antiemesis; sympathomimetic effects characterized by tachycardia; anticholinergic effects characterized by dry mouth. In addition, it produces conjunctival congestion and reduction of intraocular pressure whose physiological mechanisms are not well understood. It is known, however, that there are specific neuroreceptors (cannabinoid receptors) of the G-protein coupled superfamily that mediate the effects of THC. THC is extensively metabolized by the liver microsomal enzymes. The major metabolic route involves rapid hydroxylation at C-11 followed by further oxidation to the carboxylic acids. Minor routes involve hydroxylation at 8a- or 8b-positions, or in the side chain single or in combination with the major routes. The following metabolites and their psychoactive potency have been identified: 11-hydroxy-Δ-THC, equipotent to the parent compound; 8a-Δ-THC, inactive; 11-nor-Δ-THC-9-carboxylic acid, inactive. 11-Δ9-THC-9-carboxylic acid is the major metabolite of THC found in plasma, urine and feces. Its determination in urine is used for legal and forensic purposes to identify prior exposure to *Cannabis* preparations. Determinations of the amount of THC and its metabolites excreted during the 72 hours following THC administration (either orally, intravenously or by smoke inhalation) reveal that approximately 15% of the dose is excreted in the urine and 35% in the feces. The biological half-life of THC ranges from 24 to 33 hours. *See also* CANNABINOIDS; CANNABIS SATIVA; MARIHUANA.

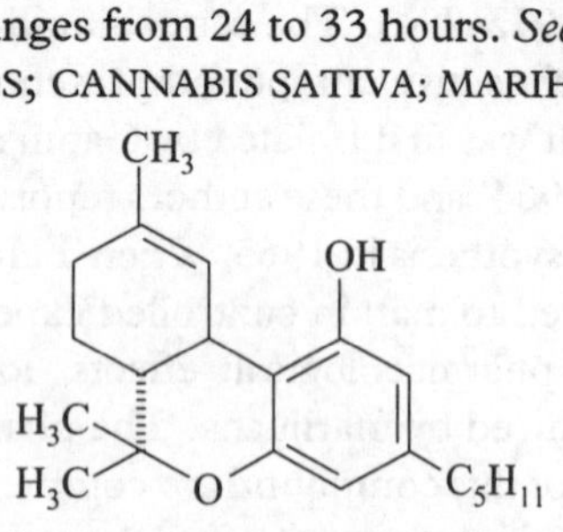

Δ⁹-Tetrahydrocannabinol (THC)

tetrahydroisoquinolines. Compounds that are toxicologically important for several reasons. Benzyltetrahydroisoquinolines, such as papaverine, are natural alkaloids found in the opium poppy. In addition, various substituted 1,2,3,4-tetrahydroisoquinolines can be formed by non-enzymatic Pictet–Spengler reactions whereby aldehydes can condense with catecholamines, indoleamines or their amine precursors or metabolites. Some of the compounds of interest formed by this reaction include: salsolinol (1-methyl-6,7-dihydroxy-1,2,3,4-tetrahydroisoquinoline) formed from dopamine and acetaldehyde; 3-carboxysalsolinol (1-methyl-3-carboxy-6,7-dihydroxy-1,2,3,4-tetrahydroisoquinoline) formed from L-dopa and acetaldehyde; and tetrahydropapaveroline (1-[3,4-(dihydroxyphenyl)methyl]-6,7-dihydroxy-1,2,3,4-tetrahydroisoquinoline), formed from dopamine and dopaldehyde. It has been hypothesized that tetrahydropapaveroline (or a related compound) may play a particular toxicological role in the etiology of alcoholism, where *in vivo* formation may lead to neurotoxicity in some people seen as loss of normal control of voluntary ethanol consumption. However, although many of these compounds have untoward effects on the nervous system when given at high doses, their role in mediating the toxicity of ethanol, or in causing alcoholism, is uncertain. *See also* β-CARBOLINES; OPIUM; PAPAVERINE.

tetrahydropapaveroline. *See* TETRAHYDROISOQUINOLINES.

tetramethyl lead. *See* TETRAALKYL LEAD.

tetrodotoxin (TTX). CAS number 4368-28-9. A toxin contained in the ovary and liver of puffer fish, in the eggs of the California newt and in some other animals. It is used as a chemical tool for the study of ion channels. The s.c. LD50 in mice is 10 mg/kg. It is a toxicant of nerve and muscle by blocking sodium channels, this action causing nerve and muscle paralysis. Symptoms include weakening of voluntary muscles, respiratory failure from paralysis of the diaphragm and hypotension. There is no antidote. Therapy involves artificial respiration.

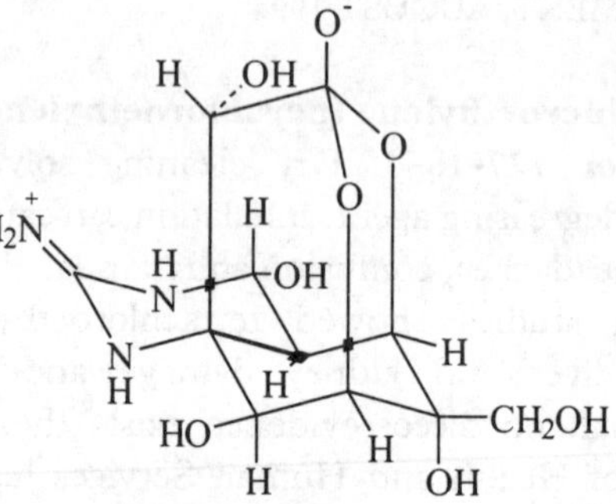

Tetrodotoxin

6-TG. *See* 6-THIOGUANINE.

thalidomide (2-(2,6-dioxo-3-piperidinyl)-1H-isoindole-1,3(2H)-dione). CAS number 50-35-1. Formerly used therapeutically as a sedative hypnotic; currently used to treat leprosy. Thalidomide is a teratogen; major morphological abnormalities result from exposure during the first trimester of pregnancy. Its mode of action involves the formation of a toxic arene oxide metabolite.

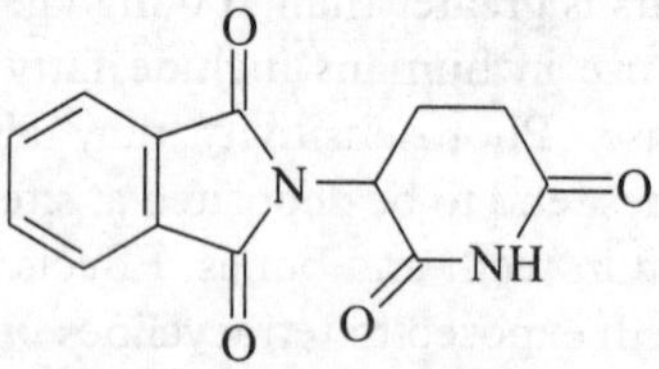

Thalidomide

thallium. CAS number 7440-28-0. A naturally occurring heavy metal used in organic syntheses, to form alloys with other metals, as a rodenticide and in superconductor research. Thallium was also used historically as a depilatory. Acute toxicity from thallium includes nausea, vomiting, diarrhea, polyneuritis, coma, convulsions and death. Chronic toxicity includes reddening of the skin, polyneuritis, alopecia and cataracts. Neural, hepatic and renal damage, as well as deafness and loss of vision, have been documented after chronic exposure. The mechanism associated with such toxic effects is thought to involve complexing of thallium with sulfhydryl groups in mitochondria and consequent interference with oxidative phosphorylation. The oral LD50 in rats is about 30 mg/kg, although 8–12 mg/kg is the estimated lethal dose in humans. Thallium is also teratogenic in rats.

THC. *See* Δ^9-*TRANS*-TETRAHYDROCANNABINOL.

theobromine (3,7-dihydro-3,7-dimethyl-1H-purine-2,6-dione; 3,7-dimethylxanthine). CAS number 83-67-0. One of the methylxanthine central stimulants that is the principal alkaloid of the cacao bean and is also present in cola nuts and tea. It has pharmacological actions and mechanisms are similar to those of caffeine. *See also* CAFFEINE; METHYLXANTHINES; PURINES.

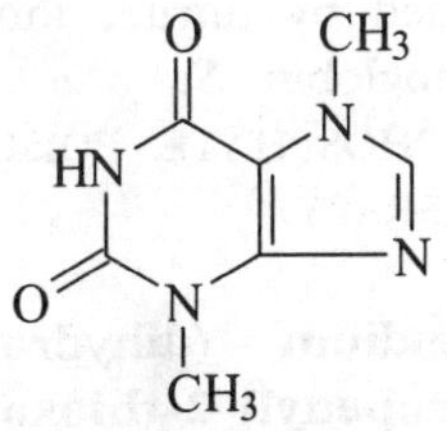

Theobromine

theophylline (3,7-dihydro-1,3-dimethyl-1H-purine-2,6-dione; 1,3-dimethylxanthine). CAS number 58-55-9. One of the methylxanthine central stimulants that is found in small amounts in tea. It has pharmacological actions and mechanisms similar to those of caffeine. It is used in over-the-counter and prescription drugs as a vasodilator and smooth muscle relaxant. Complexed with ethylenediamine (ethane-1,2-dione), it is marketed as the drug aminophylline. *See also* METHYLXANTHINES.

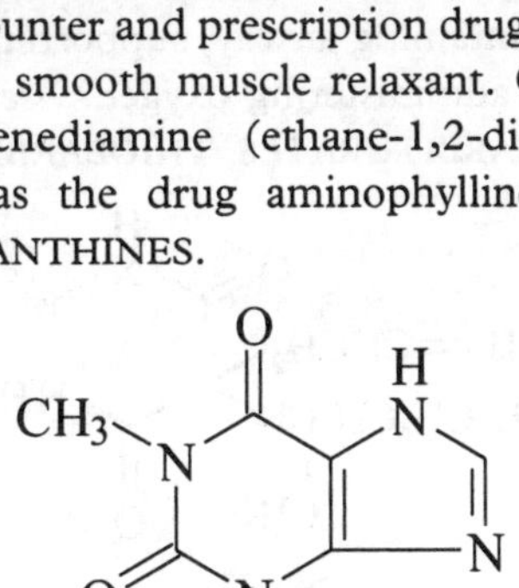

Theophylline

therapeutic index (TI). A numerical estimate of the relationship between the toxic dose of a drug and its therapeutic dose. The most commonly used value is the relationship between the median lethal dose (LD50) and the median effective dose (ED50) (i.e., TI = LD50/ED50). The principal disadvantage is that, since the slope of the dose-response curves may vary, the TI as defined above tells little of the same comparison at different dose levels. *See also* MARGIN OF SAFETY.

Therapeutic Substances Act. UK legislation that controls the manufacture, supply and sale of certain drugs (e.g., antibiotics, corticosteroids, curare, blood, heparin, insulin, vaccines and sera). The provisions of this are similar to those of the Poisons Act. *See also* POISONS ACT.

Therapeutic Substances Regulations. UK regulations that stipulate the maximum levels of antibiotics (e.g., chlortetracycline, erythromycin, bacitracin, penicillin) in feeds given to poultry, rabbits, pigs, calves and lambs. Levels of antibiotics (e.g., streptomycin, oxytetracycline) permitted in horticultural preparations for the treatment of bacterial and mycotic diseases of plants are also stipulated.

therapy. Poisoning therapy may be non-specific or specific. Non-specific therapy is treatment for poisoning that is not related to the mode of action of the particular toxicant. It is designed to prevent further uptake of the toxicant and to maintain vital signs. Specific therapy, on the other hand, is that related to the mode of action of the toxicant and not simply to the maintenance of vital signs by treatment of symptoms. Specific therapy may be based on activation and detoxication reactions, on mode of action or on elimination of the toxicant. In some cases, more than one antidote, with different modes of action, is available for the same toxicant. *See also* THERAPY, NON-SPECIFIC; THERAPY, SPECIFIC.

therapy, non-specific. Treatment for poisoning that is not related to the mode of action of a particular toxicant. Non-specific therapy is designed to prevent further uptake of the toxicant and to maintain vital signs. *Compare* THERAPY, SPECIFIC. *See also* CATHARSIS; DIALYSIS; EMESIS; GASTRIC

LAVAGE; GASTROTOMY; INTESTINAL LAVAGE; MAINTENANCE THERAPY; POISONING, EMERGENCY TREATMENT; POISONING, LIFE SUPPORT.

therapy, specific. Specific therapy is that related to the mode of action of the toxicant, and not simply to the maintenance of vital signs by treatment of symptoms, the latter being characterized as non-specific therapy. Specific therapy may be based on activation and detoxication reactions, on the mode of action or on elimination of the toxicant. In some cases, more than one antidote, with different modes of action, is available for the same toxicant. Unfortunately, there are many toxicants for which specific antidotes are not known, and it is often not clear which toxicant, or mixture of toxicants, is involved. Even with known toxicants for which a specific antidote is available, the damage may have proceeded to the point that the antidote is no longer effective. *Compare* THERAPY, NON-SPECIFIC. *See also* THERAPY, SPECIFIC: DIRECT EFFECT ON TOXICANT; THERAPY, SPECIFIC: EFFECT ON RECEPTOR SITE; THERAPY, SPECIFIC: EXCRETION; THERAPY, SPECIFIC: METABOLISM OF TOXICANT; THERAPY, SPECIFIC: REPAIR.

therapy, specific: direct effect on toxicant. Some therapeutic agents interact directly with the toxicant to render it less toxic or more readily excretable. Complexing agents such as CaEDTA or pencillamine fall into this category. *See also* CHELATING AGENTS; EDTA; PENICILLAMINE.

therapy, specific: effect on receptor site. Some therapeutic agents compete with the toxicant for the receptor site, thus preventing the toxicant from exerting its effect. In some cases, such as the use of excess oxygen for the treatment of carbon monoxide poisoning, the therapeutic agent is the normal ligand. In others, such as atropine treatment of carbamate poisoning, it serves to protect the acetylcholine receptor from the effects of excess acetylcholine resulting from carbamate-induced inhibition of acetylcholinesterase.

therapy, specific: excretion. Some specific therapeutic agents act by causing enhanced excretion of the toxicant. For example, excess chloride is rapidly excreted and, since the chloride excretory mechanism cannot distinguish between chloride and bromide, excretion of the latter is enhanced.

therapy, specific: metabolism of toxicant. Specific therapeutic agents may affect metabolism in several ways, principally by inhibiting activation or stimulating detoxication. Ethanol therapy for methanol poisoning is an example of the former, and thiosulfate treatment of cyanide poisoning an example of the latter. *See also* CYANIDE POISONING, THERAPY; METHANOL POISONING, THERAPY.

therapy, specific: repair. Specific therapeutic agents may directly repair the lesion induced by the toxicant. For example, 2-PAM dephosphorylates acetylcholinesterase inhibited by organophosphates, and methylene blue reduces methemoglobin formed by nitrite, thus regenerating functional hemoglobin. *See also* METHEMOGLOBIN; ORGANOPHOSPHATE POISONING, SYMPTOMS AND THERAPY.

thiamylal, sodium (dihydro-5-(1-methylbutyl)-5-(2-propenyl)-2-thioxo-4,6(1H,5H)-pyrimidinedione; 5-allyl-5-(1-methylbutyl)-2-thiobarbituric acid; Surital; thioseconal). CAS number 77-27-0. An ultra-short-acting barbiturate anesthetic that is used in conjunction with inhalational anesthetics. It acts on the barbiturate-binding site in the GABA receptor complex. Excessive doses cause respiratory depression, apnea or hypotension. Therapy includes establishing and maintaining airway, supporting the circulation, and administering oxygen. *See also* ANESTHETICS; BARBITURATES; THIOBARBITURATES.

Thiamylal

Thimenoz. *See* PHORATE.

Thimet. *See* PHORATE.

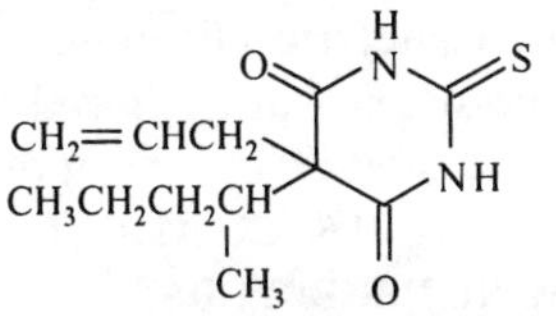

Thiamyl

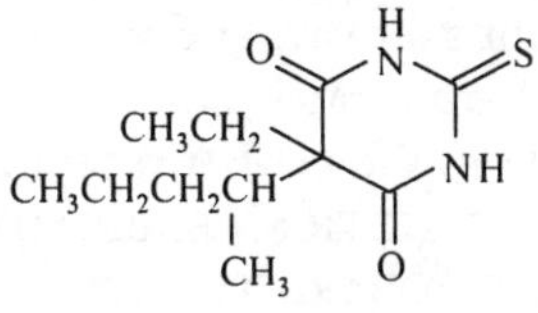

Thiopental

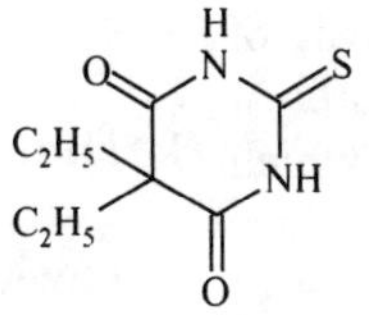

Thiobarbital

Thiobarbiturates

thin-layer chromatography (TLC). *See* CHRO-MATOGRAPHY, THIN-LAYER.

thioacetamide. CAS number 62-55-5. Experimental evidence for carcinogenesis. IARC has designated this compound as a probable human carcinogen. *See also* LEWIS, HCDR, NUMBER TFA000.

thiobarbiturates. Drugs in which the oxygen at position 2 of the barbituric acid (2,4,6-(1H,3H,5H)-pyrimidinetrione) moiety is replaced by sulfur. The thiobarbiturates are more lipid-soluble than the corresponding oxybarbiturates, and disposition rather than metabolism is important in the termination of their action. They tend to be of high potency, rapid onset and short duration of action. *See also* ANESTHETICS; BARBITURATES; BARBITURIC ACID.

thiocarbamate herbicides. *See* CARBAMATE AND THIOCARBAMATE HERBICIDES.

6-thioguanine (6-TG; 2-amino-6-mercapto-purine). CAS number 154-42-7. An antineoplastic metabolic antagonist that inhibits DNA synthesis by being metabolically converted to 6-thioGMP. This inhibits purine biosynthesis at multiple steps, and may be phosphorylated and incorporated into DNA. In humans, it causes bone marrow depression and gastrointestinal toxicity. *See also* ABNORMAL BASE ANALOGS; CHEMO-THERAPY.

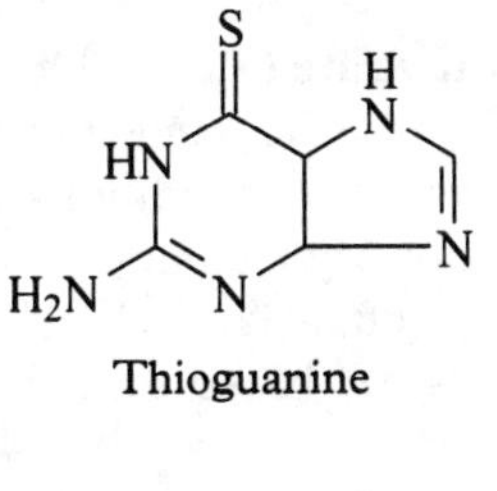

thiols. *See* MERCAPTANS.

thiol S-methyltransferase. *See* S-METHYLATION.

thiopental, sodium (5-ethyldihydro-5-(1-methylbutyl)2-thioxo-4,6(1H,5H)-pyrimidinedione monosodium salt; 5-ethyl-5-(1-methylbutyl)-2-thiobarbituric acid sodium salt; Pentothal). CAS number 71-73-8. A short-acting anesthetic that causes a rapid onset of sleep, making it suitable for induction of anesthesia. Because it causes relatively poor analgesia, its use alone is limited to situations that involve little pain. It can also be used to promote light sleep during regional local anesthesia, and it also quietens excitement and controls convulsions. Its i.p. LD50 in mice is 149 mg/kg, and its i.v. LD50 in mice is 78 ng/kg. Like the other barbiturates, acute toxicity results from respiratory depression and a fall in blood pressure. Physiological support is a key therapy, including establishing and

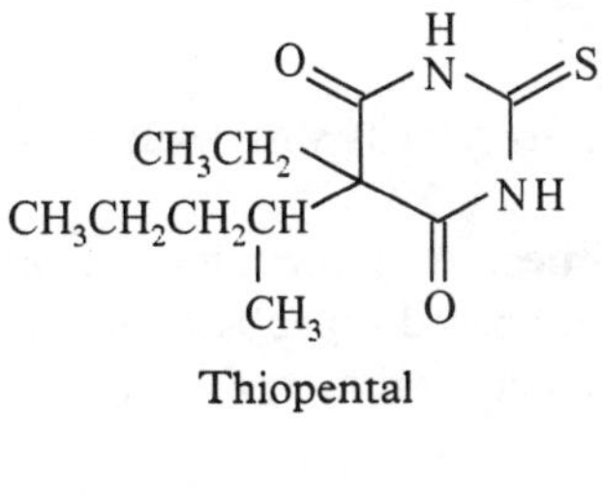

Thioguanine

Thiopental

maintaining a patient's airway, and administering oxygen. Like other barbiturates, it acts on the barbiturate binding site in the GABA receptor complex. *See also* ANESTHETICS; BARBITURATES; BARBITURIC ACID; THIOBARBITURATES.

thioridazine (10-[2-(1-methyl-2-piperidinyl) ethyl]-2(methylthio)phenothiazine; Mellaril). CAS number 50-52-2. An antipsychotic drug of the phenothiazine class. It is of particular interest because of its "atypical" properties, some of which may be due to its extensive bioconversion to active metabolites. The therapeutic and side effects of thioridazine and its metabolites involve blockade of brain dopamine receptors, but also actions mediated via blockage of muscarininc cholinergic and α-adrenergic receptors. *See also* ANTIPSYCHOTIC DRUGS; DOPAMINE RECEPTORS.

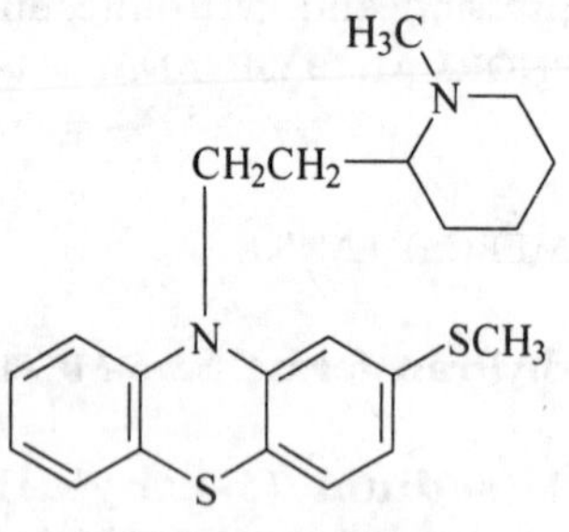

Thioridazine

Thioseconal. *See* THIAMYLAL.

thiosulfate, sodium ($Na_2S_2O_3$; sodium hyposulfite). An inorganic compound with many industrial uses, such as the removal of chlorine from solution, the extraction of silver from ores, in dyeing, leather making, photography and bleaching. It displays little toxicity and is poorly absorbed from the digestive tract. It has been used as an antidote in cyanide poisoning, since it combines enzymatically with cyanide to form thiocyanate. *See also* CYANIDE.

thiotepa. *See* TRIS(1-AZIRIDINYL)PHOSPHINE SULFIDE.

thiouracil. *See* ABNORMAL BASE ANALOGS.

thioxanthenes. A major class of antipsychotic drugs that are based on substituents of the thioxanthene (dibenzothiopyran), rather than the phenothiazene, tricyclic moiety. Drugs of this class (e.g., thiothixene) are believed to be antagonists of both the D_1 and D_2 classes of dopamine receptors. *See also* ANTIPSYCHOTIC DRUGS; DOPAMINE; DOPAMINE RECEPTORS.

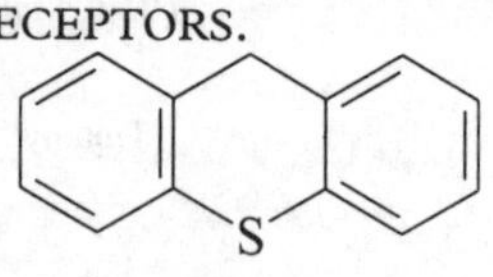

Thioxanthene

Thorazine. *See* CHLORPROMAZINE.

Three Mile Island. *See* ENVIRONMENTAL DISASTERS.

threshold. In toxicology, the lowest dose of a toxicant at which a specified adverse effect can be determined and below which it cannot be determined. The more controversial definition is that dose of a toxicant above which a specified adverse effect may occur but below which it does not occur. The controversy revolves around the assumption, used by regulatory agencies such as the US EPA, that there is no threshold dose for carcinogens.

threshold, for air pollutants. The minimum concentration of an air pollutant that will cause injury in a population in a specified time.

threshold dose. The dose of a chemical below which no adverse effect occurs. The existence of such a threshold is based on the fundamental tenet of toxicology that, for any chemical, there exists a range of doses over which the severity of the observed effect is directly related to the dose. The threshold level represents the lower limit of this dosage range and is dictated by the intrinsic potency of the chemical. Practical thresholds are considered to exist for most non-carcinogenic adverse effects. Since, theoretically, a single molecule of a genotoxic carcinogen can induce cancer, it is widely believed that there is no threshold dose for carcinogens.

threshold limit value (TLV). The upper permissive limits of airborne concentrations of substances. They represent conditions under which it is believed that nearly all workers may be repeatedly exposed day after day without adverse effect. Threshold limits are based on the best available information from industrial experience, from experimental human and animal studies and, when possible, from a combination of the three.

threshold limit value, biological. A TLV based on measurements of a biological parameter in exposed individuals that is known to be related to exposure levels. As yet too little information is available to derive other than tentative TLVs in this way. *See also* BIOLOGICAL MONITORING; THRESHOLD LIMIT VALUE.

threshold limit value, ceiling (TLV-C). The concentration that should not be exceeded even momentarily. For some substances (e.g., irritant gases) only one TLV category, the TLV-C, may be relevant. For other substances, two or three TLV categories may need to be considered.

threshold limit value, short-term exposure limit (TLV-STEL). The maximal concentration to which workers can be exposed for a period of up to 15 minutes continuously without suffering from (1) irritation, (2) chronic or irreversible tissue change or (3) narcosis of sufficient degree to increase accident proneness, impair self-rescue or materially reduce work efficiency, provided that no more than four excursions per day are permitted, that at least 60 minutes elapse between exposure periods and that the daily TLV-TWA is not exceeded. *See also* THRESHOLD LIMIT VALUE, TIME-WEIGHTED AVERAGE.

threshold limit value, time-weighted average (TLV-TWA). The time-weighted average concentration for a normal eight-hour working day or a 40-hour working week to which nearly all workers may be repeatedly exposed, day after day, without adverse effect. Time-weighted averages allow certain permissible excursions above the limit provided they are compensated for by equivalent excursions below the limit during the working day. In some instances, the average concentration is calculated for a working week rather than for a working day.

thrombocytes (platelets). The smallest of the formed elements in the blood. They are fragments of megakaryocytes, giant precursor cells. Platelets adhere to collagen fibers exposed at points of blood vessel injury. Additional platelets aggregate at this point to form a platelet plug, which is the first step in hemostasis. They release factors to promote coagulation. A typical platelet count is 250,000 per cubic millimeter. Aspirin interferes with platelet aggregation and may be useful in preventing clot formation. *See also* THROMBOCYTOPENIA.

thrombocytopenia. A condition of low platelet (thrombocyte) concentrations, resulting in excessive bruising and bleeding from wounds. This can result from an autoimmune reaction following the combination of such agents as aspirin, digoxin, antihistamines or sulfonamides with platelet proteins to form antigens.

thyme. *See* ESSENTIAL OILS.

thymidine kinase locus. *See* TK LOCUS.

thymus. A lymphoid organ; in humans it is located in the thorax, behind the sternum. It appears to be the site of maturation of T cells. *See also* LYMPHATIC SYSTEM; T CELLS.

thymus-dependent lymphocytes. *See* T CELLS.

thymus-derived lymphocytes. *See* T CELLS.

thyroid. An endocrine gland, located in the neck region, that produces three hormones: thyroxine (tetraiodothyronine, T4); triiodothyronine (T3); thyrocalcitonin (calcitonin). The former two are the classic "thyroid hormones." Thyroxine (O-(4-hydroxy-3,5-diiodophenyl)-3,5-diiodotyrosine) is the cleavage product of thyroglobulin found in the thyroid gland colloid. Thyroxine represents the predominant circulating form. The L-form is the thyroid hormone, whereas the D-form has an anticholesteremic action. Thyroxine is metabolized within target cells to T3 (O-(4-hydroxy-3-iodophenyl)-3,5-diiodo-L-tyrosine), which is five times more active than T4. T3 binds to nuclear receptors where it activates genes. Its primary actions are to increase metabolism, to increase protein synthesis, stimulate basal metabolic rate and increase heat production. Thyroid hormone synthesis and secretion are under the control of thyroid-stimulating hormone from the adenohypophysis. Hypothyroidism in the infant causes cretinism and in the adult myxedema. Hyperthyroidism leads to Graves' disease. The third hormone from the thyroid gland, calcitonin, decreases blood calcium levels and acts antagonistically to parathyroid hormone in calcium homeostasis. Calcitonin secretion is controlled by blood calcium levels and not by thyroid-stimulating hormone. *See also* THYROID GLAND TOXICITY.

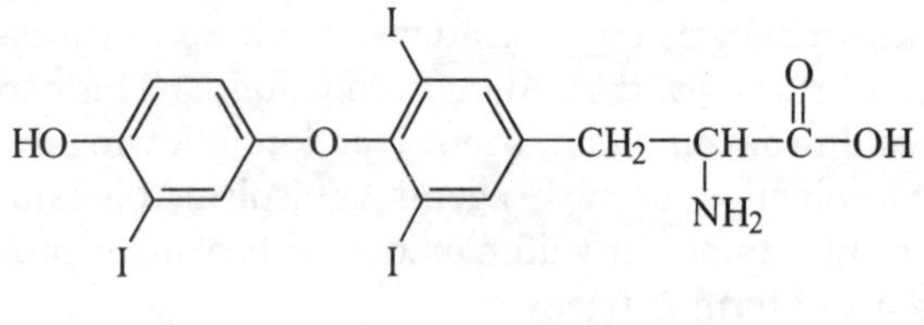

Triidothyronine

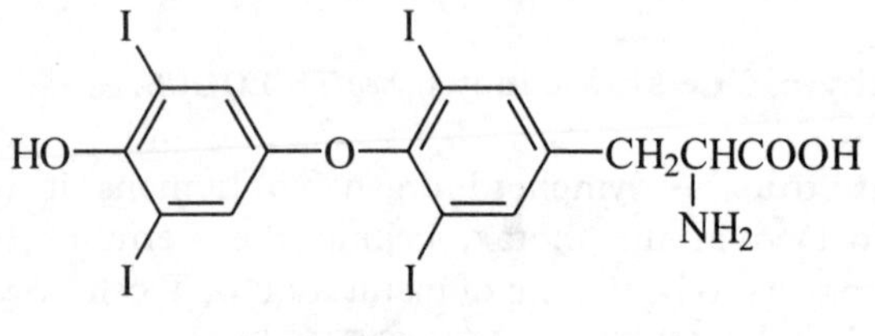

Thyroxine

thyroid gland toxicity. Hypersecretion of the thyroid hormones (thyroxine and triiodothyronine) leads to Graves' disease (toxic goiter). The excess of thyroxine leads to increased basal metabolic rate, increased heart rate, loss of weight, nervousness, sweating and, frequently, exophthalmos. Hyperthyroidism may be the result of excess thyroid-stimulating hormone (TSH) from tumors or from an autoimmune condition in which antibodies act like TSH to stimulate the thyroid.

thyroid-stimulating hormone. *See* THYROTROPIN.

thyrotropin (thyroid-stimulating hormone, TSH). A tropic hormone from the adenohypophysis that causes the thyroid gland to proliferate, absorb more iodine and synthesize and secrete the thyroid hormones thyroxine and triiodothyronine, but not thyrocalcitonin. TSH secretion is under the control of thyrotropin-releasing factor (TRF) from the hypothalamus. Thyrotropin is a glycoprotein, consisting of two large peptide units (one of which is similar to LH and FSH). *See also* THYROID.

thyroxine (T4). *See* THYROID.

TI. *See* THERAPEUTIC INDEX.

tidal volume. The volume of gas inspired or expired during each respiratory cycle. It is an indicator of the depth of breathing.

Times Beach. *See* ENVIRONMENTAL DISASTERS.

Timet. *See* PHORATE.

time-to-tumor. *See* LOW-DOSE EXTRAPOLATION.

time-weighted average (TWA). *See* THRESHOLD LIMIT VALUE, TIME-WEIGHTED AVERAGE.

tin (Sn). Metallic tin and inorganic tin compounds are not toxic to humans. Some organotin compounds are toxic. *See also* ORGANOTINS.

tinnitis. An abnormality of hearing in which an apparent persistent ringing sound is heard when in fact no such sound is present. Commonly known as "a ringing in the ears," tinnitis occurs in some cases of poisoning, but is not a reliable indication due to its considerable variation. *See also* DIAGNOSTIC FEATURES, EARS.

titanum dioxide. CAS number 13463-67-7. White pigment used in paints. Human skin irritant. Questionable evidence of animal carcinogenicity. No evidence of human carcinogenicity. *See also* LEWIS, HCDR, NUMBER TGG760.

titanium tetrachloride. CAS number 7550-45-0. Not found naturally in the environment. Manufactured from titanium-containing minerals and is used to make metallic titanium, titanium dioxide and other titanium compounds. An irritant to skin, eyes, mucus membranes and lungs due to its interaction with water to form hydrochloric acid, excessive exposure can result in chemical bronchitus, pneumonia and death. Severe burns may result from contact with liquid titanium tetrachloride. Although long-term, high-dose studies caused lung tumors in rodents, IARC and other agencies have not classified titanium tetrachloride for its potential as a human carcinogen. *See also* ATSDR DOCUMENT, JUNE 1994; LEWIS, HCDR, NUMBER TGH350.

tissue sampling. *See* SAMPLING, TISSUE.

TK locus (thymidine kinase locus). The TK locus allows cultured mammalian cells to incorporate pyrimidines from the medium so that these pyrimidines may be converted into nucleic acids. A mutation at this locus prevents uptake of pyrimidines, both normal and toxic, such as bromodeoxyuridine or trifluorothymidine; with toxic pyrimidines, such a mutation allows growth of the cultured cells since they can produce pyrimidines by de novo synthesis. This concept is utilized in some mutagenicity tests in which cultured mammalian cells are exposed to toxic pyrimidines in addition to possible mutagens; growth of these cells indicates that a mutation in the TK locus has occurred. *See also* CHINESE HAMSTER OVARY CELLS; EUKARYOTE MUTAGENICITY TESTS; MAMMALIAN CELL MUTATION TESTS; MOUSE LYMPHOMA CELLS.

TLC. *See* CHROMATOGRAPHY, THIN-LAYER.

TLV. *See* THRESHOLD LIMIT VALUE.

TLV-C. *See* THRESHOLD LIMIT VALUE, CEILING.

TLV-Ceiling. *See* THRESHOLD LIMIT VALUE, CEILING.

TLV-STEL. *See* THRESHOLD LIMIT VALUE, SHORT-TERM EXPOSURE LIMIT.

TLV-TWA. *See* THRESHOLD LIMIT VALUE, TIME-WEIGHTED AVERAGE.

T lymphocytes. *See* T CELLS.

tobacco. *Nicotiana tabacum*, the cultured tobacco of commerce, is widely used either by inhaling the smoke derived by burning the cured leaf in cigarettes, cigars or pipes, by chewing the cured leaf or by sniffing dried preparations of the leaf. Although the native leaf contains 1–6% of the toxic alkaloid, nicotine, blending of different varieties is used to maintain a concentration of 1–2% nicotine in tobacco products. Tobacco smoke contains numerous toxic chemicals including organic carcinogens such as polycyclic aromatic hydrocarbons and aromatic amines, inorganic carcinogens such as polonium 210 and arsenic and toxic alkaloids such as nicotine. Nicotine extracted from tobacco has also been used as an insecticide. *See also* NICOTINE; POLYCYCLIC AROMATIC HYDROCARBONS.

tobacco smoke. Smoke produced by burning tobacco products in cigarettes, cigars, pipes, etc. *See also* MAIN-STREAM SMOKE; SECONDHAND SMOKE; SIDE-STREAM SMOKE.

TOCP (tri-o-cresyl phosphate; TCP; tri-o-tolyl phosphate; TOTP). A plasticizer in lacquers and varnishes, an additive in lubricants and gasoline, and a flame retardant. It has low acute toxicity, but acts as a neurotoxicant producing delayed neuropathy after activation to *O*-2-tolyl *O,O*-saligenin cyclic phosphate. It is a neurotoxic esterase inhibitor and cholinesterase inhibitor, causing typical delayed neuropathy syndrome. *See also* DELAYED NEUROPATHY; MIPAFOX; NEUROTOXIC ESTERASE.

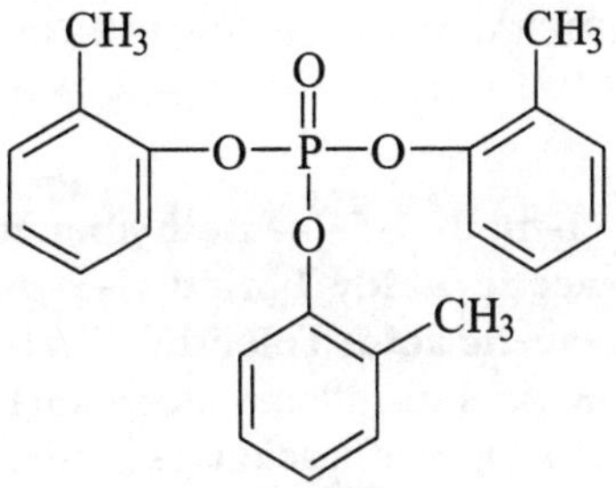

TOCP

Tofranil. *See* IMIPRAMINE.

Tolectin. *See* TOLMETIN.

tolerance. (1) An adaptational state when, after repeated exposure, a given dose of an agent produces a decreased effect or, conversely, when increasingly larger doses are necessary to obtain the effects observed with the original dose. Acute or rapid tolerance development may also occur following the administration of ethanol or benzodiazepines. Two mechanisms of acquired pharmacological tolerance are generally recognized: (a) dispositional; (b) pharmacodynamic. Dispositional tolerance results from alterations in the pharmacokinetic properties of the agent. Pharmacodynamic tolerance results from adaptive changes within affected systems, such that the response is reduced in the presence of the same concentration of the agent. Tolerance may not develop uniformly to all the actions of an agent. The toxicological manifestation of tolerance development is typically expressed as a progressive increase in the LD50 for a given agent, although it should be recognized that tolerance development is not absolute. (2) The amount of pesticide residue permitted on agricultural products in the USA under the Federal Insecticide, Fungicide and Rodenticide Act (FIFRA). If no detectable residues of a particular pesticide are permitted, it is said to have a zero tolerance. (3) For medicines "tolerance" of the marketed dosage form is established as well as consideration of the potential toxicity of the components and the whole. Tolerance is usually demonstrated in the "target species" (man for human medicines) at several (at least three, possibly up to five) times the normal maximum dose. Besides systemic effects, such aspects as local irritation, injection site reaction, etc., will be checked for. *See also* ADAPTATION TO TOXICANTS; FEDERAL INSECTICIDE, FUNGICIDE AND RODENTICIDE ACT.

tolmetin (1-methyl-5-(4-methylbenzoyl)-1H-pyrole-2-acetic acid; 1-methyl-5-*p*-toluoyl-pyrrole-2-acetic acid; Tolectin). CAS number 26171-23-3. An anti-inflammatory, analgesic and antipyretic that is as efficacious as moderate doses of aspirin and better tolerated. Tolmetin produces a number of adverse effects including epigastric pain, dyspepsia, nausea and vomiting. Tolmetin is approximately 99% plasma protein bound, yet does not interfere with concurrent treatment with oral hypoglycemics. Tolmetin has been found to be effective in the treatment of osteoarthritis and rheumatoid arthritis. *See also* ANALGESICS; ANTI-INFLAMMATORY AGENTS.

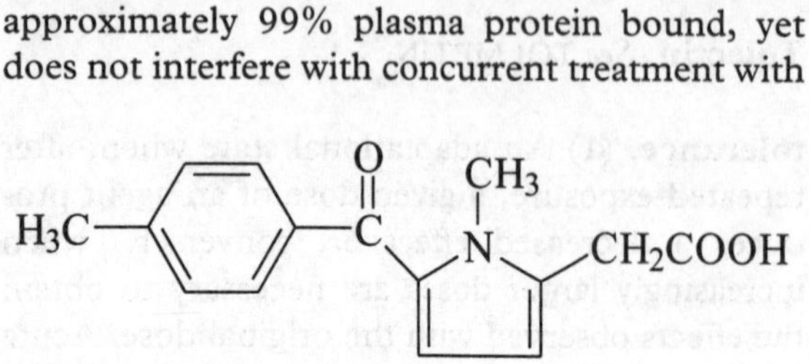

toluene (methylbenzene). CAS number 108-88-3. A colorless flammable liquid used in the synthesis of toluene diisocyanate, phenol, nitrotoluenes, saccharin and a variety of benzyl, benzoyl and benzoic acid derivatives. It is also used as a paint solvent and as a component of fuels. Toluene can enter the body by inhalation of the vapor or by ingestion or percutaneous absorption of the liquid. Locally, toluene can cause irritation of skin, eyes and mucous membranes. Systemically, it can cause CNS depression leading, in severe cases, to coma. Toluene has been shown in animal experiments to have deleterious effects on the male reproductive system and on the respiratory system. It is also known to inhibit the metabolism of benzene to toxic metabolites and thus, in this case, may exert a protective effect. No evidence for animal or human carcinogenicity. *See also* ATSDR DOCUMENT, MAY 1994.

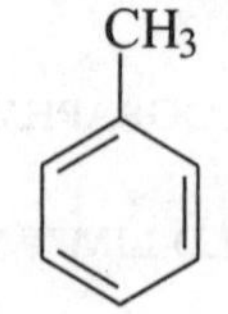

Toluene

toluene diisocyanate (TDI). CAS number 26471-62-5. A designated hazardous waste (EPA). It is a colorless to yellow solid, melting at about 20 °C. TDI and MDI (diphenylmethane diisocyanate) are used in the manufacture of polyurethane foams by reaction with polyhydroxy compounds. These foams are used for insulation, upholstering, etc. Exposure is commonly by inhalation of the vapor. Both TDI and MDI can cause irritation of eyes and mucous membranes, in

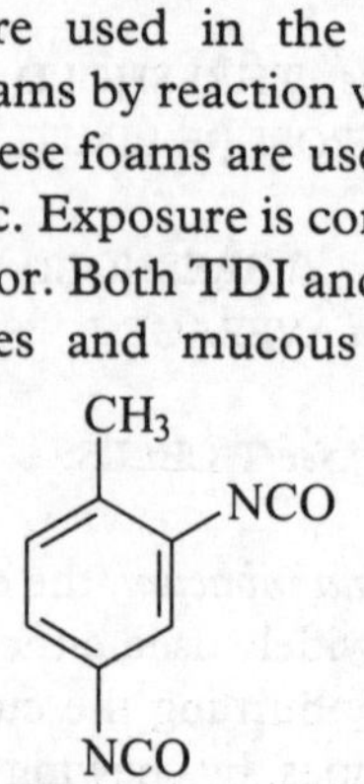

Toluene diisocyanate

Tolmetin

severe cases leading to pulmonary edema. Sensitization to TDI is common and frequently rapid, leading to an allergic reactions and some loss of lung function. In the UK, the threshold limit value is 0.02 ppm for not more than 20 minutes, or 0.005 ppm for 8 hours.

***m*-toluidine (3-methylbenzamide, 3-aminotoluene, 3-methylaniline). CAS number 10844-1.** *See* LEWIS, HCDR NUMBER TGQ500; DATABASES, TOXICOLOGY.

***o*-toluidine (*o*-aminotoluene; *o*-methylaniline). CAS number 95-53-4.** A designated suspected human carcinogen (IARC) and a hazardous waste (EPA). It is a colorless to pale yellow liquid with a slight aromatic odor. *o*-Toluidine is used as an intermediate in the synthesis of dyes and drugs, as well as in the rubber industry. It can enter the body by inhalation, dermal absorption or ingestion, the symptoms being anoxia, cyanosis, drowsiness, etc. However, the principal concern over *o*-toluidine use is its probable carcinogenicity. *See also* LEWIS, HCDR NUMBER TGQ750; DATABASES, TOXICOLOGY.

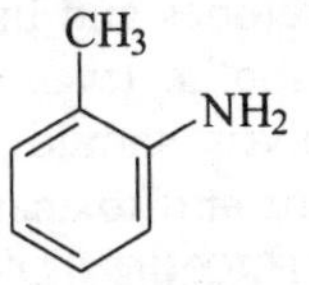

o-Toluidine

***p*-toluidine (4-methylbenzamide, 4-aminotoluene, 4-methylaniline). CAS number 106-49-0.** *See* LEWIS, HCDR NUMBER TGR000; DATABASES, TOXICOLOGY.

tonic. The body rigidity that is characteristic of a generalized tonic-clonic seizure. This body rigidity (tonic) often alternates with involuntary muscle contractions (clonic) during the course of such a seizure. The generalized tonic-clonic convulsions (grand mal) and focal convulsions are usually controlled by such drugs as carbamazepine or diphenylhydantoin. *See also* CLONIC; CONVULSIONS; SEIZURES.

Torrey Canyon. *See* ENVIRONMENTAL DISASTERS.

TOTP. *See* TOCP.

toxalbumin. *See* ABRIN.

toxaphene (polychlorocamphene). CAS number 8001-35-2. A complex mixture of more than 100 individual chlorinated camphene compounds and isomers. Recent research, however, has shown that most of the insecticidal activity is attributable to a few compounds, primarily two octachlorocamphenes. Once widely used on a variety of crops, and to a lesser extent on livestock, all registrations of toxaphene in the USA have now been cancelled. The mode of action of toxaphene is not clearly known, but is probably the same as that of the chlorinated cyclodienes (e.g., dieldrin, endrin). The oral LD50 in rats is 69 mg/kg toxicant. Based on animal studies has been designated by the EPA as a probable human carcinogen. Based on marginal effects in animal studies and cancellation of registration, is unlikely to represent a health risk. *See also* ATSDR DOCUMENT, AUGUST 1996; DATABASES, TOXICOLOGY; POISON.

toxicant. Any chemical, of natural or synthetic origin, capable of causing a deleterious effect on a living organism. The term toxin should never be used as a synonym for toxicant, being properly reserved for only those toxicants synthesized metabolically by a living organism.

toxicant administration. *See* ADMINISTRATION OF TOXICANTS.

toxicant–receptor interactions. The mechanism of toxic action of many toxicants can be shown to require an initial step where there is a binding of the toxicant to one or more populations of relatively high-affinity specific biological sites or receptors. In such cases, these interactions can be modeled by the law of mass action, and studied using enzyme kinetics or radioreceptor methods. Although the receptor site at which a toxicant acts is frequently one for which there is an endogenous ligand (e.g., an enzyme substrate or neurotransmitter), it is not obligatory that a toxicant receptor site serves a role in physiological regulation or intermediary metabolism. *See also* ENZYME KINETICS; RADIORECEPTOR ASSAYS; RECEPTORS.

toxic elements. *See* TOXIC METALS.

toxic endpoint, critical. That toxic endpoint that occurs at the lowest dose when a given chemical chemical causes more than one toxic effect. The critical endpoint is of importance in regulatory toxicology as it is used in the estimation of risk reference doses.

toxic endpoints. Although the information required from subchronic and chronic tests varies somewhat from one regulatory agency to another, the requirements are basically similar. Despite the fact that the data collected may be limited to that required for a particular regulatory purpose, additional information can be obtained from a more complete test. The data are of two types: (1) interim data which can be obtained from living animals during the course of the test; (2) termination data which are obtained from animals sacrificed either during or at the end of the test period. Many of the tests performed on living animals are first carried out before the test begins to provide a baseline for comparison to subsequent measurements. In subchronic tests, treated animals can be removed from the treated food at the end of the test period and returned to the control diet for 21–28 days while various endpoints are followed to establish whether or not the effects noted are reversible. Autopsies are performed on all animals found dead or moribund during the test. *See also* CHRONIC TOXICITY TESTING; SUBCHRONIC TOXICITY TESTING; TOXIC ENDPOINTS, INTERIM TESTS; TOXIC ENDPOINTS, TERATOLOGY; TOXIC ENDPOINTS, TERMINATION TESTS.

toxic endpoints, interim tests. Tests carried out before the study to establish baselines, at intervals during the study, and at the end of the study, prior to sacrifice. The timing will depend on whether the test is chronic or subchronic and on the predicted length of the test. Appearance, mortality and morbidity, as well as the condition of the skin, fur, mucous membranes and orifices, are checked daily and the presence of palpable masses or external lesions noted. Ophthalmological examination of

both cornea and retina is carried out at the beginning and end of the study. Food consumption is measured daily, as is body weight. Neurological response and behavioral abnormalities can also be measured, but generally at longer intervals. Rate and regularity of respiration may be noted daily. Electrocardiogram and electroencephalogram can also be monitored, particularly with larger animals. Hematological examination should ideally be carried out pretest and monthly thereafter. Hemoglobin, hematocrit, red and white cell and differential counts, platelets, reticulocytes and clotting parameters are noted. Blood chemistry should also be carried out pretest and monthly. Electrolytes and electrolyte balance, acid/base balance, glucose, urea nitrogen, serum lipids, serum proteins (albumin:globulin ratio), enzymes indicative of organ damage such as transaminases and phosphatases, as well as plasma and RBC cholinesterase, are measured. Ideally toxicant and metabolite levels are determined, but this is often done in a separate metabolism study, using a radiolabeled toxicant. Urinalysis again should be carried out pretest and monthly. Microscopic appearance (sediment, cells, stones, etc.), pH, specific gravity, chemical analysis for reducing sugars, proteins, ketones and bilirubin, as well as toxicant and metabolite levels should be determined. Fecal analysis should determine occult blood, fluid content and toxicant and metabolite levels. *See also* CHRONIC TOXICITY TESTING; SUBCHRONIC TOXICITY TESTING; TESTING VARIABLES, BIOLOGICAL; TESTING VARIABLES, NON-BIOLOGICAL.

toxic endpoints, teratology. Teratological anomalies may be variations that do not adversely affect the fetus or have a fatal outcome, or they may be malformations having adverse effects on the fetus. The distinction is difficult to define and may be academic, since any dose-related increase, even in variations known to occur in controls, is generally regarded as evidence of teratogenic potential. An example of such a variation is the number of ribs in the rabbit. Common external anomalies are determined by examination of the fetuses fixed in Bouin's fixative or by the method of Staples and by hand sectioning by the method of Wilson. Common visceral anomalies are also determined. Skeletal anomalies are examined by first fixing and clearing the fetus and then staining with Alizarin Red. Although there are numerous skeletal variations that are not uncommon in controls and may not have an adverse effect on the fetus, their frequency of occurrence may be dose-related and is evaluated. Almost all chemically related malformations have been seen in control animals, and essentially all such malformations are known to be produced by more than one cause, thus great care and a conservative approach are necessary in the interpretation of teratology studies. It has been suggested that some of the offspring born to dams treated for teratology evaluation be allowed to survive and later be subjected to behavioral tests as they develop, thus detecting functional deficits either not apparent morphologically or that appear later in development. Physiological functions such as growth rate, kidney function, liver function, EEG and EKG could also be examined. *See also* TERATOGENIC FACTORS; TERATOGENIC MECHANISMS.

toxic endpoints, termination tests. Tests that are carried out at the end of the test period following sacrifice of the animals. Since the number of tissues that may be sampled is large and the number of microscopic methods is also large (*see* Table 9), all previous results are considered before carrying out the pathological examination. Clinical tests or blood chemistry analyses may indicate that a particular target organ should be examined in greater detail. All control and high-dose animals are examined and if lesions are found, the next-lowest-dose group is examined for these lesions, and this is continued until a no-effect group is reached. Since pathology as utilized in chronic toxicity tests is largely a descriptive science that has a complex terminology, it is critical that the terminology be defined at the beginning of the study and that the same pathologist(s) examine the slides from both treated and control animals. Quality control, slide identification and data recording are also critical. Many tissues are examined, each yielding a number of tissue blocks to be sectioned. Since all of the slides are to be stained, comparable quality of staining and accurate correlation of a particular slide with its parent block, tissue and animal are critical. The necropsy must be conducted with care to avoid post-mortem damage to the specimens. Tissues are removed, weighed and examined closely for gross lesions, masses, etc. Tissues are then fixed for subsequent histological examination, usually in neutral buffered formalin or Millonigs phosphate-buffered formalin. The tissues listed in Table 9 plus any lesions, masses or abnormal tissues are embedded, sectioned and stained for light microscopy. Paraffin embedding and staining with hematoxylin and eosin are the routine methods, but special stains may be used for particular tissues or for certain lesions. Electron microscopy is also used for more specific examination of lesions or cellular changes after their initial localization by more routine methods. *See also* CARCINOGENICITY TESTING; CHRONIC TOXICITY TESTING; SUBCHRONIC TOXICITY TESTING; TESTING VARIABLES, BIOLOGICAL; TESTING VARIABLES, NON-BIOLOGICAL.

Table 9 Tissues and organs to be examined histologically in carcinogenicity; chronic and subchronic toxicity tests.

Adrenals	Mesenteric lymph
Bone, including bone	node
marrow	Nasal cavity
Brain	Ovaries
Cecum	Pancreas
Colon	Parathyroids
Cartilage	Pituitary
Duodenum	Prostate
Esophagus	Rectum
Eyes	Salivary gland
Gallbladder	Sciatic nerve
Heart	Seminal vesicles
Ileum	Skin
Jejunum	Spleen
Kidneys	Spinal cord
Larynx	Stomach
Liver	Testes
Lungs and Bronchi	Thigh muscle
Lymph nodes	Thyroid
Mammary glands	Thymus
Mandibular lymph	Urinary bladder
node	Uterus

toxicity. The ability of a chemical to cause a deleterious effect when the organism is exposed to the chemical. *See also* ACUTE TOXICITY, CHRONIC TOXICITY.

toxicity, acute. *See* ACUTE TOXICITY.

toxicity assessment. A summation of the toxic properties of a chemical including its absorption, metabolism, excretion and mechanism of action. Used in the risk assessment process.

toxicity, chronic. *See* CHRONIC TOXICITY.

toxicity, subchronic. *See* SUBCHRONIC TOXICITY.

toxicity classes. Both toxicity and toxicants have been classified in many different ways. All of these systems have some utility, but none are entirely satisfactory. Some examples are: (1) mode of action (e.g., carcinogens, mutagens, teratogens, hepatotoxicants, etc.); (2) origin (e.g., mycotoxins, botanicals, etc.); (3) chemical class (e.g., alcohols, polycyclic aromatic hydrocarbons, glycols, etc.); (4) use class (e.g., pesticides, drugs of abuse, therapeutic drugs, industrial solvents, etc.); (5) distribution (e.g., water pollutants, air pollutants, soil contaminants, etc.). Since any mode of action can be brought about by chemicals from many different classes, and chemical and use classes all include chemicals capable of causing numerous different delerious effects, it is apparent that the classification suited to the particular task at hand must be used, with the use of different classifications for different purposes.

toxicity testing. The determination of the potential of a substance to act as a poison and the conditions under which this potential is realized. Risk assessment, on the other hand, is a quantitative assessment of the probability of deleterious effects. Both are involved in the regulation of toxic chemicals, which is the control, by statute, of the manufacture, transportation, sale or disposal of chemicals deemed toxic under criteria laid down under the law in question. Tests are generally *in vivo* for acute, subchronic or chronic effects and *in vitro* for genotoxicity or cell transformation, although other tests are also used. Chemicals introduced into commerce or being developed for introduction into commerce are subject to toxicity testing in one or more countries with appropriate regulations, as are those in the waste products of industrial processes. Although routine, toxicity testing is often controversial. Among the areas of controversy are the use of animals for testing and the welfare of the animals used, extrapolation from experimental animals to humans, extrapolation from high- to low-dose effects, choice of animals and genetic strains, and the increasing cost and complexity of testing protocols relative to the benefits expected. *See also* ACUTE TOXICITY TESTING; BEHAVIORAL TOXICITY TESTING; CHRONIC TOXICITY TESTING; COVALENT-BINDING TESTS; DELAYED NEUROPATHY TESTS; HUMAN TEST DATA; HUMAN TOXICITY TESTING; IMMUNOTOXICITY TESTING; METABOLISM TESTS; NEUROTOXICITY TESTING; POTENTIATION TESTS; SUBCHRONIC TOXICITY TESTING.

toxicity test sequences. *See* TESTING SEQUENCES.

toxic metals. Metals or compounds of metals that are toxic in nature. Recently, the term toxic elements has been used. *See also* CADMIUM; HEAVY METALS; LEAD; MERCURY; THALLIUM; TRIETHYLLEAD; TRIETHYLTIN; TRIMETHYLTIN.

toxicodynamics. The relationship between toxicant concentration and effect, with specific emphasis on mechanism(s) of action. In particular, toxicodynamics deals with the study of physiological, biochemical and molecular effects of toxicants, and the underlying mechanisms of action. Toxicodynamics allows the generation of models of toxicant action and the testing of these models according to basic chemical principles of mass action. Elucidation of basic toxicokinetic parameters allows the most accurate understanding and prediction of toxicity. *See also* TOXICODYNAMICS, IN TOXICITY TESTING; TOXICOKINETICS.

toxicodynamics, in toxicity testing. A knowledge of both the toxicodynamics and toxicokinetics of a compound or mixture under study is required both to gain insight into how a toxicant effects a given system and to ensure more efficient and reliable testing. Usually, the study of toxicokinetics and toxicodynamics cannot be separated, but must be conducted interactively. By elucidating sites of action, and underlying biochemical and molecular mechanisms, toxicodynamic studies permit construction of predictive models that can be tested experimentally. In addition, they assist in prediction of possible therapeutic modalities, other sites of action for the same toxicant, factors to consider in cross-species comparisons, etc. *See also* ENZYME KINETICS; TOXICOKINETICS, IN TOXICITY TESTING.

toxicokinetics. The study of the absorption, distribution and elimination of toxic compounds in the living organism. Typically, doses of a substance known to possess toxic properties are administered and, in addition to observation for potential toxic effects, the concentration of the substance in blood or other biological tissues is measured. The kinetic parameters determined from these studies are then used to predict the concentrations expected by exposure to other single doses, to chronic doses or exposure by other routes. With sufficient data, it may be possible to perform inter-species comparisons and predictions. *See also* CLEARANCE; COMPARTMENT; FIRST-PASS EFFECT; FIRST-ORDER KINETICS; KINETIC EQUATIONS; KINETIC EQUATIONS, ELIMINATION; KINETIC EQUATIONS, HEPATIC CLEARANCE; KINETIC EQUATIONS, NONLINEAR; KINETIC EQUATIONS, PLASMA PROTEIN BINDING; KINETIC EQUATIONS, RENAL CLEARANCE; KINETIC EQUATIONS, UPTAKE; MULTI-COMPARTMENT MODELS; ONE-COMPARTMENT MODEL; PHARMACOKINETICS; PROBIT/LOG TRANSFORMS; PROBITS; TWO-COMPARTMENT MODEL; VOLUME OF DISTRIBUTION.

toxicokinetics, in toxicity testing. A knowledge of the toxicokinetics and metabolism of a potential toxicant can give valuable insight and provide for more efficient and more informative testing, providing the necessary background to make the most appropriate selection of test animal species, dose levels and method for extrapolating from animal studies to human hazard. Furthermore, such tests may provide information on possible reactive intermediates, as well as information on induction or inhibition of the enzymes of xenobiotic metabolism. Toxicokinetic studies are designed to measure the amount and rate of the absorption, distribution, metabolism and excretion of a xenobiotic. These data are used to construct predictive mathematical models so that the distribution and excretion of other doses can be simulated. Such studies

are generally carried out using radiolabeled compounds to facilitate the measurement and total recovery of the administered dose, although modern chromatographic and detection methods allow such studies with the unlabeled compound. They can be done entirely *in vivo* with examination of blood levels of the compound administered and its metabolites in expired air, feces and urine or tissue levels measured by sequential sacrifice and analysis of organ levels. *See also* METABOLISM TESTS; TOXICODYNAMICS, IN TOXICITY TESTING.

toxicology. The science that deals with poisons (toxicants) and their effects. A poison is defined as any substance that causes a harmful effect, either by accident or design, when administered to a living organism. There are difficulties, both in bringing more precise definition to the meaning of poison, and in the definition and measurement of toxic effect. Broader definitions of toxicology such as the study of the detection, occurrence, properties, effects and regulation of toxic substances, although more descriptive, do not resolve these difficulties. The attempts at their resolution do, however, circumscribe the perimeter of the science of toxicology.

toxicology computer databases. There are a number of both bibliographic and factual databases devoted in whole or in part to toxicology and available for on-line searches. Two of the most important are Toxline and Toxicology Database. *See also* DATABASES, TOXICOLOGY; TOXLINE.

Toxicology Database. An on-line factual computer database containing reviewed information on the toxicology of chemicals. Information on nomenclature, threshold limit values, pharmacology/toxicology and physical and chemical properties is compiled for each chemical from the peer-reviewed literature. It is made available for on-line search by the National Library of Medicine, Bethesda, Maryland. *See also* DATABASES, TOXICOLOGY; TOXLINE.

toxicology databases, electronic. *See* DATABASES, TOXICOLOGY, ELECTRONIC.

toxicology databases, printed. *See* DATABASES, TOXICOLOGY, PRINTED.

Toxicology Study Section. Formerly a part of the Division of Research Grants of the National Institutes of Health (USA), with responsibility for reviews of applications for research grants in all aspects of toxicology, but especially those with implications for human health.

toxicovigilance. Monitoring for suspected deleterious reactions (in man, animals and the environment) to medicines, pesticides, contaminants or other chemicals. Includes all activity tending to provide indications of probable causal links between chemical usage (when applied at the normal rate, for the designated purpose) and adverse reactions in a population of man or of animals. Pharmacovigilance is the term used specifically for clinical drugs.

Toxic Substances Control Act (TSCA). A US act enacted in 1976. It provides the EPA with the authority to require testing and, where necessary, regulate chemicals, both old and new, entering the environment. It was intended to supplement sections of several existing laws—Clean Air Act, Clean Water Act and Occupational Safety and Health Act—already providing for regulation of chemicals. TSCA requires manufacturers to submit information to allow the EPA to identify and evaluate the potential hazards of a chemical prior to its introduction into commerce. Where necessary, the act also provides for the regulation of production, use, distribution and disposal of chemicals.

toxic waste. See HAZARDOUS WASTE.

toxin. A toxicant produced by a living organism.

Toxline. A bibliographic computer database made available for on-line searches by the National Library of Medicine, Bethesda, Maryland. Formed by merger of several pre-existing files, this is probably the major bibliographical database for toxicological literature in that it contains over one million references. See also TOXICOLOGY DATABASE.

trachea. The tubular structure in mammals that passes from the larynx to the point at which it bifurcates into the bronchi; part of the airway to the lungs. It is lined with ciliated mucus-secreting epithelium and is supported by rings of cartilage that prevent collapse during respiration. Since gas exchange does not occur in the trachea, it is part of the "anatomical dead space."

tracheobronchial clearance. See NASOPHARYNGEAL CLEARANCE.

transcription. RNA synthesis from a DNA template. Transcription is catalyzed by RNA polymerases and is nuclear in eukaryotic cells except in the cases of mitochondrial and chloroplast transcription. Distinct species of RNA polymerase are responsible for the transcription of ribosomal RNA genes, transfer RNA and 5S RNA genes, and genes coding for protein. During transcription, the polymerase first recognizes the promoter sequence, which lies upstream of the coding sequence, then moves down past the initiation codon, assembling an RNA polynucleotide chain with precise complementary base pairing to the sense strand of the DNA double helix. In prokaryotes some polycistronic messages exist and transcription may proceed along a considerable length of DNA without interruption. In this case a number of genes are included in one transcription unit. See also TRANSLATION.

transferases. See ENZYMES.

transformation. See CELL TRANSFORMATION.

translation. Synthesis of protein with an amino acid sequence dictated by the code of base triplets on the messenger RNA (mRNA). Ribosomes are the sites of translation, at which the mRNAs to be translated and the transfer RNA (tRNA) molecules charged with amino acids are brought together. The anticodon triplet on the tRNA molecule aligns with a codon triplet on the mRNA, thus bringing its associated amino acid into line. Peptide bonds formed between amino acids allow polymerization of the growing polypeptide chain. One mRNA molecule is normally associated with numerous ribosomes, which together form a polysome. The mRNA is read from the 5'- to the 3'-terminus, and the synthesis of the protein proceeds from the amino end to the carboxyl end.

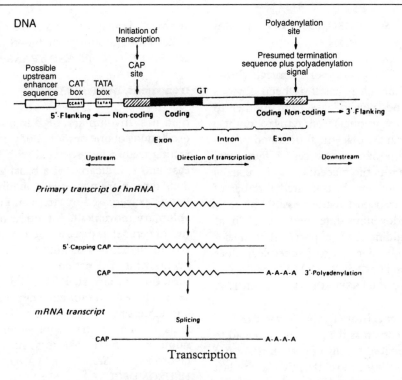

Transcription

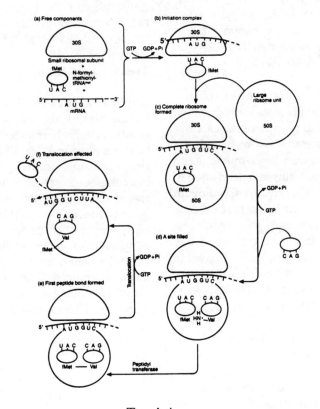

Translation

translocation. *See* CHROMOSOME ABERRATIONS.

transplacental. The passage of chemicals across the placenta. Although it has long been obvious that nutrients and oxygen pass from mother to fetus and excretory products from fetus to mother, it was believed that the placenta functioned to protect the fetus from toxic substances. In fact, toxic materials pass across the placenta readily, usually by passive diffusion, or, in a limited number of cases, by active transport made possible by their similarity to endogenous intermediates such as purines or pyrimidines. It is apparent that the so-called "placental barrier" for toxic chemicals does not exist. *See also* PLACENTA; TRANSPLACENTAL CARCINOGENESIS; TRANSPLACENTAL TOXICITY.

transplacental carcinogenesis. A few carcinogenic chemicals can cross the placenta and lead to neoplastic conversion in cells of certain tissues of the fetus, usually those most sensitive in the last trimester of the pregnancy. High dosages of certain hormones (e.g., diethylstilbestrol) can affect the development of the endocrine system and lead to neoplasms in the offspring, often at puberty, in specific endocrine-sensitive tissues.

transplacental toxicity. Toxicity due to chemicals transported across the placenta is the principal cause of teratogenicity and transplacental carcinogenesis, although the latter may not be manifested until long after birth. However, pre-implantation and early implantation mortality are clearly due to toxic effects on the germinal cells, fertilized ovum or the early stages of differentiation that precede placenta formation. Although the xenobiotic enzyme activity of the fetus and embryo is low compared with that of adults, it is becoming increasingly obvious that activation reactions are of importance in teratogenesis. *See also* PLACENTA; TERATOGENIC MECHANISMS.

Transportation Act. *See* HAZARDOUS MATERIALS TRANSPORTATION ACT.

transport of toxicants. The mechanisms that bring about movement of toxicants and their metabolites from one site in the organism to another. Transport usually involves binding to either blood albumins or blood lipoproteins. *See also* BINDING SITES AND TRANSPORT.

treatment. *See* THERAPY.

tremors. Involuntary, high-frequency rhythmical oscillations of one or more body parts. In humans, resting tremor is associated with Parkinson's disease and is indicative of a basal ganglia disorder. This type of tremor usually involves the extremities, is exacerbated by stress and is suppressed by voluntary movement. Intention tremor is indicative of cerebellar disease and occurs during voluntary movements, but not at rest. Postural tremor occurs while the patient is assuming a fixed posture, but not at rest. Parkinsonian tremor can be seen following treatment with antipsychotic and antidepressant drugs. Tremor in laboratory animals is one of the sequelae of exposure to a number of neurotoxicants such as DDT and chlordecone. *See also* DIAGNOSTIC FEATURES, NEUROMUSCULAR SYSTEM; 1-METHYL-4-PHENYL-1,2,3,6-TETRAHYDROPYRIDINE; NEUROBEHAVIORAL TERATOLOGY; NEUROBEHAVIORAL TOXICOLOGY; POSTNATAL BEHAVIORAL TESTS.

Trexan. *See* NALTREXONE.

triazine herbicides. A class of herbicides used for the control of annual grasses and broadleaf weeds. Triazine herbicides are based on a symmetrical triazine structure. This class includes atrazine, prometon, prometryn, propazine and simazine compounds which have acute oral LD50s in rats in the range 1780–7000 mg/kg. These compounds function as herbicides by inhibiting the Hill reaction in photosynthesis. Overdose in humans may cause abdominal pain, impaired adrenal function, anemia, dermatitis, diarrhea, eye irritation, mucous membrane irritation, nausea, disturbed thiamine and riboflavin function or vomiting. Therapy consists of: washing the skin

Triazine herbicides, general formula

with soap and water (dermal contact); flushing eyes with water for 15 minutes (eye contact); inducing vomiting (except with petroleum solvent formulations) (oral).

triaziquone. *See* 2,3,5-TRIS(1-AZIRIDINYL-*P*-BENZOQUINONE).

tributyltin (bis(tributyltin) oxide; TBTO; OTBE; Biomet TBTO; Butinox; hexabutyldistannoxane). An alkyltin compound used as a fungicide and molluscicide. The oral LD50 in male rats is 55 mg/kg for bis(tributyltin) oxide. There is currently a lack of data on the toxic effects of tributyltin, although it is suspected to affect the immune system and the nervous system. It is also a suspected teratogen. The mechanism of action is unknown. Symptoms in humans include headaches, stomach aches, dizziness, fatigue, blurred vision and chronic skin inflammation. There is no specific antidote; treatment is therefore symptomatic. *See also* ORGANOTINS.

trichlofos. *See* CHLORAL DERIVATIVES.

trichloroacetic acid (TCA). CAS number 76-03-9. A colorless, hygroscopic solid, used as a herbicide (sodium trichloroacetate) and as an intermediate in pesticide manufacture. TCA is also used in *in vitro* laboratory studies to stop enzyme reactions by precipitation of proteins. It is corrosive to the skin and eyes, but is not otherwise hazardous.

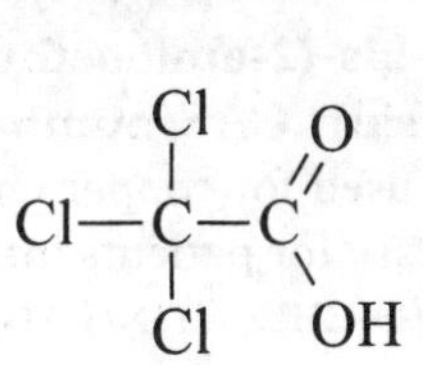

TCA

1,1,1-trichloro-bis(*p*-chlorophenyl)ethane. *See* DDT.

1,1,1-trichloroethane. *See* DRY-CLEANING SOLVENTS; METHYLCHLOROFORM.

2,2,2-trichloroethanol. CAS number 115-20-8. A hypnotic and anesthetic that is the active compound formed *in vivo* from chloral

hydrate and other chloral derivatives. The oral LD50 in rats is 600 mg/kg. *See also* CHLORAL DERIVATIVES; MICKEY FINN.

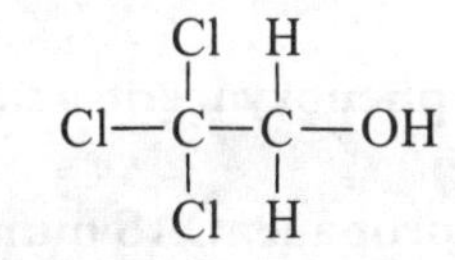

2,2,2-Trichloroethanol

trichloroethylene. CAS number 79-01-6. A compound formerly used as an anesthetic agent, and now sometimes used as a dry-cleaning solvent. Although less toxic than chloroform, it produces many of the same toxic effects. No evidence of teratogenic or carcinogenic effects. *See also* CHLOROFORM; DRY-CLEANING SOLVENTS; ATSDR DOCUMENT, APRIL 1993.

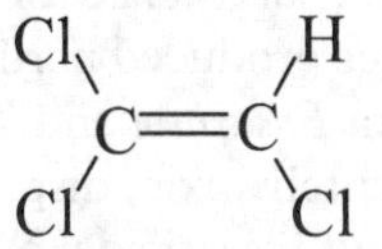

Trichloroethylene

trichlorogalactosucrose. *See* SWEETENING AGENTS.

trichloromethane. *See* CHLOROFORM.

trichlorophenols. Six isomers of trichlorophenol exist. They have been designated hazardous substances and priority toxic pollutants (EPA). The 2,4,5- and 2,4,6-isomers are designated hazardous wastes, and the 2,4,6-isomer is a designated potential carcinogen (EPA). 2,4,5-Trichlorophenol is used in the synthesis of the herbicide 2,4,5-T. 2,4,6-Trichlorophenol is used in the synthesis of pentachlorophenol and is also used directly as a bacteriocide, wood preservative and for mildew control. One of the principal toxicological problems associated with trichlorophenol is that at high temperatures two molecules of 2,4,5-trichlorophenol can combine to form a molecule of TCDD. The trichlorophenols

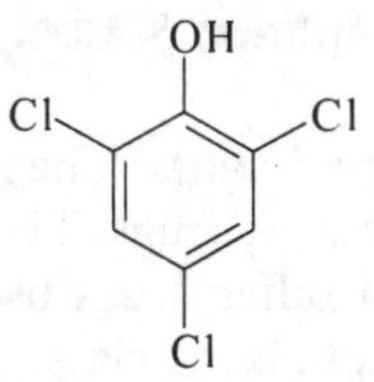

2,4,6-Trichlorophenol

themselves do not appear particularly toxic. How-ever, acute toxicity of the 2,4,5-isomer can lead to motor weakness and seizures. *See also* TCDD.

2,4,5-trichlorophenoxyacetic acid. *See* 2,4,5-T.

1,2,3-trichloropropane. CAS number 96-18-4. Synthetic intermediate, industrial solvent, paint remover and cleaner. Eye, skin and mucus mem-brane irritant on exposure to high ambient levels in air. Animal carcinogen, not known to be a human carcinogen. *See also* ATSDR DOCUMENT, SEPTEM-BER 1992; HCDR, NUMBER TJB600.

Triclos. *See* CHLORAL DERIVATIVES.

tricothecenes. A large class of sesquiterpenoid fungal metabolites produced particularly by mem-bers of the genera *Fusarium* and *Tricoderma*. They are frequently acutely toxic, displaying bacterioci-dal, fungicidal and insecticidal activity, as well as causing a variety of clinical symptoms in mam-mals, including diarrhea, anorexia and ataxia. They have been implicated in natural intoxications in both humans and animals, such as Abakabi dis-ease in Japan and stachybotryotoxicosis in the USSR, as well as being the center of a continuing controversy concerning their possible use as chemical warfare agents. The structure of T-2 toxin, most frequently suggested as a chemical warfare agent, is shown below. *See also* VOMI-TOXIN.

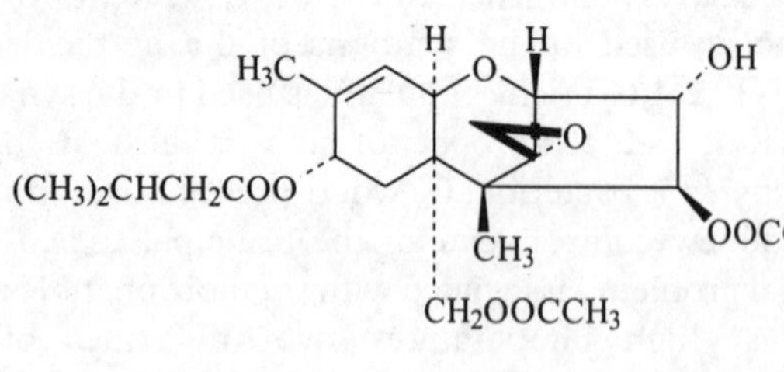

$(CH_3)_2CHCH_2COO$

CH_2OOCCH_3

T-2 toxin

tri-*o*-cresylphosphate. *See* TOCP.

tricyclic antidepressants. The most widely used class of antidepressant drugs. They share a tricyc-lic structure with other drugs used in psychiatry such as the phenothiazine class of antipsychotics. Full therapeutic effects often take several weeks to occur. The most important biochemical effect is believed to be potentiation of biogenic amine func-tion by inhibition of biogenic amine uptake in nerve terminals. As a result of this biochemical action, they interact with other drugs that affect synaptic function, such as amphetamine. Chronic use causes alterations in noradrenergic and seroto-nergic receptors, but the significance of this is uncertain. The tertiary amines in use (e.g., imi-pramine, amitriptyline, doxepin) are more potent in inhibiting serotonin uptake, whereas the secon-dary amines (e.g., desimipramine, nortriptyline) are better inhibitors of norepinephrine uptake. Many of the tricyclics have active metabolites that contribute to pharmacological and toxicological effects. The major side effects of the tricyclics are due to their inhibition of amine uptake, and their intrinsic anticholinergic properties. Cardiovascu-lar effects may occur, even at therapeutic doses, and anticholinergic side effects (e.g., dry mouth, epigastric distress, dizziness, tachycardia, urinary retention and confusion or delirium) also occur. Because of the potential cardiotoxicity, small quantities are usually prescribed to minimize the use of these drugs in suicide attempts. *See also* IMI-PRAMINE.

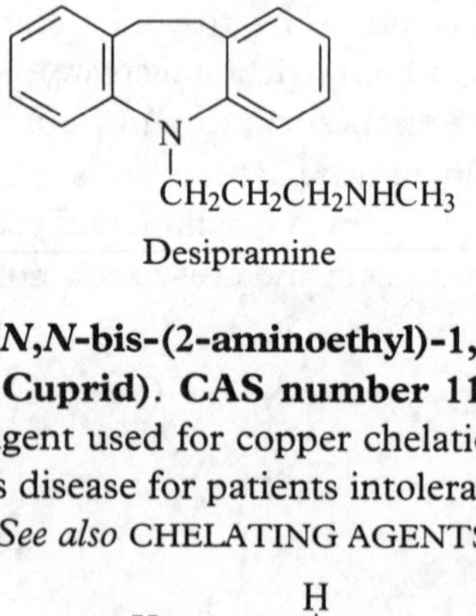

$CH_2CH_2CH_2NHCH_3$

Desipramine

trientine (*N*,*N*-bis-(2-aminoethyl)-1,2-ethane-diamine; Cuprid). CAS number 112-24-3. A chelating agent used for copper chelation therapy in Wilson's disease for patients intolerant of peni-cillamine. *See also* CHELATING AGENTS.

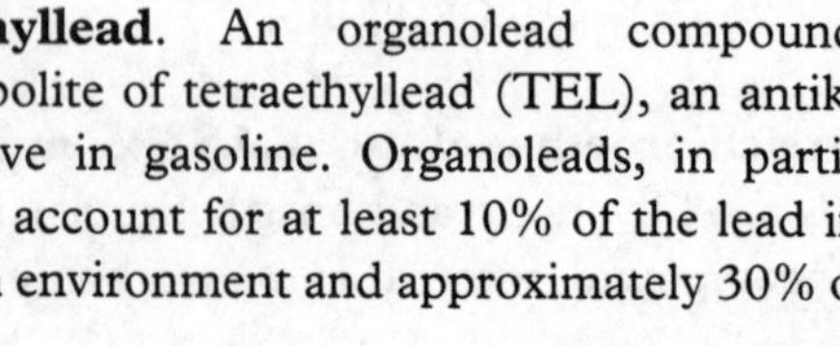

Trientine

triethyllead. An organolead compound; a metabolite of tetraethyllead (TEL), an antiknock additive in gasoline. Organoleads, in particular TEL, account for at least 10% of the lead in the urban environment and approximately 30% of the total lead in the human brain. There is also evidence that inorganic lead in the biosphere can be alkylated under appropriate conditions to more toxic organolead species. Triethyllead is a highly lipid-soluble neurotoxicant in both laboratory animals and man that causes extensive encephalopathy. TEL produces a different profile of toxicity and is more toxic on a mg/kg basis than inorganic lead and has been shown to preferentially affect the nervous system. The i.p. LD50 in male rats is 5 mg/kg for the chloride salt. The mode of action is unknown, but TEL may act primarily via effects on oxidative metabolism which then cause secondary effects such as on protein synthesis. Treatment of experimental animals with TEL does not cause the edema of white matter which is a hallmark of triethyltin. However, both TEL and trialkyltins, when administered during development, severely inhibit myelinogenesis. Clinical accounts of organolead poisonings have described a syndrome consisting of motor hyperexcitability, disorientation and a transient psychotic state involving hallucinations and paranoid ideation, with other symptoms including loss of appetite, nausea, vomiting, diarrhea, impotence and memory impairment. It has been reported that triethyllead intoxication results in decreased responses in behavioral tests of nociception, measures that have been considered to be an index of analgesia, possibly involving opioid peptide mechanism. The psychotic symptoms caused by triethyllead are attenuated by haloperidol, a dopamine receptor blocker, suggesting that dopaminergic hyperactivity (either at the neuronal or receptor level) may be caused by TEL intoxication. Chelation therapy is controversial. *See also* LEAD.

triethyltin (TET). An alkyltin compound occurring as an impurity in the manufacture of other alkyltin compounds. TET is neurotoxic, and in humans causes severe and persistent headache, nausea, vomiting, vertigo, visual disturbances, photophobia, transient paresis, permanent paralysis, meningial signs, papilloedema and convulsions. TET causes extensive myelinopathy characterized by intramyelin edema and damage to nerve terminals. There is actually a catabolism of myelin so that the concentrations of myelin-specific components (such as cerebroside and sulfatide) are decreased in whole brain. The myelin edema is relatively specific to the CNS, and even drastic pretreatment produces only minor changes in the peripheral nervous system. Newly forming CNS myelin is preferentially susceptible to degradation. The loss of myelin in adult rats brought about by TET intoxication is, to a large extent, reversible, in that myelin is readily synthesized after cessation of the toxicant treatment. In developing animals, administration of TET causes white matter edema, but few clinical signs, presumably because the open cranial fissures in the young rat prevent the development of increased intracranial pressure. The oral LD50 in male rats is approximately 10 mg/kg for TET sulfate. There is no specific antidote; treatment is therefore symptomatic. TET is a potent inhibitor of mitochondrial ATPases and of chloride/hydroxide exchange across membranes, and it affects the respiratory activity of tissue slices from various organs of the rat, with greatest effects in the nervous system. There does not seem to be any selective accumulation of TET in brain, although the TET that does enter brain could be enriched in a specific compartment.

triglycerides. Neutral fat comprises three fatty acids esterified to glycerol. The fatty acids may be saturated or unsaturated, and the most common ones are stearic, oleic and palmitic acids. This is the primary storage form of lipid as an energy reserve. Triglycerides are synthesized in adipose tissue from glycerol phosphate, derived from glucose, and from fatty acids, either derived from acetyl CoA formed from glucose or absorbed from the plasma after they are released from lipoproteins. Triglyceride synthesis in adipose cells is dependent upon insulin-stimulated uptake of plasma glucose. Whereas the amount of glycogen that can be stored as an energy reserve is limited, the amount of triglyceride stored appears to be essentially unlimited.

triiodothyronine (T3). *See* THYROID.

trimethylene. *See* CYCLOPROPANE.

trimethyltin. An alkyltin compound occurring as an impurity in manufacturing processes. The oral LD50 in male rats is 10 mg/kg for the chloride salt. Trimethyltin is a neurotoxicant that causes neuronal damage to sensory neurons of both the central and peripheral nervous systems. Trimethyltin also causes damage to the limbic system, specifically the hippocampus. The mode of action is, at present, unknown, although in the hippocampus damage to the machinery associated with neurotransmission may be preferentially affected. Symptoms in humans include headaches, fatigue, weakness, loss of libido and motivation, sleep disturbances, depression, fits of rage and seizures. There is no specific antidote; treatment is therefore symptomatic.

tripelennamine (*N,N*-**dimethylamino-***N'*-**(phenylmethyl)-***N'*-**2-pyridinyl-1,2-ethanediamine; 2-[benzyl(2-dimethylaminoethyl) amino]pyridine).** CAS number 91-81-6. An antihistamine with properties similar to those of diphenhydramine and related compounds. In a 1982 survey of police toxicology laboratories, this drug was one of the six most frequently detected analytes. The s.c. LD50 in mice is 210 mg/kg. *See also* ANTIHISTAMINES.

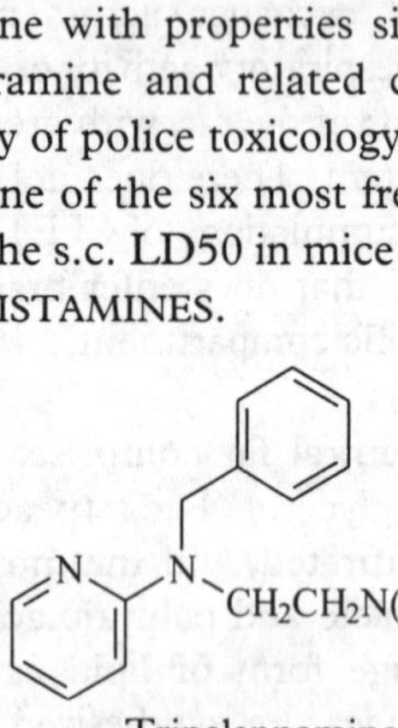

Tripelennamine

2,3,5-tris(1-aziridinyl)-benzoquinone (triaziquone). CAS number 68-76-8. An antineoplastic agent related to thiotepa. It has considerable acute toxicity and is a probable carcinogen. *See also* 2,3,5-TRIS(1-AZIRIDINYL)PHOSPHINE SULFIDE

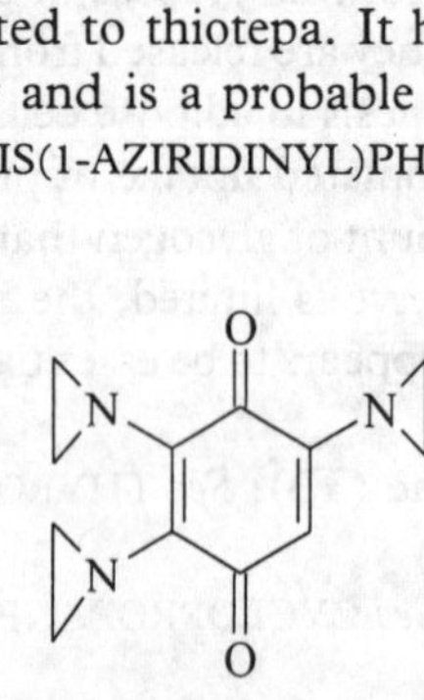

Tris(1-aziridinyl)-*p*-benzoquinone

2,3,5-tris(1-aziridinyl)phosphine sulfide (thiotepa). An antineoplastic agent. It is also used experimentally as an insect sterilant. It has been designated a carcinogen by EPA and IARC.

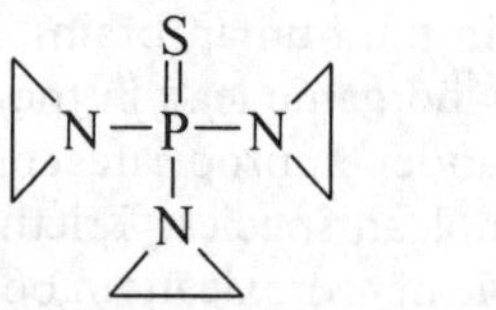

Tris(1-aziridinyl)phosphine sulfide

tris (2-chloroethyl) phosphate. A relatively high volume chemical used as a flame retardant in plastics and synthetic fibers. Does not appear to be either mutagenic or carcinogenic. Some mortality in subchronic (16 week) feeding studies in rats with lesions observed in the hippocampus.

trisomy. The state of having three representatives of a given chromosome instead of the usual pair, as in trisomy 21 (Downs syndrome).

tritium (^{3}H). A radioactive isotope of hydrogen, with mass number 3 and atomic mass 3.016. It occurs in natural hydrogen as one part in 10^{17}, but it can be made artificially in nuclear reactors. Its half-life is 12.5 years. Tritium is used extensively as a radiolabel tracer in toxicity studies.

tri-*o*-**tolylphosphate.** *See* TOCP.

tropan alkaloids. Constituents of such plants as *Atropa belladonna* (deadly nightshade), *Hyoscyamus niger* (henbane) and *Datura strammmonium* (thorn apple). Many are esters of tropine. *See also* TROPINE; ATROPINE; HYOSCYAMINE; HYOSCINE.

tropine (3-tropanol). CAS number 12-29-6. Obtained by hydrolysis of atropine. A *meso*-compound (mp 63 K, *pK*$_a$ 10.33), with secondary hydroxyl (oxidizable to ketone), tertiary amine with no double bonds.

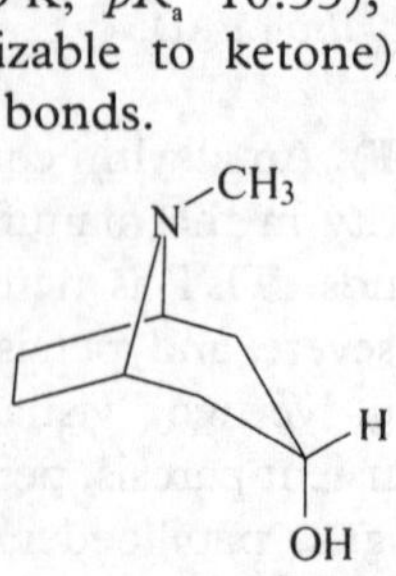

Tropine

trypan blue. CAS number 72-57-1. A vital dye that is used to determine the viability of isolated cells. Living cells exclude the dye, whereas nonviable cells do not.

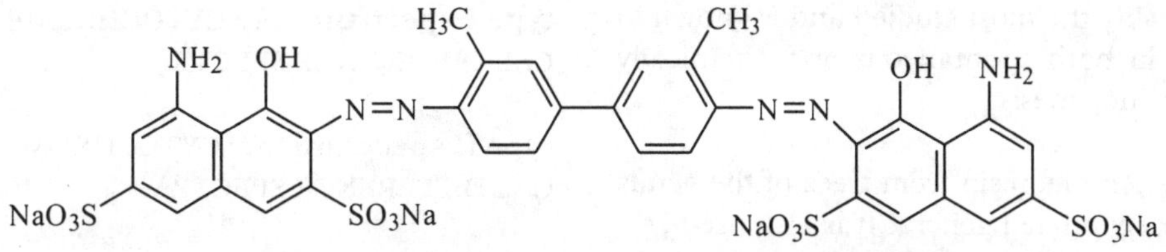

H₃C   CH₃

Trypan blue structure

Trypan blue

tryptophan hydroxylase (EC 1.14.16.4). An enzyme that is located in indoleamine-synthesizing cells and hydroxylates tryptophan at the 5-position to form 5-hydroxytryptophan (5-HTP), which is then decarboxylated by an L-aromatic amino acid decarboxylase to form 5-hydroxytryptamine (5-HT or serotonin). This enzyme requires oxygen and a tetrahydrobiopterin as a cofactor. The K_m has been estimated to be about 5×10^{-5}M. Because the substrate is not present in saturating concentrations, precursor availability is thought to influence significantly 5-HT concentrations in brain.

TSCA. *See* TOXIC SUBSTANCES CONTROL ACT.

TSH. *See* THYROID-STIMULATING HORMONE.

TTX. *See* TETRODOTOXIN.

tubocurarine. CAS number of chloride is 57-94-3. The active principle of curare, extracts of South American plants of the genus *Chondrodendron*. In addition to the use of crude extracts as arrow poisons by certain South American natives, purified tubocurarine was once widely used as a skeletal muscle relaxant during surgery. The natural agent has now largely been replaced by synthetic curarimimetics. The mode of action is a highly selective blockade of acetylcholine nicotinic receptors. Because penetration of the blood–brain barrier is negligible, peripheral application of tubocurarine results selectively in paralysis of striated skeletal muscle. The i.p. LD50 in mice is 0.63 mg/kg.

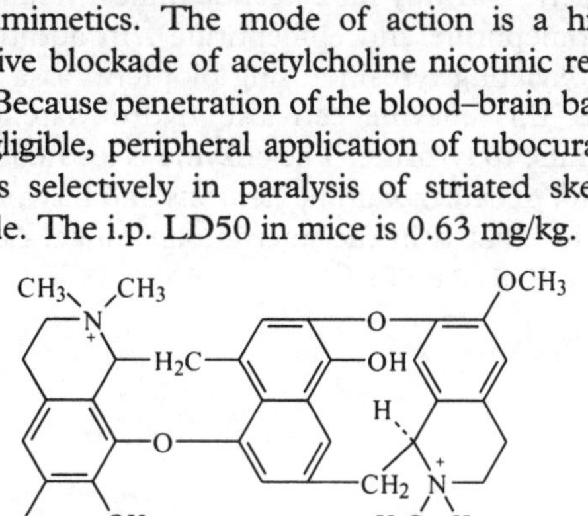

d-Tubocurarine

tubular reabsorption. *See* EXCRETION, RENAL.

tubular secretion. *See* EXCRETION, RENAL.

tubule. *See* EXCRETION, RENAL; NEPHRON; NEPHROTOXICITY.

tubulin (colchicine-binding protein). The protein subunit of microtubules in eukaryotic cells. Tubulin exists in the cell as a dimer of α- and β-tubulin, each with a molecular weight of about 55,000 daltons as determined by electrophoresis. α-tubulin contains 450 amino acids, with a very acidic C-terminal sequence. β-Tubulin has 445 amino acids with about 42% sequence identity with the α-subunit, which suggests a common ancestral origin. The tubulin dimer is associated with two moles of ATP, one at an exchangeable site and the other at a non-exchangeable site. Under appropriate conditions of temperature, pressure, ionic strength and calcium concentration, tubulin dimers self-assemble to form the cytoplasm microtubule complex of interphase cells and the spindle of dividing cells.

Tullidora. *See* BUCKTHORN TOXINS.

tumor. An overt neoplasm, either benign or malignant. *See also* CARCINOGENESIS; NEOPLASM.

tumorigen. *See* CARCINOGEN.

tumor suppressor genes. The protein products of tumor suppressor genes inhibit the progression of cells in the division cycle. Mutations in tumor suppressor genes may bring about the formation of proteins that cannot suppress cell division. Inactivating mutations in the germ cells bring about a predisposition to certain form of cancer, for example familial retinoblastoma, familial polyposis, etc. Somatic mutations in tumor suppressor genes may also play a role in tumor progression. The p53 gene is probably the most studied and is known to play a role in both spontaneous and chemically induced carcinogenesis.

turpentine. An oleoresin from trees of the genus *Pinus* or closely related genera. It is also used as a synonyn for oil of turpentine or spirits of turpentine which is the volatile oil distilled from the oleoresin. The resin itself is used primarily as a source of oil and is toxic, affecting skin, gastrointestinal tract and nervous system, although it has been used in the past for both human and veterinary medicine as a rubefacient and counterirritant. The oil is used as a solvent for paints, waxes, resins, etc. and has been used in the same way in clinical and veterinary practice as the resin. Its importance in toxicology is due to its frequent involvement in accidental or suicidal acute poisoning episodes in the home and the workplace.

TWA. *See* THRESHOLD LIMIT VALUE, TIME-WEIGHTED AVERAGE.

two-compartment model. A pharmacokinetic model in which a substance is introduced into the body and is simultaneously subjected to processes of elimination and distribution. It is usually assumed that elimination occurs from the central compartment. The blood or plasma concentration declines in a biexponential manner when plotted against time. The terminal exponential phase provides a measure of the functional half-life for this model. *See also* COMPARTMENT; KINETIC EQUATIONS; MULTI-COMPARTMENT MODELS; ONE-COMPARTMENT MODEL; PHARMACOKINETICS; TOXICOKINETIGS.

Tylenol. *See* ACETAMINOPHEN.

type I error. *See* NULL HYPOTHESIS.

type II error. *See* NULL HYOPOTHESIS.

type I spectrum. *See* CYTOCHROME P450, OPTICAL DIFFERENCE SPECTRA.

type II spectrum. *See* CYTOCHROME P450, OPTICAL DIFFERENCE SPECTRA.

type III spectrum. *See* CYTOCHROME P450, OPTICAL DIFFERENCE SPECTRA.

tyramine   (4-(2-aminoethyl)phenol).   **CAS number 51-67-2**. A decarboxylation product of tyrosine found in various fermentation products, including cheeses and some wines. It causes sympathomimetic effects by acting as an indirect agonist, causing the release of endogenous catecholamines. Because it is metabolized principally by monoamine oxidase, patients taking monoamine oxidase inhibitors may have a hypertensive crisis if they ingest foods containing significant amounts of tyramine. *See also* MONOAMINE OXIDASE INHIBITORS.

Tyramine

tyrosine hydroxylase (EC 1.14.3). An enzyme that is located in catecholamine-synthesizing cells and is responsible for the hydroxylation of L-tyrosine to L-3,4-dihydroxyphenylalanine (L-dopa). This is the initial and rate-limiting step in the biosynthetic pathway for catecholamines (dopamine, norepinephrine and epinephrine). In addition to hydroxylating tyrosine using biopterin as a coenzyme, this enzyme can also hydroxylate phenylalanine to tyrosine. The enzyme is located in the cytosol of catecholamine neurons and has a K_m for tyrosine that is in the micromolar range. *See also* CATECHOLAMINES.

U

UDPG. *See* URIDINE DIPHOSPHATE GLUCOSE.

UDPGA. *See* URIDINE DIPHOSPHATE GLUCURONIC ACID.

UDPG dehydrogenase. *See* URIDINE DIPHOSPHATE GLUCURONIC ACID.

UDPG phosphorylase. *See* URIDINE DIPHOSPHATE GLUCOSE; URIDINE DIPHOSPHATE GLUCURONIC ACID.

UDPG pyrophosphorylase. *See* URIDINE DIPHOSPHATE GLUCOSE; URIDINE DIPHOSPHATE GLUCURONIC ACID.

UDS test. *See* UNSCHEDULED DNA SYNTHESIS TEST.

UKAEA. *See* UNITED KINGDOM ATOMIC ENERGY AUTHORITY.

UK Environmental Mutagen Society. *See* UNITED KINGDOM ENVIRONMENTAL MUTAGEN SOCIETY.

UKEMS. *See* UNITED KINGDOM ENVIRONMENTAL MUTAGEN SOCIETY.

ultimate carcinogen. *See* CARCINOGEN, ULTIMATE.

ultraviolet radiation (UV radiation). Electromagnetic radiation in the wavelength range of about 4×10^{-5} to 5×10^{-9} m, placing it between visible light and X-rays in the spectrum. The UV spectrum is divided further by wavelengths into A, B and C bands, and certain wavelengths that affect cells are known in the USA as DUV (damaging UV). Much of the UV radiation from the sun is absorbed in the ozone layer of the Earth's atmosphere. UV radiation, in the skin of some animals, including humans, acts on ergosterol to produce Vitamin D. UV is non-ionizing radiation but within cells it can cause chromosome breaks. In nature, most organisms are protected against the effects of UV. In humans, the radiation is absorbed by melanin in the skin, causing the melanin to darken, but excessive exposure of fair-skinned people can cause non-melanoma skin cancers.

ultraviolet spectrophotometry. *See* SPECTROMETRY, ULTRAVIOLET/VISIBLE.

uncertainty factor. *See* SAFETY FACTOR.

unconditioned behavior. An archaic term referring to behavior that is not acquired by conditioning or learning. *See also* NEUROBEHAVIORAL TERATOLOGY; NEUROBEHAVIORAL TOXICOLOGY.

uncouplers, oxidative phosphorylation. *See* OXIDATIVE PHOSPHORYLATION, INHIBITORS.

UNEP. *See* UNITED NATIONS ENVIRONMENT PROGRAM.

unit cancer risk. The probability of an individual developing cancer as a result of lifetime (70 yr) exposure to a specified unit concentration of a carcinogen. The unit usually used is 1 $\mu g/m^3$ for ambient air or 1 mg/L for water.

United Kingdom Atomic Energy Authority (UKAEA). The statutory body in the UK that is responsible for all aspects of atomic energy and for the commercial and scientific use of radioisotopes. The UKAEA is also involved in more general research into energy use and resources. It was established under the Atomic Energy Act, 1946.

United Kingdom Environmental Mutagen Society (UKEMS). Learned body that publishes guidelines on minimal professional criteria that should be applied to mutagenicity testing. (Basic Mutagenicity Tests: UKEMS Recommended Procedures; Supplementary Tests; and Statistical Evaluation of Mutagenicity Test Data. Cambridge University Press).

United Nations Environment Programme (UNEP). A United Nations agency with headquarters in Nairobi, Kenya charged with the coordination of intergovernmental measures for environmental monitoring and protection. It was formed after the 1972 United Nations Conference on the Human Environment. UNEP operates the Earthwatch program, which includes the Global Environmental Monitoring System and the Global Resource Information Database, and funds Earthscan.

United States Department of Agriculture (USDA). A large, diverse agency involved in all aspects of the production and utilization of food and fiber. Many of its programs impact on toxicology including the Food Safety and Inspection Service, the Animal and Plant Health Inspection Service, the Food Quality Assurance Program and the Food and Nutrition Service. It is concerned with the safe and effective use of pesticides and other agricultural chemicals.

unscheduled DNA synthesis test (UDS test). A test for mutagenicity that monitors the repair of DNA following DNA damage by a mutagen. The amount of repair, as monitored autoradiographically by the incorporation of ^{3}H-thymidine into the nuclei of cultured cells, is proportional to the amount of damage. The *in vitro* test involves the exposure of cultured primary hepatocytes from adult male rats to the test chemical. The *in vivo* test involves exposure of the intact animal to the test chemical, followed by the primary hepatocyte culture. One limitation of the test is that it cannot discern whether or not DNA repair is accurate. *See also* EUKARYOTE MUTAGENICITY TESTS.

upper bound cancer risk assessment. Since cancer risk assessments usually involve conservative assumptions and the use of a statistical upper confidence limit, the actual risk is likely to be much lower, possibly close to zero. To make this clear, cancer risk assessment may carry a qualifying statement that the risk estimate is likely to overstate the actual risk.

upper confidence limit. *See* CONFIDENCE LIMIT.

uptake. *See* KINETIC EQUATIONS.

uptake of toxicants. *See* PENETRATION, RATE; PENETRATION ROUTES, DERMAL; PENETRATION ROUTES, GASTROINTESTINAL; PENETRATION ROUTES, PULMONARY.

uracil mustard (5-[bis(2-chloroethyl)amino] uracil). **CAS number 66-75-1**. An antineoplastic agent. *See also* ANTINEOPLASTIC AGENTS.

Uracil mustard

uranium (U). **CAS number 7440-61-1**. Three isotopes (^{234}U, ^{235}U, ^{238}U) exist, and a large number of uranium salts are known. They present both toxic and radiological hazards. The most important use of uranium is in the nuclear energy industry, but uranium compounds are also used in ceramics, as catalysts and in certain alloys. Entry into the body can occur during a variety of processes involved with the mining, processing or use of uranium and its compounds, and is probably largely by inhalation of dusts, fumes, etc. or by ingestion. Acute uranium toxicity is primarily nephrotoxicity. About 50& of plasma uranium is bound, as the uranyl ion, to bicarbonate $\left(HCO_3^- \right)$, which is filtered by the glomerulus. As a result of acidification in the proximal tubule, the bicarbonate complex dissociates followed by reabsorption of the HCO_3^-; the released UO^{2+} then becomes attached to the membrane of the proximal tubule cells. Loss of cell function follows, as evidenced by increased concentration of glucose, amino acids and proteins in the urine. 2,3-Mercapto-1-propanol (British anti-Lewisite, BAL) is ineffective as a therapeutic agent for uranium poisoning; CaEDTA is recommended. Chronic uranium toxicity appears to be radiation-related, the effects being similar to those of ionizing radiation. In humans, cancer of the lung, bone and lymphatic system are all known to occur.

urea herbicides. A class of substituted urea herbicides used for the control of germinating broadleaf and grass weeds, having the general structure shown. This class includes diuron, flumeturon, linuron and monuron, with oral LD50s in rats in the range 3400–8000 mg/kg. Their herbicidal mode of action is as inhibitors of photosynthesis. In mammals, overdose causes abdominal distress, anemia, dermal irritation, diarrhea, eye irritation, mucous membrane irritation, nausea and vomiting, although the mode of action is unknown. The therapy consists of washing the skin with soap and water (dermal), flushing eyes for 15 minutes with water (ocular) or inducing vomiting (oral) except in the case of petroleum solvent formulations. Hallenbeck, W.H. & Cunningham-Burns, K.M. (eds) Pesticides and Human Health (Springer-Verlag, New York, 1985). *See also* AGRICULTURAL CHEMICALS; HERBICIDES; MONURON.

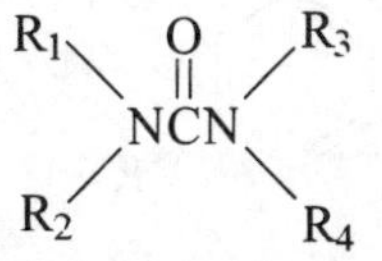

Urea herbicide, general formula

urea nitrogen. *See* BLOOD UREA NITROGEN.

urethane (carbamic acid ethyl ester; Urethan). **CAS number 51-79-6**. A synthetic intermediate used in the preparation of amino resins and in the pesticide industry as a solubilizing agent. It was developed as an antineoplastic agent; it is a direct-acting carcinogen, a hepatotoxicant, causing liver necrosis, and an immunosuppressive agent.

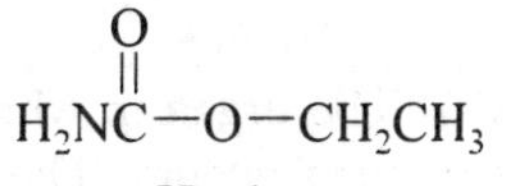

$$H_2NC-O-CH_2CH_3$$

Urethane

uric acid. **CAS number 69-93-2**. A nitrogenous end product and the principal excretory product of purine metabolism in mammals. In birds and reptiles, it is the principal end product of nitrogen metabolism in general. Defects in uric acid metabolism and excretion appear to be associated with a number of disease states, and it frequently occurs as a component of renal calculi. It has not been associated closely with toxic insults except in the case of lead poisoning. Lead causes an elevation in blood uric acid concentration (uric acidemia) and a decrease in uric acid excretion.

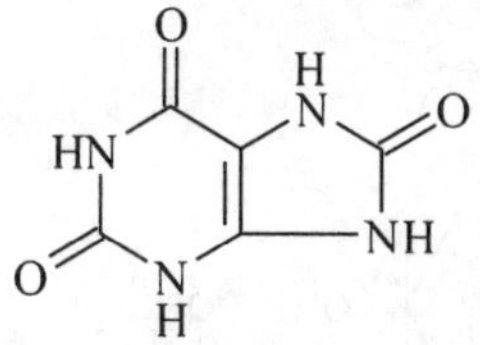

Uric acid

uridine diphosphate glucose (UDPG). **CAS number 133-89-1**. An intermediate in the phase II reaction that results in the formation of glucose conjugates of xenobiotics which contain substituents such as hydroxyl, amino or sulfhydryl groups, the O-, N- and S-glucosides, respectively. UDPG is formed from uridine triphosphate and glucose-1-phosphate in a reaction catalyzed by the enzyme UDPG pyrophosphorylase. Glucoside formation is common in insects and plants, whereas animals other than insects utilize uridine diphosphate glucuronic acid to form glucuronides. *See also* GLUCOSIDE FORMATION; PHASE II REACTIONS.

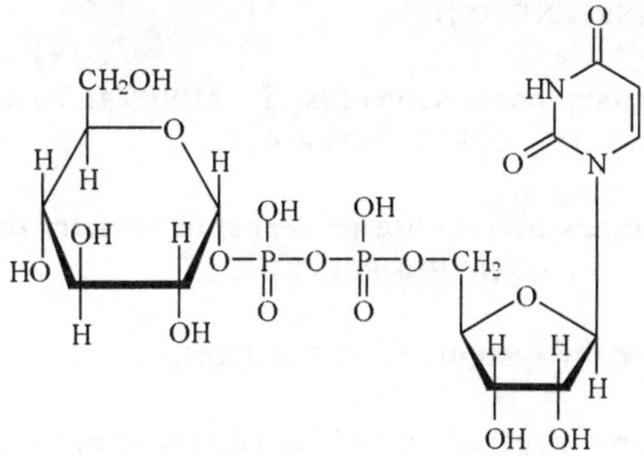

Uridine diphosphate glucose (UDPG)

uridine diphosphate glucuronic acid (UDPGA). An intermediate in the phase II reaction that results in the formation of glucuronic acid conjugates of xenobiotics which contain substituents such as hydroxyl, amino or sulfhydryl groups, forming the *O*-, *N*- and *S*-glucuronides, respectively. UDPGA is formed by two reactions: (1) the formation of UDPG from UTP and glucose-1-phosphate; (2) the formation of UDPGA from UDPG. The two reactions are catalyzed by UDPG pyrophosphorylase and UDPG dehydrogenase, respectively, whereas glucuronide formation is catalyzed by glucuronosyltransferase. Glucuronide formation from xenobiotics is common in all animal groups except insects. *See also* GLUCURONIDE FORMATION; PHASE II REACTIONS.

Uridine diphosphate glucuronic acid (UDPGA)

urinalysis. *See* CHRONIC TOXICITY TESTING; PHARMACOKINETICS; SUBCHRONIC TOXICITY TESTING.

urinalysis, in chronic toxicity testing. *See* TOXIC ENDPOINTS.

urinalysis, in subchronic toxicity testing. *See* TOXIC ENDPOINTS.

urinary corticosteroids. *See* ADRENAL GLAND TOXICITY; CORTICOSTEROIDS.

urinary metabolite patterns, in toxicity testing. *See* TOXIC ENDPOINTS.

urinary system. *See* EXCRETION, RENAL.

urine. The fluid filtered from the blood by the kidneys, modified by the kidneys, stored in the urinary bladder and discharged, normally voluntarily, through the urethra; one of two primary routes of excretion for the products of endogenous metabolism and also the products of xenobiotic metabolism. The composition of the urine is important in

diagnosis of poisoning and renal disfunction. *See also* DIAGNOSTIC FEATURES, URINARY TRACT; EXCRETION, RENAL.

urobilinogen (stercobilinogen). A derivative of bilirubin formed by the gut microflora; this compound is colorless.

urushiol. A 1-(alkyl)- or 1-(alkenyl)-2,3-dihydroxybenzene, where the alkyl/alkenyl group is C15–C17 with one to three double bonds. Urushiol is a mixture of several catechol derivatives that are the main constituents of the irritant oil of plants of the *Toxicodendron* species, such as poison ivy, poison oak and the Asiatic lacquer tree. It is responsible for the dermatitis condition commonly known as poison ivy. Urushiol can cause hypersensitivity in a large percentage of the population by dermal contact, or more seriously, through inhalation of burning vegetation. Prompt removal of the toxin by swabbing of the skin (e.g., with methanol or commercial organic solvents) can prevent or minimize dermal toxicity when contact is certain. Once the characteristic urticaria, blistering and itching develop, therapy is symptomatic (compresses or calamine lotion), or in severe cases corticosteroids like prednisolone can be given.

$R = (CH_2)_{14}CH_3$
$= (CH_2)_7CH=CH(CH_2)_5CH_3$
$= (CH_2)_7CH=CHCH_2CH=CH(CH_2)_2CH_3$
$= (CH_2)_7CH=CHCH_2CH=CHCH=CHCH_3$
$= (CH_2)_7CH=CHCH_2CH=CHCH_2CH=CH_3$

Urushiols

USDA. *See* UNITED STATES DEPARTMENT OF AGRICULTURE.

USEPA. *See* ENVIRONMENTAL PROTECTION AGENCY.

uterus (womb). The organ in which embryonic and fetal development occurs. The inner layer is the endometrium, a glandular layer that is responsive to estrogens and progesterone, which produces "uterine milk" for the early nourishment of the embryo and which deteriorates and is sloughed off (menstrual cycle) or resorbed (estrous cycle) if there is no pregnancy. The myometrium is a smooth muscle layer that responds to the hormone oxytocin at the time of parturition.

UV/visible spectrometry. *See* SPECTROMETRY, ULTRAVIOLET/VISIBLE.

V

V-agents. Persistent (war gas) nerve agents (e.g., VX; sarin).

Valium. *See* DIAZEPAM.

valproic acid. *See* ANTICONVULSANTS.

van der Waals forces. Very weak forces acting between the nucleus of one atom and the electrons of another atom (i.e., between dipoles and induced dipoles). The attractive forces arise from slight distortions induced in the electron clouds surrounding each nucleus as two atoms are brought close together. The binding force is critically dependent upon the proximity of interacting atoms and diminishes rapidly with distance. However, when these forces are summed over a large number of interacting atoms that fit together spatially, they can play a significant role in determining specificity of toxicant–protein interactions. *See also* BINDING.

Vapona. *See* DICHLORVOS.

variance. A measure of the variability in a set of observations. The sample variance is defined as the sum of the squared deviations from the sample mean divided by the number of observations in the sample. The square root of this estimate yields the standard deviation. *See also* STATISTICS, FUNCTION IN TOXICOLOGY.

vasoconstriction. Narrowing of a blood vessel with resultant decrease in blood flow.

vasopressin (antidiuretic hormone; ADH). A hormone synthesized primarily in the supraoptic and paraventricular nuclei of the hypothalamus and released by nerve endings in the neurohypophysis. It has two main actions: increasing water retention in the kidney (antidiuretic hormone) and increasing vasoconstriction and thereby blood pressure (vasopressin). It is secreted in response to low blood pressure. A lack of vasopressin results in diabetes insipidus.

$$Cys-Tyr-Phe-Gln-Asn-Cys-Pro-Arg-GlyNH_2$$

Arginine vasopressin

vector. In molecular biology a vector is a plasmid or other self-replicating DNA molecule that transfers DNA between cells in nature or in recombinant DNA technology. In the latter case it may be called a cloning vector or cloning vehicle. In medicine or parasitology a vector is an organism responsible for parasite transmission between hosts.

vehicle. The solvent or other inert material used in the administration of toxicants during toxicity testing. In pharmacology, it is used primarily with reference to drug delivery.

venom. A toxin produced by an animal specifically for the poisoning of other species via a mechanism designed to deliver the toxin to its prey. Examples include the venom of bees and wasps, delivered by a sting, and the venom of snakes, delivered by fangs. *See also* BLACK WIDOW SPIDER VENOM; COBRA VENOM; SCORPION VENOM; SNAKE VENOM.

Venom-X. Along with somin, sarin, and tabun, one of the four major organophosphate nerve agents. *See also* G GAS; SOMIN; SARIN; TABUN.

ventilation. Movement of air between lungs and the ambient air.

Versalide. *See* ACETYLETHYLTETRAMETHYL-TETRALIN.

vesicant. A chemical that causes blisters on contact with the skin. Gases such as mustard gas are vesicants and have been used as chemical warfare agents. *See also* MUSTARD GAS.

Veterinary Medicines Directorate (VMD). An executive agency within the UK Ministry of Agriculture Fisheries and Food, responsible for the licensing of veterinary medicines.

Veterinary Poisons Information Service (VPIS). A UK information service operating from the London and Leeds centers of the National Poisons Information Service, giving similar information to veterinary practitioners as is provided to physicians by the NPIS. *See also* CENTRE NATIONAL D'INFORMATIONS TOXICOLOGIQUES VETERINAIRES.

Veterinary Products Committee (VPC). Review and advisory committee for veterinary medicines, under the UK's Medicines Acts.

veterinary toxicology. The diagnosis and treatment of the poisoning of animals other than humans, particularly livestock and companion animals, but not excluding feral species. An important concern of veterinary toxicology is the possible transmission of toxicants to the human population in meat, fish, milk and other foodstuffs.

viability index. An expression of survival of offspring in reproductive toxicity tests. Numerically it is the number of young surviving at a particular time expressed as a percentage of those born alive. In experiments involving culling to a constant litter size, at times after culling it is expressed as the percentage of the culled litter. *See also* FERTILITY INDEX; GROWTH INDEX; REPRODUCTIVE TOXICITY TESTING; SEX RATIO; WEANING INDEX.

vibrio. Microorganism, a member of the *Vibrionidae* that is responsible for a food-borne disease in humans.

vinblastine. **CAS number 865-21-4**. An alkaloid derived from the periwinkle (*Vinca rosea*) commonly used as an antitumor drug. It binds to the microtubule subunit, tubulin, at a site distinct from that of colchicine and podophyllotoxin. This binding is reversible, temperature-dependent and rapid, and results in large tubulin aggregates of highly ordered structure (vinblastine paracrystals).

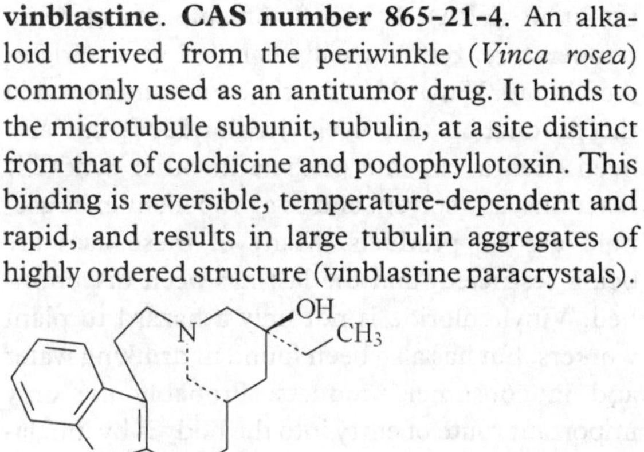

Vinblastine

vincristine. **CAS number 57-22-7**. The aldehyde derivative of the plant alkaloid vinblastine. It competitively inhibits the binding of vinblastine to tubulin and, therefore, probably binds at the same site. It results in microtubule disassembly and the formation of tubulin paracrystals. Roberts, K. & Hyams, J.S. (eds) Microtubules (Academic Press, New York, 1979). *See also* VINBLASTINE.

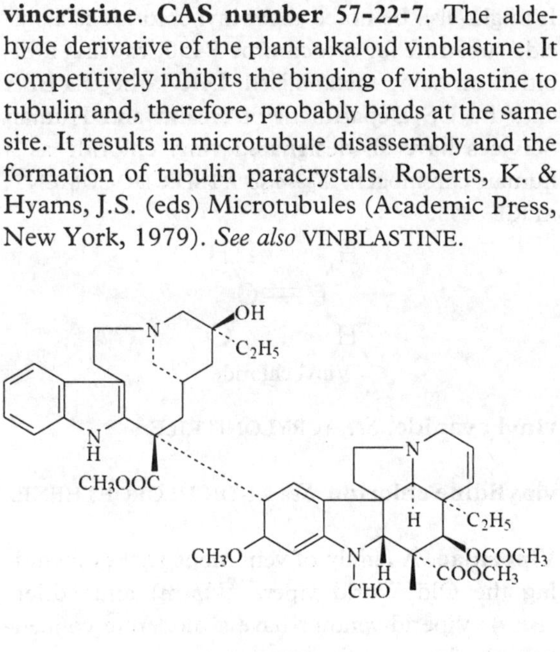

Vincristine

vinylbenzene. *See* STYRENE.

vinyl chloride (chloroethylene). **CAS number 75-01-4**. A designated human carcinogen (IARC), hazardous waste (EPA) and priority toxic pollutant (EPA). It is a flammable gas at room temperature, but is usually handled as a refrigerated liquid. Vinyl chloride is the monomer used in the production of polyvinyl chloride. It has also been used as an intermediate in other synthetic reactions, as a solvent and as a propellant in household aerosol products. Many of these uses are being restricted, and the last has been discontinued. Vinyl chloride is not only a hazard to plant workers, but has also been found in drinking water and in consumer products. Probably the only important route of entry into the body is by inhalation. Locally vinyl chloride is an irritant, and acute poisoning causes CNS depression and hepatotoxicity. The principal toxicological concern, however, is that chronic poisoning with vinyl chloride leads to angiosarcoma of the liver in humans. It is mutagenic, affects reproduction in both males and females and, in experimental animals, causes cancer at several sites. The active metabolite appears to be an epoxide formed by the cytochrome P450-dependent monooxygenase system. It might also be noted that vinyl chloride is a suicide substrate for cytochrome P450, causing inhibition on being metabolized. IARC, the US EPA and the US Department of Health and Human Services have all designated vinyl chloride as a human carcinogen. *See also* ATSDR DOCUMENT, APRIL 1993.

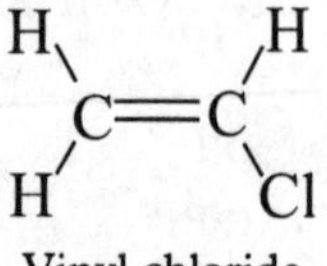

Vinyl chloride

vinyl cyanide. *See* ACRYLONITRILE.

vinylidine chloride. *See* 1,1-DICHLOROETHENE.

Viperidae. A family of venomous snakes including the Old World vipers (*Vipera*) and adders (*Bitis*). Viperid venoms have a moderate concentration of proteolytic enzymes.

viruses. Obligate intracellular parasites composed of either DNA or RNA as genetic information, protein and occasionally lipid. Virtually all living cells are capable of being infected by viruses. These unique forms of life code for some of their own necessary proteins, use many native cellular enzymes and occasionally modify pre-existing cellular proteins for their own benefit.

viscotoxin. *See* MISTLETOE.

vital capacity. The volume of gas that can be forcibly exhaled after a maximum inhalation or, conversely, forcibly inhaled after a maximum exhalation. Loss of vital capacity is characteristic of restrictive defects. It may result from pulmonary fibrosis or pneumonia, either of which may be the result of chemical insult.

vitamin A vitaminosis. *See* HYPERVITAMINOSIS A.

vitamin C. *See* ASCORBIC ACID.

vitamin deficiencies. The direct effects of vitamin deficiency, or the chronic dietary intake of a suboptimal amount of one or more vitamins, are not usually of direct concern to toxicologists. Such deficiencies can, however, affect the metabolism of xenobiotics and hence their toxicity, for example, by bringing about a reduction in monooxygenase activity. *See also* NUTRITIONAL EFFECTS ON METABOLISM, MICRONUTRIENTS.

vitamin K. A general term referring to a group of naphthoquinone derivatives required in the diet for blood clotting. Vitamin K_5 or medadione (CAS number 83-70-5) and its derivatives are synthetic, lipid soluble compounds.

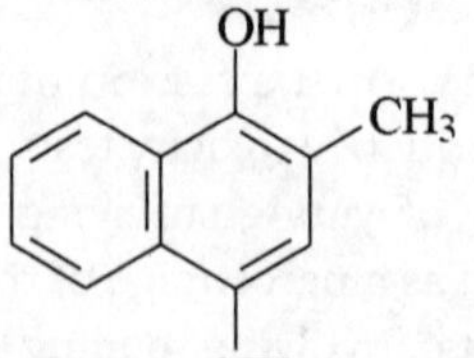

Vitamin K_5

vitamin K antagonists. Hydroxycoumarins, such as warfarin, are antimetabolites for vitamin K and therefore suppress prothrombin synthesis. They are commonly used as rodenticides. Over a period of multiple exposures to the rodenticide in a bait, the prothrombin levels become sufficiently low that the rodent dies of hemorrhage. Accidental poisonings can result in internal bleeding and hematomas, and ultimately hemorrhagic shock and death. Therapy consists of vitamin K administration.

vitaminosis. *See* HYPERVITAMINOSIS A.

vitamins. Substances required in small amounts in the diet of animals, including humans. Because of variations in the ability of organisms to synthesize essential metabolites, the number and type of compounds that are defined as vitamins vary from one animal to another although the requirements are broadly similar. They include the following water-soluble vitamins: B1, thiamine; B2, riboflavin; folic acid; B6, pyridoxine; B12, cyanocobalamine; *p*-aminobenzoic acid; choline; biotin; meso-inositol; lipoic acid; nicotinamide; pantothenic acid; C, ascorbic acid; as well as the following fat-soluble vitamins: A, retinol; D, calciferol; E, alpha-tocopherol; K1, phylloquinone. Excessive doses of vitamins often have a deleterious effect, such toxic overdoses being known by the general term, hypervitaminosis.

VLDLP (very-low-density lipoprotein). *See* LIPOPROTEINS.

V_{max}. The term representing the theoretical maximum velocity of an enzymatic assay. It usually is determined experimentally from a Lineweaver–Burk, Eadie–Hofstee or similar plot. *See also* EADIE–HOFSTEE PLOT; ENZYME KINETICS; K_D; K_M; LINEWEAVER–BURK PLOT.

VMD. *See* VETERINARY MEDICINES DIRECTORATE.

volume of distribution. A proportionality constant relating the amount of drug in the body to the concentration in a biological fluid, typically blood or plasma. It is an apparent volume which rarely corresponds to a real physiological volume. The magnitude of the volume of distribution is dependent upon the physiochemical properties of the drug and its binding characteristics to tissues and components of blood. Several volumes of distribution have been described and include the one-compartment volume of distribution (usually expressed as V or V_d), and several volumes of distribution for multi-compartment models including the volume of the central compartment (V_c), the β-phase volume of distribution (V_a) and the volume of distribution at steady state (V_{ss}). *See also* COMPARTMENT; KINETIC EQUATIONS; PHARMACOKINETICS; TOXICOKINETICS.

vomiting. *See* EMESIS; MAINTENANCE THERAPY, GASTROINTESTINAL TRACT.

vomitoxin. **CAS number 51481-10-8**. A tricothecene mycotoxin from *Fusarium roseum*. A claim was made that this mycotoxin had been used as a biological warfare agent in South-East Asia but, to date, this is not supported by objective evidence. *See also* TRICOTHECENES.

VPC. *See* VETERINARY PRODUCTS COMMITTEE.

VPIS. *See* VETERINARY POISONS INFORMATION SERVICE.

W

Wagner–Nelson method. *See* BIOAVAILABIL-
ITY.

Wallerian degeneration. The degeneration of
myelinated and unmyelinated axons that occurs in
a nerve distal to a transection or crush of the nerve.
Myelin sheaths also degenerate in the distal nerve
stump as a consequence of the loss of their underlying axon. Axonal degeneration due to other
causes (e.g., neurotoxicants) is often referred to as
"Wallerian-like" or "Wallerian-type" if the axonal
degeneration is morphologically similar to Wallerian degeneration. Landon, D.N. (ed) The
Peripheral Nerve (Chapman and Hall, London,
1975).

warfarin. *See* RODENTICIDES.

water pollution. Water pollution is of concern in
almost all parts of the world, although the nature
of the pollution varies widely, particularly between
industrialized and non-industrialized nations.
Chemical contamination is most common in
industrialized nations, whereas microbial contamination is more important in non-
industrialized areas. Surface water contamination
has been the primary cause for concern, but since
the discovery of insecticides (e.g., aldicarb) and
soil fumigants (e.g., ethylene dibromide) in
ground water drawn from wells, contamination of
water from this source is also recognized as a problem. Water pollution may arise from run-off of
agricultural chemicals, from sewage or from specific industrial sources such as refineries, smelters
or chemical plant. Some sources are diffuse and
difficult to control, whereas others are from specific point sources and can be controlled at the
point of origin. Agricultural chemicals found in
water include insecticides such as chlorinated
hydrocarbons, organophosphates and carbamates,
as well as other pesticides including herbicides,
fungicides and nematocides. The chlorinated
hydrocarbons such as DDT, chlordane and
dieldrin, previously of most concern because of
their persistance, are now less important because
of curtailed use. Fertilizers, although less of a toxic
hazard, contribute to such environmental problems as eutrophication. Low-molecular-weight
halogenated hydrocarbons such as chloroform,
dichloroethane and carbon tetrachloride may
enter water directly or may be formed as a result of
the chlorination of precursors during water purification. Chlorinated aromatics such as the polychlorinated biphenyls (PCBs), chlorophenols and
even the highly toxic 2,3,7,8-tetrachloro-
dibenzo-*p*-dioxin (TCDD) are commonly found
in water, as are the phthalate ester plasticizers,
di-(2-ethylhexyl) phthalate and di-*n*-butyl phthalate. Detergents, such as the alkylbenzene sulfonates, are common contaminants of water that
arises from domestic effluent. A number of toxic
inorganics have also been found in water. *See also*
POLLUTION.

water sampling. *See* SAMPLING, WATER.

weaning index. An expression of survival of offspring to weaning in reproductive toxicity tests.
The number of offspring surviving to weaning
(i.e., 21 days in the rat) as a percentage of those
alive at four days. *See also* FERTILITY INDEX;
GROWTH INDEX; REPRODUCTIVE TOXICITY
TESTING; VIABILITY INDEX.

Weibull distribution. *See* LOW-DOSE EXTRAPO-
LATION.

Weibull model. *See* LOW-DOSE EXTRAPOLA-
TION.

weight change, in chronic toxicity testing. *See* TOXIC ENDPOINTS.

weight change, in subchronic toxicity testing. *See* TOXIC ENDPOINTS.

weight-of-evidence. A determination of whether several experimental determinations of adverse effect, none of which are definitive alone, can, taken together, be regarded as definitive that a particular toxicant causes the adverse effect in question. Weight-of-evidence determinations are almost always controversial, in large part because they permit the use of inadequate or inappropriate experiments.

well water. *See* GROUND WATER.

Western blotting. Method for identifying proteins in complex mixtures. The proteins are separated by electrophoresis through a slab gel and then blot transferred onto a sheet of nitrocellulose by electrophoresis at 90° to the gel surface. The proteins bound on the nitrocellulose membrane can be then be identified by reaction with specific reagents such as radioactive or fluorescent-labelled antibodies. *See also* NORTHERN BLOTTING; SOUTHERN BLOTTING.

wheat gluten. *See* GLUTEN, WHEAT.

white blood cells. *See* LEUKOCYTES.

white phosphorus. *See* PHOSPHORUS.

WHO/OMS. *See* WORLD HEALTH ORGANIZATION.

Wilcoxon rank-sum test. A distribution-free, non-parametric test for two independent groups. The data from both groups are combined and ranked with the lowest value assigned a rank of 1. The ranks assigned to each group are then summed, with the test statistic T' being the sum of the ranks for the smaller group. For small groups ($n < 10$), the critical value for T' can be obtained from special tables. If $n > 10$ for both groups, the distribution approximates normal, and the

obtained value for T' can be assessed using the normal curve table. *See also* NON-PARAMETRIC; STATISTICS, FUNCTION IN TOXICOLOGY.

wildlife criterion. In risk assessment a level of a toxicant exposure which is considered not to cause an adverse effect in a particular wildlife species. The wildlife criterion will vary with individual species.

Wilson's disease. *See* COPPER.

womb. *See* UTERUS.

Woolf plot. A way to linearize enzyme- or receptor-binding data based on derivations of the law of mass action. The Woolf plot is particularly useful for radioreceptor assays because it is less subject to effects of experimental outliers. For receptor assays, the Woolf equation is:

$$\frac{[F]}{B} = \left(\frac{1}{B_{max}}\right) \cdot [F] + \frac{K_D}{B_{max}}$$

where a plot of $[F]/B$ versus $[F]$ yields a straight line where the Y intercept is K_D/B_{max} and the slope is $1/B_{max}$. A similar equation exists for enzyme kinetics, except that B (amount bound) is equivalent to v (initial velocity), $[F]$ (concentration of free ligand) to $[S]$ (concentration of substrate), K_D (dissociation constant) to K_m (Michaelis constant) and B_{max} (theoretical number of sites) to V_{max} (maximal theoretical velocity). *See also* ENZYME KINETICS; K_D; K_M; LINEWEAVER–BURK PLOT; METABOLITE INHIBITORY COMPLEXES; MICHAELIS–MENTEN EQUATION; RADIORECEPTOR ASSAYS; XENOBIOTIC METABOLISM, INHIBITION.

workplace, toxicants. In industrial societies the number of chemicals that may be found in the workplace is extremely high, and many are known to have deleterious biological effects. Regulation and control of industrial chemicals are the subject of many laws and regulations. Among the typical inorganic chemicals are metals such as lead, copper, mercury, zinc, cadmium and beryllium, as well as fluorides, carbon monoxide, etc. The organic compounds include aliphatic hydrocarbons (e.g., hexane), aromatic hydrocarbons (e.g., benzene, toluene, xylene), halogenated hydrocarbons (e.g., dichloromethane, trichloroethane, trichloroethylene, vinyl chloride), alcohols (e.g., methanol, ethylene glycol), esters (e.g., methyl methacrylate, di-(2-ethylhexyl) phthalate), organo-metallics (e.g., tributyltin acetate), amino compounds (e.g., aniline), nitro derivatives (e.g., nitrobenzene) and many others. In addition, many manufactured products, as well as the intermediates in their synthesis, are also found in the workplace. *See also* HEALTH AND SAFETY COMMISSION; OCCUPATIONAL SAFETY AND HEALTH ADMINISTRATION.

World Health Organization (WHO). The health agency of the United Nations, WHO is based in Geneva, Switzerland. It coordinates international health activities, emphasizing the health needs of developing countries.

X

xanthine oxidase (EC 1.2.3.2). An enzyme that is closely related to aldehyde oxidase (EC 1.2.3.1). Both are metalloflavoproteins of about 300,000 daltons. They consist of two subunits of equal size and contain molybdenum, FAD and iron (as Fe/S) in a ratio of 1:1:4 per subunit. These enzymes are widely distributed and catalyze a reaction in which the substrate is hydroxylated by an oxygen atom derived from water and electrons from the substrate are transferred to a variety of acceptors. These two enzymes have a broad overlapping substrate specificity including many purines, pyrimidines and pteridines. However, xanthine, the best known substrate for xanthine oxidase, is not a substrate for aldehyde oxidase, whereas the reverse is true for quaternary pyridinium compounds, such as N-methylnicotinamide. The role of oxygen as an electron acceptor with its production of hydrogen peroxide and the intermediate superoxide anion (both potential toxicants) may not be important *in vivo* since there is evidence that these enzymes are NAD-dependent dehydrogenases *in vivo* and become oxidases as a result of modification during purification. However, they are probably important in two types of detoxication. The

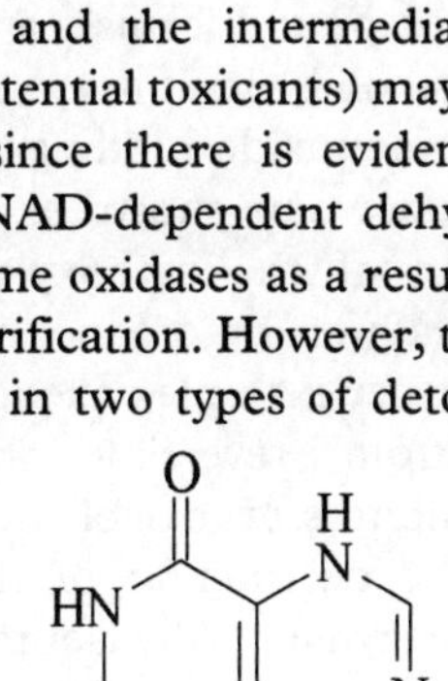

Xanthine

$$R' + H_2O \longrightarrow R'OH + 2e^- + 2H^+$$

$$R'' + 2e^- + 2H^+ \longrightarrow R''H_2$$

(R' is the oxidizable substrate and R'' the electron acceptor)

Xanthine oxidase

first of these is the hydroxylation of exogenous aldehydes, purines, pyrimidines and other heterocyclic compounds, and the second involves the utilization of exogenous componds as electron acceptors. Examples of the latter include the conversion of organic nitro compounds to hydroxyamino derivatives and the reduction of N-oxides to the free base. *See also* ALDEHYDE OXIDASE.

xenobiotic. A general term used to describe any chemical interacting with an organism that does not occur in the normal metabolic pathways of that organism. The use of this term in lieu of foreign compound, etc., is gaining wide acceptance.

xenobiotic metabolism (xenobiotic biotransfomation). The overall effect of the metabolism of xenobiotics is an increase in water solubility. Most xenobiotics enter the body because they are lipophilic, a property that facilitates penetration of lipid membranes and distribution by lipoproteins in the blood. Without metabolism to water-soluble products such products could not be readily excreted and would accumulate to toxic concentrations. Such metabolism consists of two phases: (1) phase I, in which a reactive, polar group is introduced into the molecule; (2) phase II, in which such polar groups are conjugated with water-soluble endogenous metabolites. Although the process brings about an incease in water solubility and a decrease in $T_{0.5}$ *in vivo*, it is not always a detoxication mechanism, since reactive intermediates may be formed which are more toxic than the parent compound. *See also* ACTIVATION; DETOXICATION; PHASE I REACTIONS; PHASE II REACTIONS; REACTIVE INTERMEDIATES; XENOBIOTIC METABOLISM, CHEMICAL EFFECTS; XENOBIOTIC METABOLISM, EFFECTS OF INDUCTION; XENOBIOTIC METABOLISM, INHIBITION;

XENOBIOTIC METABOLISM, IRREVERSIBLE INHI-
BITION; XENOBIOTIC METABOLISM, REVERSIBLE
INHIBITION.

xenobiotic metabolism, chemical effects. The
effect of one exogenous chemical on the metabolism of another is of critical importance in toxicology since organisms are seldom, if ever, exposed to
one such compound at a time. Stimulation of activation reactions can increase toxicity, whereas
their inhibition can cause a decrease, the reverse
situation being true of detoxication reactions. *See
also* BIPHASIC EFFECTS ON METABOLISM;
INDUCTION, INHIBITION; XENOBIOTIC METABO-
LISM, EFFECTS OF INDUCTION; XENOBIOTIC
METABOLISM, EFFECTS OF INHIBITION.

xenobiotic metabolism, effects of induction.
As with inhibition, the effects of induction can be
at the level of *in vivo* symptoms, *in vivo* metabolism or *in vitro* metabolism by enzyme preparations
from induced animals. For example, treatment of
rats with benzo[*a*]pyrene can reduce the zoxazolamine paralysis time from 11 hours to 17 minutes.
Exposure of humans to DDT doubles the rate at
which they metabolize antipyrine. *In vitro* effects
are also well known. Microsomes from polycyclic
aromatic hydrocarbon-treated animals have
increased aryl hydrocarbon hydroxylase activity,
whereas microsomes from animals treated with
inducers such as phenobarbital have an increased
ability to carry out many oxidative reactions,
including benzphetamine *N*-demethylation,
p-nitroanisole *O*-demethylation, *N*-demethylation
of ethylmorphine and aldrin epoxidation. *See also*
INDUCTION.

xenobiotic metabolism, effects of inhibition.
Inhibition of xenobiotic metabolism can be demonstrated in a number of ways. *In vivo* symptoms
can be affected, as in the prolongation of the pentobarbital sleeping time by SKF-525A. Distribution and blood levels can also be affected as in the
higher levels of pentobarbital that are maintained
following the above treatment with SKF-525A.
Effects can also be seen on *in vitro* metabolism following *in vivo* treatment or when both inhibitor
and substrate are administered to enzyme preparations *in vitro*. *See also* XENOBIOTIC METABOLISM,

INHIBITION; XENOBIOTIC METABOLISM, IRRE-
VERSIBLE INHIBITION; XENOBIOTIC
METABOLISM, REVERSIBLE INHIBITION.

xenobiotic metabolism, inhibition. The primary considerations in inhibition kinetics are
reversibility and selectivity. Although the biochemistry of reversible inhibition has been intensively studied and can give much insight into reaction mechanisms, it is less important in xenobiotic
interaction than irreversible inhibition. *See also*
INHIBITION; METABOLITE INHIBITORY COM-
PLEX; XENOBIOTIC METABOLISM, IRREVERSIBLE
INHIBITION; XENOBIOTIC METABOLISM, REVER-
SIBLE INHIBITION.

**xenobiotic metabolism, irreversible inhibi-
tion**. Irreversible inhibition is important in toxicology and can arise from several causes, usually
either covalent binding or disruption of the
enzyme structure. Neither effect can be reversed *in
vitro* either by dialysis or by dilution. Covalent
binding usually involves the prior formation of a
metabolic intermediate that then interacts with the
enzyme. This type of inhibition occurs when
piperonyl butoxide interacts with the microsomal
cytochrome P450-dependent monooxygenase
system. This compound forms a stable inhibitory
complex (metabolite inhibitory complex) that
blocks carbon monoxide binding to cytochrome
P450 and also prevents substrate oxidation. The
phosphorylation of the carboxylesterase which
hydrolyzes malathion by organophosphates such
as EPN, is a further example of xenobiotic interaction resulting from irreversible inhibition. Other
irreversible inhibitors of toxicological significance
bring about the destruction of the xenobiotic-
metabolizing enzymes. Allylisopropylacetamide,
for example, causes the breakdown of cytochrome
P450 and the release of the heme moiety. *See also*
INHIBITION; METABOLITE INHIBITORY COM-
PLEXES; XENOBIOTIC METABOLISM, INHIBI-
TION; XENOBIOTIC METABOLISM, REVERSIBLE
INHIBITION.

xenobiotic metabolism, nutritional effects.
See NUTRITIONAL EFFECTS ON XENOBIOTIC
METABOLISM, CARBOHYDRATE; NUTRITIONAL
EFFECTS ON XENOBIOTIC METABOLISM, LIPIDS;
NUTRITIONAL EFFECTS ON XENOBIOTIC

METABOLISM, MICRONUTRIENTS; NUTRITIONAL EFFECTS ON XENOBIOTIC METABOLISM, PROTEINS; NUTRITIONAL EFFECTS ON XENOBIOTIC METABOLISM, STARVATION AND DEHYDRATION.

xenobiotic metabolism, physiological effects. *See* PHYSIOLOGICAL EFFECTS ON XENOBIOTIC METABOLISM, AGING; PHYSIOLOGICAL EFFECTS ON XENOBIOTIC METABOLISM, DEVELOPMENTAL; PHYSIOLOGICAL EFFECTS ON XENOBIOTIC METABOLISM, DISEASE; PHYSIOLOGICAL EFFECTS ON XENOBIOTIC METABOLISM, HORMONES; PHYSIOLOGICAL EFFECTS ON XENOBIOTIC METABOLISM, PREGNANCY; PHYSIOLOGICAL EFFECTS ON XENOBIOTIC METABOLISM, SEX; XENOBIOTIC .

xenobiotic metabolism, reversible inhibition. Reversible inhibition is divided into competitive inhibition, uncompetitive inhibition and noncompetitive inhibition, although intermediate classes have also been described. All three are known for xenobiotic-metabolizing enzymes. Competitive inhibition is due to two substrates competing for the same active site. Type I ligands for cytochrome P450 which often appear to bind as substrates, but do not bind to the heme iron, frequently appear to be competitive inhibitors. Examples are the inhibition of aldrin epoxidation by dihydroaldrin and *N*-demethylation of aminopyrine by nicotinamide. Uncompetitive inhibition, which has seldom been reported in studies of xenobiotic metabolism, is seen when an inhibitor interacts with an enzyme–substrate complex, but cannot interact with the free enzyme. Simple noncompetitive inhibitors bind to both enzyme and enzyme–substrate complex to form either an enzyme–inhibitor complex or an enzyme–inhibitor–substrate complex. Metyrapone is a noncompetitive inhibitor of monooxygenase reactions, although it can, in some cases, stimulate metabolism. In either case, the effect is noncompetitive, in that the K_m does not change, whereas V_{max} decreases with inhibition and increases with stimulation. *See also* INHIBITION; METABOLITE INHIBITORY COMPLEX; XENOBIOTIC METABOLISM, INHIBITION; XENOBIOTIC METABOLISM, IRREVERSIBLE INHIBITION.

Xenopus. *See* FETAX.

xeroderma pigmentosum. A rare disease of the skin resulting from a inherited sensitivity to the carcinogenic effects of ultraviolet light. Fibroblasts obtained from xeroderma pigmentosum patients have been used in the development of mutation assays based on the HGPRT locus. *See also* HGPRT LOCUS.

xylenes. Usually used as a mixture of the three forms, 2-, 3- and 4-xylene or ortho-, meta- and para-xylene. It is a high-volume industrial chemical used in the synthetic fiber, chemical and plastics industries and as a solvent, cleaning agent and thinner for paints and varnishes. An irritant to the skin and mucus membranes. Teratogenic to animals but no evidence of carcinogenicity. *See also* ATSDR DOCUMENT, OCTOBER 1993.

xylitol. *See* SWEETENING AGENTS.

Y

yeast mutation tests. *In vitro* test systems used to detect mutagenicity that have been developed with strains of the yeast *Saccharomyces cerevisiae* which are capable of detecting forward mutations, reverse mutations and recombinant events such as reciprocal or non-reciprocal mitotic recombination. Because of the limited metabolic capacity of yeast for xenobiotics, the S-9 fraction from induced rat liver is frequently included in the assay system to ensure activation of promutagens. *See also* EUKARYOTE MUTAGENICITY TESTS; S-9 FRACTION.

yew. *Taxus brevifolia*, the Western yew, is a tree of the family Taxaceae found in the western US and *T. canadensis* in the eastern US. *T. cuspidata*, the Japanese yew, and *T. baccata*, a European yew, are grown as ornamentals. The principal toxic constituents of yew are the alkaloids taxine A and B, both capable of causing digitalis-like poisoning (i.e., hypotension, bradycardia and depressed myocardial contractility and conduction delay). Various yew preparations have been used in folk medicine and an anti-cancer agent, taxol, extracted from yew, has been shown to be clinically effective. *See also* TAXOL.

yohimbine. CAS number 146-48-5. Obtained from leaves and bark of *Corynanthe johimbe*. Formerly used as an aphrodisiac in veterinary medicine, yohimbine works primarily by acting as an antagonist at α2-adrenergic receptors.

Yohimbine

Z

zearalenone. A mycotoxin produced by *Fusarium* which is estrogenic and causes hyperestrogenic effects. It is found on corn, barley, wheat, hay, oats and other agricultural commodities. It can cause adverse effects on reproduction in domestic animals, particularly swine.

zero tolerance. *See* TOLERANCE.

zinc (Zn). An essential nutrient that serves as cofactor for a large number of enzymes. Zinc deficiency is, therefore, serious. Zinc toxicity, on the other hand, is not common and is important only in the industrial setting, with metal fume fever being the most significant effect commonly associated with inhalation of zinc oxide. The symptoms are a delayed onset of chills, fever, sweating and muscular weakness. *See also* ATSDR DOCUMENT, MAY 1994.

Zovirax. *See* ACYCLOVIR.

ZPP (zinc protoporphyrin). *See* FREE ERYTHROCYTE PROTOPORPHYRIN.

References

Aizawa, H. Metabolic Maps of Pesticides (Academic Press, New York, 1982).

Alberts, B., Bray, D., Lewis, J., Raff, M., Roberts, K. & Watson, J.D. Molecular Biology of the Cell, 3rd Edn (Garland Publishing, New York, 1994).

Allaby, M. Macmillan Dictionary of the Environment, 3rd Edn. (Macmillan Reference Books, London, 1989).

Anderson, K. & Scott, R. Fundamentals of Industrial Toxicology (Ann Arbor Science Publishers, Ann Arbor, 1980).

Arbuckle, J.G., Brown, M.A., Bryson, N.S., Frick, G.W., Hall, R.M. Jr, Miller, J.G., Miller, M.L., Sullivan, T.F.P., Vanderver, T.A. Jr & Wegman, L.N. Environmental Law Handbook 8th edn (Government Institutes, Rockville, 1985).

Ashby, John (ed). Evaluation of Short-Term Tests for Carcinogens. (Cambridge University Press, Cambridge, 1988).

Ashford, R.D. Ashford's Dictionary of Industrial Chemicals: Properties, Production, Uses; (Wavelength Publications Ltd., ACS Books, Columbus, 1994).

Ballantyne, B., Marrs, T. and Turner, P. (eds) General and Applied Toxicology, 2 vols. (Macmillan Press, London 1993). (A new edition is due in 1999 in 3 volumes).

Balls, M., Riddell, R.J. & Worden, A.N. (eds) Animals and Alternatives in Toxicity Testing (Academic Press, London, 1983).

Caldwell, J. & Jakoby, W.B. Biological Basis of Detoxication (Academic Press, New York, 1983).

Ceccarelli, B. & Clementi, F. Neurotoxins: Tools in Neurobiology (Raven Press, New York, 1979).

Chambers, J.E. & Yarbrough, J.D. (eds) Effects of Chronic Exposures to Pesticides on Animal Systems (Raven Press, New York, 1982).

Chemical Manufacturers Association. Risk Management of Existing Chemicals (Government Institutes, Rockville, 1984).

Coats, J.R. (ed) Insecticide Mode of Action (Academic Press, New York, 1982).

Congress of the United States. Technologies and Management Strategies for Hazardous Waste Control (Office of Technology Assessment, Washington, DC, 1983).

Coombs, J., Dictionary of Biotechnology 2nd edn (Macmillan Press, London, 1992).

Cooper, A. R., Sr., Cooper's Toxic Exposure (CRC Press, Boca Raton FL, 1991)

Cooper, J. R., Bloom, F. C. and Roth, R. H. The Biochemical Basis of Neuropharmacology, 7th edn. (Oxford University Press, New York, 1997)

Dorner, F. and Drews, J. (eds) International Encyclopedia of Pharmacology and Therapeutics. (Pergamon Press, Oxford, 1986).

Dreisbach, R.H. and Robertson W.O. Handbook of Poisoning 12th edn (Lange Medical Publications, Los Altos, 1987).

Duffus, J.H. and Worth, H.G.F. (eds) Fundamental Toxicology for Chemists. (The Royal Society of Chemistry, London, 1996).

Ecobichon,D.J., The Basis of Toxicity Testing. (CRC Press, Boca Raton, 1992).

Ellenhorn, M.J., and Barceloux, D.G. Medical Toxicology: Diagnosis and Treatment of Human Poisoning. (Elsevier Science Publishing Co., New York, 1988).

Environ Corporation. Elements of Toxicology and Chemical Risk Assessment (Washington DC, 1988).

Environmental Protection Agency. Toxicology Handbook (Government Institutes, Rockville, MD 1986).

Environmental Protection Agency. Glossary of Terms Related to Health, Exposure and Risk Assessment. (Washington, DC 1989).

Fan, A.M. and Chang, L.W. Toxicology and Risk Assessment: Principles, Methods and Applications. (Marcel Dekker, New York, 1996).

Feldman, R.S., Meyer, J.S., and Quenzer, L.F. Principles of Neuropsychopharmacology. (Sinauer: Sunderland, 1997)

Fox, S.I. Human Physiology, 5th edn (Wm C. Brown, Dubuque, 1996).

Friberg, L., Nordberg, G.F. & Vouk, V.B. (eds) Handbook of the Toxicology of Metals (2 vols) (Elsevier Science Publishers, Amsterdam, 1986).

Gorrod, J.W. (ed) Testing for Toxicity (Taylor & Francis, London, 1981).

Gosselin, R.E., Smith, R.P., Hodge, H.C. & Braddock, J.E. Clinical Chemistry of Commercial Products, (Williams & Wilkins, Baltimore/London, 1984).

Guthrie, F.E. & Perry, J.J. Introduction to Environmental Toxicology (Elsevier Science Publishers, New York, 1980).

Guyton, A.C. Textbook of Medical Physiology 9th edn (W.B. Saunders, Philadelphia, 1996).

Hardman, J.G., Limbird, L.E., Molinoff, P.B., Ruddon, R.W., and Gilman, A.G. (eds) Goodman & Gilman's The Pharmacological Basis of Therapeutics, 9th edn (McGraw-Hill, New York, 1996).

Haschek, W. M. and Rousseaux. Fundamentals of Toxicologic Pathology (Academic Press, San Diego,1998) .

Hayes, A.W. (ed) Principles and Methods of Toxicology 3rd edn. (Raven Press, New York, 1994).

Hayes, W. J. Jr., and Laws, E. R. Jr. Handbook of Pesticide Toxicology, 3 vols. (Academic Press, San Diego, 1991).

Hazardous Chemicals Data Book Environmental Health Review No. 4 (Noyes Data Corp, Park Ridge, 1980).

Hibbert D.B. and A.M. James, Macmillian Dictionary of Chemistry. (Macmillan Reference Books, London, 1987).

Hodgson, E. (ed) Reviews in Environmental Toxicology Vols. 1-3 (Elsevier Science Publishers, Amsterdam, 1984, 1986, 1987).

Hodgson, E. (ed) Reviews in Environmental Toxicology Vols 4-5 (Toxicology Communications, Raleigh NC, 1990, 1993)

Hodgson E. and Levi, P.E. (eds) Introduction to Biochemical Toxicology, 2nd edn (Appleton and Lange, Norwalk, CT, 1994).

Hodgson, E. and Levi, P.E. (eds) A Textbook of Modern Toxicology, 2nd edn (Appleton and Lange, Norwalk, CT, 1997).

Hodgson, E., Bend, J.R. & Philpot, R.M. (eds) Reviews in Biochemical Toxicology Vol. 1-9, (Elsevier Science Publishers, New York, 1979 - 88).

Hodgson, E., Bend,J.R., and Philpot, R.M. (eds) Reviews in Biochemical Toxicology Vol. 11, (Toxicology Communications, Raleigh, NC, 1995)

Hoel, D.G., Merrill, R.A. & Perera, F.P. Risk Quantitation and Regulatory Policy Banbury Report No. 19 (Cold Spring Harbor Laboratory, 1985).

Homburger, F. Safety Evaluation and Regulation of Chemicals Vol. 2 (Karger, Basel, 1985).

Homburger, F., Hayes, J.A. & Pelican, E.W. A Guide to General Toxicology (Karger, Basel, 1983).

IARC Monographs on the Evaluation of the Carcinogenic Risk of Chemicalsto Humans. A series of monographs, started in 1972, summarizing the carcinogenic risks associated with various classes of chemicals. Includes occasional supplements with cumulative indexes.(IARC, Lyons, France, 1972 to date).

Jacobs, B. L. (ed) Hallucinogens: Neurochemical, Behavioral and Clinical Perspectives (Raven Press, New York, 1984).

Jakoby, W.B. Enzymatic Basis of Detoxication (2 vols) (Academic Press, New York, 1980).

Jakoby, W.B., Bend, J.R. and Caldwell, J. Metabolic Basis of Detoxication (Academic Press, New York, 1982).

Khera, K.S. & Munro, I..C. A Review and Specifications and Toxicity of the Food Colors Permitted in Canada. CRC Critical Reviews in Toxicology (1979).

King, D.W., Fenoglio, C.M. and Lefkowtich, J.H. General Pathology: Principles and Dynamics (Lea & Feabiger, Philadelphia, 1983).

Klaasen, C.D. (ed) Casarett and Doull's Toxicology 5th edn. (McGraw-Hill, New York, 1996).

Lehninger, A.L., Nelson, D.L. and Cox, M.M. Principles of Biochemistry 2nd edn (Worth Publishers, New York, 1993).

Lewis, R.J. Carcinogenically active chemicals (Van Nostrand Reinhold, NewYork, 1991).

Lewis, R.J. Hazardous Chemicals Desk Reference. 4th edn (Van Nostrand Reinhold, New York, 1997).

Lewis, R.J. Rapid Guide to Hazardous Chemicals in the Workplace, 2nd ed. (Van Nostrand Reinhold, New York, 1990).

Lu, F.C. Basic Toxicology (Hemisphere Publishing, Washington, DC, 1985).

Maclean, N., Macmillan Dictionary of Genetics and Cell biology (Macmillan Press, London, 1987).

Manahan, S.E. Toxiological Chemistry, 2nd edn. (Lewis Publishers, Chelsea, Michigan, 1992).

Matsumura, F. Toxicology of Insecticides, 2nd ed. (Plenum Press, New York, 1985).

McKenna and Cuneo, and Technology Services Group, Inc., Pesticide Regulation Handbook, 3rd edn. (McKenna and Cuneo, Washington DC, 1991).

Meister, R. T. and Sine, C. Farm Chemicals Handbook '95 (Meister Publishing Company, Willoughby, 1995)

Merck Index, 12th edn., (Merck, Rahway, 1996).

National Academy of Sciences Principles and Procedures for Evaluating the Toxicity of Household Substances (National Academy of Science, Washington DC, 1977).

Neckers, D.C. & Doyle, M.P. Organic Chemistry (John Wiley & Sons, New York, 1977).

Neidle,S. & Waring, (eds) Molecular Aspects of Anti-cancer Drug Action (Macmillan Press, London, 1983).

O'Neill, I.K., Von Borstel, R.C., Miller, C.T., Long, J. & Bartsch, H. N-Nitroso Compounds: Occurrence, Biological Effects and Relevance to Human Cancer. IARC Scientific Publications, No. 547 (IARC, Lyons, 1984).

Physicians' Desk Reference 52nd edn (Medical Economics, Oradell, 1998).

Pitot, H. C. Fundamentals of Oncology 3rd edn (Marcel Dekker, New York & Basel, 1986).

Roberts, J. J. & Pera, M. in Molecular Aspects of Anti-cancer Drug Action (eds Neidle, S. & Waring, M.) 183-232 (Macmillan Press, London, 1983).

Roberts, K. & Hyams, J. S. Microtubules (Academic Press, London, 1979).

Salmon, E. O. et al. J. Cell Biol. 99, 1066-1075 (1984).

Russell, F.E. Snake Venom Poisoning (Scholium International, Great Neck, 1983).

Salmon, S.E. & Sartorelli, A.C. Basic and Clinical Pharmacology (Lange Medical Publications, Los Altos, 1984).

Sax, N.I. & Lewis, R.J. Rapid Guide to Hazardous Chemicals in the Workplace (Van Nostrand Reinhold, New York, 1986).

Sell, S., Berkower, I. & Max, E.E. Immunology, Immunopathology & Immunity. (Appleton & Lange, Norwalk,1996).

Siegel, G.J., Agranoff, B.W., & Albers,R.W. Basic Neurochemistry: Molecular, Cellular, and Medical Aspects, 6th Edn (Lippincott-Raven, Philadelphia, 1998).

Sipes, I. G., McQueen, C. A. and Gandolfi, A. J. Comprehensive Toxicology, 13 vols. (Pergamon, Elsevier Science Ltd., Oxford, 1997)

Sittig, M. Handbook of Toxic and Hazardous Chemicals and Carcinogens, 2nd Edn, (Noyes Publications, Park Ridge, 1981).

Sorokin, S. P. Histology: Cell and Tissue Biology (Elsevier Biomedical Publications, New York, 1983).

Spencer, P.S. & Schaumburg, H.H. (eds) Experimental and Clinical Neurotoxicology (Williams & Wilkins, Baltimore/London, 1980) (a new edition is due in 1999).

Stryer, L. Biochemistry, 4th edn, (W.H. Freeman, New York, 1995).

Target Organ Toxicity Series (Raven Press, New York, 1981). (This series includes separate volumes on each of the mammalian organ systems).

Thomas, C.L. Tabers Cyclopedic Medical Dictionary 15th (F.A. Davis, Philadelphia, 1985).

Timbrell, J.A. Principles of Biochemical Toxicology 2nd edn (Taylor & Francis, London, 1991).

Toxicological Profiles. Agency for Toxic Substances and Disease Registry (ATSDR), US Public Health Service. A series of comprehensive toxicological profiles, each of a single compound or a small group of related compounds, produced by ATSDR as mandated under the Superfund Amendments and Reauthorization Act (SARA) of 1986. They appear in several forms: drafts for public comment; toxicological profiles; updates of toxicological profiles.

The following is, in each case, the most advanced version available to the editors.

Toxicological Profiles – Drafts for Public Comment
    Benzene, August 1995 (Update)
    2-Butoxyethanol and 2 butoxyethanol Acetate, August 1996
    Chlorfenvinphos, August 1995
    Chloroform, August 1995
    Chlorpyrifos, August 1995
    Cyanide, August 1995 (Update)
    Dichlorvos, August 1995
    Diisopropymethylphosphonate, August 1996
    Di-N octylphthalate, June 1994
    Ethylene Glycol/Propylene Glycol, May 1993
    Hexachloroethane, June 1994
    Hexamethylene Diisocyanate, August 1996
    HMX, June 1994
    Hydraulic Fluids, June 1994
    Hydrazines, June 1994

Jet Fuels (JP-5 and JP 8), August 1996
Methylenedianiline, August 1996
Mineral-Based Crankcase Oil, June 1994
Nickel, August 1995 (Update)
Polychlorinated Biphenyls, August 1995 (Update)
Tetrachloroethylene, August 1995 (Update)
Titanium Tetrachloride, June 1994
Trichloroethylene, August 1995 (Update)
Vinyl Chloride, August 1995 (Update)
White Phosphorus, June 1993

Toxicological Profiles
Acetone, May 1994
Aldrin/Dieldrin, April, 1993
Antimony, September 1992
Arsenic, April 1993
Asbestos, August 1995 (Update)
Automotive Gasoline, June 1995
Benzidine, August 1995 (Update)
2,3-Benzofuran, September 1992
Beryllium, April 1993
Bromomethane, September 1992
Cadmium, April 1993
Carbon Disulfide, August 1996 (Update)
Carbon Tetrachloride, May 1994 (Update)
Chlordane, May 1994 (Update)
Chlordecone - See Mirex and chlordecone
Chlorodibenzofurans, May 1994
Chromium, April 1993
Chreosole, August 1996 (Update)
4,4'-DDT, 4,4'-DDE, 4,4'-DDD, May 1994 (Update)
Diazinon, August 1996 (Update)
1,2-Dibromo-3-chloropropane, September 1992
1,2-Dichlorobenzene, April 1993 (Update)
1,2-Dichloroethane, May 1994 (Update)
1,1-Dichloroethene, May 1994 (Update)
1,2-Dichloroethene, August 1996 (Update)
1,3-Dichloropropene, September 1992
Di(2 ethylhexyl) Phthalate, April 1993 (Update)
Diethyl Phthalate, June 1995
1,3-Dinitrobenzene and 1,3,5-Trinitrobenzene, June 1995
Dinitrocresols, August, 1995
Dinitrophenols,. August 1995
Disulfoton, August, 1995
Endosulfan, April 1993

Endrin and Endrin Aldehyde, August 1996 (Update)
Fluorides, Hydrogen Fluoride and Fluorine, April 1993
Fuel Oils, June 1995
Heptachlor/Heptachlor Epoxide, April 1993
Hexachlorobenzene, August 1996 (Update)
Hexachlorobutadiene, May 1994 (Update)
Alpha, Beta-, Gamma-, and Delta-Hexachlorocyclohexane, May 1994
2-Hexanone, September 1992
Jet Fuels (JP4 and JP7), June 1995
Lead, April 1993 (Update)
Mercury, May 1994 (Update)
Methoxychlor, May 1994
Methyl t Butyl Ether, August 1996
Methylene Chloride, April 1993 (Update)
Methylene bis-(2 Chloroaniline) (MBOCA), May 1994
Methyl Mercaptan, September 1992
Methyl Parathion, September 1992
Mirex and Chlordecone, August 1995
Naphthalene, August 1995 (Update)
N-Nitrosodiphenylamine, April 1993
Otto Fuels II, June 1995
Pentachlorophenol, May 1994 (Update)
Polyborminated Biphenyls (PBBS), August 1995
Polycyclic Aromatic Hydrocarbons (PAHS), August 1995 (Update)
Pyridine, September 1992
RDX, June 1995
Selenium, August 1996 (Update)
Stoddard Solvent, June 1995
Styrene, September 1992
1,1,2-Tetrachloroethane, August 1996 (Update)
1,2,3 Trichloropropane, September 1992
Tetryl, June 1995
TIN, September 1992
Toluene, May 1994 (Update)
Toxaphene, August 1996 (Update)
Trichloroethane, August 1995 (Update)
2,4,6-Trinitrotoluene, June 1995
Xylenes, August 1995 (Update)
Zinc, May 1994 ((Update)

Tu, A.T. Venoms: Chemistry and Molecular Biology (John Wiley, New York, 1977).

Wexler, P. Information Resources in Toxicology (Elsevier, New York, 1988).

Wexler, P. Encyclopedia of Toxicology (3 volumes) (Academic Press, San Diego, 1998).

Zakrzewski, S.F.   Principles of Environmental Toxicology, 2nd ed. (ACSMonograph Series No. 190; Columbus, 1997).